Acute Medicine

A Practical Guide to the Management of Medical Emergencies

Edited by

Mridula Rajwani, Leila Vaziri, and Ivie Gbinigie
Oxford University Hospitals NHS Foundation Trust, Oxford, UK

SIXTH EDITION

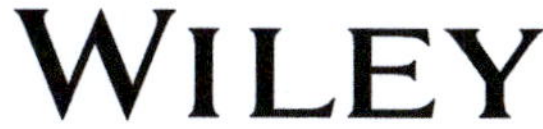

This edition of *Acute Medicine* is dedicated to John Chambers, who died in April 2024.

John and I wrote the first edition of the book in the late 1980s, following our experience as medical registrars on take – a role which then, as now, required competence in medicine across the board and grace under pressure. Further editions followed. John went on to become an internationally recognised expert in heart valve disease and echocardiography, yet remained a firm believer in the importance of the skills and outlook of the generalist. We were proud to learn that a sixth edition of *Acute Medicine* had been commissioned, with the baton passed to new editors, and despite illness, John contributed chapters to this.

John's kindness, high standards and outstanding breadth of knowledge will be remembered by his many friends.

David Sprigings

To my mother, my strength, my guide, my heart, whose love made everything possible.
— Mridula Rajwani

To my beloved sister Kome, the joy of my life.
— Ivie Gbinigie

To my loved one, and to whom challenges are not barriers but stepping stones—who remain true to themselves, follow their hearts, and never stop until they succeed.
— Leila Vaziri

Contents

List of Contributors

Basma A.A. Abdelsalam
Senior Leadership and Clinical Fellow in Ambulatory Medicine, Oxford University Hospitals NHS Foundation Trust, Oxford, UK

Lynn Affarah
Gastroenterology Registrar, Guy's and St Thomas' Hospital, London, UK

Rand Alkaissy
Clinical Fellow in Ambulatory and Emergency Medicine, Oxford University Hospitals NHS Foundation Trust, Oxford, UK

Mustafa Alsahab
Consultant Geriatrician, Oxford University Hospitals NHS Foundation Trust, Oxford, UK

Noor Al-Zubaidi
Haematology Specialist Registrar, Guy's and St Thomas' NHS Foundation Trust, London, UK

Christopher Ambrose
Specialist Registrar in General Internal Medicine and Geriatrics, Oxford University Hospitals NHS Foundation Trust, Oxford, UK

Simon Anderson
Consultant Gastroenterologist, Guy's and St Thomas' Hospital NHS Foundation Trust, London, UK

Sally Aziz
Specialty Registrar, St. Johns Institute of Dermatology, Guy's and St Thomas' NHS Foundation Trust, London, UK

Anil Babar
Speciality Trainee in Medical Oncology, Oxford University Hospitals Foundation Trust, Oxford, UK

Soma Banerjee
Consultant Stroke Physician, Imperial College Healthcare NHS Trust, London, UK

Grace Barnes
Internal Medicine Trainee in Acute General Medicine and Gastroenterology, Oxford University Hospitals NHS Trust, Oxford, UK

Mike Beadsworth
Consultant in Tropical and Infectious Diseases, Royal Liverpool University Hospital, and Hon. Senior Lecturer, Liverpool School of Tropical Medicine, Liverpool, UK

Nick Beeching
Emeritus Professor of Tropical and Infectious Diseases, Department of Clinical Sciences, Liverpool School of Tropical Medicine, Liverpool, UK

Roberto Bellanti
Clinical Research Training Fellow & Neurology Specialty Registrar, Nuffield Department of Clinical Neurosciences, University of Oxford & Oxford University Hospitals NHS Foundation Trust, Oxford, UK

Ajay Bhalla
Consultant Stroke Physician, Guy's and St Thomas' NHS Foundation Trust, London, UK

Shivam Bhargava
Neurology Registrar, Oxford University Hospitals NHS Foundation Trust, Oxford, UK

Geetha Bhat
Assistant Professor of Medicine, Division of Endocrinology, Cooper Medical School of Rowan University and Cooper University Hospital, Camden, New Jersey, USA

Jonathan J.H. Bray
Internal Medicine Trainee in Cardiology, Oxford University Hospitals NHS Foundation Trust, Oxford, UK

Matthew Brook
Consultant Nephrologist & Transplant Physician, Oxford University Hospitals NHS Foundation Trust, Oxford, UK

Katherine R. Bull
Honorary Consultant Nephrologist, Oxford University Hospitals NHS Foundation Trust - Principal Investigator, Centre for Human Genetics Nuffield Department of Medicine, University of Oxford, Oxford, UK

Alex Bunn
Chief Registrar in Ambulatory Medicine, Oxford University Hospitals NHS Trust, Oxford, UK

John Chambers
Consultant Cardiologist and Professor of Clinical Cardiology at Guy's and St Thomas' Hospitals, London, UK

Mas Chaponda
Senior Consultant Infectious Diseases, Hamad Medical Corporation and Qatar University, Doha, Qatar

Tom Cibulskas
Consultant Physician in Acute Medicine, Oxford University Hospitals NHS Foundation Trust, Oxford, UK

Mia Cokljat
Specialty Trainee in Respiratory Medicine, Wexham Park Hospital, NHS Frimley Health Foundation Trust, Slough, UK

Vincent Connolly
Consultant Physician, South Tees Hospitals NHS Trust, Middlesbrough, UK

John Corcoran
Consultant in Respiratory Medicine, University Hospitals Plymouth NHS Trust, Plymouth, UK

Adele Crapnell
Specialty Registrar in Respiratory Medicine, University Hospitals Plymouth NHS Trust, Plymouth, UK

Martin Crook
Consultant in Clinical Biochemistry and Metabolic Medicine, Guy's and St Thomas' Hospital, Lewisham Greenwich Trust, London, UK

Alexandra Croom
Consultant Allergist, Queen's Medical Centre, Nottingham University Hospitals NHS Trust, Nottingham, UK

Abhijit Das
Consultant Neurologist, Royal Preston Hospital. Clinical Lead, Functional Neurological Disorder Service, Lancashire and South Cumbria. Honorary Associate Professor, University of Central Lancashire (UCLan), Preston, UK

Charlotte David
Internal Medical Trainee, Barts Health Trust, London, UK

Joel David
Consultant Rheumatologist & Senior Lecturer, Oxford University Hospitals NHS Foundation Trust, Oxford, UK

Nemesha Desai
Consultant Dermatologist, St. Johns Institute of Dermatology, Guy's and St Thomas' NHS Foundation Trust, London, UK

Eilish Donnelly
Specialty Trainee in Acute Internal Medicine, Guy's and St Thomas' NHS Foundation Trust, London, UK

Edward Droscher
Speciality Trainee in Renal and General (Internal) Medicine, Oxford University Hospitals NHS Foundation Trust, Oxford, UK

Nathan Eager
Speciality Trainee in Acute Medicine, Oxford University Hospitals NHS Foundation Trust, Oxford, UK

Alguili Elsheikh
Pleural Research Fellow, Oxford Centre for Respiratory Medicine and Oxford Respiratory Trials Unit, Oxford University Hospitals NHS Foundation Trust, Oxford, UK

Sarah Fellows
Speciality Trainee in Cardiology, Oxford University Hospitals NHS Foundation Trust, Oxford, UK

William Flowers
Consultant in Adult Cystic Fibrosis, Bronchiectasis, NTM & Respiratory Medicine, Oxford University Hospitals NHS Foundation Trust, Oxford, UK

Matthew C. Frise
Consultant in Acute Medicine and Intensive Care, Royal Berkshire NHS Foundation Trust, Reading, UK

William Fowkes
Speciality Trainee in Cardiology, Royal Berkshire Hospital, Reading, UK

Joseph Gaied
Speciality Registrar in Renal and General Medicine, Imperial College NHS Trust, London, UK

James Gamble
Consultant Cardiologist, Oxford University Hospitals NHS Foundation Trust, Oxford, UK

Michelle Goonasekera
Specialty Trainee in Renal and General Internal Medicine, Oxford University Hospitals NHS Trust, Oxford, UK

Gina Hadley
Multiple Sclerosis Clinical Fellow, Post CCT (Geriatrics and General Internal Medicine), Oxford University Hospitals NHS Foundation Trust, Oxford, UK

Rob Hallifax
Consultant in Respiratory Medicine, Oxford University Hospitals NHS Foundation Trust, and Senior Clinical Lecturer University of Oxford, Oxford, UK

Carl Hartelius
Speciality Trainee in Acute Medicine, Oxford University Hospitals NHS Foundation Trust, Oxford, UK

Carolyn Hemsley
Infectious Diseases and Microbiology Consultant, Lead for Outpatient Parenteral Antibiotic Therapy Service (OPAT), Department of Infectious Diseases, Guy's & St Thomas' NHS Foundation, London, UK

Sandeep S. Hothi
Consultant Cardiologist, Heart & Lung Centre, Royal Wolverhampton NHS Trust, Honorary Associate Clinical Professor, University of Birmingham, NIHR West Midlands Research Scholar, Birmingham, UK

Zaw Ye Htet
Consultant Physician in Endocrinology and Diabetes, Wexham Park, NHS Firmley Health Foundation Trust, London, UK

Arif Hussenbux
Consultant Gastroenterologist and PB Endoscopist, Buckinghamshire Healthcare Trust, Buckinghamshire, UK

Anne-Catherine M.L. Huys
Consultant Neurologist, Cambridge University Hospitals NHS Foundation Trust, Cambridge, UK

Hannah Irvine
Obstetric Medicine Clinical Fellow/Rheumatology SpR, Oxford University Hospitals NHS Foundation Trust, Oxford, UK

Bahram Jafar-Mohammadi
Consultant Endocrinologist, Oxford Centre for Diabetes, Endocrinology and Metabolism, Oxford, UK

Nicola Jones
Consultant Physician in Infectious Diseases and Acute General Medicine, Lead Physician for Antimicrobial Stewardship, Oxford University Hospitals NHS Foundation Trust, Oxford, UK

Nimrath Kainth
Specialist Trainee in Ophthalmology, University Hospitals of Northamptonshire, Northampton, UK

Rachel Kesse-Adu
Consultant Haematologist, Guy's and St Thomas' NHS Foundation Trust, London, UK

Sanna Khawaja
Consultant Physician in Acute Internal Medicine, Guy's and St Thomas' NHS Foundation Trust, London, UK

Sung-Hee Kim
Speciality Trainee in Rheumatology, Oxford University Hospitals NHS Foundation Trust, Oxford, UK

Jamie Kitt
Honorary Cardiology and GIM Consultant OUH NHS Foundation Trust and Post-Doctoral Research Fellow RDM Cardiovascular Medicine, London, UK

John L. Klein
Consultant Microbiologist and Training Lead, Trust Lead for Endocarditis, St Thomas' Hospital, London, UK

Ruth Lamb
Consultant Dermatologist, Guy's and St Thomas' NHS Foundation Trust and St Georges NHS Foundation Trust, London, UK

Kezia Lange
Consultant Psychiatrist, Emergency Department Psychiatric Service, Oxford Health NHS FT- Honorary Senior Clinical Lecturer | University of Oxford, Oxford, UK

Nigel Langford
Consultant Physician in Clinical Pharmacology and Therapeutics and Acute and General Internal Medicine, University Hospitals of Leicester, Leicester, UK

Daniel Lasserson
Clinical Lead, Acute Hospital at Home, Dept of Geratology OUH NHS FT and Professor of Acute Ambulatory Care, University of Warwick, Coventry, UK

Clement Lau
Associate Consultant, National Heart Research Institute Singapore, National Heart Centre Singapore, Singapore

Doreen Lee
Speciality Trainee in Acute Medicine, Oxford University Hospitals NHS Foundation Trust, Oxford, UK

M. Isabel Leite
Associate Professor, Nuffield Department of Clinical Neurosciences, University of Oxford, Honorary Consultant Neurologist, Oxford University Hospitals NHS Foundation Trust, Oxford, UK

Jeremy Levy
Consultant Nephrologist, Imperial College NHS Trust, London, UK

Bernard Liem
Speciality Registrar in Neurology, Oxford University Hospitals NHS Foundation Trust, Oxford, UK

Ruth Lithgow
Senior Clinical Fellow in Ambulatory Medicine, Oxford University Hospitals NHS Foundation Trust, Oxford, UK

Boyang Liu
Consultant Cardiologist at Wythenshawe Hospital, Manchester, UK

Gabriele C. De Luca
Professor of Clinical Neurology and Experimental Neuropathology, Consultant Neurologist and Clinical Lead for Multiple Sclerosis Disease Modifying Therapy Service, Oxford University Hospitals NHS Foundation Trust, Oxford, UK

Lucy Mackillop
Consultant Obstetric Physician, Honorary Senior Clinical Lecturer, Oxford University Hospitals NHS Foundation Trust, Oxford, UK

Samuel W. Mackrill
Speciality Registrar in Neurology and Internal Medicine, Oxford University Hospitals NHS Foundation trust, Oxford, UK

Arti Mahto
Consultant Rheumatologist, Clinical Lead for Vasculitis, Kings' College Hospital NHS Trust, London, UK

Swapna Mandal
Consultant Respiratory Physician, Royal Free London NHS Foundation Trust/University College London, UK

Priyadarshini Marathe
Consultant in Emergency Medicine, Oxford University Hospitals NHS Foundation Trust, Oxford, UK

Shani A.D. Mathara Didhenipothage
Post CCT Fellow Endocrinology, Oxford Centre for Diabetes, Endocrinology and Metabolism, Oxford, UK

Irene Mathias
Foundation Doctor, Oxford University Hospitals Foundation Trust, Oxford, UK

Aye Chan Maung
Specialty Registrar in Endocrinology and Diabetes, Oxford University Hospitals NHS Foundation Trust, Oxford, UK

Christine J.H. May
Consultant Endocrinologist, Oxford Centre for Diabetes, Endocrinology and Metabolism, Oxford, UK

Andrew McCallum
Consultant in Clinical Infection and Acute General Medicine|TB Lead|Sepsis Lead|OXMID Secretary, Oxford University Hospitals NHS Foundation Trust, Oxford, UK

Tristan McMullan
Consultant Oculoplastic and Ophthalmic Surgeon, Northampton General Hospital, Northampton, UK

Ajmal Memon
Leadership Fellow in Acute General Medicine, Oxford University Hospitals NHS Trust, Oxford, UK

Mary Miller
Consultant in Palliative Medicine & End of Life Care Lead, Oxford University Hospitals NHS Foundation Trust, Oxford, UK

Ben Millette
Consultant in Anaesthesia and Intensive Care Medicine, Trust Lead for Point of Care Ultrasound, Buckinghamshire Healthcare NHS Trust, Buckinghamshire, UK

Alexandra Montagu
Consultant Geriatrician, Oxford University Hospitals NHS Foundation Trust, Oxford, UK

Muhammad Owais Musani
Senior Clinical Fellow in Pulmonary Hypertension, Royal Brompton Hospital NHS Trust, London, UK

Vishal Nathwani
Research Fellow in Interstitial Lung Disease, c, UK

Roshan Navin
Consultant Physician in Acute Internal Medicine, Guy's and St Thomas' NHS Foundation Trust, London, UK

Khizr Nawab
Specialty Trainee in Renal Medicine, Oxford University Hospitals NHS Trust, Oxford, UK

Sue Anne Ng
Clinical Fellow in Haematology, UK

David O'Brien
Consultant Physician in Intensive care Medicine and Acute Medicine, Oxford University Hospitals NHS Foundation Trust, Oxford, UK

Julian O.M. Ormerod
Consultant Cardiologist, Oxford University Hospitals NHS Foundation Trust, Lecturer in Medicine|Jesus College, Oxford University, Oxford, UK

Claire van Nispen tot Pannerden
Public Health, GGD Rotterdam – Rijnmond, Rotterdam, Netherlands

Keisha Patel
Specialty Trainee in Geriatric & General Internal Medicine, Leicester Royal Infirmary, University Hospitals of Leicester NHS Trust, Leicester, UK

Ojaswini Pathak
Consultant Geriatrician, Clinical Director, Care of the Older Adult Team, Shrewsbury and Telford Hospital NHS Trust, Telford, UK

Yani Perera
Speciality Registrar in Emergency Medicine, Oxford University Hospitals NHS Foundation Trust, Oxford, UK

Nayia Petousi
Consultant Respiratory Physician & Senior Clinical Research Fellow, Nuffield Department of Medicine, University of Oxford, Oxford, UK

Su Latt Phyu
Respiratory Registrar, Thames Valley Deanery, Oxford, UK

Kapil Mohan Rajwani
Post-CCT Fellow in Neurosurgery, Oxford University Hospital NHS Foundation Trust, Oxford, UK

Shvaita Ralhan
Consultant Geriatrician, Oxford University Hospitals NHS Foundation Trust, Oxford, UK

Maheshi N. Ramasamy
Consultant Physician in Infectious Diseases and Acute General Medicine, Oxford University Hospitals NHS Foundation Trust- Clinician Scientist, Oxford Vaccine Group, Oxford, UK

Jo Riley
Respiratory and Home Oxygen Service Lead, Oxford Health NHS Foundation Trust, Oxford, UK

Simon Rinaldi
Associate Professor of Neurology & Honorary Consultant Neurologist, Nuffield Department of Clinical Neurosciences, University of Oxford & Oxford University Hospitals NHS Foundation Trust, Oxford, UK

Pramith Ruwanpathirana
Registrar in Medicine, National Hospital of Sri Lanka, Sri Lanka

Kirn Sandhu
Consultant Paediatric Gastroenterologist, King's College Hospital NHS Trust, London, UK

Peter Saunders
Consultant in Interstitial Lung Disease, Oxford University Hospitals NHS Foundation Trust, Oxford, UK

Silvia Sbardella
Specialty Registrar in Acute Medicine and Point of Care Ultrasound Fellow at Buckinghamshire Healthcare NHS Trust, Buckinghamshire, UK

Susan Shapiro
Consultant Haematologist, Oxford University Hospitals NHS Foundation Trust and Associate Professor, Oxford University, Oxford, UK

Robert H. Shaw
Clinical Research Fellow, Oxford Vaccine Group, Centre for Clinical Vaccinology and Tropical Medicine, University of Oxford, Oxford, UK

Udi Shmueli
Consultant Gastroenterologist, Northampton General Hospital NHS Trust UK, Northampton, UK

Eleanor Smith
Consultant in Acute General Medicine/Ambulatory Medicine/Nephrology, Oxford University Hospitals NHS Foundation Trust, Oxford, UK

Nathan Spence
Acute Surgical Physician, Oxford University Hospitals NHS Foundation Trust, Oxford, UK

Laura Spiers
Speciality Trainee in Medical Oncology, Oxford University Hospitals NHS Foundation Trust, Oxford, UK

David Sprigings
Locum Consultant Cardiologist, Oxford University Hospitals NHS Foundation Trust, Oxford, UK - Previously Consultant Physician, Northampton General Hospital, Northampton, UK

Michelle Stefanelli
Clinical Fellow in Endocrinology, Department of Medicine, Cooper Medical School of Rowan University and Cooper University Hospital, Camden, New Jersey, USA

Gagandeep Sukhija
Speciality Trainee in Rheumatology, Kings' College Hospital NHS Trust, London, UK

Kehinde Sunmboye
Consultant Rheumatologist, Honorary Associate Professor in Medical Education, University Hospitals of Leicester, Leicester, UK

Connor Sweeney
Consultant Haematologist, Oxford University Hospitals NHS Foundation Trust, Oxford, UK

Nick Talbot
Consultant in Respiratory Medicine, Oxford University Hospitals NHS Foundation Trust, Supernumerary Fellow and College Lecturer, University College, Oxford, UK

Ivan Tang
Speciality Trainee in Respiratory Medicine, Intensive Care Medicine, and General Medicine, Health Education Thames Valle, Oxford, UK

Ann Thompson
Senior Resuscitation Officer, Oxford University Hospitals NHS Foundation Trust, Oxford, UK

Sanja Thompson
Consultant Geriatrician, Bermuda Hospitals Board, Bermuda, UK

Christopher Turnbull
Consultant Physician in Respiratory Medicine and Honorary Researcher, Department of Respiratory Medicine, Oxford University Hospitals NHS Foundation Trust, Oxford, UK

Martin R. Turner
Professor of Clinical Neurology & Neuroscience, Nuffield Department of Clinical Neurosciences, University of Oxford, Oxford, UK

Michael Turner
Speciality Trainee in Renal and General (Internal) Medicine, Oxford University Hospitals NHS Foundation Trust, Oxford, UK

Vimal Venugopal
Consultant in Diabetes&Endocrinology/General Internal Medicine, University Hospitals Leicester, Leicester, UK

Ben Warner
Consultant Gastroenterologist, Guy's and St Thomas' Hospital, London, UK

Edmund Watson
Haematology Registrar and Clinical Training Research Fellow, Oxford University Hospitals NHS Trust, Oxford, UK

Praveen Weeratunga
Consultant in Acute General Medicine, Oxford University Hospitals Foundation NHS Trust, Oxford, UK

Stephen Woolley
Consultant in Tropical Medicine and Medical Microbiology, Liverpool University Hospitals NHS Foundation Trust and Senior Clinical Lecturer in Medical Parasitology and Microbiology, Department of Clinical Sciences, Liverpool School of Tropical Medicine, Liverpool, UK

S. John Wort
Consultant in Pulmonary Hypertension, Clinical Lead for Pulmonary Hypertension, National Pulmonary Hypertension Service at the Royal Brompton Hospital- Professor of Practice at Imperial College, London, UK

Ahmed Yousuf
Consultant in Respiratory Medicine, Glenfield Hospital, Leicester, UK

Zainab Zafar
Consultant Physician in Acute Medicine, Oxford University Hospitals NHS Foundation Trust, Oxford, UK

Sabrina Zulfikar
Research Fellow in Interstitial Lung Disease, Oxford University Hospitals NHS Foundation Trust, Oxford, UK

Introduction

Dear Readers,

Welcome to the new edition of *Acute Medicine: A Practical Guide to the Management of Acute Medical Emergencies*. This essential resource is designed for anyone training in this dynamic and rapidly evolving specialty. It serves as a comprehensive guide for practitioners, including physicians, trainees, nurses, nurse practitioners, and physician associates, and can also be a valuable revision aid for both undergraduate and postgraduate students.

This guide addresses a wide array of acute medical emergencies affecting various organ systems, incorporating the latest guidelines and evidence-based practices. It discusses the principles of ambulatory and same-day emergency care, as well as the diverse services available in the community, such as the Hospital at Home model. These topics have become critical priorities for clinicians, healthcare managers, and patient advocacy groups alike. We also delve into the growing role of point-of-care ultrasound in frontline medicine and its applications in clinical assessment.

Designed as a quick reference, the book features concise, user-friendly sections that cover common presentations in Acute Medicine. It adopts a unique approach to clinical assessment by outlining key priorities during acute critical periods, along with ongoing management considerations after diagnosis and initial treatment. Each section includes summary boxes that highlight essential learning points.

Our contributors are leading experts in their fields, sharing the latest and most innovative clinical practices. Many are currently practicing in Acute Medicine and have drawn on their real-life experiences to enrich this content.

The field of Acute Medicine has witnessed significant advancements over the years, further solidifying its importance in the education and development of healthcare professionals and in the provision of acute care. Research in this specialty is gaining traction, promising to shape future clinical practices.

With these developments in mind, we are pleased to present this revised edition as a valuable educational resource. We hope you find it as engaging and informative as we found the process of compiling it.

Happy reading!
Mridula, Leila and Ivie

Emergency Presentations

CHAPTER 1

Cardiorespiratory arrest in hospital

Ann Thompson

This chapter summarises the management of cardiac arrest in hospitals following the 2021 Resuscitation Council UK (RCUK) guidelines. All hospital medical staff should know how to respond to cardiac arrest and should receive regular training in the management of emergency events.

The appropriateness of a resuscitation attempt should be considered and discussed with patients in order that resuscitation is NOT attempted where this would be inappropriate and futile.

Background

The incidence of in-hospital cardiac arrest (IHCA) is 1–1.5 per 1000 hospital admissions annually.

The majority of in-hospital cardiopulmonary arrests present with a non-shockable rhythm: pulseless electrical activity (PEA) – 52% and asystole – 21%. Only 17% of cardiopulmonary arrests present with a shockable rhythm (ventricular fibrillation (VF) or pulseless ventricular tachycardia (pVT)). Not surprisingly the majority of these in-hospital events occur in ward areas (85%) in patients admitted with a medical complaint. It is important to recognise that signs of deterioration prior to cardiac arrest are seen in 50–80% of patients; thus, the recognition of deterioration and prevention of cardiopulmonary arrest is important.

Many NHS Trusts submit data regarding cardiopulmonary arrest to the National Cardiac Arrest Audit (NCAA) that provides quarterly reports on the incidence of confirmed cardiac arrest in patients over the age of 28 days, who were subject to a cardiac arrest call and received chest compressions and/or defibrillation. This audit compares the hospitals' observed cardiac arrest rates with all other hospitals participating in NCAA.

Initial management

Figure 1.1 shows the algorithm for advanced life support in adults. The initial response ensuring early chest compressions and early defibrillation if appropriate is key to patient survival.

Use the DRS ABC approach (Danger, Response, Shout for help).

The airway should be opened using Head Tilt, Chin Lift manoeuvre. No more than 10s should be taken to confirm cardiopulmonary arrest by a look, listen and feel for signs of normal breathing and any other signs of life. A central pulse may be palpated but must be done in conjunction with breathing checks.

Please note that agonal breathing should be considered a sign of cardiopulmonary arrest.

Once cardiopulmonary arrest is confirmed, an emergency call via 2222 should be made and resuscitation equipment accessed. If alone, leave the patient to get help and equipment.

Acute Medicine: A Practical Guide to the Management of Medical Emergencies, Sixth Edition.
Edited by Mridula Rajwani, Leila Vaziri, and Ivie Gbinigie.
© 2026 John Wiley & Sons Ltd. Published 2026 by John Wiley & Sons Ltd.

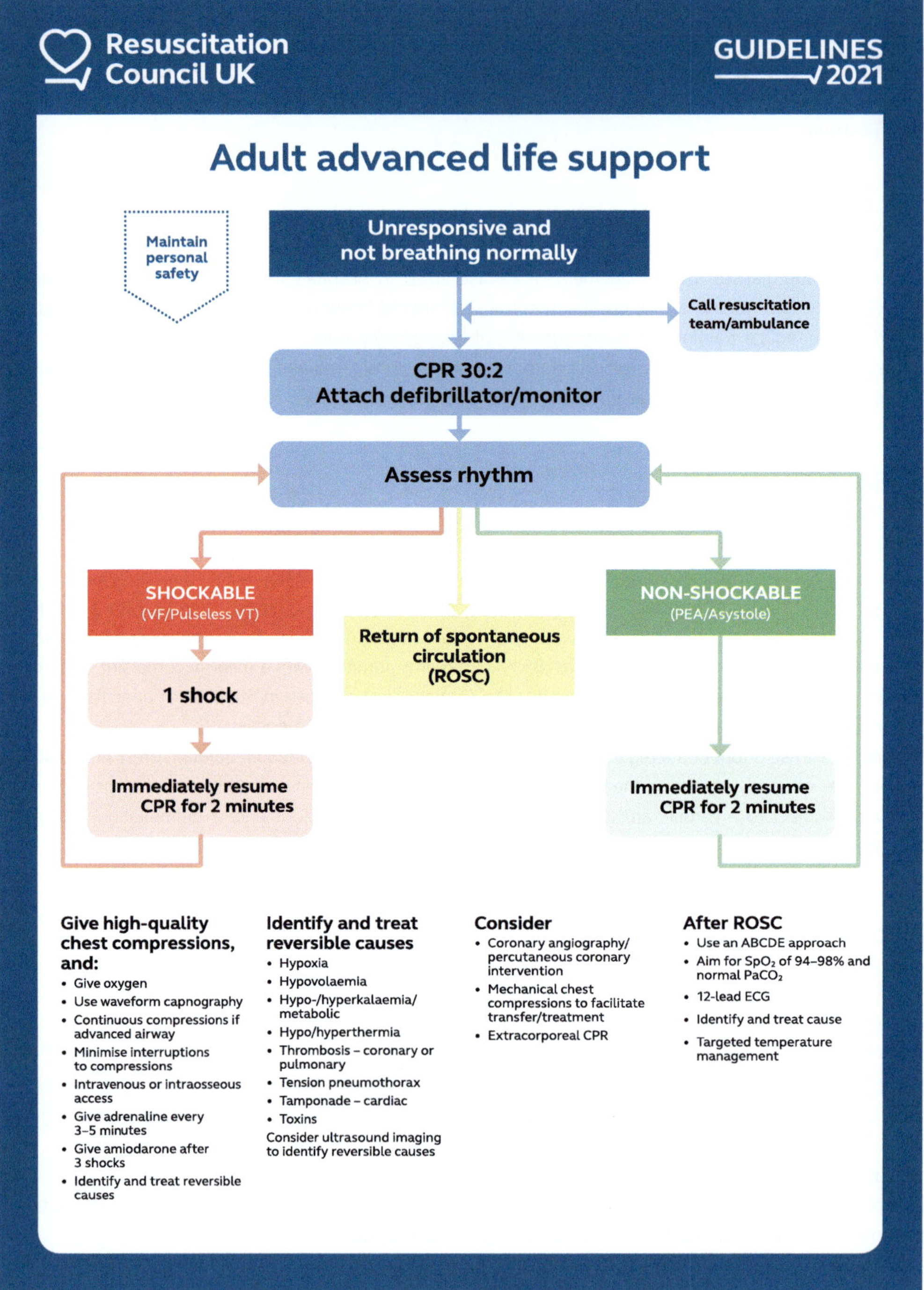

Figure 1.1 Algorithm for adult advanced life support. Source: Resuscitation Council. Reproduced with permission of the Resuscitation Council (UK).

Chest compressions

Chest compressions should commence as soon as cardiopulmonary arrest is confirmed.

Hands should be placed in the middle of the lower half of the sternum ('centre of the chest').

Chest compressions should be delivered at a rate of 100–120/min at a depth of 5–6 cm. The chest should be allowed to recoil to its normal resting position between each compression.

Once 30 compressions have been delivered, a pause should be made to allow for 2 breaths to be given if colleagues are ready with a bag-valve-mask device.

Any pause in chest compressions should be limited to less than 5 s.

Personnel delivering chest compressions must swap at least every 2 min to maintain high-quality chest compressions. If available, a cardiopulmonary resuscitation (CPR) feedback device should be used so the quality of the chest compressions can be monitored. Any pauses should be planned and limited to 5 s or less. A mechanical chest compression device should be accessed if available.

Airway and ventilation

See Chapter 105 for further information.

Use head tilt and chin lift or jaw thrust to open the airway. Use suction to clear the mouth of secretions if required.

A bag-valve-mask should be accessed, and the tubing attached to 15 L of oxygen. This is a two-person technique. One operator should secure the mask to the patient's face, pushing down to establish a seal between the mask and the face, and then with fingers along the jawline lift the face into the mask while opening the airway.

The second airway assistant should squeeze the bag to deliver breaths following every 30 compressions. The breaths should be delivered over approx. 1 s and the bag only squeezed enough to provide chest rise. Over-inflation should be avoided to prevent gastric insufflation or barotrauma.

An oropharyngeal airway should be inserted if required to support airway opening.

Once resuscitation is underway, the team should consider the insertion of a supraglottic airway device (e.g. Igel) if the team is skilled in its insertion.

Endotracheal intubation should only be attempted by those with airway expertise. The decision to intubate should be made by the airway expert in conjunction with the team leader.

Once the airway has been secured with a supraglottic airway or an endotracheal tube, compressions and ventilation can be asynchronous, with compressions continuing at a rate of 100–120 min and ventilation at 10–12 breaths per minute.

Waveform capnography should be attached to the tube (Igel or endotracheal tube [ETT]), so this can be monitored during the resuscitation attempt.

Management of cardiac arrest rhythms

Once chest compressions are established, the priority is the application of a defibrillator to analyse and treat the cardiac arrest rhythm.

Defibrillator pads should be placed on dry skin; along with correct placement, it is important to ensure good skin contact taking a moment to ensure the pad is smooth and well adhered to the skin. Place one defibrillator electrode to the right of the sternum, below the clavicle. Place the second electrode in the mid-axillary line, clear of any breast tissue. Follow the pictures provided on the defibrillator pad packaging.

The defibrillator should be turned on, and as soon as a rhythm is established, chest compressions should be paused to allow for rhythm analysis.

The rhythm should be analysed as either shockable – VF, pVT or non-shockable – PEA, asystole. PEA is the most common presenting cardiac arrest rhythm in hospital.

Ventricular fibrillation/pulseless ventricular tachycardia

Once the defibrillator is attached, chest compressions should be paused to confirm the cardiac arrest rhythm, and the team leader should confirm the rhythm and verbalise this to the team.

If the rhythm is shockable and a manual defibrillator is being used, the following sequence should be followed:

Chest compressions are restarted immediately. The team leader will hand control to the defibrillator operator to deliver a safe shock.

The defibrillator operator and the person performing chest compressions should be able to see each other.

The defibrillator operator will instruct chest compressions to continue and everyone else to stand clear, ensuring that oxygen is removed (if free flowing via bag-valve-mask). The charge button is pressed, and once pressed the defibrillator operator should keep their hands away from the defibrillator until chest compressions are stopped and that person has stood clear.

Once the defibrillator is charged, the instruction is given for chest compressions to stop and that person to stand clear. A final check that all personnel are away from the patient should be made before the shock is delivered.

Once the shock is delivered, chest compressions should immediately restart.

CPR should continue for 2 min; the team leader should prepare the team for the next pause in chest compressions.

At 2 min the rhythm should be analysed again, and if the rhythm remains shockable, a further shock is delivered using the sequence mentioned earlier. Once the shock has been delivered, CPR continues for a further 2 min.

At the end of 2 min, the rhythm is analysed, and if this remains shockable, a further shock should be given repeating the sequence above. Once the third shock has been delivered and CPR recommenced, 1 mg of adrenaline 1 : 10000 IV/IO and 300 mg of amiodarone IV/IO should be delivered.

Adrenaline should be repeated every 3–5 min (alternate cycles of CPR) and a further 150 mg of amiodarone can be considered following the fifth shock.

Defibrillators and pulse checks

Staff should familiarise themselves with the type of defibrillators in use in order that these can be used safely and efficiently in cardiac arrest. Defibrillators can be used in automated external defibrillator (AED) mode or in some instances a standalone AED may be used. The emergency team and team leader should listen to the instructions provided by the AED; the delivery of the shock will depend on the shock button being pressed, so safety checks are essential prior to this action. Please note that the confirmation of cardiopulmonary arrest as described earlier is essential, once confirmed.

VF is not compatible with a pulse, so there should be no delay for a pulse check before a shock is delivered. A pulse check should only be undertaken if the rhythm is compatible with life. There should be no pause to check a rhythm or pulse following the delivery of a shock.

Pulseless electrical activity (PEA)/asystole

Once defibrillator pads are attached and the device is turned on, pause chest compressions. If the rhythm is confirmed as PEA or asystole chest compressions should immediately restart and continue for 2 min.

Adrenaline 1 mg 1 : 10000 IV/IO should be administered as soon as possible or as soon as vascular access is established. Adrenaline should be repeated every 3–5 min or every other cycle of CPR. A rhythm check must always precede the administration of adrenaline.

Pulse checks should only be undertaken if the rhythm is compatible with life.

Once the first dose of adrenaline is given in a cardiac arrest, it should be repeated every 3–5 min (every other cycle of CPR) regardless of the rhythm. Amiodarone is given after 3 shocks whether these occur sequentially or are staggered.

Reversible causes of cardiac arrest

Once cardiopulmonary resuscitation is underway, the patients' medical notes and information regarding events prior to the cardiac arrest should be ascertained by the team leader to determine the possible cause of cardiopulmonary arrest. The reversible causes are commonly referred to as the 4H's and 4T's:

Hypoxia

Hypovolaemia

Hyperkalaemia, hypokalaemia and other metabolic disorders

Hypothermia

Thrombosis (coronary or pulmonary)

Tension pneumothorax

Tamponade – cardiac

Toxins

If a potential reversible cause of the cardiopulmonary arrest is identified, appropriate treatment for this should commence promptly while advance life support continues. In the event of a prolonged resuscitation attempt (e.g. administration of thrombolysis for a Pulmonary Embolus [P.E.]) then a mechanical chest compression device should be sought to ensure effective chest compressions are maintained over a long period of time. It is important to ensure that staff are trained in the application of the device to ensure minimal interruption to chest compressions.

Ultrasound may be useful in the identification of some reversible causes (e.g. cardiac tamponade, P.E.). The use of this investigative technique requires training and skills in order that the operator can obtain views during a rhythm check and within 10 s.

Following return of spontaneous circulation (ROSC)

A full ABCDE assessment should be carried out.

Saturations should be maintained at 94–98%; if the patient requires ongoing airway management, endotracheal intubation should be considered if not already present. Waveform capnography should continue with ventilation to achieve normocapnia.

Ensure the patient has reliable vascular access, and further lines may be needed prior to transfer. Continuous monitoring should be in place and a 12-lead ECG carried out. Fluid replacement should continue to achieve normovolaemia and achieve an systolic blood pressure (SBP) >100 mmHg.

The patient's temperature should be maintained at 32–36°. It should be noted that patients are often cool following ROSC, so take time to cover the patient and warm them if needed. Shivering should be avoided.

Any identified reversible cause should continue to be treated. The team should refer to the appropriate specialist teams (e.g. cardiology or surgeons) in order that definitive management can be provided. A discussion about the most appropriate place for ongoing management of the patient should be decided, and if transferring, this should be done by a skilled team ensuring all appropriate equipment is in place.

The team should be supported in a debrief, and the event should be documented in the patients' notes by a member of the attending resuscitation team.

Duration of a resuscitation attempt

The duration of any resuscitation attempt should be based on each individual patient case. It is important that the team leader gathers appropriate information while resuscitation attempts are ongoing to ensure that a decision is made based on the circumstances of the cardiopulmonary arrest, the patients' best interests and the likelihood of a successful outcome, achieving not only a return of spontaneous circulation but longer-term survival and quality of life.

The team leader should share their thoughts with the team, seeking agreement from all those in the resuscitation team. It is important that all members of the team are warned of the plan to stop resuscitation attempts and are given the opportunity to ask questions if needed.

In all circumstances, those people most important to the patient should be informed of the events and given the opportunity to have time with the patient. There should be a clear plan for speaking to the patients' significant others and meeting them if they are travelling to the hospital.

Decisions regarding cardiopulmonary resuscitation

The NCAA reports a survival to hospital discharge rate of 23.9% based on information collected from 175 hospitals in the United Kingdom. Patients who experience a cardiac arrest in hospital often have significant comorbidities or a disease process that will be life-limiting. CPR is not without harm; its delivery in certain patients can result in an undignified death and the delivery of a treatment that will not work. The Recommended Summary Plan for Emergency Care and Treatment (ReSPECT) is an initiative from the RCUK. ReSPECT provides a framework that enables shared decision-making in relation to emergency treatments including CPR. This plan can evolve and change over time but provides information on the patient's wishes when the person is unable to participate in decision-making. This is replacing the previous Do Not Attempt Cardiopulmonary Resuscitation (DNACPR) process in many hospitals across the United Kingdom.

Further reading

National Cardiac Arrest Audit (NCAA) Welcome to the National Cardiac Arrest Audit. https://ncaa.icnarc.org/Home.

Resuscitation Council UK ReSPECT – ReSPECT for healthcare professionals|resuscitation Council UK. https://www.resus.org.uk/respect/respect-healthcare-professionals.

Resuscitation Council UK Resuscitation guidelines 2021. Adult advanced life support guidelines|resuscitation Council UK. https://www.resus.org.uk/library/2021-resuscitation-guidelines/adult-advanced-life-support-guidelines.

CHAPTER 2

The critically ill patient

David O'Brien and Nathan Eager

General

Key features of the critically ill patient are severe respiratory, cardiovascular or neurological derangement, often in combination, reflected in abnormal physiological observations (Table 2.1 and Charts 1–3). Principles of management are summarised in Box 2.1 and Figure 2.1.

Priorities

Make a rapid but systematic assessment using the Airway, Breathing, Circulation, Disability, Exposure (ABCDE) approach.

While doing this, collect information about the patient, the current problem, the context and co-morbidities. Attach monitoring (electrocardiogram (ECG) and oxygen saturation) and secure venous access.

Airway and breathing

Ensure the airway is clear. If the patient is unconscious, remove dentures if loose, conduct airway opening manoeuvres, airway suction under direct vision and consider the use of airway adjuncts. See Chapter 105 for detailed advice on airway management.

If there is a reduced conscious level, significant respiratory compromise or a respiratory rate less than 8/min then endotracheal intubation should be considered. Before this is done, ventilate the patient using a bag-mask system or a supraglottic airway device with 100% oxygen.

What is the respiratory rate? Rates <8 or >30/min signify potential critical illness. Is there respiratory distress, shown by dyspnoea, tachypnoea, ability to speak only in short sentences or single words, agitation and sweating? Is arterial oxygen saturation <90% despite supplemental oxygen? This indicates severe impairment of gas exchange. See Chapter 30 for management of respiratory failure.

Circulation

Remember that a 'normal' blood pressure may be maintained by vasoconstriction and does not mean that organ perfusion is adequate. Signs of low cardiac output include confusion and agitation, cold extremities, sweating, oliguria and metabolic acidosis.

Acute Medicine: A Practical Guide to the Management of Medical Emergencies, Sixth Edition.
Edited by Mridula Rajwani, Leila Vaziri, and Ivie Gbinigie.
© 2026 John Wiley & Sons Ltd. Published 2026 by John Wiley & Sons Ltd.

Table 2.1 Nine key observations in suspected critical illness.

Observation	Signs of critical illness	Action
Airway	Evidence of upper airway obstruction (Table 2.2)	See Table 2.2 and Chapter 105 for management of the airway
Respiratory rate	Respiratory rate <8 or >30/min	Give oxygen Connect a pulse oximeter Check arterial oxygen saturation and blood gases See Chapter 30 for management of respiratory failure
Arterial oxygen saturation	SaO_2 <90%	Give oxygen Check arterial blood gases (Chapter 7)
Heart rate	Heart rate <40 or >130/min with signs of impaired organ perfusion	Give oxygen Connect an ECG monitor and obtain IV access See Chapter 13 for management of cardiac arrhythmias
Blood pressure	Systolic BP <90 mmHg, a MAP <65 mmHg or a drop of systolic BP by >40 mmHg with signs of impaired organ perfusion.	Give oxygen Connect an ECG monitor and obtain IV access
Perfusion	Signs of impaired organ perfusion: cool mottled skin; capillary refill time >2 s; agitation/reduced conscious level; oliguria; lactate >4	Give oxygen Connect an ECG monitor and obtain IV access
Conscious level	Reduced conscious level (Less than 'alert' on an ACVPU scale)	Stabilise airway, breathing and circulation Consider urgent endotracheal intubation if less than 'responsive to voice' on ACVPU scale Exclude/correct hypoglycaemia Give naloxone if opioid poisoning is possible See Chapter 3 for further management of the patient with a reduced consciousness level
Temperature	Core temperature <36 °C or >38 °C, with hypotension, hypoxaemia, oliguria or agitation/reduced conscious level	See Chapter 5 for further management of sepsis
Blood glucose	Blood glucose <4 mmol/L with signs of hypoglycaemia (sweating, abnormal behaviour, reduced conscious level, seizures)	Give 100 mL of 20% glucose or 200 mL of 10% glucose over 15–30 min IV, or glucagon 1 mg IV/IM/SC, see Chapter 81

GCS, Glasgow Coma Scale score.
ACVPU scale with approximate GCS: alert = GCS 15; confused = GCS 14; voice responsive = GCS 12; pain responsive = GCS 8; unresponsive = GCS 3.

Heart rates <40 or >130/min with life threatening features require urgent correction: see Chapter 13 for management of arrhythmias.

If systolic BP is <90 mmHg, the mean arterial pressure (MAP) is <65 mmHg or the systolic has fallen by more than 40 mmHg and there are signs of low cardiac output, urgent correction is needed. Look carefully at the jugular venous pressure (JVP), which may provide an important clue to the diagnosis.

If there are no signs of pulmonary oedema, give IV fluid (500 mL crystalloid over 15 min). If hypovolaemia or vasodilatation is likely (suspect vasodilatation if the pulses are bounding), lay the patient flat and elevate the foot of the bed.

Table 2.2 Assessment and stabilisation of the airway.

	Signs of acute upper airway obstruction	Causes of acute upper airway obstruction	Action if you suspect upper airway obstruction
Conscious patient	Respiratory distress* Inspiratory stridor Suprasternal retraction Abnormal voice Coughing/choking	Foreign body Anaphylaxis (Chapter 4) Angioedema (Chapter 100)	Sit the patient up Give high-flow oxygen Call for urgent help from someone trained in endotracheal intubation and an ENT surgeon Specific management of the cause of obstruction, e.g. Adrenaline in the case of anaphylaxis
Unconscious patient	Respiratory arrest Inspiratory stridor Gurgling Grunting/snoring	Above causes as well as laxity of the tongue and soft tissues of the oropharynx, inhalation of a foreign body, secretions, blood or vomitus	Head-tilt/chin-lift manoeuvre Remove dentures if loose and suction under direct vision Call for urgent help from someone trained in endotracheal intubation See Chapter 105 for management of the airway Specific management of cause of obstruction, e.g. adrenaline in the case of anaphylaxis

* Respiratory distress is shown by dyspnoea, tachypnoea, ability to speak only in short sentences or single words, agitation and sweating.

Chart 1 The NEWS2 scoring system.

Physiological parameter	3	2	1	Score 0	1	2	3
Respiration rate (per minute)	$\leq$8		9–11	12–20		21–24	$\geq$25
SpO_2 Scale 1 (%)	$\leq$91	92–93	94–95	$\geq$96			
SpO_2 Scale 2 (%)	$\leq$83	84–85	86–87	88–92 $\geq$93 on air	93–94 on oxygen	95–96 on oxygen	$\geq$97 on oxygen
Air or oxygen?		Oxygen		Air			
Systolic blood pressure (mmHg)	$\leq$90	91–100	101–110	111–219			$\geq$220
Pulse (per minute)	$\leq$40		41–50	51–90	91–110	111–130	$\geq$131
Consciousness				Alert			CVPU
Temperature (°C)	$\leq$35.0		35.1–36.0	36.1–38.0	38.1–39.0	$\geq$39.1	

Source: Reproduced from RCP, 2017/Royal College of Physicians.

Chart 2 NEWS2 thresholds and triggers.

NEW score	Clinical risk	Response
Aggregate score 0–4	Low	Ward-based response
Red score Score of 3 in any individual parameter	Low–medium	Urgent ward-based response*
Aggregate score 5–6	Medium	Key threshold for urgent response*
Aggregate score 7 or more	High	Urgent or emergency response†

* Response by a clinician or team with competence in the assessment and treatment of acutely ill patients and in recognising when the escalation of care to a critical care team is appropriate.
† The response team must also include staff with critical care skills, including airway management.
Source: Reproduced from RCP, 2017/Royal College of Physicians.

Chart 3 Clinical response to the NEWS2 trigger thresholds.

NEW score	Frequency of monitoring	Clinical response
0	Minimum 12 hourly	• Continue routine NEWS monitoring
Total 1–4	Minimum 4–6 hourly	• Inform registered nurse, who must assess the patient • Registered nurse decides whether increased frequency of monitoring and/or escalation of care is required
3 in single parameter	Minimum 1 hourly	• Registered nurse to inform medical team caring for the patient, who will review and decide whether escalation of care is necessary
Total 5 or more urgent response threshold	Minimum 1 hourly	• Registered nurse to immediately inform the medical team caring for the patient • Registered nurse to request urgent assessment by a clinician or team with core competencies in the care of acutely ill patients • Provide clinical care in an environment with monitoring facilities
Total 7 or more emergency response threshold	Continuous monitoring of vital signs	• Registered nurse to immediately inform the medical team caring for the patient – this should be at least at specialist registrar level • Emergency assessment by a team with critical care competencies, including practitioner(s) with advanced airway management skills • Consider transfer of care to a level 2 or 3 clinical care facility, i.e. higher-dependency unit or ICU • Clinical care in an environment with monitoring facilities

Source: Reproduced from RCP, 2017/Royal College of Physicians.

Box 2.1 The critically ill patient: principles of management (Resuscitation Council [UK]).

Use the Airway, Breathing, Circulation, Disability, Exposure (ABCDE) approach to assess and treat the patient.

Do a complete initial assessment and re-assess regularly.

Treat life-threatening problems before moving to the next part of the assessment.

Assess the effects of treatment.

Recognize when you will need extra help. Call for appropriate help early.

Use all members of the team. This enables interventions (e.g. assessment, attaching monitors and intravenous access), to be undertaken simultaneously.

Communicate effectively – plan approach.

The aim of the initial treatment is to keep the patient alive and achieve some clinical improvement. This will buy time for further treatment and making a diagnosis.

Remember: it can take a few minutes for treatments to work, so wait a short while before reassessing the patient after an intervention.

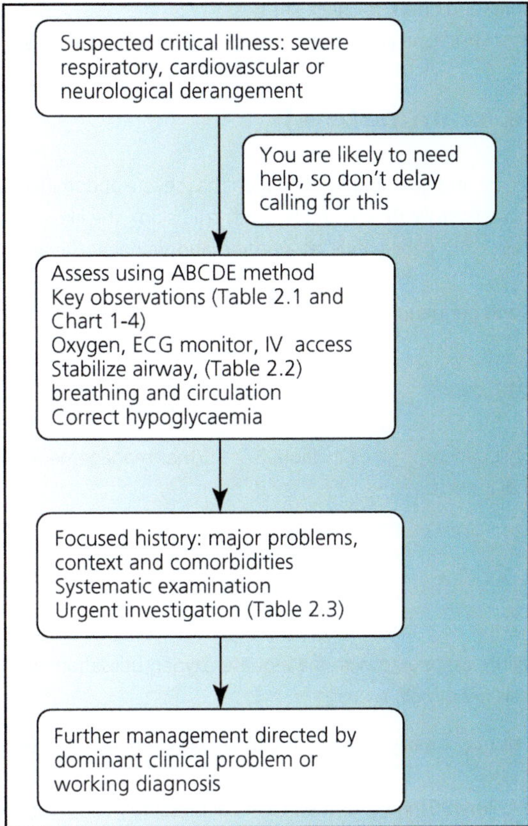

Figure 2.1 Approach to the patient with suspected critical illness.

Neurological status ('disability')

What is the conscious level (assessed using the 'ACVPU' scale)? If the patient is unresponsive to voice then contact someone with advanced airway skills as the patient may need urgent endotracheal intubation.

If the conscious level is reduced, you must exclude hypoglycaemia by immediate stick test. If blood glucose is <4.0 mmol/L, give 100 mL of 20% glucose or 200 mL of 10% glucose over 15–30 min IV, or glucagon 1 mg IV/IM/SC. Recheck blood glucose after 10 min, if still below 4.0 mmol/L, repeat the above IV glucose treatment. In patients with malnourishment or alcohol-use disorder, there is a remote risk of precipitating Wernicke encephalopathy by a glucose load: prevent this by giving thiamine 100 mg IV before or shortly after glucose administration. See Chapter 46 for further management of hypoglycaemia.

If the respiratory rate is <12/min or the pupils are pinpoint, or there is another reason to suspect opioid poisoning, give naloxone. Give up to 1 dose of 400 μg IV, then 800 μg at 1-min intervals if there is no response, and then give 2 mg for 1 dose if there is still no response. The aim is to achieve a respiratory rate of 12–16/min. Doses can be given IM but only if the IV route is not available. Until the respiratory rate is around 15/min.

Further doses or an infusion may be needed.

If there are recurrent or prolonged major seizures, treat with buccal midazolam, IV lorazepam or rectal diazepam, see Chapter 57 for management of seizures.

Examine the eyes and pupils, and check for neck stiffness.

Make a rapid assessment of limb tone and power: is there lateralized weakness?

Exposure (entire examination)

Check for abdominal tenderness and guarding. If the patient has severe abdominal pain or generalised abdominal tenderness, and is shocked (systolic BP <90 mmHg with cold skin), the likely diagnosis is generalised peritonitis, mesenteric infarction, severe pancreatitis or ruptured abdominal aortic aneurysm; for further reading, please see Chapter 32.

Examine the limbs, spine and perineum for evidence of ischaemia or a septic focus.

Further management

Investigation of the critically ill patient is given in Table 2.3. Further management is directed by the dominant clinical problem or working diagnosis.

Shock

General

Shock is acute circulatory failure associated with inadequate oxygen utilisation by the cells, resulting in organ dysfunction and lactic acidosis (>2 mmol/L).

- Compensatory mechanisms may initially maintain the blood pressure, but hypotension is usually present and is defined by:
  - Systolic blood pressure (SBP) <90 mmHg or mean arterial pressure (MAP) <65 mmHg or
  - Fall in systolic BP >40 mmHg
- Causes of shock are given in Table 2.4. Up to one-third of patients admitted to ICU have shock predominantly caused by sepsis. Clinical signs that may indictae the underlying cuase are shown in Table 2.5.

Table 2.3 Investigation of the critically ill patient.

Immediate

Arterial blood gases, pH and lactate

ECG

Blood glucose

Plasma sodium, potassium, urea and creatinine

Full blood count

Urgent

Chest X-ray

Echocardiography if hypotension/shock

Cranial CT if reduced conscious level or focal neurological signs

Coagulation screen if low platelet count, suspected coagulation disorder, jaundice or purpura

Biochemical profile

Amylase if abdominal pain or tenderness

C-reactive protein

Blood culture if suspected sepsis

Urine stick test

Toxicology screen (serum 10 mL and urine 50 mL) if suspected poisoning

Table 2.4 Differential diagnosis of hypotension and shock.

Hypovolaemia
Haemorrhage
Urinary loss
Gastrointestinal fluid loss
Cutaneous loss (e.g. burns)
Third-space sequestration (e.g. acute pancreatitis)

Cardiac obstruction
Pulmonary embolism (Chapter 31)
Cardiac tamponade (Chapter 6)
Tension pneumothorax (Chapter 28)

Cardiac pump failure
Acute myocardial infarction (usually associated with pulmonary oedema, except when due to right ventricular infarction)
Acute myocardial ischaemia (usually associated with pulmonary oedema)
Myocarditis, postpartum cardiomyopathy or Takotsubo cardiomyopathy
Arrhythmia (especially when associated with valve disorder, e.g. severe aortic stenosis, or impaired left ventricular function, in which case usually associated with pulmonary oedema)
Acute aortic or mitral regurgitation (due to endocarditis, aortic dissection, papillary muscle or chordal rupture) (always associated with pulmonary oedema)
Ventricular septal rupture complicating myocardial infarction (often associated with pulmonary oedema)

Vasodilatation
Sepsis
Drugs and toxins
Anaphylaxis
Acute adrenal insufficiency (Addisonian crisis)

Table 2.5 Clinical signs pointing to the cause of hypotension.

Cause of hypotension	Pulse volume	Skin temperature	Jugular venous pressure
Hypovolaemia	Low	Cool	Low
Cardiac obstruction or pump failure	Low	Cool	Normal or raised
Vasodilatation	Normal or increased	Warm	Low

Blood culture
Urine stick test

- Monitor vital signs in patients at risk (e.g. acute coronary syndrome and pneumonia) to detect the first signs of developing shock and take prompt action to reverse this.
- Consider early echocardiography in unexplained shock or shock that is suspected to be a result of a cardiogenic origin. Table 2.6 gives a summary of these indications.

Priorities

Initial management is summarised in Figure 2.2.

1 If hypovolaemia or vasodilatation is likely, lay the patient flat and elevate the foot of the bed.

2 Give oxygen. Place an IV cannula. Attach an ECG monitor. Check oxygen saturation. Make a rapid clinical assessment (Figure 2.1). Look carefully at the JVP, and assess skin temperature and perfusion. Investigations needed urgently are given in Table 2.3.

Table 2.6 Indications for urgent echocardiography in the hypotensive patient.

Suspected cardiac tamponade
- Hypotension and breathlessness following placement of central venous cannula or pacing lead, or in a patient with known cancer
- Raised jugular venous pressure
- Pulsus paradoxus >10 mmHg

Suspected acute major pulmonary embolism
- Risk factors for venous thromboembolism
- Raised jugular venous pressure
- Hypoxaemia

Hypotension with pulmonary oedema

Unexplained severe hypotension

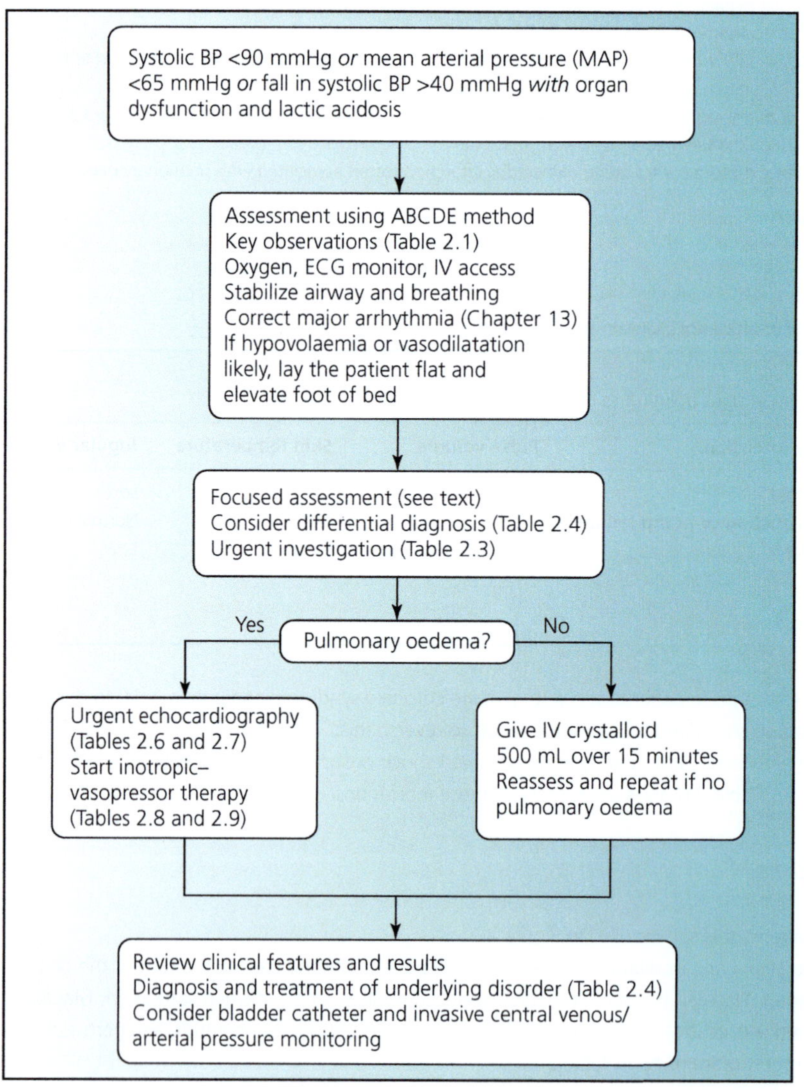

Figure 2.2 Management of hypotension and shock.

Questions to ask yourself include:
- Is there obvious haemorrhage from the gastrointestinal tract (Chapters 38 and 39) or another site (e.g. abdominal aortic aneurysm [Chapter 18]).
- Is there a major arrhythmia (Chapter 39).
- Is there ECG evidence of an acute coronary syndrome (ST segment elevation or depression, new left bundle branch block) (Chapter 12).
- Is there associated pulmonary oedema, indicating cardiogenic shock (see below).
- Is there fever, or other features pointing to sepsis (Chapter 5).
- Is pulmonary embolism possible (Chapter 31). Hypotension and hypoxaemia without pulmonary oedema suggest pulmonary embolism or sepsis; in this setting, a raised JVP would favour pulmonary embolism and a low JVP sepsis.
- Is tension pneumothorax a possibility (e.g. recent central vein cannulation) (Chapter 28).
- Could this be anaphylaxis (Chapter 4)? If the patient has recently been exposed to a potential allergen, and has urticaria, erythema, angio-oedema or wheeze, treat as anaphylaxis and give adrenaline 0.5–1 mg IM (0.5–1 mL of 1 in 1000 solution). Further management is detailed in Chapter 4.

3 If hypotension does not respond promptly, put in a bladder catheter so that urine output can be monitored. The urine output is a rough guide to renal blood flow and cardiac output; the target is >0.5 mL/kg/h.

If there is obvious haemorrhage

Get help from a gastroenterologist (if you are dealing with suspected upper gastrointestinal haemorrhage) or a surgeon (see Chapters 38 and 39).

Place a second large-bore IV cannula (e.g. grey Venflon).

Activate the local Major Haemorrhage Protocol.

Rapidly transfuse crystalloid until the systolic BP is around 100 mmHg. Start transfusing blood as soon as it is available via the major haemorrhage protocol.

Aim for a haemoglobin concentration of 80 g/L.

- Correct clotting abnormalities. If the prothrombin time is >1.5× control, give vitamin K 10 mg IV and 2 units of fresh frozen plasma. If the platelet count is <50 × 10^{12}/L, give platelet concentrate. Recheck the platelet count if >4 units of blood have been transfused. If fibrinogen is <1.5 g/L, give cryoprecipitate.
- Consider tranexamic acid.
- Correct hypocalcaemia by maintaining ionised Ca >1.13 mmol/L.

Cardiogenic shock

Cardiogenic shock is the second most common cause of shock and accounts for nearly 20% of all cases of shock. It has an in-hospital mortality rate approaching 60% and therefore it is important to prioritise early recognition and treatment. Clinically, it is often characterised by hypotension in combination with pulmonary oedema and is primarily due to left ventricular failure. The treatment for this form of shock is often more distinct from other forms of shock and therefore warrants specific attention.

Priorities

- Correct major arrhythmias (Chapter 13).
- If there is ECG evidence of ST-segment-elevation acute coronary syndrome, consider primary angioplasty if feasible (Chapter 12).
- Arrange urgent echocardiography to assess right and left ventricular function and to exclude ventricular septal rupture, pericardial tamponade and acute aortic or mitral regurgitation (Table 2.7).

Table 2.7 Echocardiographic findings in hypotension.

Cause of hypotension	IVC	LV size	LV contraction	RV size	RV contraction
Hypovolaemia	Flat	Small	Increased	Small	Increased
Sepsis	Flat	Normal or large	Normal, reduced or increased	Normal or large	Normal or reduced
LV dysfunction due to ischaemia	Normal or dilated	Large	Reduced regionally or globally	Normal	Normal (unless associated RV infarction)
Acute major pulmonary embolism	Dilated	Normal or small	Normal or increased	Large	Reduced
Cardiac tamponade	Dilated	Normal or small	Normal or increased	Normal or small	Diastolic free wall collapse
RV infarction	Dilated	Normal or large if associated LV inferior infarction	Normal or reduced if associated inferior infarction	Large	Reduced

IVC, inferior vena cava; LV, left ventricular; RV, right ventricular.

Table 2.8 Choice of inotropic/vasopressor therapy.

Cause of hypotension	Choice of therapy
Left ventricular failure	Dobutamine or Milrinone if systolic BP is >90 mmHg
	Digoxin
Right ventricular infarction	Dobutamine if systolic BP is 80–90 mmHg
Pulmonary embolism	Noradrenaline if systolic BP is <80 mmHg
Cardiac tamponade while awaiting pericardiocentesis	Noradrenaline
Septic shock	Noradrenaline
	Dobutamine should be added if cardiac output is low
Anaphylactic shock	Adrenaline

Table 2.9 Inotropic/vasopressor therapy: dosages.

Drug	Dosage (μg/kg/min)	Effect
Adrenaline	0.05	Beta-1 inotropism and beta-2 vasodilatation
	0.05–5	Beta-1 inotropism and alpha-1 vasoconstriction
Dobutamine	5–40	Beta-1 inotropism and beta-2 vasodilatation
Dopamine	5–10	Beta-1 inotropism
	10–40	Alpha-1 vasoconstriction
Noradrenaline	0.05–5	Alpha-1 vasoconstriction and beta-1 inotropism
Milrinone	0.375–0.75	Phosphodiesterase inhibitor; inotropy and vasodilatation

- Increase the inspired oxygen, aiming for an oxygen saturation of >90%/arterial PO_2 >8 kPa. If these targets are not met despite an inspired oxygen concentration of 60%, consider the use of a continuous positive airway pressure system (Chapter 113). Intubation and mechanical ventilation may be appropriate in some patients: discuss this with an intensivist and cardiologist.
- Consider starting inotropic/vasopressor therapy (Tables 2.8 and 2.9).
- Diuretics are relatively ineffective in patients with cardiogenic shock, but can be used in case of fluid overload once the cardiac output has increased (as shown by improvement in the patient's mental state and skin perfusion): if renal function is normal, give Furosemide 40 mg IV.

- Providing the systolic BP has increased to at least 100 mmHg systolic, start a nitrate infusion, initially at low dose (e.g. isosorbide dinitrate 2 mg/h).
- If the patient is not improving, consider haemodynamic monitoring using pulse contour or thermodilution techniques to allow more accurate titration of therapy. Adjust the doses of inotrope/vasopressor +/nitrate, aiming for normalisation of tissue perfusion parameters (serum lactate, urine output and skin perfusion).
- Discuss management with a cardiologist if you suspect a surgically correctable cause (e.g. papillary muscle rupture) or if there is evidence of acute myocardial ischaemia without infarction (Chapter 12).
- If appropriate discuss early with extracorporeal membrane oxygenation (ECMO) centre as venous-to-arterial ECMO or another form of mechanical cardiac support may be required.

Further management

The key points in the management of hypotension/shock are to:
- Make a diagnosis and give specific treatment (e.g. pericardiocentesis for tamponade, PCI for ACS, cardiac surgery for ruptured papillary muscle). Seek help from an intensivist and, in the case of cardiogenic shock, a cardiologist.
- Correct cardiac arrhythmias.
- Correct hypovolaemia while avoiding fluid overload.
- Correct hypoxia and biochemical abnormalities.
- Use inotropic/vasopressor therapy if there is refractory hypotension.

Summary

1 Make a diagnosis and give specific treatment
- Consider the causes in Table 2.4.
- Echocardiography is indicated if the diagnosis remains unclear.
- Give hydrocortisone 200 mg IV if the patient has been on previous long-term steroid treatment (prednisolone >7.5 mg daily) or you suspect acute adrenal insufficiency (Chapter 47).

2 Correct cardiac arrhythmias
- Ventricular tachycardia or supraventricular tachycardia with life-threatening features (shock, syncope, myocardial ischaemia, severe heart failure) should be treated with DC cardioversion (Chapter 106).
- Acute atrial fibrillation: consider DC cardioversion if the ventricular rate is >140 min, after correction of hypoxia and electrolyte disorders. Otherwise, give amiodarone IV (via a central line; 300 mg in glucose 5% over 60 min, followed by 900 mg over 24 h). Most drugs used to control the ventricular rate in atrial fibrillation are contraindicated in hypotension. Digoxin is largely ineffective when sympathetic drive is high. If there are life-threatening features present then treat urgently with DC cardioversion.
- If there is severe bradycardia (heart rate < 40 min), give atropine 0.6–1.2 mg IV, with further doses at 5-min intervals up to a total dose of 3 mg if the heart rate remains below 60 min. If there is little response to atropine, use an external transcutaneous pacing system or place a temporary pacing wire (Chapter 107).

3 Correct hypovolaemia
- If there is obvious hypovolaemia (appropriate clinical setting; low JVP with flat neck veins), give IV fluid (blood, colloid or crystalloid as appropriate to the cause). There is no role for a central line unless the patient needs inotropic medication.
- If the evidence for hypovolaemia is less certain, but there are no clinical signs of fluid overload, give a fluid challenge, especially if the JVP is difficult to assess.
- If systolic BP remains <90 mmHg or MAP <65 mmHg despite correction or exclusion of hypovolaemia, search for and treat other causes of hypotension, of which sepsis is the most likely. In patients with acute bleeding, relative hypotension can be accepted until the bleeding is stopped surgically. In sepsis with prior systemic hypertension, a MAP >65 mmHg may be needed to prevent acute kidney injury.

- There is no single value of LV filling pressure or CVP that should guide fluid replacement; instead, multiple methods should be used, including dynamic measures (e.g. pulse-pressure variability on the arterial line or the change in IVC diameter on leg raising).
- Even in fluid-responsive patients, titrate fluid carefully to avoid hypervolaemia.
- If BP remains low, inotropic–vasopressor therapy will be needed.

4 Correct hypoxia and biochemical abnormalities
- Maintain $PaO_2 > 8$ kPa (60 mmHg), arterial saturation $> 90\%$.
- Severe metabolic acidosis may contribute to hypotension. It is crucial to identify the cause of metabolic acidosis so that the correct treatment can be initiated. Causes of metabolic acidosis are given in Chapter 7. If arterial pH is <7.1 and falling, consider giving 50 mL of 8.4% sodium bicarbonate whilst waiting for a response to treatment of the underlying disease. Recheck arterial pH after 30 min.

5 Use inotropic/vasopressor therapy if there is refractory hypotension
- If systolic BP remains <90 mmHg (MAP <65 mmHg) with signs of hypoperfusion (associated with low central venous oxygen saturation) despite correction of hypovolaemia, start inotropic/vasopressor therapy whilst searching for the underlying cause.
- Inotropes are not indicated for a low LV ejection fraction on echocardiography without signs of low cardiac output.
- Invasive central venous and arterial pressure monitoring is recommended.
- Choice of therapy and dosages are summarised in Tables 2.8 and 2.9.
- Discuss with a cardiologist whether intra-aortic balloon counterpulsation (balloon pump) or left ventricular assist device is indicated as a bridge to definitive treatment (e.g. surgery for a ruptured papillary muscle).

Further reading

Francis GS, Bartos JA, Adatya S. (2014) Inotropes. *J Am Coll Cardiol* 63, 2069–2078.

Harjola V-P, Mebazaa A, Celutkiene J. (2016) Contemporary management of acute right ventricular failure: a statement from the Heart Failure Association and the Working Group on Pulmonary Circulation and right ventricular function of the European Society of Cardiology. *Eur J Heart Fail* 18, 226–241.

Levy B, Bastien O, Bendjelid K. (2015) Experts' recommendations for the management of adult patients with cardiogenic shock. *Ann Intensive Care* 5, 17. (Open access). doi: 10.1186/s13613-015-0052-1.

Mackenzie DC, Noble VE. (2014) Assessing volume status and fluid responsiveness in the emergency department. *Clin Exp Emerg Med* 1, 67–77. doi: 10.15441/ceem.14.040.

Roshdy A, Francisco N, Rendon A, *et al.* (2014) Critical care echo rounds: haemodynamic instability. *Echo Res Pract* 1(1), D1–D8. doi: 10.1530/ERP-14-0008.

Royal College of Physicians (2017). National Early Warning Score (NEWS) 2: standardising the assessment of acute-illness severity in the NHS. Updated report of a working party. London: RCP. https://www.rcp.ac.uk/improving-care/resources/national-early-warning-score-news-2.

Soar, J., Deakin, C. D., Nolan, J. P., Perkins, G. D., Yeung, J., Couper, K., Hall, M., Thorne, C., Price, S., Lockey, A., Wyllie, J., & Hampshire, S. (2021). Adult advanced life support guidelines. Resuscitation Council UK. https://www.resus.org.uk/library/2021-resuscitation-guidelines/adult-advanced-lifesupport-guidelines.

Task force of the European Society of Intensive Care Medicine. (2014) Consensus on circulatory shock and hemodynamic monitoring. *Intensive Care Med* 40, 1795–1815. doi: 10.1007/s00134-014-3525-z.

Van Herck JL, Claeys MJ, De Paep R, *et al.* (2015) Management of cardiogenic shock complicating acute myocardial infarction. *Eur Heart J Acute Cardiovasc Care* 4, 278–297.

Weiss SL, Peters MJ, Alhazzani W, *et al.* (2020) Surviving sepsis campaign international guidelines for the management of septic shock and sepsis-associated organ dysfunction in children. *Intensive Care Med* 46(Suppl 1), 10–67. doi: 10.1007/s00134-019-05878-6.

CHAPTER 3

The unconscious patient

SIMON RINALDI AND ROBERTO BELLANTI

Unconsciousness is a state of absent awareness and responsiveness. The three most common causes of reduced or absent conscious level in patients under 40 years of age are traumatic brain injury, poisoning (drug, alcohol or carbon monoxide intoxication) and seizures. Stroke is the most common cause in those >60. Other causes are listed in Table 3.1. Akinetic mutism, functional unresponsiveness, neuromuscular paralysis and the locked-in syndrome may mimic a reduced conscious level. However, in all of these, awareness is usually preserved.

Priorities

1 **Stabilize airway, breathing and circulation**
2 **Exclude or correct hypoglycaemia**
   - If blood glucose (BG) is <4.0 mmol/L, give 100 mL of 20% glucose or 200 mL of 10% glucose over 15–30 min IV, or glucagon 1 mg IV/IM/SC, then recheck BG after 10 min: if still below 4.0 mmol/L, repeat the above IV glucose treatment.
   - In patients with malnourishment or alcohol-use disorder, there is a risk of precipitating Wernicke's encephalopathy by a glucose load. This can be prevented by giving thiamine 100 mg IV before or shortly after glucose administration.
3 **Treat prolonged or recurrent major seizures**
   - Take into account prehospital treatment. Give IV lorazepam 0.1 mg/kg (typically 4–8 mg) over 5–10 min, buccal midazolam 10 mg, IV diazepam 10–20 mg IV at a rate of <2.5 mg/min (faster injection rates carry the risk of sudden apnoea), or rectal diazepam.
   - If the seizure does not terminate within 5 min, give a second dose, to a maximum total IV dose of lorazepam 8 mg or diazepam 40 mg.
   - In case of status epilepticus (prolonged seizure lasting >5 min) not responding to two doses of benzodiazepines, give IV levetiracetam or IV phenytoin (with cardiac monitoring) or IV sodium valproate.
4 **Give naloxone if opioid poisoning is suspected**
   - If the respiratory rate is <12/min, or the pupils are pinpoint, or there is another reason to suspect opioid poisoning, give IV naloxone 800 μg every 2–3 min up to a total dose of 3.2 mg or until the respiratory rate is >15/min.
   - If there is a response to bolus naloxone, start an IV infusion: add naloxone 2 mg to 500 mL glucose 5% or normal saline (4 μg/mL) and titrate against respiratory rate and conscious level. The plasma half-life of naloxone is 1 h, shorter than that of most opioids. In patients who have taken partial opioid agonists such as buprenorphine, methadone and tramadol, repeated large (1.2 mg) doses of naloxone may be required to achieve a satisfactory response. If there is no response to naloxone, opioid poisoning is excluded.

Acute Medicine: A Practical Guide to the Management of Medical Emergencies, Sixth Edition.
Edited by Mridula Rajwani, Leila Vaziri, and Ivie Gbinigie.
© 2026 John Wiley & Sons Ltd. Published 2026 by John Wiley & Sons Ltd.

Table 3.1 Causes of loss of consciousness.

Without meningism or localizing signs	With meningism (+/− localizing signs)	With localizing signs
Trauma		
Concussion	—	Subdural haematoma (SDH) Extradural haematoma (EDH) Other traumatic brain injury
Toxic		
Alcohol/drugs/carbon monoxide	—	—
Metabolic/endocrine		
Hypoxia, hypercapnia	Pituitary apoplexy	Wernicke's encephalopathy
Hypoglycaemia and diabetes-associated emergencies (DKA/HHS)		Hypo/hyperglycaemia
Hypo/hypernatremia, hypercalcaemia, uraemia, hepatic encephalopathy		Hypo/hypernatremia
Addisonian crisis		
Dysthyroidism (thyrotoxicosis, severe hypothyroidism)		
Hypo/hyperthermia		
Wernicke's encephalopathy		
Vascular		
Shock	Subarachnoid haemorrhage	Brainstem infarction
Hypertensive encephalopathy		Cerebral infarction with mass effect
Eclampsia		CVST
Cerebral venous sinus thrombosis (CVST)		Posterior fossa haemorrhage
Inflammatory		
Autoimmune encephalitis	—	Bickerstaff's brainstem encephalitis (BBE)
Hashimoto's encephalopathy		Acute disseminated encephalomyelitis (ADEM)
		Autoimmune encephalitis
Infective		
Sepsis/severe systemic infection	Bacterial meningitis	Herpes simplex encephalitis
	Viral meningoencephalitis	Subdural empyema
	Cerebral malaria	Abscess
		Septic embolism
Epileptic		
• Post-ictal state		• Post-ictal state
• Status epilepticus (convulsive or non-convulsive)		• Status epilepticus
Neoplastic		
Paraneoplastic CNS involvement	Carcinomatous meningitis	Brain tumour (space occupying lesion)
Acute hydrocephalus		

DKA, diabetic ketoacidosis; HHS, hyperglycaemic hyperosmolar state

5 Give flumazenil in case of benzodiazepine-induced coma in hospital
- Give flumazenil 200 μg IV over 15 s; if needed, further doses of 100 μg can be given at 1-min intervals up to a total dose of 2 mg.

6 Once the patient is stabilized, make a full clinical assessment and arrange urgent investigation
- Document the level of consciousness using the Glasgow Coma Scale (Table 3.2).
- Check for neck stiffness and examine for signs of head injury (e.g. scalp laceration, bruising, bleeding from an external auditory meatus or from the nose). If there are signs of head injury, assume additional cervical spine injury until proven otherwise: the neck must be immobilized in a collar and X-rayed before you check for neck stiffness and the oculocephalic response.
- Record the size of pupils and their response to bright light. Examine the fundi.
- Check the oculocephalic response to assess the integrity of the brainstem. Rotate the head to left and right. In an unconscious patient with an intact brainstem, both eyes rotate in the opposite direction from the movement of the head.
- Examine the limbs: tone, response to a painful stimulus (nailbed pressure), tendon reflexes and plantar responses.
- Table 3.3 outlines the key elements to consider in a focused assessment of patients with reduced level of consciousness.

7 Make a diagnosis
- The differential diagnosis for unconsciousness depends on the presence or absence of focal signs and meningism (Table 3.1 and Figure 3.1).
- **If bacterial meningitis or viral meningoencephalitis are suspected** (fever and meningism), empirical antimicrobial therapy with ceftriaxone and acyclovir should be started as soon as possible, *after* taking blood for culture and polymerase chain reaction (PCR) testing. If ceftriaxone is contraindicated, consider cefotaxime. Give intravenous amoxicillin in addition to ceftriaxone or cefotaxime for people over 55 or

Table 3.2 Glasgow Come Scale (GCS).

	Rating	Score
Eye opening (E)		
Open before stimulus	Spontaneous	4
After spoken of shouted request	To sound	3
After fingertip stimulus	To pressure	2
No opening at any time, no interfering factor	None	1
Closed by local factors	Non-testable	NT
Verbal response (V)		
Gives name, place and date correctly	Orientated	5
Disorientated but able to communicate coherently	Confused	4
Intelligible single words	Words	3
Only moans/groans	Sounds	2
No audible response, no interfering factor	None	1
Factors interfering with communication	Non-testable	NT
Best motor response (M)		
Obeys two-stage commands	Obeys commands	6
Brings hand above clavicle to stimulus on head/neck	Localising	5
Bends arm at elbow rapidly but features not predominantly abnormal	Normal flexion	4
Bends arm at elbow, features clearly predominantly abnormal	Abnormal flexion	3
Extends arm at elbow	Extension	2
No movement in arms/legs, no interfering factors	None	1
Paralysed or other limiting factors	Non-testable	NT

Table 3.3 Focused assessment of the patient with reduced conscious level.

History

History will usually need to be obtained from third-party sources such as family or friends, paramedics, GPs and existing medical records. It is important to establish:

- Tempo and pattern of onset (sudden, gradual and fluctuating)
- Prodromal fever, headache, nausea/vomiting, altered behaviour, seizure, focal neurological deficits
- History of trauma (head injury and neck manipulation) or alcohol/drug intoxication
- History (systemic, neurological and psychiatric)
- Current medications/immunosuppression/anticoagulants
- History of exposure or foreign travel

Examination

- Vital signs (respiratory rate, pulse, blood pressure, temperature and oxygen saturation)
- Conscious level (using GCS [Table 3.2])
- Meningism? Focal signs?
- Signs of trauma? Skin colour, rash?
- Eye signs, pupillary size, light reflex, corneal reflex
- Disc swelling? If present, it may indicate raised ICP (papilledema)
- Spontaneous venous pulsations? Absence may be a sign of raised ICP
- Eye movements (tracking, spontaneous, oculocephalic response (OCR) to passive head turn, conjugate or dysconjugate gaze deviation?)
- Breath odour (uraemic, hepatic and ketotic)
- General examination (murmur, bruit, pulmonary disease, liver disease, peritonism and urinary retention)

with risk factors for Listeria monocytogenes. Empirical antibiotic treatment should be continued until the results of blood and cerebrospinal fluid (CSF) tests suggest an alternative treatment is needed or there is an alternative diagnosis. If CSF testing suggests bacterial meningitis, but blood culture and diagnostic PCR do not identify specific organisms, continue antibiotics for 10 days. After 10 days, antibiotics should be stopped if the patient has recovered; otherwise, advice from Infectious Diseases or Microbiology should be sought.

- **If acute adrenal insufficiency is possible,** give hydrocortisone 200 mg IV. Fludrocortisone is not required in addition as this dose of hydrocortisone has sufficient mineralocorticoid action.
- **If CT shows a mass lesion or hydrocephalus, seek urgent advice from Neurosurgery.**

Further management

- Patients with a reduced conscious level should be nursed in a high-dependency or intensive-care unit.
- In all patients, regular reassessment of the depth of coma, eye signs and neurology is required to establish any progression or resolution.
- Some patients, for example those with a malignant middle cerebral artery (MCA) territory infarct, may require close monitoring and repeat neuroimaging if neurosurgical intervention/decompressive craniectomy is being considered.
- Induced hypothermia can improve the neurological prognosis for coma after cardiac arrest.
- In some patients, no cause is apparent for their reduced conscious level. It is important to remember that the history and toxicology may not disclose the ingestion of all relevant drugs, that hepatic encephalopathy can occur with normal liver function tests, and that CSF PCR does not detect all cases of viral encephalitis. Investigations to consider in patients with cryptogenic unconsciousness are listed in Table 3.4.

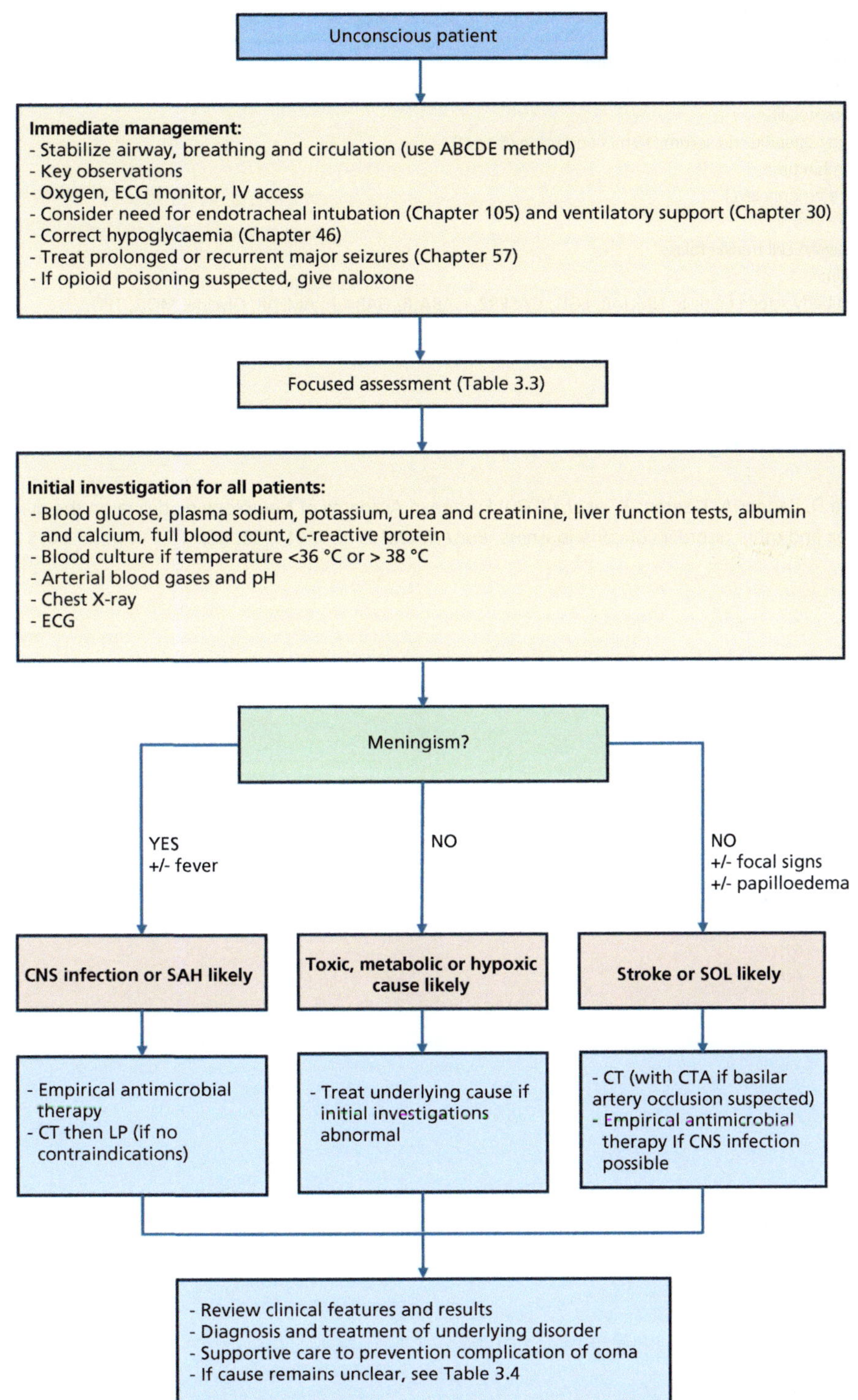

Figure 3.1 Assessment and management of patients with a reduced conscious level.

Table 3.4 Investigations to consider in unconsciousness of unclear cause.

If cause remains unidentified, consider:
- CT/LP (if not yet done)/MRI brain/EEG
- Plasma osmolality
- Toxicology screen (send serum (10 mL) and urine (50 mL))
- Prothrombin time
- Arterial ammonia level
- Cortisol
- Thiamine/red cell transketolase
- Blood film
- Autoantibody screen (initially, NMDAR, LGI1, CASPR2, $GABA_AR$, $GABA_BR$, AMPAR, Glycine, MOG, TPO, paraneoplastic, and GQ1b)

Further reading

Kondziella D, Bender A, Diserens K, *et al.* (2020) European Academy of Neurology guideline on the diagnosis of coma and other disorders of consciousness. *Eur J Neurol* 27(5), 741–756. doi: 10.1111/ene.14151.

CHAPTER 4

Anaphylaxis

ALEXANDRA CROOM

Suspect anaphylaxis if, after an IV or IM injection, insect sting or exposure to an ingested potential food or drug allergen, the patient rapidly develops breathlessness and wheeze, or hypotension/shock. The potential manifestations of anaphylaxis are shown in Table 4.1; not all features will occur in every patient.

Causes of anaphylactic reaction are given in Table 4.2. Symptoms usually start within minutes of exposure to a trigger, and most reactions will occur within 60 minutes. The route of allergen exposure influences the rapidity of symptom onset; allergens given intravenously and insect stings produce a more rapid clinical deterioration than ingested allergens, for example food and oral drugs.

The management of anaphylaxis is summarized in Figure 4.1. Prompt recognition and administration of adrenaline IM is essential to effective treatment.

Recognition

The rapid onset of breathlessness (due to upper airway obstruction or bronchospasm) or hypotension/shock, associated with itch, flushing or urticaria, suggest anaphylaxis and immediate treatment with adrenaline IM should be considered. Skin changes are absent in 20% and are not essential to the diagnosis of anaphylaxis.

Table 4.1 Manifestations of anaphylaxis.

Cutaneous
Itch, flushing, urticaria (hives), angioedema

Respiratory
Dyspnoea, cough, hoarse voice, stridor, wheeze, respiratory arrest

Cardiovascular
Dizziness, syncope, confusion, chest pain (due to myocardial ischaemia, even with normal coronary arteries), arrhythmia, cardiac arrest

Gastrointestinal
Nausea and vomiting, diarrhoea, abdominal cramping

Others
Fear of impending doom, uterine contractions ('period pain')

Acute Medicine: A Practical Guide to the Management of Medical Emergencies, Sixth Edition.
Edited by Mridula Rajwani, Leila Vaziri, and Ivie Gbinigie.
© 2026 John Wiley & Sons Ltd. Published 2026 by John Wiley & Sons Ltd.

Table 4.2 Causes of anaphylactic reactions.

Drugs*

For example, antibiotics – most commonly of beta-lactam group, non-steroidal inflammatory drugs (NSAIDs), neuromuscular blocking agents (NMBAs), cytotoxic agents, contrast media (iodinated radiocontrast media and gadolinium-based contrast media), therapeutic monoclonal antibodies

Foods†

Insect venom‡

Other causes

Exercise (with or without food allergy)

Chlorhexidine

Latex

Plasma expanders

Blood products

Idiopathic (20%)

* 50% of fatal anaphylaxis in the United Kingdom is iatrogenic.

† Milk, peanuts and tree nuts are the commonest causes of food anaphylaxis.

‡ Responsible insect varies worldwide – bee and wasp in the United Kingdom.

- There should be a high index of suspicion if there has been exposure to a possible allergen, for example administration of IV medication, or after ingestion of food.
- The differential diagnosis of anaphylaxis includes any condition that can cause the rapid onset of dyspnoea or hypotension, as well as those that cause urticaria and angioedema (Chapter 100). See Table 4.3 for a list of the most common differential diagnoses.

Suspected severe anaphylactic reaction (anaphylactic shock)

1 Call for assistance. If there is cardiorespiratory arrest, start resuscitation.

2 Remove the trigger allergen if possible (e.g. disconnect IV infusion of antibiotic; remove the stinger after a bee sting). Do not induce vomiting.

3 Position the patient. Lay the patient flat and raise the foot of the bed. This position should be maintained particularly when transferring patients; resuming an upright position before the volume shifts in shock have improved can lead to cardiac arrest. If breathless keep the patient seated upright. If pregnant lie on the left side to avoid aortocaval obstruction.

4 Adrenaline IM is the first-line drug in anaphylaxis; absent or delayed use is associated with fatal outcome.

- Administration should be IM in the middle-third anterolateral aspect of the thigh. A 23 G needle (blue – length 25 mm) should be used to ensure that muscle is reached; in the morbidly obese consider a 21 G (green – needle length 38 mm) or administration into the calf. Subcutaneous or deltoid muscle administration is NOT recommended. A dose of 500 µg adrenaline should be given IM.
- If no clinical improvement after 5 min a second dose should be given. It should be given at a separate site, for example the contralateral thigh.

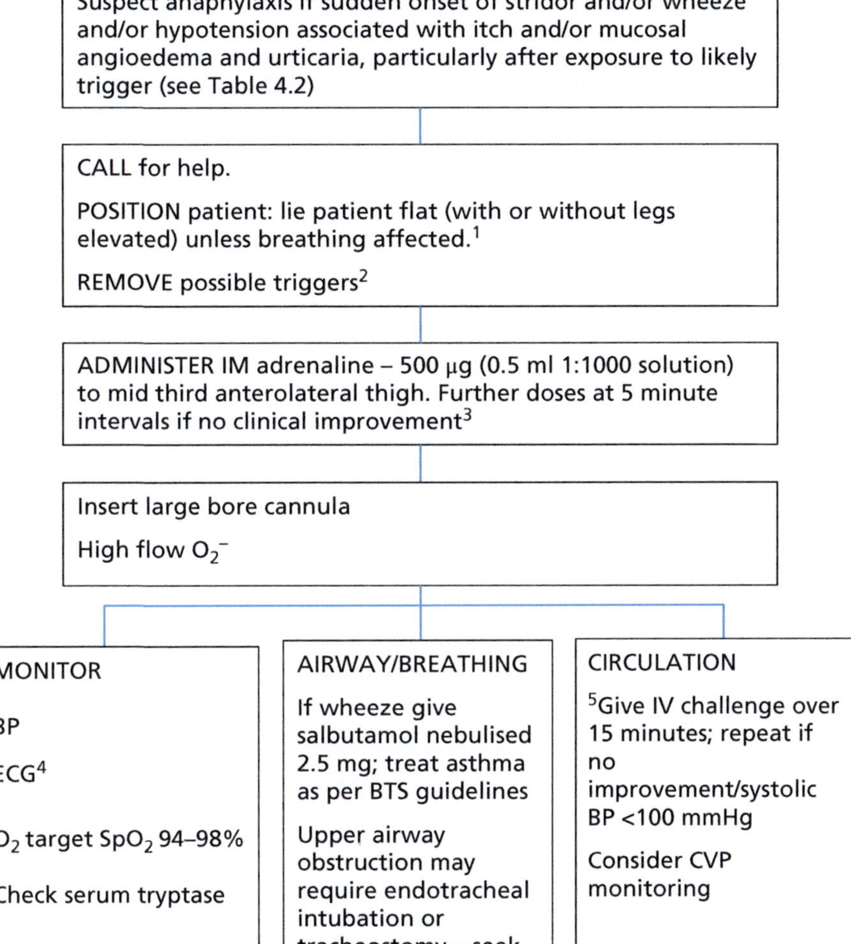

Figure 4.1 The management of anaphylaxis.

Table 4.3 Differential diagnosis of anaphylaxis.

Diagnosis	Comment
Chronic spontaneous urticaria and angioedema	Background of symptoms daily for >6 weeks Stridor may develop due to laryngeal oedema Hypotension and wheeze not typical
ACE-inhibitor-induced angioedema	Swelling affects head and neck only; no itch, urticaria or hypotension; episodic, lasting 24–72 hours Swelling resistant to antihistamines and/or adrenaline Stridor may develop due to laryngeal oedema; if life-threatening airways obstruction consider treatment with icatibant. Seek Immunology advice May develop days to years after starting ACE-inhibitor; may persist for up to 3 months after ACE-inhibitor discontinuation
Hereditary angioedema	Urticaria and hypotension absent Swelling resistant to anti-histamines and/or adrenaline Stridor (due to laryngeal oedema) rather than wheeze
Acute asthma	Typically, airway symptoms only: hypotension late feature of severe asthma
Acute heart failure	No itch, urticaria or angioedema
Scombrotoxin poisoning	Symptoms appear within 30 min of eating spoiled fish, typically tuna, mackerel: urticaria, nausea, vomiting, diarrhoea, headache, metallic taste
Inducible laryngeal obstruction	Transient upper airway obstruction due to vocal cord adduction
Vasovagal reaction	No itch, urticaria or angioedema
Acute panic disorder	No itch, urticaria, angioedema, hypoxia or hypotension

ACE, angiotensin-converting enzyme.

Table 4.4 Serum mast cell tryptase in anaphylaxis.

Take samples at onset of symptoms then 1–2 h and >24 h (baseline) thereafter; label sample time clearly on request form

May be of use post-event when diagnostic uncertainty

Peaks at 60–120 min after onset of symptoms – falls to baseline by 24 h

Peak value >1.2 × baseline + 2 µg/L (even within the reference range) indicative of anaphylaxis

Poor negative predictive value – rise often absent in food anaphylaxis

Baseline elevated >20 µg/L may be due to mast cell disorders including mastocytosis

5 If there is respiratory distress call an anaesthetist. Upper airway obstruction can be due to either oedema of the larynx or epiglottis, and may require endotracheal intubation or emergency tracheostomy.
- Give high-flow oxygen as soon as available – target SpO_2 94–98%
- Treat bronchospasm, with nebulized salbutamol 2.5 mg. IV aminophylline (Chapter 22) can be added if needed.
- Nebulized adrenaline (5 mL of 1:1000 solution) may be of benefit where there is significant laryngeal obstruction due to angioedema (but not in lieu of IM adrenaline).

6 Hypovolaemia due to extravascular fluid shifts can be considerable. Start an IV infusion of crystalloid, e.g. 0.9% sodium chloride, Hartmann's solution, 500 mL to 1000 mL over 15 min (the higher rate if systolic BP is <90 mmHg). If there is heart failure, give 250 mL over 15 min. Monitor for signs of fluid overload. Use IO route if IV access is delayed.

7 Antihistamines are not recommended for initial emergency treatment in anaphylaxis; they may be used if persistent cutaneous symptoms e.g. urticaria or itch; corticosteroids are not recommended for initial treatment of anaphylaxis.

8 Using the patient's own adrenaline autoinjector (Epipen or Jext) is discouraged as delivers adrenaline 300 µg versus recommended 500 µg dose.

9 Take timed blood samples for mast cell tryptase testing (see Table 4.4).

Refractory anaphylaxis

Anaphylaxis is considered refractory if there is no sustained improvement after two doses of IM adrenaline.

- Critical care input is essential for airway management and administration of IV adrenaline. Consider low-dose adrenaline infusion via *dedicated* peripheral line: 0.5–1.0 mg/kg/h, opposite side to BP cuff. Titrate against clinical response. If infusion is not available continue with 500 µg adrenaline IM at 5 min intervals until infusion is established.
- Continue IV crystalloid infusion, giving a further 500 mL over 30 min. When the patient's condition is stable, put in a CVP line to guide fluid management (Chapter 2).
- Consider arterial line for continuous BP monitoring (Chapter 114).
- If the patient has been taking a non-cardioselective beta blocker and is resistant to adrenaline, give glucagon (1 mg IV bolus followed by an infusion of 1–2 mg/h).
- Consider corticosteroids if asthma exacerbation (Chapter 22).

Further management

1 In up to 20% of cases, biphasic reactions occur between 1 and 8 h after the onset of symptoms; rarely the second phase of the reaction may be more severe than the first. There are no features of anaphylaxis predictive of a biphasic reaction occurring, other than the individual having had one during a previous episode. Treatment is as per initial treatment of the reaction.
2 If ongoing cutaneous symptoms, e.g. urticaria or angioedema, treat with oral non-sedating antihistamine, for example cetirizine 10–20 mg.
3 If drug allergy is suspected update allergy alerts on drug chart/electronic prescribing system and patient records. Hospital allergy alert wristband should be issued, if available.

On discharge

- Inform the patient of the allergen responsible or suspected of having been responsible for the reaction. The advice given by non-specialists on allergen avoidance should be over-inclusive (e.g. avoid all nuts when only one type appears implicated): this can be revised in specialist care.
- Signpost to patient support groups (e.g. Anaphylaxis UK and Allergy UK) for information about allergen avoidance and use of adrenaline autoinjectors (AAIs).
- AAIs should be prescribed where an allergen is not predictably avoidable or is unknown; they are not usually required when a drug has been the trigger. Prescription should not be deferred until specialist review. Prescribing and training for AAIs is device-specific and should be given prior to discharge.
- If a drug is implicated, mark clinical notes clearly; inform the patient's GP and other involved health professionals.
- Poorly controlled asthma increases the risk of life-threatening and fatal anaphylaxis. Assess ongoing asthma control (nocturnal disturbance, frequency of use of rescue medication and oral corticosteroid use) and intensify treatment as appropriate.
- Beta-blockers will antagonize the effects of adrenaline and may make anaphylaxis difficult to treat. Risk assess their continued use and discontinue if the benefit does not outweigh that risk.
- Refer to an allergy clinic for specialist assessment if new presentation; also consider referral if previously diagnosed and taking high-risk behaviour or if a new allergen is implicated.

Further reading

National Institute for Health and Care Excellence (2016) Anaphylaxis: assessment and referral after emergency treatment. Clinical guideline (CG134). https://www.nice.org.uk/guidance/cg134?un lid=639094620201610645435.

Resuscitation Council UK (2021) Emergency treatment of anaphylaxis: Guidelines for healthcare providers. https://www.resus.org.uk/sites/default/files/2021-05/Emergency%20Treatment%20of%20Anaphylaxis %20May%202021_0.pdf.

CHAPTER 5

Sepsis

ANDREW MCCALLUM

- Make a working diagnosis of sepsis (Box 5.1) if a patient has **organ dysfunction** in the context of **suspected or proven infection**. Because infection may be occult consider the diagnosis whenever organ dysfunction is unexplained.

Box 5.1 Definitions and criteria.

Term	Definition	Clinical criteria
Sepsis	Life-threatening organ dysfunction caused by a dysregulated host response to infection	Suspected or proven infection with total SOFA score ≥ 2
Septic shock	Subset of sepsis in which underlying circulatory, cellular and metabolic abnormalities are associated with a greater risk of mortality than sepsis alone	Sepsis with persisting hypotension requiring vasopressor therapy to maintain mean arterial pressure ≥ 65 mmHg and having a serum lactate level > 2 mmol/L, despite adequate volume resuscitation
Organ dysfunction	Organ dysfunction is identified using SOFA score. If previous baseline organ dysfunction is not known, for the purposes of the initial diagnosis baseline SOFA could be assumed as 0.	Please refer to Table 5.1
qSOFA	Consists of three variables. Presence of two or more of these abnormalities in patients with suspected infection identifies higher risk of developing adverse outcomes often associated with sepsis.	Systolic blood pressure < 100 mmHg Acute change in mentation (GCS ≥ 13) Respiratory rate > 22/min
Red Flag Sepsis	Pragmatic, operational solution to sepsis identification on the wards. Patients with suspected infection meeting the criteria should be treated as a case of 'suspected sepsis'	Suspected or proven infection with NEWS2 score of ≥ 7 OR Suspected or proven infection with NEWS2 score of 5 or 6 AND • Lactate >2 mmol/L • Chemotherapy in the last 6 weeks • Other organ failure evident (e.g. acute kidney injury [AKI]) • Patient looks extremely unwell • Patient is actively deteriorating

Definition refers to the illness concept and clinical criteria refers to the clinical variables used to identify a case of sepsis or septic shock.

SOFA, Sequential Organ Failure Assessment.

Acute Medicine: A Practical Guide to the Management of Medical Emergencies, Sixth Edition.
Edited by Mridula Rajwani, Leila Vaziri, and Ivie Gbinigie.
© 2026 John Wiley & Sons Ltd. Published 2026 by John Wiley & Sons Ltd.

Table 5.1 Sequential (sepsis-related) organ failure assessment score.

Organ system	Variable (units)	Dysfunction			Failure	
		0	1	2	3	4
Respiratory system	PaO_2/FiO_2 ratio (kPa)	≥53.3	<53.3	<40	<26.7 and ventilation	<13.3 and ventilation
Cardiovascular system	MAP (mmHg) or vasoactive drugs µg/kg/min	MAP ≥70	MAP <70	Dopamine <5 or Dobutamine	Epinephrine or norepinephrine ≤0.1 or dopamine 5.1–15	Epinephrine or norepinephrine >0.1 or dopamine >15
Central nervous system	Glasgow Coma Score	15	13–14	10–12	6–9	<6
Coagulation	Platelets	≥150	<150	<100	<50	<20
Renal	Creatinine (µmol/L) OR	<110	110–170	171–299	300–440	>400
	Urine output (mL/24 h)				<500 mLs/24 h	<200 mLs/h
Liver	Bilirubin µmol/L	<20	20–32	33–101	102–204	>204

- Septic shock (Box 5.1) is a subset of sepsis in which underlying circulatory, cellular and metabolic abnormalities are associated with a greater risk of mortality than sepsis alone.
- *Escherichia coli* and other Enterobacterales, *Staphylococcus aureus*, *Streptococcus pneumoniae* (pneumococcus), *Neisseria meningitidis* (meningococcus) and *Streptococcus pyogenes* (Group A Strep) are the most common pathogens.
- A good outcome depends on prompt diagnosis, timely administration of appropriate initial antibiotic therapy, adequate fluid resuscitation and drainage of any infected collection (source control).

Clinical assessment of the patient with suspected sepsis

Patients with suspected sepsis require prompt and focussed clinical history and examination. Consider risk factors for sepsis:
- Exposure to pathogens
  - Typically, commensal pathogens in the United Kingdom
  - Consider outbreaks and recent travel
- Impaired immunity – anatomical
  - Loss of epithelial barrier – wounds, ulcers, surgery, lines, perforated viscus, injecting drug use
  - Loss of normal drainage – urinary/biliary obstruction, lung disease, lymphoedema
  - Prosthetic material – lines, catheters, endotracheal tubes
- Impaired immunity – cellular or humoral
  - Iatrogenic – chemotherapy, deliberate immunosuppression
  - Chronic illness – diabetes, liver/renal failure, malignancy, malnutrition
  - Haematological malignancy/marrow failure
  - Splenectomy/hyposplenism

Table 5.2 Clinical assessment of the patient with suspected sepsis.

History

Context: age, sex, comorbidities, medications, hospital or community acquired

Current major symptoms and their time course

Risk factors for sepsis? Consider immunosuppressive therapy, HIV infection, cancer, renal failure, liver failure, diabetes, malnutrition, splenectomy, IV drug use, prosthetic heart valve, other prosthetic material, peripheral IV cannula, central venous cannula, bladder catheter

Recent culture results?

Recent surgery or invasive procedures?

Recent foreign travel?

Contact with infectious disease? Any risk of exposure to a High Consequence Infectious Disease (HCID)?

Passed urine in the past 18 h?

Examination

Physiological observations

Head and neck: Neck stiffness? Jaundice? Mouth, teeth and sinuses: focus of infection? Lymphadenopathy?

Chest: Focal lung crackles/bronchial breathing? Pleural/pericardial rub? Heart murmur? Prosthetic heart valve? Pacemaker/implantable cardioverter defibrillator (ICD)?

Abdomen and pelvis: Distension? Ascites? Tenderness/guarding? Bladder catheter? Perineal/perianal abscess?

Limbs: Acute arthritis? Prosthetic joint? Abscess?

Skin and soft tissues: Rash/purpura? Pressure ulceration? Cellulitis? Soft-tissue infection? IV cannula/tunnelled line?

- HIV infection
- Congenital immunodeficiency syndromes
- Pre-existing organ dysfunction
  - Heart failure, chronic lung disease, renal failure, liver failure
  - Reduced physiological reserve increases the risk of more severe infection
- Extremes of age and pregnancy
  - Risks are greater in babies and the elderly. Reflects reduced reserve and immune immaturity or senescence
  - Pregnancy, including the peripartum, and up to 4 weeks post birth/loss
  An overview of clinical assessment is shown in Table 5.2.
- Prioritise observations for a NEWS2 score and measure lactate.
- Remember that some patients with sepsis may not develop a fever – including those at extremes of age, with spinal cord injuries, or those on some anticancer treatments.
- The clinical setting may make it obvious, for example signs of pneumonia (Chapters 25) or meningitis (Chapter 73) or recent instrumentation of the urinary or biliary tract.
- Check for neck stiffness, focal lung crackles or bronchial breathing, heart murmur, abdominal tenderness or guarding, acute arthritis, cellulitis, soft tissue abscess and signs of infection at the site of IV lines.
- Obtain a surgical opinion if you suspect an abdominal or pelvic source of sepsis.
- Many patients with neutropenic sepsis (Chapter 74) have no detectable clinical focus.

Evaluating severity

Scoring systems (Table 5.3) should be used to stratify the risk of death from sepsis to inform urgency of response. These guidelines apply to adult patients (>16 years) who are not pregnant or have not recently been pregnant (past 4 weeks).

- **HIGH RISK** of severe illness or death from sepsis:
  - NEWS2 ≥ 7 OR

- NEWS2 5 or 6 AND one of:
  - Any one NEWS2 parameter with a score of 3
  - Mottled or ashen appearance
  - Non-blanching petechial or purpuric rash
  - Cyanosis of skin, lips or tongue
  - Deterioration since the last assessment
  - Deterioration since any recent intervention
  - Lactate >2 mmol/L OR known AKI
- **MODERATE RISK** of severe illness or death from sepsis:
  - NEWS2 5 or 6 OR
  - NEWS2 1–4 AND one of:
    - Any one NEWS2 parameter with a score of 3
    - Mottled or ashen appearance
    - Non-blanching petechial or purpuric rash
    - Cyanosis of skin, lips or tongue
    - Deterioration since the last assessment
    - Deterioration since any recent intervention
- **LOW RISK** of severe illness or death from sepsis
  - NEWS2 1–4

Table 5.3 The NEWS2 scoring system (Royal College of Physicians, 2017).

Physiological parameter	Score						
	3	**2**	**1**	**0**	**1**	**2**	**3**
Respiratory rate (per minute)	≤8		9–11	12–20		21–24	≥25
SpO$_2$ Scale 1 (%)	≤91	92–93	94–95	≥96			
SpO$_2$ Scale 2 (%)	≤83	84–85	86–87	88–92 ≥93 on room air	93–94 on oxygen	95–96 on oxygen	≥97
Air or oxygen?		Oxygen		Air			
Systolic blood pressure (mmHg)	≤90	91–100	101–110	111–219			≥220
Pulse (per minute)	≤40		41–50	51–90	91–110	111–130	≥131
Consciousness				Alert			CVPU
Temperature (°C)	≤35.0		35.1–36.0	36.1–38.0	38.1–39.0	≥39.1	

C, confusion; V, voice; P, pain; U, unresponsive.

Use SpO$_2$ Scale 2 if target oxygen range 88–92% (typically those at risk of hypercapnic respiratory failure).

Table 5.4 NEWS2 trigger thresholds.

National Early Warning Score (NEWS2)	Frequency of monitoring
0	Minimum 12 hourly
Total 1–4	Minimum 4–6 hourly
3 in a single parameter	Minimum 1 hourly
Total 5 or more (urgent response threshold)	Minimum 1 hourly
Total 7 or more (emergency response threshold)	Continuous monitoring of vital signs

Priorities

Manage patients with sepsis according to a sepsis bundle, for example the 'Sepsis 6'.

1 **Obtain senior help:**
   Typically, a specialty registrar doctor or equivalent.
   Involve relevant specialties early (ICU, Infectious Diseases/Microbiology, Radiology, Surgery) – allows for judgement around antibiotics, targeted diagnostics, source control. May help to seek alternative diagnoses or de-escalate care.

2 **Give oxygen if required:**
   Give targeted oxygen therapy if saturations are <92% – aiming for $SpO_2 \geq 94\%$, or 88–92% in patients at risk of hypercapnic respiratory failure.

3 **Send bloods including cultures:**
   - Full blood count – the white cell count may be low in overwhelming bacterial sepsis; a low platelet count may reflect disseminated intravascular coagulation (DIC).
   - U&Es – acute kidney injury (AKI)?
   - LFTs – transaminitis? Evidence of biliary obstruction?
   - Clotting – DIC?
   - Blood glucose – hypoglycaemia can complicate sepsis, especially in patients with liver disease.
   - Amylase – pancreatitis may be a sepsis mimic.
   - Venous blood gas – acidosis? Hyperlactataemia? A raised lactate is an important marker of septic shock and is associated with increased mortality (other causes include liver dysfunction, seizures, metformin and salbutamol).
   - Blood cultures and microbiology samples – see Table 5.5. Early confirmation of infection is from microscopy or Gram staining or PCR panels or antigen detection tests. Take blood cultures and cultures from other relevant sites urgently in sepsis.

4 **Give IV antibiotics and consider source control:**
   Empiric broad spectrum, maximum dose. Where there is a clear source, use targeted antibiotics according to local guidelines (Table 5.6). Consider allergy status and need for antivirals.
   Start prompt antibiotic therapy as soon as blood is taken for culture:
   - Within 1 h in patients at HIGH RISK of severe illness or death
   - Within 3 h in patients at MODERATE RISK of severe illness or death
   - Within 6 h in patients at LOW RISK of severe illness or death
   If the source is amenable to drainage, this should occur within 12 h.

5 **Give IV fluids:**
   If systolic blood pressure is <90 mmHg and/or the serum lactate is >2 mmol/L, give crystalloid IV 500 mL over 15 min using one, if necessary two, large bore (16 G or larger) cannulae. Give further IV fluid up to at least 30 mL/kg if hypotension or hyperlactataemia persists.

6 **Monitor:**
   Sepsis is dynamic – is your patient improving?
   Aim for a urine output >0.5 L/kg/h and consider a urinary catheter.
   Recheck lactate – aiming for <2 mmol/L.
   Serial monitoring of NEWS2 score (Tables 5.3 and 5.4).
   If patients meeting the high-risk criteria do not respond within 1 h of any intervention, discuss with critical care and ensure senior review in person.

Imaging should be included as part of your assessment: a chest X-ray should be performed, and consideration of further cross-sectional imaging if no likely source of infection identified after clinical examination and initial tests. An ECG should be performed if aged >50, history of cardiac disease or suspicion of arrhythmia.

Table 5.5 Microbiological tests in suspected sepsis.

Sample type	First-line tests	Second-line tests (required in specific cases)
Blood	Peripheral blood cultures Two sets (before antimicrobials provided it will not lead to significant delays). Positive in 30–50% and then associated with a worse outcome. Volume is important – 8–10 ml/bottle HIV serology	For example, malaria if travel history
Intravenous catheter	Catheter blood culture (each lumen) paired with peripheral. Consider removal of catheter and MC&S of tip if the patient is in septic shock and deteriorating	
Urine	Urinalysis Microscopy, culture and sensitivity. If catheterised, consider changing catheter and sending catheter-specimen of urine from new catheter.	Urine legionella antigen
Cerebrospinal fluid	—	Microscopy, culture and sensitivity Pneumococcal/meningococcal PCR
Nose and throat	—	Respiratory viral PCR panel SARS-CoV-2/influenza PCR or point-of-care tests
Sputum	—	Microscopy, culture and sensitivity Once intubated a deep, non-directed or bronchoscopic-directed washing has greater sensitivity and specificity Acid-fast bacilli
Pus/tissue	—	Microscopy, culture and sensitivity
Stool	—	Bacterial culture/PCR *Clostridioides difficile* testing

Antimicrobials and stewardship

Principles of good antibiotic practice are given in Table 5.7. The antibiotic used should be guided by a hospital protocol or an infection specialist based on the likely organism, taking account of the source of sepsis if known (Table 5.6), whether the infection is community or hospital-acquired, results of previous isolates from the patient and the local pattern of antibiotic resistance in patients.

Antibiotics should be given promptly, ideally after blood cultures are taken. Data from large observational studies of patients with sepsis and shock have shown increased mortality with every hour delay in antibiotic administration. **Current guidelines recommend that antibiotics are administered within 1 h (of first NEWS2 score on Emergency Department (ED) presentation or ward deterioration) in patients at HIGH RISK of severe illness or death, within 3 h in patients at MODERATE RISK of severe illness or death, and within 6 h in patients at LOW RISK of severe illness or death**. This encourages rapid treatment of the most unwell patients, and more focussed treatment in clinically stable patients by using this time to gather information for a more specific diagnosis.

Once the source of infection is confirmed or microbiological results are available the spectrum should be narrowed. Change to oral therapy once the patient is improved, has been apyrexial for >24 h, is eating and drinking and there is no evidence of a deep-seated infection. Review the need for continuing antibiotics early and repeatedly: if the diagnosis of sepsis/infection is refuted the antibiotic should be stopped. Some antibiotics

Table 5.6 The example of initial antibiotic therapy regime for adult sepsis (excludes penicillin-allergic patients). Always seek local guidance and check doses in the *British National Formulary*.

Suspected source of sepsis	Initial antibiotic therapy (IV, high dose if septic shock)
Bacterial meningitis	Ceftriaxone 2 g IV BD. If immunocompromised or age > 60 y, consider amoxicillin 2 g IV q 4-hourly to cover listeria
Community-acquired pneumonia	Severe (CURB 65 ≥ 2): co-amoxiclav 1.2 g IV tds plus clarithromycin 500 mg PO/IV
Hospital-acquired pneumonia	Co-amoxiclav 1.2 g IV tds
Infective endocarditis	Take 3 sets of cultures, ideally 2–4 h apart. Discuss with ID/micro prior to starting antibiotics (see Table 5.5)
Urinary tract infection	Complicated/healthcare-associated/pyelonephritis: co-amoxiclav 1.2 g IV tds plus gentamicin 5 mg/kg IV
Intra-abdominal sepsis, for example appendicitis, peritonitis Seek advice for other conditions, for example spontaneous bacterial peritonitis.	Co-amoxiclav 1.2 g IV tds plus metronidazole 500 mg IV tds
Suspected vascular catheter-related bloodstream infection Remove suspected infected line after alternative vascular access established	Vancomycin IV plus flucloxacillin 2 g IV qds plus stat gentamicin 5 mg/kg IV
Septic arthritis (native joint) Seek advice for prosthetic joint or metalwork infection	Co-amoxiclav 1.2 g IV tds
Cellulitis	Flucloxacillin 2 g IV qds
Necrotising fasciitis Discuss urgently with infection/plastic surgeon	Co-amoxiclav 1.2 g IV tds plus clindamycin 900 mg IV qds plus vancomycin IV (in MRSA-positive patients)
No localising signs: neutropenic	Piperacillin-tazobactam 4.5 g IV qds Meropenem 1 g IV tds in patients on high-dose methotrexate protocols (≥ 1 g/m^2)
No localising signs: not neutropenic	Amoxicillin 1 g IV tds plus gentamicin 5 mg/kg IV

Table 5.7 Good practice in antimicrobial prescribing for sepsis.

Antibiotics should be administered promptly (within 1, 3 or 6 h depending on severity)

Antibiotics should target the likely source of infection (Table 5.6)

Empiric 'broad spectrum' antibiotics should be used when the source is unknown

Consider whether the infection is community-acquired or healthcare-associated, any previously known culture results and the patient's allergy status when selecting antimicrobials

The first dose should be prescribed as a timed 'stat' and the need for urgent administration should be communicated to nursing staff

The indication for the antibiotics should be documented as well as a review and stop date

Antibiotics should be focussed as soon as it is safe to do so by narrowing the spectrum and converting to oral therapy

require drug-level monitoring, for example gentamicin or vancomycin (in severe penicillin allergy or for treatment of methicillin-resistant *S. aureus* [MRSA] infection).

Duration of antibiotics will depend on the source of sepsis. Shorter courses (e.g. five days) are often safe if clinical resolution has occurred. In some situations, prolonged courses are necessary, for example infective endocarditis, lung abscess or bone infection: seek advice from an infection specialist.

To avoid the development of resistance and the development of healthcare-associated infection (e.g. *Clostridioides difficile* diarrhoea) antibiotics should not be overused: document the indication for the drug and review the need for continuing antibiotics early and repeatedly.

Further management

Hypotension and organ dysfunction (see Chapter 2)

Management requires invasive monitoring and critical care expertise.

Arterial and central venous monitoring will be required if the patient is in septic shock or once in the ICU but placement should not delay initial priorities.

The first priority is adequate fluid resuscitation, using a balanced crystalloid (e.g. Hartmann's solution). Aim for at least 30 mL/kg of IV crystalloid in the first 3 h of resuscitation. This will be guided by a clinical assessment of the circulation and tissue perfusion. Dynamic measures can guide adequacy of fluid resuscitation: cardiac output monitoring (stroke volume, stroke volume variation and pulse pressure variation), response to passive leg raising, echocardiography.

If the patient remains hypotensive despite adequate fluid correction, start norepinephrine (dose range 0.05–1.0 µg/kg/min). This must be administered via a central line. Aim for mean arterial pressure > 65 mmHg. The goal is to restore tissue perfusion. Monitor with:

- Vital signs, capillary refill time, pulse and skin findings
- Urine output (aim for >0.5 mL/kg/h)
- Arterial lactate (aim for normalization)
- Central venous O_2 saturation ($ScvO_2$) (aim for >70%)

If evidence of end-organ hypoperfusion persists, perform a bedside echocardiogram and/or measure the cardiac output. Consider measures to improve oxygen delivery, such as transfusion of packed red cells or adding inotropic therapy, for example dobutamine.

Respiratory support

Mechanical ventilation in sepsis is indicated for:

- Severe acidosis
- Multi-organ failure
- Reduced consciousness
- Respiratory failure, for example due to pneumonia or acute respiratory distress syndrome (ARDS). ARDS is characterised by acute-onset hypoxia and bilateral pulmonary infiltrates in the absence of a cardiac cause (excluded by pulmonary artery occlusion pressure measurement or echocardiography).

The principles of ARDS management include:

- Mechanical ventilation with positive end expiratory pressure (PEEP) and low tidal volumes (6 mL/kg predicted body weight)
- A conservative fluid regimen
- Ventilation in the prone position for moderate or severe ARDS
- Neuromuscular blocking drugs for severe ARDS

High-flow nasal oxygen (HFNO) therapy may be used in sepsis-induced hypoxaemic respiratory failure and may be available outside HDU/ICU on some wards. This can achieve airflows as high as 60 L/min and inspired oxygen fractions of 95–100%.

Acute kidney injury (see Chapter 86)

AKI is common in sepsis and is associated with a worse outcome.

The principles of treatment of AKI in sepsis are:

- Rule out additional obstruction
- Optimise fluid replacement and correction of tissue perfusion
- Consider renal replacement (usually with continuous veno-venous haemofiltration or intermittent haemodialysis) for refractory oliguria, fluid overload, acidosis, hyperkalaemia or azotaemia

Source control

When a persisting source of sepsis exists, it is unlikely that antibiotics alone will be effective. Consider empyema, appendicitis, pyelonephrosis, necrotizing fasciitis. Indwelling cannulae, especially central venous lines, should be removed (and the tip sent for culture). Involve surgical teams/interventional radiology early if the source of infection is amenable to intervention.

Problems

Sepsis in the neutropenic patient (see Chapter 74)

Consider neutropenic sepsis in people who become unwell and have had systemic anticancer treatment in the last 30 days or are receiving some immunosuppressive treatments. Patients with some haematological malignancies (e.g. acute lymphoblastic leukaemia (ALL) or acute myeloid leukaemia (AML) or a bone marrow failure syndrome e.g. myelodysplastic syndrome) or recipients of haematopoietic stem cell transplants are at risk of neutropenic sepsis.

Patients with neutrophil counts $<0.5 \times 10^9$/L are at high risk of bacterial infection, particularly from Gram-negative rods and *S. aureus* and *epidermidis*. If the neutropenic patient has a temperature of $>37.5\,°C$ or other features compatible with sepsis (including, but not limited to, tachycardia, hypothermia, hypotension, confusion and diarrhoea) consider neutropenic sepsis and start empiric broad spectrum antibiotic therapy. Search for a focus of infection. Examination should include the entire skin including the perineum and perianal region, indwelling IV lines and other IV sites, and the mouth, teeth and sinuses. Investigations required urgently are given in Table 5.5.

Sepsis associated with IV drug use

Several causes of fever must be considered (Table 5.8). Right-sided endocarditis may not give rise to abnormal cardiac signs. Antibiotic therapy must cover *Staphylococci*.

Disseminated intravascular coagulation

DIC is a complication of sepsis (as well as a number of non-infective disorders). This should be suspected in patients with sepsis and in patients with septic shock who develop purpura, prolonged oozing from puncture sites, bleeding from surgical wounds or bleeding from the gastrointestinal and respiratory tracts. Confirm by a

Table 5.8 Possible causes of fever associated with IV drug use.

Infection at injection sites
Thrombophlebitis
Endocarditis (especially right-sided) (which may be complicated by septic pulmonary embolism)
Pulmonary tuberculosis
Hepatitis B or C
Septic arthritis
Pyrogen reaction
HIV-related infection, for example cryptococcal meningitis, *Pneumocystis carinii* pneumonia

low platelet count ($<100 \times 10^{12}$/L), prolonged prothrombin and activated partial thromboplastin times, and a high plasma concentration of fibrin degradation products. Ask for advice on management from a haematologist.

If there is active bleeding or a significant invasive procedure (i.e. surgery or radiological drainage) is needed, give fresh frozen plasma and platelet concentrate, although this is not usually necessary for invasive lines in the ICU (seek specialist advice). There is no conclusive evidence for the use of heparin in the treatment of DIC, but this should be considered if there is thromboembolism. Give vitamin K 10 mg IV to reverse possible vitamin K deficiency which may contribute to the coagulopathy, although there is no evidence base addressing this specific question in sepsis.

Further reading

Evans L, Rhodes A, Alhazzani W, *et al.* (2021) Surviving sepsis campaign: international guidelines for management of sepsis and septic shock 2021. *Crit Care Med* 49, e1063–e1143.

National Institute for Health and Care Excellence (NICE) (2024) Suspected sepsis: recognition, diagnosis and early management. NICE guideline NG51. https://www.nice.org.uk/guidance/ng51.

Royal College of Physicians (2017) National Early Warning Score (NEWS) 2: standardising the assessment of acute-illness severity in the NHS. Updated report of a working party. https://www.rcplondon.ac.uk/file/8636/download.

Seymour CW, Liu VX, Iwashyna TJ, *et al.* (2016) Assessment of clinical criteria for sepsis: for the Third International Consensus definitions for sepsis and septic shock (Sepsis-3). *JAMA* 315, 762–774.

Shankar-Hari M, Phillips GS, Levy ML, *et al.* (2016) Developing a new definition and assessing new clinical criteria for septic shock: For the Third International Consensus definitions for sepsis and septic shock (Sepsis-3). *JAMA* 315, 775–787.

Singer M, Deutschman CS, Seymour CW, *et al.* (2016) The Third International Consensus definitions for sepsis and septic shock (Sepsis-3). *JAMA* 315, 801–810.

Standards Unit, Specialised Microbiology and Laboratories, UK Health Security Agency (2023) UK Standards for Microbiology Investigations: Sepsis and systemic or disseminated infections. https://www.rcpath.org/static/aae2df9a-72c9-4bf3-8e686eaa4d9d5ef9/a14bbad5-1638-46d0-82fd84d122d4abd2/uk-smi-s-12i1-review-of-users-comments-sepsis-and-systemic-or-disseminated-infections-january-2023-pdf.pdf.

UK Health Security Agency (2024) Start smart then focus: antimicrobial stewardship toolkit for inpatient care settings. https://www.gov.uk/government/publications/antimicrobial-stewardship-start-smart-then-focus/start-smart-then-focus-antimicrobial-stewardship-toolkit-for-inpatient-care-settings.

CHAPTER 6

Cardiac tamponade

DAVID SPRIGINGS AND DOREEN LEE

Consider cardiac tamponade in the breathless patient who has distended neck veins or pulsus paradoxus. Pulsus paradoxus is an exaggeration of the normal inspiratory fall in systolic blood pressure of >10 mmHg and may be palpable in the radial artery, with the radial pulse disappearing on inspiration. Have a high index of suspicion in the presence of predisposing conditions (Table 6.1), notably after percutaneous cardiac intervention, central vein cannulation or cancer. The blood pressure may be normal until the late stage of tamponade, maintained by sympathetic vasoconstriction.

The speed of accumulation of pericardial fluid determines whether the presentation of cardiac tamponade is acute or subacute. Urgent echocardiography is the key investigation.

Table 6.1 Causes of cardiac tamponade.

Bleeding into the pericardial space	• Penetrating and blunt chest trauma, including external cardiac compression • Bleeding from a cardiac chamber or coronary artery caused by perforation or laceration as a complication of cardiac catheterisation, percutaneous coronary or valve intervention, implantation of cardiac device with transvenous lead, pericardiocentesis or central venous cannulation • Bleeding after cardiac surgery • Cardiac rupture after myocardial infarction • Aortic dissection (proximal, type A) with retrograde extension into pericardial space • Anticoagulant therapy for atrial fibrillation or other indication in the presence of pericarditis • Thrombolytic therapy given (inappropriately) for acute pericarditis
Serous or sero-sanguinous pericardial effusion	• Neoplastic involvement of the pericardium (most commonly in carcinoma of breast or bronchus, lymphoma or cardiac angiosarcoma) • Pericarditis complicating autoimmune diseases (e.g. systemic lupus erythematosus, rheumatoid arthritis) • Post-cardiac injury syndrome • Tuberculous and viral pericarditis • Uraemic pericarditis • Idiopathic pericarditis (tamponade is a rare complication)
Purulent pericarditis	Pyogenic bacterial infection, usually due to spread of intrathoracic infection, e.g. following thoracic surgery or trauma or complicating bacterial pneumonia

Acute Medicine: A Practical Guide to the Management of Medical Emergencies, Sixth Edition.
Edited by Mridula Rajwani, Leila Vaziri, and Ivie Gbinigie.
© 2026 John Wiley & Sons Ltd. Published 2026 by John Wiley & Sons Ltd.

Table 6.2 Echocardiography in suspected cardiac tamponade.

Is there a pericardial effusion?	Note the presence, size and distribution (circumferential or loculated) of pericardial fluid; small effusions are <10 mm thick at end-diastole, moderate 10–20 mm thick, and large >20 mm
	Be aware that a pleural effusion or dilated right ventricle may be misdiagnosed on echocardiography as a pericardial effusion
Are there echocardiographic signs of cardiac tamponade?	Prolonged and widespread diastolic collapse of the free wall of the right ventricle
	Fall in transmitral E wave and aortic velocities during inspiration by >25%
	Dilated inferior vena cava (>20 mm) with inspiratory collapse <50%
	Decrease in LV cavity size on inspiration
	Increase in trans-tricuspid E wave during inspiration by >40%
Is pericardiocentesis feasible and safe?	The risks of pericardiocentesis are lowest when the pericardial effusion is >20 mm thick. The subcostal approach is usually the preferred route.
	Drainage may be difficult if the fluid is dense or there are multiple loculations.

Priorities

1 Give oxygen if there is hypoxaemia, attach an electrocardiogram (ECG) monitor and place an IV cannula. Your examination should include careful inspection of the neck veins and assessment for pulsus paradoxus.

2 Obtain an ECG and chest X-ray and perform bedside echocardiography. The ECG typically shows tachycardia, and may show low QRS voltages and electrical alternans. Echocardiographic findings are summarised in Table 6.2.

3 If a pericardial effusion with clinical and echocardiographic signs of tamponade is confirmed, contact a cardiologist urgently to discuss pericardiocentesis. If systolic pressure is <90 mmHg and the effusion cannot be drained immediately, treat with IV fluids together with an infusion of noradrenaline via a central line.

4 Causes of cardiac tamponade needing urgent surgical management include proximal (type A) aortic dissection with haemopericardium, ventricular free wall rupture after acute myocardial infarction, severe chest trauma and iatrogenic haemopericardium when bleeding cannot be controlled percutaneously. Give blood products as needed to treat coagulopathy, reverse anticoagulation and correct anaemia.

Further management

This is directed at the underlying cause (Table 6.1).

Consider purulent pericarditis if the patient is unwell with signs of sepsis. Take blood cultures and start antibiotic therapy (e.g. IV vancomycin and ceftriaxone). Seek urgent advice from a microbiologist.

Patient with malignant effusions will usually require further intervention to prevent recurrent tamponade, for example chemotherapy or creation of a pericardial window.

If the patient has pericardial effusion with tamponade complicating autoimmune disease, start prednisolone 30–40 mg PO daily, with gastroprotection.

Problems

1 **Signs of tamponade but only small pericardial effusion (echo separation < 10 mm).**

This can occur with effusive-constructive pericarditis in malignancy, autoimmune disease and after viral infection. Percutaneous drainage is potentially hazardous and may not relieve the symptoms. Seek urgent advice from a cardiologist.

2 **Tamponade early after cardiac surgery**

Discuss management with a cardiac surgeon. It may be more appropriate to drain the effusion surgically.

3 **Tamponade with severely impaired left ventricular function**

Total pericardiocentesis may lead to further ventricular dilatation. Limit drainage to 1 L. Seek urgent advice from a cardiologist.

Echocardiography should be used to guide pericardiocentesis by confirming the position of the needle tip from the presence of intra-pericardial bubbles by injecting up to 10 mL of agitated saline.

Pericardial fluid should be drained slowly over time to prevent pericardial decompression syndrome.

Further reading

Alerhand S, Adrian RJ, Long B, Avila J. (2022) Pericardial tamponade: a comprehensive emergency medicine and echocardiography review. *Am J Emerg Med* 58, 159–174.

CHAPTER 7
Acid–base disorders

Nick Talbot and Ivan Tang

Arterial pH is tightly regulated (Box 7.1). Disorders of arterial pH are commonly encountered in acute medicine; arterial blood gases and pH should be measured in any patient with critical illness. Abnormalities of acid–base balance can be identified as acidosis or alkalosis, noting the nature and severity of the disturbance (Tables 7.1 and 7.2; Figure 7.1). The physiological and pathological consequences of acid–base disorders are summarized in Table 7.3.

- An effective approach to understanding an acid–base disorder is to look at the relationship between arterial pH (or hydrogen ion concentration) and PCO_2 (Table 7.1, Figure 7.1). When the primary disturbance is metabolic, the PCO_2 will generally be either normal or out of keeping with the pH, that is, low in metabolic acidosis and high in metabolic alkalosis. When the primary disturbance is respiratory, the PCO_2 will be in keeping with the pH, that is, high in respiratory acidosis, and low in respiratory alkalosis.

Box 7.1 Compensation for acid–base disturbances.

Several homeostatic mechanisms defend against extracellular pH disturbance:

- Excess plasma hydrogen ions are buffered rapidly by other blood constituents. In particular, negatively charged proteins such as albumin and haemoglobin have a large capacity for binding hydrogen ions. The concentration of these proteins therefore influences the buffering capacity of the blood.
- Hydrogen ions may be taken up across cell membranes, often in exchange for potassium ions.
- Through sensing of the hydrogen ion concentration by arterial and central chemoreceptors, metabolic acid–base disturbances often result in respiratory compensation. This typically starts within minutes and can lead to profound changes in alveolar ventilation, particularly in the setting of acidosis.
- Metabolic compensation for acid–base disturbance can be mediated through changes in bicarbonate handling within the kidney. Changes in the plasma bicarbonate concentration may begin within hours, but typically progress over several days, so the presence of significant metabolic compensation is a marker of chronicity in acid–base disturbances.

In some cases, compensation for acid–base disturbance will be partial, such that the pH remains abnormal. Alternatively, a disturbance may be fully compensated. The latter is common, for example, in patients with longstanding type 2 respiratory failure due to chronic obstructive pulmonary disease (COPD), in whom the arterial partial pressure of CO_2 (PCO_2) is likely to be chronically elevated, but the pH normal, due to a compensatory rise in plasma bicarbonate. Beware of attributing any pH disturbance to overcompensation, which is much less likely than a mixed disturbance.

Acute Medicine: A Practical Guide to the Management of Medical Emergencies, Sixth Edition.
Edited by Mridula Rajwani, Leila Vaziri, and Ivie Gbinigie.
© 2026 John Wiley & Sons Ltd. Published 2026 by John Wiley & Sons Ltd.

Table 7.1 Classification and examples of acid–base disorders according to arterial hydrogen ion concentration/pH and PCO_2 (Figure 7.1).

Arterial PCO_2 (kPa)	Arterial pH or hydrogen ion concentration (nmol/L)		
	pH<7.35 [H+]>45	7.35–7.45 35–45	>7.45 <35
<4.7	Metabolic acidosis with partial respiratory compensation *or* Metabolic acidosis plus respiratory alkalosis, for example: • Pulmonary oedema • Salicylate poisoning (late) • Hepatorenal syndrome	Respiratory alkalosis with metabolic compensation	Respiratory alkalosis *or* Respiratory alkalosis plus metabolic alkalosis, for example: • Acute liver failure with vomiting or nasogastric drainage • Peritoneal dialysis for chronic renal failure
4.7–6.0	Metabolic acidosis	Normal acid–base status	Metabolic alkalosis
>6.0	Respiratory acidosis *or* Respiratory acidosis plus metabolic acidosis, for example: • Cardiopulmonary arrest • COPD complicated by circulatory failure or sepsis • Severe pulmonary oedema • Combined respiratory and renal failure • Severe tricyclic poisoning	Respiratory acidosis with metabolic compensation, for example: • COPD with chronic CO_2 retention*	Metabolic alkalosis plus respiratory acidosis, for example: • Diuretic therapy plus chronic CO_2 retention

COPD, chronic obstructive pulmonary disease.

* Chronic CO_2 retention (hypercapnia) is a feature with multiple chronic pathologies. COPD is the most widely described, but consider chronic hypercapnia in patients with other severe lung diseases, including bronchiectasis, cystic fibrosis, or fibrotic lung disease, and in those with systemic disease impacting ventilatory capacity, such as obesity hypoventilation, motor neuron disease or chest wall deformities.

Table 7.2 Grading of severity of acid–base disorders.

Arterial pH	Acid–base status	Arterial hydrogen ion concentration (nmol/L)
<7.2	Severe acidosis	>60
7.2–7.3	Moderate acidosis	50–60
7.3–7.35	Mild acidosis	45–50
7.35–7.45	Normal range	35–45
7.45–7.5	Mild alkalosis	30–35
7.5–7.6	Moderate alkalosis	20–30
>7.6	Severe alkalosis	<20

• Hyperkalaemia commonly accompanies both acute and chronic extracellular acidosis, so the plasma potassium concentration should be measured early in acidotic patients. Hyperkalaemia often results from impaired potassium excretion in renal failure, but extracellular acidosis of any cause may also lead to hyperkalaemia through the uptake of hydrogen ions into cells, in exchange for potassium. In extracellular alkalosis, the direction of exchange is reversed, so hypokalaemia may result.

Table 7.3 Consequences of acid–base disorders.

Acidosis	Alkalosis
Physiological	**Physiological**
Systemic vasodilatation	Peripheral vasoconstriction
Pulmonary vasoconstriction	Pulmonary vasodilatation
Hyperventilation	Hypoventilation
Renal ammoniagenesis	Renal bicarbonate secretion
Pathological	**Pathological**
Hyperkalaemia	Hypokalaemia
Impaired cardiac contractility/arrythmia	Reduced coronary blood flow
Bone demineralization	Reduced cerebral blood flow
Increased cerebral blood flow	Decreased ionized plasma calcium
Drowsiness and coma	Paraesthesia and muscle cramps

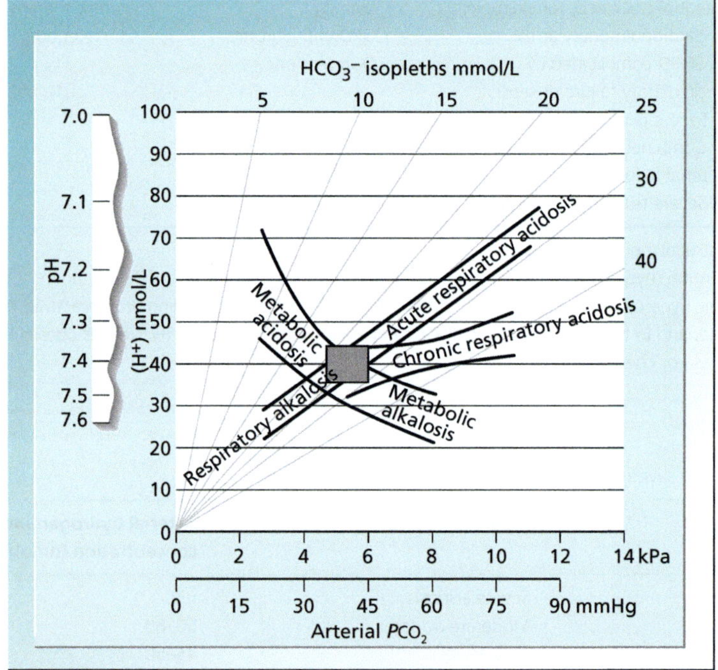

Figure 7.1 Acid–base diagram relating arterial pH or hydrogen ion concentration to arterial PCO_2. The shaded rectangle is the normal range. The 95% confidence limits of hydrogen ion concentration/PCO_2 relationships in single disturbances of acid–base balance are shown. Source: Flenley DC (1971) *Lancet* 1, 961. Reproduced with permission of Elsevier.

- Causes of metabolic acidosis can be subdivided according to the size of the so-called 'anion gap'. This value represents the difference between the sum of the concentration of major plasma cations (sodium and potassium), and the sum of the concentration of major plasma anions (chloride and bicarbonate):

$$\text{Anion gap} = \left(\left[Na^+\right]+\left[K^+\right]\right)-\left(\left[Cl^-\right]+\left[HCO_3^-\right]\right)$$

- A normal anion gap is around 10–18 mmol/L, but the reference range can vary considerably according to laboratory. It is an estimate of the unmeasured anions in the plasma. A high anion gap implies excess unmeasured plasma anions, which may be the cause of metabolic acidosis.
- Common causes of the four primary acid–base disturbances are given in Tables 7.4–7.7.
- The base excess is a calculated parameter that may provide further insight into the nature of an acid–base disorder. It represents the amount of strong acid that would need to be added or removed to bring the plasma pH to 7.4, with the temperature and PCO_2 normalised to 37.0 °C and 5.3 kPa, respectively. Acidosis in the presence of normal base excess on venous blood gas analysis, for example, suggests a respiratory cause and arterial blood gas analysis should be considered to characterise this further.
- When the primary pathology is not clear, consider a mixed disturbance, with two or more contributing factors (Table 7.1). This is distinct from a single disturbance with compensation (Box 7.1). Common examples include respiratory and metabolic acidosis in the setting of severe pneumonia and sepsis or combined metabolic alkalosis and metabolic acidosis in a patient with vomiting and chronic renal failure.

Table 7.4 Causes of metabolic acidosis.

With increased anion gap

Ketoacidosis
- Diabetic ketoacidosis
- Alcoholic ketoacidosis*
- Starvation ketoacidosis

Lactic acidosis
- Inadequate tissue perfusion due to hypotension, low cardiac output or sepsis
- Prolonged hypoxemia
- Muscle contraction: status epilepticus
- Metformin
- β_2-adrenergic agonists

Renal failure
- Chronic uraemic acidosis
- Acute renal failure

Toxins
- Ethylene glycol
- Methanol
- Salicylates
- Toluene

With normal anion gap (hyperchloraemic acidosis)

Renal
- Renal tubular acidosis
- Carbonic anhydrase inhibitors

Gastrointestinal
- Severe diarrhoea
- Obstructed ileal conduit
- Small bowel fistula
- Uretero-enterostomy
- Drainage of pancreatic or biliary secretions
- Small bowel fistula

Others
- Recovery from ketoacidosis
- Infusion of normal saline

*Alcoholic ketoacidosis is due to alcohol binge plus starvation and is often associated with pancreatitis; hyperglycaemia may occur but is mild (<15 mmol/L).

Table 7.5 Causes of respiratory acidosis (inadequate alveolar ventilation resulting in a raised arterial PCO_2).*

Brain
Stroke
Mass lesion with brainstem compression
Encephalitis
Sedative drugs
Status epilepticus
Spinal cord
Cord compression
Transverse myelitis
Poliomyelitis
Motor neuron disease
Rabies
Peripheral nerve
Guillain–Barré syndrome
Critical illness polyneuropathy
Toxins
Acute intermittent porphyria
Vasculitis
Diphtheria
Neuromuscular junction
Myasthenia gravis
Eaton–Lambert syndrome
Botulism
Toxins
Muscle
Myotonic dystrophy
Muscular dystrophy
Hypokalaemia
Hypophosphatemia
Rhabdomyolysis
Thoracic cage and pleura
Crushed chest
Morbid obesity
Kyphoscoliosis
Ankylosing spondylitis
Large pleural effusion
Lungs and airways
Upper airway obstruction
Severe (near fatal) acute asthma
Chronic obstructive pulmonary disease
Severe pneumonia
Severe pulmonary oedema

*Ventilatory failure commonly results from a combination of factors, for example pneumonia in an obese patient with chronic obstructive pulmonary disease; see Chapter 30.

- The judicious administration of sodium bicarbonate may be appropriate in certain clinical scenarios, for example for urinary alkalinisation or for metabolic acidosis associated with hyperkalaemia. There are, however, several potential undesirable effects, including hypernatraemia, increased fluid retention, paradoxical cerebral acidosis and precipitation of hypercapnia. Seek advice from intensive care and/or renal physicians and explore alternatives such as continuous renal replacement therapy.

Table 7.6 Causes of metabolic alkalosis.

Loss of gastric acid:
- Prolonged vomiting
- Gastric aspiration

Diuretic therapy

Severe and prolonged potassium deficiency

Mineralocorticoid and glucocorticoid excess

Post-hypercapnic alkalosis*

* Typically in patients with subacute-on-chronic respiratory acidosis, in whom $PaCO_2$ is rapidly reduced through ventilatory support. The plasma bicarbonate falls back to baseline more slowly, leading to a transient metabolic alkalosis.

Table 7.7 Causes of respiratory alkalosis.

Pulmonary disorders with hyperventilation:
- Acute asthma
- Pneumonia
- Pulmonary embolism
- Pulmonary oedema

Hyperventilation syndrome

Anxiety and pain

Central nervous system disorders, for example stroke, bacterial meningitis

Liver failure

Sepsis

Salicylate poisoning (early)

Further reading

Berend K, de Vries APJ, Gans ROB. (2014) Physiological approach to assessment of acid–base disturbances. *N Engl J Med* 371, 1434–1445.

Flenley, DC. (1971) Another non-logarithmic acid-base diagram? *Lancet* 1(7706), 961–965.

Jaber S, Paugam C, Futier E, *et al*. (2018) Sodium bicarbonate therapy for patients with severe metabolic acidaemia in the intensive care unit (BICAR-ICU): a multicentre, open-label, randomised controlled, phase 3 trial. *Lancet* 392, 31–40.

Seifter JL. (2014) Integration of acid–base and electrolyte disorders. *N Engl J Med* 371, 1821–1831.

CHAPTER 8
Poisoning

Nigel Langford and Keisha Patel

- In the United Kingdom, information on poisons and their management can be found:
- On the TOXBASE website (www.toxbase.org); username and password required.
- Via the National Poisons Information Service (NPIS) for complex and severe poisoning; 24-h phone line, 0344 8920111.

Management of the unconscious patient with suspected poisoning:

1 **Stabilize the airway, breathing and circulation.**
   - See Chapters 1 and 105 for airway management, Chapters 30 and 113 for respiratory failure management and Chapter 2 for the management of hypotension and shock.
2 **Exclude and correct hypoglycaemia**
   - If blood glucose is <4.0 mmol/L, give 100 mL of 20% glucose, 200 mL of 10% glucose over 15–30 min IV, or glucagon 1 mg IV/IM/SC.
   - Recheck blood glucose after 10 min; if still <4.0 mmol/L, repeat the above IV glucose treatment (see Chapter 46).
   - In patients with malnourishment or alcohol misuse, there is a remote risk of precipitating Wernicke encephalopathy by administering a glucose load; prevent this by giving thiamine 100 mg IV concurrently.
3 **Treat prolonged or recurrent major seizures**
   - Be mindful of pre-hospital treatment already administered.
   - Give **lorazepam** (less likely to cause respiratory suppression) 0.1 mg/kg (typically 4–8 mg) IV over 5–10 min (Chapter 57), **midazolam** 10 mg buccally (NICE-recommended, but only licensed in patients <18 years), or **diazepam** 10–20 mg IV at a rate of <2.5 mg/min (faster administration carries the risk of sudden apnoea).
   - Give a second dose for ongoing seizures, to a maximum total dose of lorazepam 8 mg or diazepam 40 mg (see Chapter 57).
4 **If opioid poisoning is suspected or must be excluded, give naloxone**
   - If the respiratory rate is <12/min, pupils are pinpoint, or other indication to suspect opioid poisoning, give naloxone 800 μgm IV every 2–3 min; up to a total dose of 4000 μgm or until the respiratory rate is >15/min (aim is reversal of respiratory depression but not full reversal of consciousness).
   - If there is a response to bolus naloxone, start an IV infusion: make up a naloxone solution with 10 mg naloxone (25 vials) made up to a final volume of 50 mL with glucose 5% (200 μgm/mL); start the infusion at 60% of the initial dose required for resuscitation per hour and titrate against the respiratory rate and Glasgow Coma Scale (GCS).

Acute Medicine: A Practical Guide to the Management of Medical Emergencies, Sixth Edition.
Edited by Mridula Rajwani, Leila Vaziri, and Ivie Gbinigie.
© 2026 John Wiley & Sons Ltd. Published 2026 by John Wiley & Sons Ltd.

- In patients who have taken partial opioid agonists (e.g. buprenorphine, methadone and tramadol), repeated large (1200 µgm) doses of naloxone may be required to achieve a satisfactory response.
- A lack of response to naloxone suggests that another Central nervous System (CNS) depressant has been taken or brain injury has occurred.

5 Obtain the history from all available sources (e.g. ambulance crew, family etc.).

6 Make a systematic examination:
- Clinical features may provide clues to the poison (Tables 8.1 and 8.2), but keep in mind that mixed poisoning is common.
- There is also the possibility of multiple pathologies (e.g. poisoning followed by head injury).
- Is there evidence of IV substance use? Check for needle marks and complications of IV substance use (e.g. venous thrombosis and cellulitis).
- Check for possible complications of a coma (hypothermia, pressure necrosis of skin or muscle, corneal abrasions and inhalation pneumonia).

7 Investigations
- Should be sent/obtained urgently and may help identify poisons taken (see Table 8.3).
- Urine is preferable to blood for qualitative analysis as toxins are concentrated in the urine.

8 Discuss management with an intensivist and arrange admission to ICU if:
- The GCS<8 (may need intubation as may be unable to protect their airway), respiratory failure despite antidote administration, or there are recurrent seizures.
- There are major arrhythmias, or the patient is at high risk of arrhythmias (e.g. tricyclic poisoning with broad QRS complex).
- There is hypotension or severe acidosis (pH<7.2) not responding to fluid resuscitation.

Table 8.1 Clues to the poison (1): clinical and biochemical features.

Feature	Poisons to consider
Coma	Barbiturates, benzodiazepines, ethanol, opioids, trichloroethanol, tricyclics
Seizures	Amphetamines, cocaine, dextropropoxyphene, insulin, oral hypoglycaemics, phenothiazines, theophylline, tricyclics, lead
Miosis	Opioids, organophosphates, trichloroethanol
Mydriasis	Amphetamines, cocaine, phenothiazines, quinine, sympathomimetics, tricyclics
Arrhythmias	Anti-arrhythmics, anticholinergics, phenothiazines, quinine, sympathomimetics, tricyclics
Hypertension	Amphetamines, cocaine
Pulmonary oedema	Carbon monoxide, ethylene glycol, irritant gases, opioids, organophosphates, paraquat, salicylates, tricyclics
Ketones on breath	Ethanol, isopropyl alcohol, alcoholic or starvation ketoacidosis
Hypothermia	Barbiturates, ethanol, opioids, tricyclics
Hyperthermia	Amphetamines, MDMA (3,4-methylenedioxymethamphetamine), anticholinergics, cocaine, monoamine oxidase inhibitors
Hypoglycaemia	Insulin, oral hypoglycaemics, ethanol, salicylates
Hyperglycaemia	Theophylline, organophosphates, salbutamol
Acute kidney injury	Amanita phalloides, ethylene glycol, paracetamol, salicylates, prolonged hypotension, rhabdomyolysis
Hypokalaemia	Salbutamol, salicylates, theophylline
Metabolic acidosis	Carbon monoxide, ethanol, ethylene glycol, methanol, paracetamol, salicylates, tricyclics
Raised plasma osmolality	Ethanol, ethylene glycol, isopropyl alcohol, methanol
Rhabdomyolysis	Carbon monoxide, ethanol, opioids, solvents

MDMA, 3,4-methylenedioxy-methamphetamine ('ecstasy').

Table 8.2 Clues to the poison (2): toxidromes.

Toxidrome	HR	BP	RR	T	GCS	Pupil size	Sweat	Comments
Sympathomimetic (cocaine, cathinones, amphetamines, some novel psychoactive substances)	↑	↑	↑	↑	↑	↑	↑	Electrolyte disturbances and rhabdomyolysis
Anticholinergic (hyoscine, antidepressants, diphenhydramine, antipsychotics)	↑	(↑)	↓	↑	↓	↑	↓	Urinary retention
Cholinergic (organophosphorous sarin, VX)		—	—	(—)	(—)	↓	↑	Vomiting, diarrhoea, urinary incontinence, hypersalivation
Opioid (morphine, fentanyl, oxycodone, codeine, methadone, buprenorphine)	↓	↓	↓	↓	↓	↓	↓	Monitor GCS/AVPU as naloxone only short acting
Sedative hypnotic (benzodiazepines, 'Z' hypnotics)	↓	↓	↓	↓	↓	(↑)	↓	Monitor GCS/AVPU
Serotonin syndrome (SSRI, SNRI lithium)	↑	↑	↑	↑	↑	↑	↑	Check for myoclonus; short onset and duration of events
Neuroleptic malignant syndrome (antipsychotics)	↑	(↑)	—	↑	↓	(↑)	↑	↑ muscle tone and rhabdomyolysis; long duration of events
Alcohol withdrawal (alcohol)	↑	—	(—)	(↑)	(↑)	↑	↑	Use **CIWA-Ar/GMAWS** to objectively monitor and respond to withdrawal
Opioid withdrawal (opioids)	↑	(—)	(↑)	(↑)	(↑)	↑	↑	Consider using **COWS** to objectively monitor and respond to withdrawal

HR, heart rate; BP, blood pressure; RR, respiratory rate; T, temperature; GCS, Glasgow Coma Scale.
↓ reduction in effect, () qualified change in effect, ↑ increase in effect, − no change

Table 8.3 Urgent investigation of the patient with poisoning.

Bloods: glucose, sodium, potassium, urea, creatinine, plasma osmolality*, full blood count, paracetamol level (if indicated), arterial/venous blood gas and pH
Urinalysis (myoglobinuria due to rhabdomyolysis gives a positive stick test for blood)
Chest X-ray
ECG
If the substance ingested is not known, save serum (10 mL) and urine (50 mL) at 4 °C in case later analysis is needed

*Normal plasma osmolality 280–300 mOsmol/kg. If the measured plasma osmolality exceeds calculated osmolality (formula [2(Na + K) + urea + glucose]) by 10 mOsmol/kg or more, consider poisoning with ethanol, ethylene glycol, isopropyl alcohol or methanol.

Management of the conscious patient with poisoning

1 **Check baseline observations** including GCS and blood glucose.
2 **Establish**:
   - Which poisons were taken, when, over what time period and the quantity.
   - Current symptoms and if the patient has vomited since ingestion (unlikely to have eliminated significant amounts of poison if over an hour from ingestion).
   - Associated physical and psychiatric illness.

Table 8.4 Poisoning in which plasma levels should be measured.

Poison	Plasma level at which specific treatment is indicated	Treatment
Aspirin and other	250–500 mg/L (mild poisoning)	Fluids
Salicylates	500–750 mg/L (moderate poisoning)	Urinary alkalinization
	750–1000 mg/L (severe poisoning)	HD
	>1000 mg/L (massive poisoning)	HD
Digoxin	>4 ng/mL	Digoxin-specific antibody fragments
Ethylene glycol	>500 mg/L	Ethanol or 4-methyl pyrazole, HD
Iron*	>3.5 mg/L	Desferrioxamine
Lithium	>5 mmol/L	HD
Methanol	>500 mg/L	Ethanol or 4-methyl pyrazole, HD
Paracetamol	See Appendix 36.1	Acetylcysteine
Theophylline	>50 mg/L	RAC, HD
Carbamazepine	>40 mg/L (170 micromol/L)	MDAC, consider lipid emulsion for cardiac toxicity

HD, haemodialysis; RAC, repeated oral-activated charcoal.

NB: Always check the units of measurement used by your laboratory.

*Also measure plasma iron level if clinical evidence of severe iron toxicity (hypotension, nausea, vomiting, diarrhoea) or after massive ingestion (>20 mg elemental iron/kg body weight; one 20 mg tablet of ferrous sulphate contains 6 mg elemental iron).

3 Investigations
- Dependent upon the poisons taken – check plasma levels (Table 8.4).

4 If the patient is at risk of harm but refuses treatment

Consult and senior colleague and psychiatrist (see Chapter 104 for further information on mental capacity and consent to treatment).

Further management

Is a specific antidote or treatment indicated?

See Table 8.5 for antidotes – if you are unfamiliar with the poison/antidote, discuss the case with the Poisons Centre as some antidotes may be harmful if given inappropriately.

Reducing absorption

- **Activated charcoal**
  - 50 g mixed with 200 mL of water should be given if a significant amount of any poison has been ingested within 1 h (or longer if modified-release preparations or drugs with anticholinergic effects have been taken), and oral antidotes are not indicated (Table 8.6); unless substance is poorly absorbed by charcoal.
  - High risk of inhalation therefore it should not be given to a patient with a reduced conscious level unless the airway is protected by a cuffed endotracheal tube.
- **Gastric lavage s**hould **not** be employed in the management of poisoned patients, as the risks of complications outweigh any benefits.

Table 8.5 Specific antidotes.

Poison	Antidote
Anticholinergic agents	Physostigmine
Arsenic	Dimercaprol
Benzodiazepines	Flumazenil
Beta-blockers	Glucagon
Calcium antagonists	Calcium gluconate
Cyanide	Dicobalt edetate alone or sodium nitrite + sodium thiosulphate
Dabigatran	Idarucizumab
Digoxin	Digoxin-specific antibody fragments
Ethylene glycol	Ethanol or 4-methylpyrazole
Fluoride	Calcium gluconate
Buproprion, local anaesthetics	Lipid emulsion (Intralipid®)
Iron	Desferrioxamine
Lead and Mercury	Dimercaprol or penicillamine
Methanol	Ethanol or 4-methylpyrazole
Opioids	Naloxone
Organophosphates	Atropine
Paracetamol	Acetylcysteine (Appendix 8.1)
Thallium	Berlin blue
Warfarin	Vitamin K, fresh frozen plasma or prothrombin complex concentrate

Table 8.6 Charcoal administration after poisoning.

Repeated dosing indicated	Single dose indicated (only within the first hour after presentation)	Charcoal not indicated
Barbiturates	Antihistamines	Acids
Carbamazepine	Paracetamol	Alkalis
Dapsone	Salicylates	Carbamate
Digoxin	Tricyclics	Cyanide
Phenytoin		Ethanol
Quinine		Ethylene glycol
Sustained-release		Hydrocarbons
preparations		Iron
Theophylline		Lithium
		Methanol
		Organophosphates

Increasing elimination

- Repeated dosing with activated charcoal may help eliminate some substances (Table 8.6). Give 50 g initially then 25 g 4-hourly by mouth or nasogastric tube until recovery or until plasma drug levels have fallen to within the safe range. Laxatives may also be required.
- Other methods (e.g. haemodialysis) may be indicated in selected cases, after discussion with a Poisons Centre.

Monitoring & Supportive Care

In all patients with severe poisoning, monitor:

- GCS/level of consciousness.
- Oxygen saturations and heart rate/ECG via continuous monitoring.
- RR and BP (initially every 15 min); temperature and urine output (hourly).
- Arterial blood gases and pH (initially 2-hourly) if the poison can cause metabolic acidosis (Table 8.1) or there is suspected acute respiratory distress syndrome or after inhalation injury.
- Blood glucose if the poison may cause hypo- or hyperglycaemia (initially hourly) or in paracetamol poisoning presenting after 16 h (initially 4-hourly).
- Monitoring should be continued until the time symptoms are likely to develop has passed or until the patient has recovered. Prolonged observation may be required for patients who have taken sustained-release medication.
- Management of problems seen after poisoning is summarised in Table 8.7.

Psychiatric assessment

- All patients with deliberate self-poisoning should have a psychiatric assessment, performed when recovered from the physical effects of the poisoning. Factors to consider:
  - The circumstances of the overdose: carefully planned, indecisive or impulsive; taken alone or in the presence of another person; action taken to avoid intervention or discovery; suicidal intent admitted?

Table 8.7 Problems encountered in the patient with poisoning.

Problem	Comment and management
Coma	If associated with focal neurological signs or evidence of head injury, CT must be done to exclude intracranial haematoma.
Cerebral oedema	May occur after cardiac arrest, in severe carbon monoxide poisoning, in acute liver failure from paracetamol (Chapter 42), and in MDMA poisoning, due to hyponatraemia. Results in hypertension and dilated pupils. Give mannitol 20% 100–200 mL (0.5 g/kg) IV over 10 min, provided urine output is >30 mL/h. Check plasma osmolality: further mannitol may be given until plasma osmolality is 320 mOsmol/kg Hyperventilate to a PCO_2 of 4 kPa (30 mmHg)
Seizures	Due to toxin or metabolic complications. Check blood glucose, arterial gases and pH, plasma sodium, potassium, calcium and magnesium. Treat prolonged or recurrent major fits with diazepam IV up to 20 mg. See Chapter 57 for further management.
Respiratory depression	Half-life of most opioids is longer than that of naloxone and repeated doses or an infusion may be required. Elective ventilation may be preferable.
Inhalation pneumonia	Treatment includes tracheobronchial suction, consideration of bronchoscopy to remove particulate matter from the airways, physiotherapy and antibiotic therapy (Chapter 25).
Hypotension	Usually reflects vasodilatation, but always consider other causes (e.g. gastrointestinal bleeding). Obtain an ECG if the patient has taken a cardiotoxic poison, has known cardiac disease, and if hypotension does not respond to IV fluids.
Arrhythmias	Due to toxin or metabolic complications. Check arterial gases and pH, and plasma potassium, calcium and magnesium. See Chapter 13 for further management.
Acute kidney injury	May be due to prolonged hypotension, nephrotoxic poison, haemolysis or rhabdomyolysis. See Chapter 86 for further management.
Gastric stasis	Place a nasogastric tube in comatose patients to reduce the risk of regurgitation and inhalation.
Hypothermia	Usually managed by passive rewarming. See Chapter 9.

MDMA, 3,4-methylenedioxy-methamphetamine ('ecstasy').

- Past history of self-poisoning or self-injury; psychiatric history or contact with psychiatric services; alcohol or substance use disorder and current mental state,
  - Family history of depression or suicide.
- Patients at increased risk of suicide (Table 8.8) and those with overt psychiatric illness should be discussed with a psychiatrist. Follow-up by the primary care physician or psychiatric services should be arranged before discharge.

Paracetamol poisoning

- Hepatotoxicity may occur after a single ingestion of >150 mg/kg paracetamol taken in <1 h; and is more likely if there is hepatic enzyme induction due to chronic alcohol use or drug therapy (e.g. carbamazepine), or if there is depletion of hepatic glutathione (e.g. anorexia).
- Acetylcysteine (AC) replenishes hepatic glutathione and is the mainstay treatment (Table 8.9).
- For patients weighing >110 kg (body mass index > 30), use a body weight of 110 kg rather than actual body weight when calculating dose of paracetamol ingested in mg/kg.
- Plasma paracetamol level is a poor guide to the risk of hepatotoxicity in patients with staggered poisoning (overdose taken over a period of longer than 1 h or multiple ingestions within a 24-h period). If the total amount taken is >150 mg/kg in a 24-h period, or the patient is at increased risk of liver damage, acetylcysteine should be given empirically.
- Management (Figure 8.1) is dependent on the amount ingested over what time, and the time since ingestion that the patient presents to services.

Minor reactions to acetylcysteine (nausea, flushing, urticaria and pruritus) are relatively common, and usually settle when the peak rate of infusion is passed. If there is a severe reaction (angioedema, wheezing, respiratory distress, hypotension or hypertension), stop the infusion and give an antihistamine (chlorphenamine 10 mg IV over 10 min). Then re-start the acetylcysteine infusion at the lowest rate.

Table 8.8 Patients with self-poisoning at high risk of suicide.

Middle-aged or elderly male
Widowed/divorced/separated or living alone
Unemployed
Chronic physical illness or psychiatric illness, especially depression
Alcohol or substance abuse
Circumstances of poisoning: massive; planned; taken alone; timed – intervention or discovery unlikely
Suicide note written or suicidal intent admitted

Table 8.9 Acetylcysteine (AC) regimen in paracetamol poisoning.

Traditional 21-h Infusion
150 mg/kg in 200 mL glucose 5% IV over 1 h, then
50 mg/kg in 500 mL glucose 5% IV over 4 h, then
100 mg/kg in 1 L glucose 5% IV over 16 h

New 12-h SNAP Regimen
100 mg/kg in 200 mL glucose 5% IV over 2 h, then
200 mg/kg in 1 L glucose 5% IV over 10 h

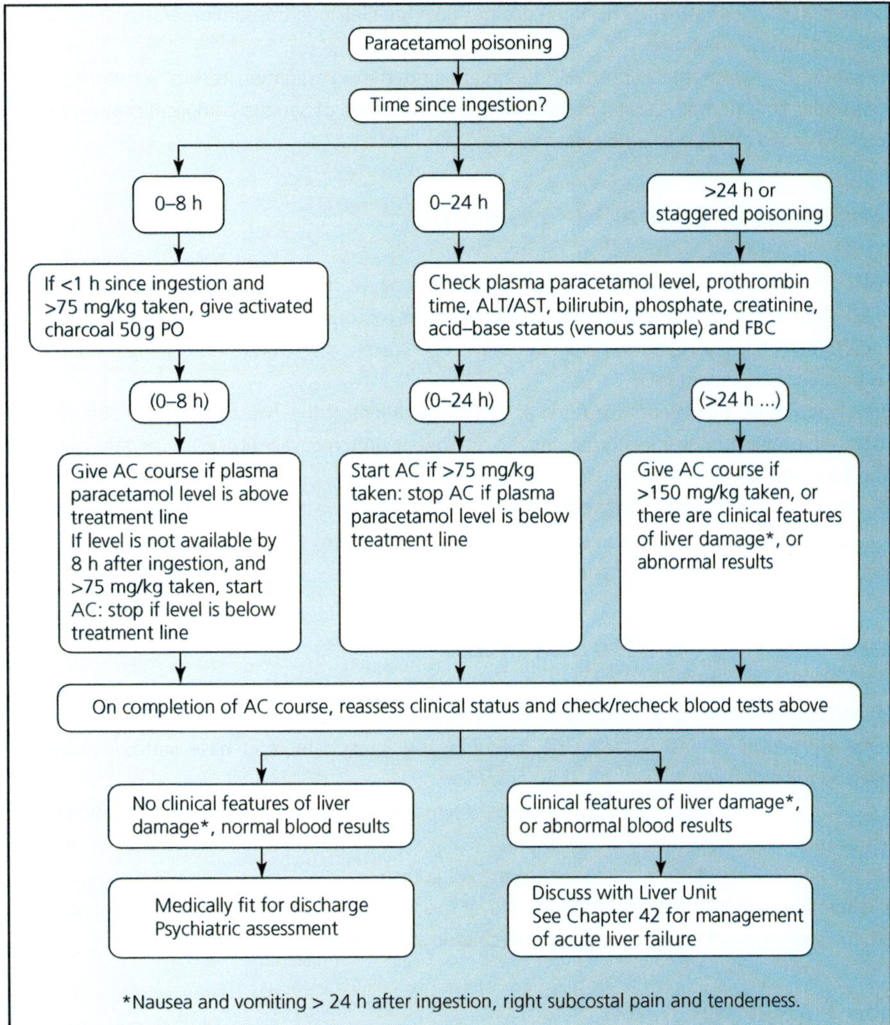

Figure 8.1 Management of paracetamol poisoning.

Patient was seen within 8h after poisoning

- Give activated charcoal 50 g if <1 h since ingestion and > 75 mg/kg paracetamol has been ingested.
- Take blood for plasma paracetamol level at or after 4 h since ingestion.
- If the plasma paracetamol concentration at four or more hours post ingestion is less than the paracetamol treatment line, the patient is asymptomatic and the investigations are normal, there is no risk of serious complications, and the patient may be discharged following psychiatric assessment.
- Start acetylcysteine (AC) if the plasma paracetamol level is above the treatment line (graph of plasma levels and treatment threshold can be found on TOXBASE).
- If the plasma paracetamol level is not available by 8h, begin AC if >75 mg/kg of paracetamol has been taken; discontinue AC if the plasma paracetamol level is then found to be below the treatment line.

- On completion of AC treatment, check the prothrombin time, alanine transaminase/aspartate transaminase activities and plasma creatinine.
- If the patient is asymptomatic post AC treatment and the investigation results are normal (INR < 1.3, ALT < 2 × upper limit normal, creatinine normal), there is no risk of serious complications, and the patient may be discharged after psychiatric assessment.

Patient seen 8–24 h after poisoning

- Take blood for plasma paracetamol level, prothrombin time, alanine transaminase/aspartate transaminase activities, plasma creatinine and bilirubin, acid–base status (venous sample) and full blood count.
- Start AC immediately if >75 mg/kg paracetamol has been taken; discontinue AC if the plasma paracetamol level is below the treatment line.
- On completion of AC treatment repeat the above investigations; if the investigations are abnormal or if the patient is symptomatic, consider continuing AC treatment until recovery (INR < 1.3, or falling on two consecutive tests and < 3.0).
- If the patient is asymptomatic following treatment and the investigation results are normal (INR < 1.3, ALT < 2 × upper limit normal, creatinine normal), there is little risk of serious complications; the patient may be discharged after psychiatric assessment.

Patient seen >24 h after overdose

- Take blood on admission for plasma paracetamol level, prothrombin time, alanine transaminase/aspartate transaminase activities, plasma creatinine, bilirubin and phosphate, acid–base status (venous sample), glucose and full blood count.
- If the patient has taken >150 mg/kg paracetamol, is symptomatic, or has abnormal investigation results, give AC treatment.
- Repeat the above investigations at the end of the AC course.
- Normal blood tests at 24 h indicate that serious liver toxicity has not occurred, and treatment can be discontinued; the patient may be discharged after psychiatric assessment.

Severe hepatotoxicity

Make early contact with a Liver Unit if the patient has evidence of severe hepatotoxicity (Table 8.10). In such patients (before transfer):

- Start a course of acetylcysteine if not previously administered.
- Give glucose 10% 1 L 12-hourly IV to prevent hypoglycaemia, and monitor blood glucose 4-hourly.

Table 8.10 Paracetamol poisoning: indications of severe hepatotoxicity.

Rapid development of grade 2 encephalopathy (confused but able to answer questions)
Prothrombin time >20 s at 24 h, >45 s at 48 h or >50 s at 72 h
Increasing plasma bilirubin
Increasing plasma creatinine
Falling plasma phosphate
Arterial pH <7.3 more than 24 h after ingestion

- Monitor conscious level 4-hourly.
- Monitor CVP and urine output: correct hypovolaemia with crystalloid.
- Check prothrombin time 12-hourly and plasma creatinine daily.
- Start prophylaxis against gastric stress ulceration with omeprazole 40 mg daily IV by mouth or by nasogastric tube.
- See Chapter 42 for other aspects of the management of acute liver failure.

Carbon monoxide poisoning

- May occur from inhalation of car exhaust fumes, fumes from inadequately maintained or ventilated heating systems, smoke from all types of fires and methylene chloride in paint strippers (by hepatic metabolism).
- The severity of poisoning depends on the concentration of carbon monoxide in the inspired air, the length of exposure and the presence of anaemia or cardiorespiratory disease. Clinical features of acute poisoning are given in Table 8.11.
- If carbon monoxide poisoning is suspected, give 100% oxygen (10 L/min) using a tightly fitting facemask with a circuit that minimizes rebreathing. Unconscious patients should be intubated and ventilated mechanically with 100% oxygen.
- Cerebral oedema may occur and is treated with mannitol and mild hyperventilation.
- Attach an ECG monitor and record a 12-lead ECG. Severe poisoning may result in myocardial ischaemia, with anginal chest pain, ST segment depression and arrhythmias. Check arterial blood gases and pH (metabolic acidosis is usually present) and arrange a chest X-ray.
- Check the carboxyhaemoglobin (COHb) level in blood (most arterial blood gas analysers will do this). If acute carbon monoxide poisoning is confirmed (COHb > 10%), recheck 2-hourly and continue 100% oxygen until two consecutive samples contain <5%.
- Although its effectiveness is disputed, generally accepted indications for hyperbaric oxygen therapy are:
  - Carboxyhaemoglobin level >40% at any time
  - Coma
  - Neurological symptoms or signs other than mild headache
  - Evidence of myocardial ischaemia or arrhythmias
  - Pregnancy
- Contact a Poisons Centre to discuss the management of severe poisoning and for the location of the nearest centre which can provide hyperbaric oxygen therapy.

Table 8.11 Acute carbon monoxide poisoning: clinical features.

Blood carboxyhaemoglobin (%)	Clinical features that may be seen
<10	No symptoms – acute poisoning excluded if exposure was within 4 h
10–50	Headache, nausea, vomiting, tachycardia, tachypnoea
>50	Coma, fits, cardiorespiratory arrest

CHAPTER 9

Hypothermia

Rand Alkaissy and Tom Cibulskas

Hypothermia is defined as a core temperature below 35 °C, causing vital functions to drop to the point of cardiac arrest. Exposure to cold (e.g. outdoor activities, homelessness and substance abuse) results in primary hypothermia, whilst illness and other external causes (e.g. elderly and multimorbidity) result in secondary hypothermia.

Severity of hypothermia can be classified based on the patient's core temperature (Table 9.1) but also on clinical signs if unable to measure the core temperature (Table 9.2). Urgent investigations to consider in hypothermia are listed in Table 9.3. Management is summarized in Figure 9.1.

Table 9.1 Classification of severity of hypothermia.

Stage	Clinical signs[*]	Core temperature
Hypothermia I (mild)	Conscious, shivering	35–32 °C
Hypothermia II (moderate)	Impaired consciousness, may be shivering	32–28 °C
Hypothermia III (severe)	Unconscious, not shivering, vital signs present	<28 °C
Hypothermia IV (severe)	Vital signs absent	Variable

[*] Clinical findings may be diminished in comorbidity or drugs regardless of core temperature.

Table 9.2 Rewarming methods.

Method	Treatment
Passive external rewarming (HT I)	Place patient in warmed room (28 °C) and remove wet clothing. Cover with blankets and other insulating materials. Give warm drinks and encourage active movement. Aim for rise of 0.5 °C/h.
Active external rewarming (HT II)	Apply forced external heat (e.g. Bair Hugger). Aim for rise of 2.0 °C/h (beware hypotension).
Active internal rewarming (HT II-III)	Give heated IV fluids (40–42 °C), apply warmed and humidified O_2 via facemask. Focus on torso first.
Extracorporeal rewarming (HT IV)	Peritoneal or haemodialysis, arteriovenous rewarming, cardiopulmonary bypass, extracorporeal membrane oxygenation (ECMO).

Table 9.3 Urgent investigation in hypothermia.

Investigations and monitoring	Comment
Continuous monitoring	
ECG (Figure 9.2)	Prolongation of PR, QRS, QT intervals, ST-elevation, T-wave inversion, Osborn J wave, atrial fibrillation or sinus bradycardia. Supraventricular arrhythmias usually resolve once core temperature returns to normal. Ventricular fibrillation may occur at core temperatures <30 °C and can be refractory to shock.
Arterial oxygenation	Hypothermia reduces the oxygen demand of the body (6–7% per 1 °C cooling) to protect vital organs from hypoxic damage. Beware that pulse oximeters placed on fingers can be slow.
Check every hour	
Vital signs	Temperature, respiratory rate, level of consciousness
Blood pressure, urine output and central venous pressure	Most hypothermic patients are volume-depleted and will need monitoring for adequate fluid therapy.
Check every 4 h	
Blood glucose	Raised levels (10–20 mmol/L) should not be treated with insulin because of the risk of hypoglycaemia on rewarming.
Full blood cell count	White blood cells and platelets may be reduced due to splenic sequestration
Electrolytes, creatinine and creatinine kinase	Renal failure due to hypovolaemia/hypotension and rhabdomyolysis
Arterial blood gases and lactate	Severe hypothermia results in metabolic acidosis
Lipase	Can be increased due to hypothermia-induced pancreatitis
Re-assess if necessary	
CRP, blood and urine cultures, thyroid function, toxicology screen	To rule out other causes of hypothermia (e.g. infection and substance abuse)
Chest radiograph	Pulmonary oedema, vascular congestion or aspiration pneumonia. Pneumonia is a common cause and complication of hypothermia: give antibiotics once cultures have been taken. Further doses need not be given until the core temperature is >32 °C.
X-pelvis and hips	If history of fall or clinical signs of femur fractures

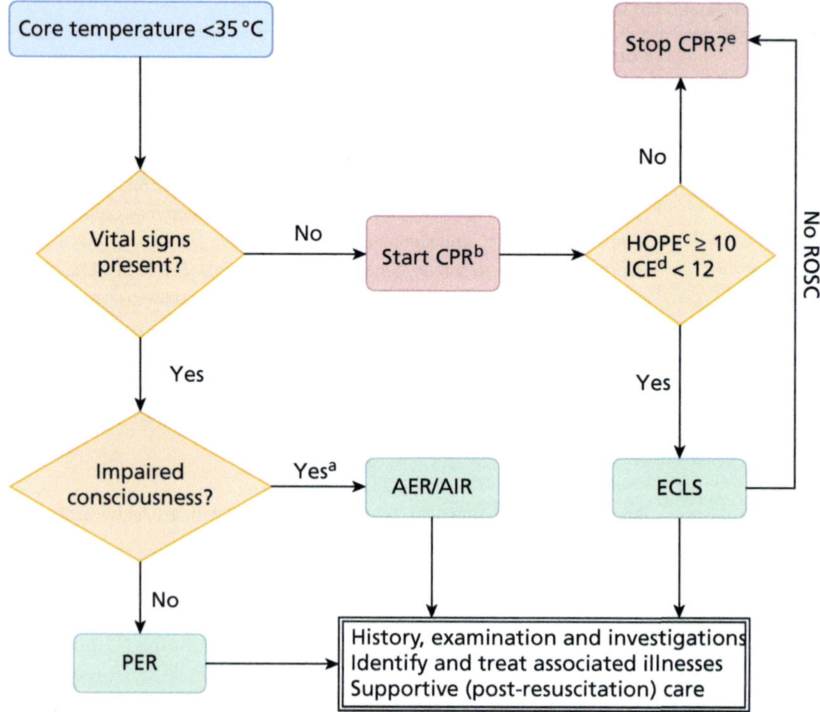

a) cardiocirculatory instability with a core temperature ≤32 °C
b) unless obvious cause of irreversible death
c) Hypothermia Outcome Prediction after ECLS
d) ICE Survival Score
e) consider if serum K>12 mmol/L or patient rewarmed to >32 °C with on-going asystole and no other causes of reversible caridac arrest

Figure 9.1 Management accidental hypothermia – figure adapted from the European Resuscitation Council Guidelines 2021: Cardiac arrest in special circumstances. CPR, cardiopulmonary resuscitation; PER, passive external rewarming; AER, active external rewarming; AIR, active internal rewarming; ECLS, extracorporeal life support.

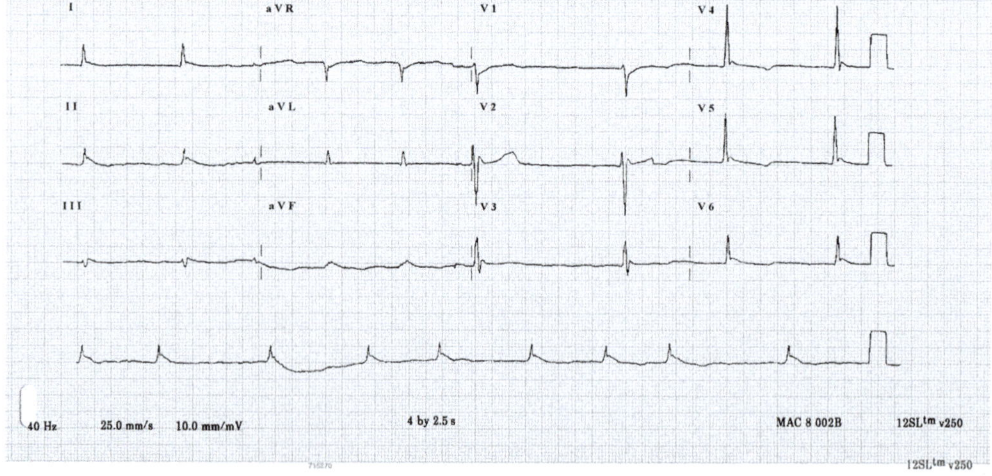

Figure 9.2 ECG in hypothermia (core temperature 30 °C) showing bradycardia, prolongation of ECG intervals, and elevation of the J point in the chest leads giving a J or Osborne wave.

Further reading

Duong H, Patel G. (2024) Hypothermia. In: StatPearls [Internet]. Treasure Island, FL: StatPearls Publishing. Available from: https://www.ncbi.nlm.nih.gov/books/NBK545239/.
European Resuscitation Council Guidelines (2021) RC guidelines. https://cprguidelines.eu/.
Zafren K, Crawford MC. (2024) Accidental hypothermia in adults. In: UpToDate, Connor RF (Ed). Wolters Kluwer.

CHAPTER 10

Drowning

CARL HARTELIUS AND TOM CIBULSKAS

Drowning is defined as a process resulting in primary respiratory impairment from submersion or immersion in a liquid medium. Submersion without respiratory impairment should be considered as water rescue. Submersion triggers laryngospasm preventing initial aspiration, but eventually hypoxia and hypercapnia stimulate gasping leading to aspiration. Water causes surfactant destruction and alveoli wash-out. In a small minority of cases, cardiac arrest occurs before aspiration. Assessment for underlying causes, associated injury and complications is important (Box 10.1 and Table 10.1).

Box 10.1 Drowning – alerts.

Pitfalls in the management of the patient after drowning include:
- Missing airway obstruction
- Missing cervical spine injury or head injury
- Missing occult haemorrhage
- Missing the cause of drowning: consider alcohol or substance use, epilepsy, acute coronary syndrome, primary arrhythmia, hypoglycaemia or attempted suicide

Priorities

- In cardiac arrest initiate treatment with five rescue breaths before following resuscitation protocols. Maintain a clear airway (Chapter 105) with endotracheal intubation if the patient is comatose (Glasgow Coma Scale score < 9).
- Treat hypoxia with 15 L of oxygen by face mask and titrate. Treat bronchospasm using a beta-agonist. If still hypoxic, consider continuous positive airway pressure (CPAP) or bilevel positive airway pressure (BiPAP) if awake and compliant (see Chapter 113).

Further management

Admit or discharge?
- Discharge following observation for 6–8 h (as acute respiratory distress syndrome may develop over this period) if:
  - Clear history of only brief immersion/submersion
  - Normal conscious level

Acute Medicine: A Practical Guide to the Management of Medical Emergencies, Sixth Edition.
Edited by Mridula Rajwani, Leila Vaziri, and Ivie Gbinigie.
© 2026 John Wiley & Sons Ltd. Published 2026 by John Wiley & Sons Ltd.

Table 10.1 Urgent investigation after drowning.

Full blood count (haemorrhage, haemolysis)
Coagulation screen
Urea, electrolytes and creatinine
Glucose (hypo- or hyperglycaemia may be present)
Creatine kinase
Urine stick test for myoglobinuria
Blood alcohol level and urine toxicology screen
ECG: may have changes due to cold (Figure 9.2), myocardial ischaemia, channelopathy (e.g. long QT syndrome, arrhythmia)
Chest X-ray (aspiration, oedema or signs of a foreign body (e.g. segmental atelectasis)), arterial blood gases and pH
CT head if there are signs of head injury, reduced conscious level or cause of drowning is unclear. Trauma imaging as indicated

- No significant injuries
- No bronchospasm, tachypnoea or dyspnoea
- Normal arterial oxygen saturation breathing air and normal arterial blood gases
- No comorbidities
  Those discharged should be advised to return if they develop cough, dyspnoea or fever.
- Patients needing oxygen should be admitted to level 1 care, whilst patients with pulmonary oedema should be admitted to ICU.

Hypoxia
- This may be due to airway obstruction, brain injury, acute respiratory distress syndrome or pneumonia.
- Consider early intubation and mechanical ventilation. High levels of positive end-expiratory pressure may be needed due to reduced lung compliance. After endotracheal intubation, insert a nasogastric or orogastric tube to decompress the stomach.
- Bronchoscopy or bronchial lavage may be required to remove foreign bodies and clear debris from the airways.
- Consider extracorporeal membrane oxygenation if adequate oxygenation cannot be achieved by ventilation.

Hypotension
Rewarming causes vasodilation and the patient is likely to require additional fluid resuscitation and may also need vasoactive therapy (Chapter 2).

Hypothermia
- Hypothermia should be corrected by rewarming (Chapter 9).

Acute kidney injury
- Caused by hypoxaemia, hypotension or rhabdomyolysis (Chapter 86).

Prophylactic antibiotic or steroid therapy?
There is no benefit from prophylactic corticosteroid or antibiotic therapy unless near-drowning occurs in highly contaminated water.

Further reading

European Resuscitation Council Guidelines (2021) European Resuscitation Council guidelines 2021: executive summary. https://www.cprguidelines.eu/assets/guidelines/European-Resuscitation-Council-Guidelines-2021-Ex.pdf

Cardiology

CHAPTER 11

Syncope and presyncope

CLEMENT LAU AND SANDEEP S HOTHI

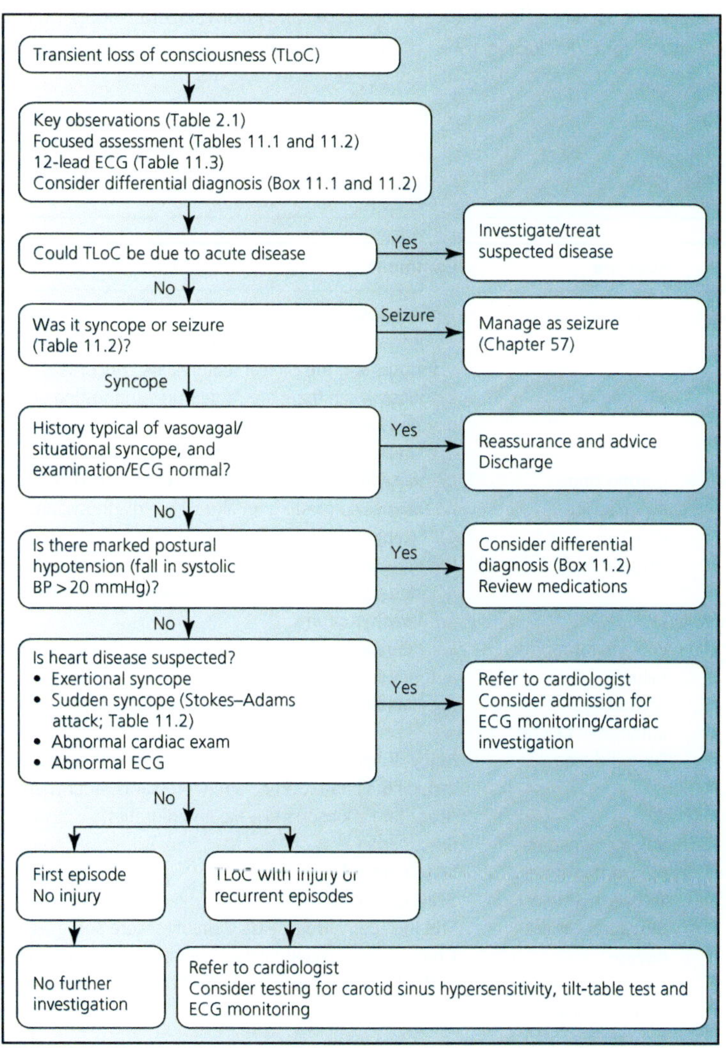

Figure 11.1 Assessment of syncope.

- Risk stratification is important, as patients at low risk of serious adverse events can be discharged from the emergency department.
- The assessment of syncope is summarized in Figure 11.1.

Priorities

1 Is TLoC related to acute disease? (See Box 11.1)
2 Was TLoC due to syncope or a seizure?
- A detailed history will usually differentiate syncope (Box 11.1) from seizure (Tables 11.1 and 11.2)
  - Involuntary movements (including tonic–clonic seizures within 30 s of cardiac arrest) are common in syncope.

Box 11.1 Causes of syncope.

Mechanism	Subtype	Comment
Reflex (neurally mediated)	Vasovagal	Typically follows pain, emotional distress or prolonged standing. Diagnose when there are no features suggesting an alternative diagnosis, and the clinical features are concordant (Table 11.2).
	Situational	Diagnose when there are no features suggesting an alternative diagnosis and syncope occurred in typical circumstances (e.g. micturition while standing or a prolonged bout of coughing).
	Carotid sinus hypersensitivity (CSH)	Diagnose in patients aged 60 and over with TLoC, when there are no features suggesting an alternative diagnosis, and testing for CSH (Table 11.4) is positive.
	Atypical form	Diagnose when there are no features suggesting an alternative diagnosis, testing for CSH is negative, and tilt-table testing provokes symptoms.
Orthostatic hypotension	Primary autonomic failure	For example in multiple system atrophy, Parkinson's disease with autonomic failure.
	Secondary autonomic failure	For example in diabetes mellitus or amyloidosis.
	Drug-induced	Many drugs may cause or contribute to orthostatic hypotension, including alpha-blockers, antidepressants, antihypertensive agents, drugs for Parkinson's disease and diuretics.
	Volume depletion	See Chapter 2.
Cardiovascular	Bradyarrhythmia	See Chapter 13.
	Tachyarrhythmia	See Chapter 13.
	Structural cardiac disease	This includes valve disease (notably severe aortic stenosis; see Chapter 20), congenital heart disease and cardiomyopathies. ECG and echocardiography typically show characteristic abnormalities.
	Acute myocardial ischaemia	See Chapter 12.
	Aortic dissection	See Chapter 18.
	Pulmonary embolism	See Chapter 31.
	Severe pulmonary hypertension	May result in exertional syncope. There may be clinical signs of right ventricular failure (e.g. elevated jugular venous pressure). ECG and echocardiography typically show characteristic abnormalities.

Table 11.1 Focused assessment after syncope.

History

Background
Any previous similar attacks
Previous significant head injury (i.e. with skull fracture or loss of consciousness)
Birth injury, febrile convulsions in childhood, meningitis or encephalitis
Family history of epilepsy
Cardiac disease associated with ventricular arrhythmia (previous myocardial infarction, hypertrophic or dilated cardiomyopathy and heart failure)
Medications
Alcohol or substance use
Sleep deprivation

Before the attack
Prodromal symptoms: were these cardiovascular (e.g. dizziness, palpitations and chest pain) or focal neurological symptoms (aura)?
Circumstances, for example exercising, standing, sitting or lying and asleep
Precipitants, for example coughing, micturition and head-turning

The attack
Were there any focal neurological features at the onset: sustained deviation of the head or eyes or unilateral jerking of the limbs?
Was there a cry (may occur in tonic phase of fit)?
Duration of loss of consciousness
Associated tongue biting, urinary incontinence or injury
Facial colour changes (pallor common in syncope, uncommon with a fit)
Abnormal pulse (must be assessed in relation to the reliability of the witness)

After the attack
Immediately well or delayed recovery with confusion or headache?

Examination
Conscious level and mental state (confirm the patient is fully oriented)
Pulse, blood pressure, respiratory rate, arterial oxygen saturation, temperature
Systolic BP sitting or lying, and after 2 min standing (a fall of >20 mmHg is abnormal; note if symptomatic or not)
Arterial pulses (check major pulses for asymmetry and bruits)
Jugular venous pressure (if raised, consider pulmonary embolism, pulmonary hypertension, heart failure or cardiac tamponade)
Heart murmurs (aortic stenosis and hypertrophic cardiomyopathy may cause exertional syncope; atrial myxoma may simulate mitral stenosis)
Neck mobility (does neck movement induce presyncope? Is there neck stiffness?)
Presence of focal neurological signs: as a minimum, check visual fields, limb power, tendon reflexes and plantar responses
Fundi (check for haemorrhages or papilloedema)

3 Admit or discharge?

   High-risk features warranting inpatient management include:

   • Suspicion of acute disease causing syncope (see Box 11.1)

   • Evidence of significant structural or ischaemic heart disease, or the presence of heart failure

   • Clinical (e.g. exertional syncope) or ECG features (Table 11.3) suggesting arrhythmic syncope

   • Abnormal physiological observations

   • Major comorbidities

4 Advice to discharged patients

Table 11.2 Features differentiating a generalized seizure from vasovagal syncope and cardiac syncope due to arrhythmia.

	Generalized seizure	Vasovagal syncope	Cardiac syncope due to arrhythmia
Occurrence when sitting or lying	Common	Rare	Common
Occurrence during sleep	Common	Does not occur	May occur
Prodromal symptoms	May occur, with focal neurological symptoms, head turning, automatisms	Typical, with dizziness, sweating, nausea, blurring of vision, disturbance of hearing, yawning	Often none; palpitation may precede syncope in tachyarrhythmias
Focal neurological features at onset	May occur, and signify focal cerebral lesion	Never occur	Never occur
Tonic–clonic movements	Characteristic, occur within 30 s of onset	May occur after 30 s of syncope (secondary anoxic seizure)	May occur after 30 s of syncope (secondary anoxic seizure)
Facial colour	Flush or cyanosis at onset	Pallor at onset and after syncope	Pallor at onset, flush on recovery
Tongue biting	Common (lateral border)	Rare	Rare
Urinary incontinence	Common	May occur	May occur
Injury	May occur	Uncommon	May occur
After the attack	Confusion common	Nauseated and 'groggy'	Usually well

Source: Stokes-Adams attack.

Table 11.3 The ECG indications for pacing after transient loss of consciousness (TLoC).

ECG feature	Comment
Sinus bradycardia (rate < 50/min) or sinus pauses	May reflect sinoatrial disorder. Pacing indicated for syncope with sinus bradycardia <40/min or sinus pauses >3 s.
Sinus tachycardia	Many possible causes. Consider: • Pulmonary embolism • Aortic dissection • Rapid blood loss and other causes of hypovolaemia
First-degree AV block	Raises the possibility of intermittent second- or third-degree AV block, but as an isolated abnormality is usually of no significance.
Second-degree AV block	Likely to be the cause of syncope: indication for pacing.
Third-degree (complete) AV block	Includes alternating right and left bundle branch block. Likely to be the cause of syncope: indication for pacing. Arrange echocardiography to check for associated structural heart disease and assess left ventricular function prior to pacing.
Atrial fibrillation	May reflect sinoatrial disorder of underlying structural heart disease.
Paced rhythm	Pacemaker failure is rare but should be excluded. Arrange for interrogation of device to determine rhythm at the time of TLoC.
Short PR interval (<120 ms)	Look for other features of Wolff–Parkinson–White (WPW) syndrome: delta wave, widened QRS complex. If WPW present, discuss management with a cardiologist.
Right-axis deviation (QRS predominantly negative in lead I and positive in lead II)	Consider pulmonary hypertension or pulmonary embolism.
Left-axis deviation (QRS predominantly positive in lead I and negative in lead II)	As an isolated abnormality, usually of no significance.

Table 11.3 (*Continued*)

ECG feature	Comment
Right bundle branch block (RBBB)	Consider pulmonary hypertension or pulmonary embolism. Consider Brugada syndrome (ECG shows RBBB pattern with ST-elevation in leads V1–V3).
Left bundle branch block (LBBB)	May reflect structural heart disease or conducting system disease. Arrange echocardiography.
Bifascicular block (RBBB or LBBB with right-axis or left-axis deviation), with or without first-degree AV block	Significantly increases the likelihood that syncope was due to intermittent AV block.
Left ventricular hypertrophy	May be seen in: • Severe hypertension • Aortic valve disease • Hypertrophic cardiomyopathy
Pathological Q waves	Usually reflect previous myocardial infarction (with associated risk of ventricular tachycardia (Chapter 13)). May also be seen in hypertrophic cardiomyopathy or WPW syndrome (pseudoinfarct pattern).
Dominant R wave in V1	May be seen in: • Right ventricular hypertrophy • RBBB • WPW syndrome • Posterior myocardial infarction • Duchenne muscular dystrophy with cardiomyopathy • Normal variant
Short QT interval	Short QT interval may reflect congenital channelopathy (short QT syndrome) or acquired disorder (e.g. due to acidosis, hyperkalaemia or hypercalcaemia), or a combination of the two. Short QT syndrome is associated with atrial and ventricular arrhythmias.
Long QT interval	Long QT interval may reflect congenital channelopathy (long QT syndrome) or acquired disorder (due to drugs (see http://www.sads.org.uk/drugs-to-avoid/)), or metabolic disorder (e.g. hypokalaemia or hypocalcaemia), or a combination of the two QT interval > 500 ms is associated with a high risk of polymorphic ventricular tachycardia (torsade de pointes) (Chapter 13).
T wave inversion	May be seen in: • Structural heart disease (e.g. severe aortic stenosis) • Cardiomyopathies • Acute coronary syndrome • Myopericarditis • Subarachnoid haemorrhage • Stress cardiomyopathy

Driving

In general, any patient with syncope must not drive until specialist assessment has been completed and they have been advised by the specialist that they may drive.

- Patients who have had typical vasovagal syncope while standing, with a reliable prodrome, may continue to drive and need not notify the DVLA.
- Consult the guidelines of the Driver and Vehicle Licensing Agency (DVLA) (available online at: www.gov.uk/dvla/fitnesstodrive).

Box 11.2 Differential diagnosis of syncope.

Transient global cerebral hypoperfusion: syncope (Box 11.1)

Metabolic disorders:

- Hypoglycaemia
- Severe hypoxia
- Hyperventilation with hypocapnia
- Poisoning with alcohol and psychoactive drugs
- Epilepsy
- Migraine
- Vertebrobasilar transient ischaemic attack
- Subclavian steal syndrome
- Subarachnoid haemorrhage

The causes of transient loss of consciousness (TLoC) (Box 11.1) can usually be differentiated by a detailed history taken from the patient and any eyewitnesses (Tables 11.1 and 11.2), supplemented by the examination findings and a careful review of the electrocardiogram (ECG) (Table 11.3). Further investigation may be needed for definitive diagnosis.

Occupational issues

- Working patients who have had TLoC should be given advice on the implications of the episode for health and safety at work and any action they must take to ensure the safety of themselves and others. They should inform their occupational health department.

Further management

Suspected cardiovascular cause

- Patients waiting for cardiovascular assessment should be advised to return to the emergency department in the event of a further episode. If TLoC occurred with high-risk features (see above) they should be advised not to exercise until the assessment has been completed, and the management plan should be discussed with a cardiologist before discharge.

Suspected epilepsy

See Chapter 57 for the advice you should give to patients after a generalized seizure.

Probable vasovagal syncope

- Give advice to the patient on avoiding action to take in the event of prodromal symptoms. Muscle clenching (leg crossing and arm tensing/hand grip) can prevent progression to syncope.
- For recurrent episodes with a significant impact on quality of life or high risk of injury, arrange a tilt-table test with cardiology follow-up: pacing may be considered for patients with a pronounced cardio-inhibitory response (typically prolonged asystole).

Table 11.4 Testing for carotid sinus hypersensitivity.

Indicated in patients aged 60 and over with unexplained syncope.
Contraindications include the presence of a carotid bruit, recent myocardial infarction, recent stroke or a history of ventricular tachycardia.
Begin with the patient lying.
Attach an ECG monitor with a printer and check the blood pressure.
The carotid sinus lies at the level of the upper border of the thyroid cartilage just below the angle of the jaw.
Perform carotid sinus massage for up to 15s whilst recording a rhythm strip. Press posteriorly and medially over the artery (first on the right, and if this is negative on the left) with your thumb or index and middle fingers.
If the test is negative, repeat with the patient sitting.
An abnormal response is defined by a sinus pause >3s or a drop in systolic blood pressure >50mmHg. If these occur, discuss with a cardiologist whether pacemaker implantation is indicated.

Suspected arrhythmic syncope

The choice of ECG monitoring depends on the frequency of episodes and the presence or absence of heart disease. Patients with high-risk features (see above) should be admitted for investigation. For those without high-risk features, recommendations for ECG monitoring are:

- TLoC at least several times a week: Holter monitoring (up to 48h if necessary)
- TLoC every 1–2 weeks: external event recorder or patch recorder
- TLoC infrequently (less than once every two weeks): implantable event recorder

Unexplained syncope

- For patients with suspected carotid sinus hypersensitivity, and for those with unexplained syncope who are aged >60 years, carotid sinus massage should be the initial investigation (Table 11.4).
- For other patients with unexplained syncope, and those with negative testing for carotid sinus hypersensitivity, ambulatory ECG monitoring should be done (see above).

Further reading

National Institute for Health and Care Excellence (2010) Transient loss of consciousness ('blackouts') in over 16s. Clinical guideline (CG109) Last updated: November 2023. https://www.nice.org.uk/guidance/cg109.
Wieling W, van Dijk N, de Lange FJ, *et al.* (2015) History taking as a diagnostic test in patients with syncope: developing expertise in syncope. *Eur Heart J* 36, 277–280. doi: 10.1093/eurheartj/ehu478.

CHAPTER 12

Acute coronary syndromes (ACS)

WILLIAM FOWKES AND JAMIE KITT

Acute coronary syndromes (ACS) represent a spectrum of conditions characterised by a sudden reduction in blood flow to the myocardium, leading to myocardial ischemia. This includes ST-segment elevation myocardial infarction (STEMI), non-ST-segment elevation myocardial infarction (NSTEMI) and unstable angina (UA). The underlying pathophysiology usually involves the disruption of atherosclerotic plaques within the coronary arteries, often due to rupture or erosion, resulting in partial or complete occlusion of the vessel.

ST-segment elevation myocardial infarction

STEMI is characterised by a complete occlusion of a coronary artery, leading to significant myocardial injury. The diagnosis is primarily based on the presence of new ST-segment elevations on the electrocardiogram (ECG) and raised troponin. STEMI requires immediate reperfusion therapy to restore blood flow and minimise myocardial damage. Spontaneous coronary artery dissection (SCAD) is a rare cause of STEMI, more common in young to middle-aged women and in pregnancy.

NSTEMI and unstable angina

NSTEMI and UA share similar pathophysiological mechanisms, typically involving partial occlusion of a coronary artery. NSTEMI and UA present similarly with a history and possible ECG changes suspicious of cardiac ischaemia, but without persistent ST-segment elevation on the ECG. NSTEMI also has evidence of myocardial injury indicated by a raised troponin, where in UA troponin is normal. UA is characterised by worsening chest pain at rest or with minimal exertion, indicating increased risk for myocardial infarction.

The widespread use of high-sensitivity troponins has made the diagnosis of UA increasingly rare, with very few cases of clinical and ECG evidence of myocardial ischaemia without a raised troponin.

Differentials for ACS

Differentiating ACS from other causes of chest pain is critical for appropriate management. Conditions that mimic ACS include (by no means an exhaustive list):

- **Pulmonary Embolism:** Sudden onset dyspnoea, pleuritic chest pain and hypoxia.
- **Aortic Dissection:** Severe, tearing chest or back pain, often with pulse deficits or differences in blood pressure between limbs.
- **Pneumothorax:** Sudden onset of sharp chest pain and shortness of breath.
- **Takotsubo cardiomyopathy:** Stress-induced cardiomyopathy with symptoms and ECG changes that can resemble ACS.

Acute Medicine: A Practical Guide to the Management of Medical Emergencies, Sixth Edition.
Edited by Mridula Rajwani, Leila Vaziri, and Ivie Gbinigie.

- **Pericarditis:** Sharp, pleuritic chest pain that may improve with sitting up and leaning forward.
- **Gastro-oesophageal Reflux Disease (GORD):** Burning chest pain, often after meals, improving with antacids.
- **Pancreatitis:** Epigastric pain radiating to the back, often after eating or drinking.
- **Musculoskeletal Pain:** Chest pain related to movement or palpation of the chest wall.

ACS management

Initial assessment, investigations and stabilisation

Upon presentation, the initial assessment of patients suspected of having ACS includes a focused history, physical examination and rapid initiation of diagnostic tests. It is important to identify patients who require immediate reperfusion therapy, i.e. percutaneous coronary intervention (PCI) or thrombolysis. Diagnosis is made on a combination of history, ECG and troponins. Key steps include:

1 **History and Physical Examination:**
   - Assess the nature, onset, duration and intensity of chest pain:
     - Site
     - Severity
     - Time of onset and duration
     - Character (e.g. 'stabbing', 'tight/gripping' or 'dull/aching')
     - Radiation (e.g. to arms, neck, jaw and back)
     - Precipitating and relieving factors (e.g. exertion/rest/GTN spray)
     - Previous episodes of similar pain, particularly on exertion
   - Associated symptoms
     - Breathlessness, nausea and vomiting, sweating, palpitations, dizziness and loss of consciousness
   - Identify risk factors such as older age, male sex, hypertension, hyperlipidaemia, diabetes, smoking, renal disease and family history of coronary artery disease. New female-specific risk factors include history of pre-eclampsia, gestational diabetes, preterm birth, use of HRT and premature ovarian insufficiency.
2 **Electrocardiogram (ECG):**
   - Look for ST-segment elevation or depression, T-wave inversions, or new left bundle branch block. The European Society of Cardiology (ESC) 2023 guideline includes an update on the finding of LBBB. ECG changes are discussed in further detail below.
3 **Cardiac Biomarkers:**
   - High-sensitivity troponin is now universally used as the standard biomarker of myocardial injury.
   - Different units will have different troponin assays and local guidelines should be used to determine timing and interpretation of levels.
4 **Echocardiography:**
   - Bedside echocardiography (ECHO) is particularly useful in suspected ACS patients presenting with shock.
   - **In shocked patients:** ECHO helps assess left ventricular (LV) and right ventricular (RV) function and detect large pericardial effusions, which can guide immediate management. It also allows evaluation for LV thrombus, LV free wall rupture +/− ventricular septal rupture, particularly relevant in late presenting infarcts.
   - **Regional Wall Motion Abnormalities (RMWAs):** ECHO can identify RMWAs that support a diagnosis of ACS, particularly if they correspond to the same territory as ECG changes.
   - **Formal departmental ECHO** should be performed in all patients while an inpatient to accurately assess LV function and identify any valvular disease, especially in patients who are considered for revascularisation. This also helps guide driving advice as per DVLA guidance.

5 Chest X-ray

- Chest X-ray to assess for other causes of chest pain (e.g. aortic dissection, pneumothorax and pneumonia), as well as for evidence of pulmonary oedema.

6 Other bloods

- Glucose and HbA1c – aim to keep glucose <11.
- U&Es and LFTs – replace potassium and magnesium if deficient.
- Lipid profile including triglyceride levels.

ECG changes in STEMI

STEMI:

STEMI diagnostic criteria: New ST-segment elevation at the J-point in two contiguous leads with the cut-off points: ≥1 mm in all leads other than V2-V3. For leads V2-V3 the following cut-off points apply: ≥2 mm in males ≥40 years, ≥2.5 mm in males <40 years, or ≥ 1.5 mm in females.

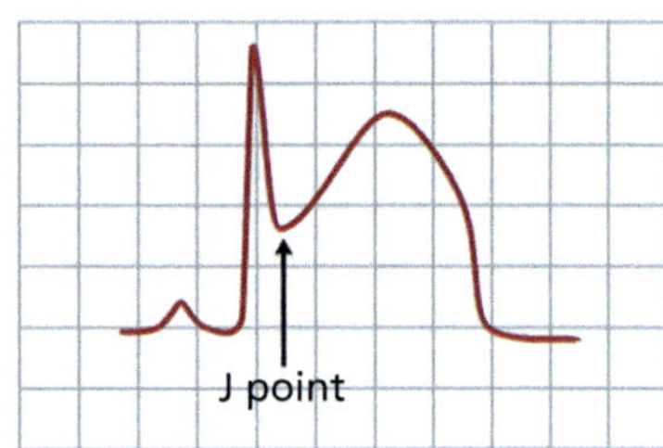

LBBB:

The ESC 2023 guideline no longer classifies new or presumably new left bundle branch block (LBBB) as a STEMI equivalent warranting planned emergent reperfusion therapy. This represents an evolving paradigm, moving away from the previous approach that considered LBBB a STEMI equivalent.

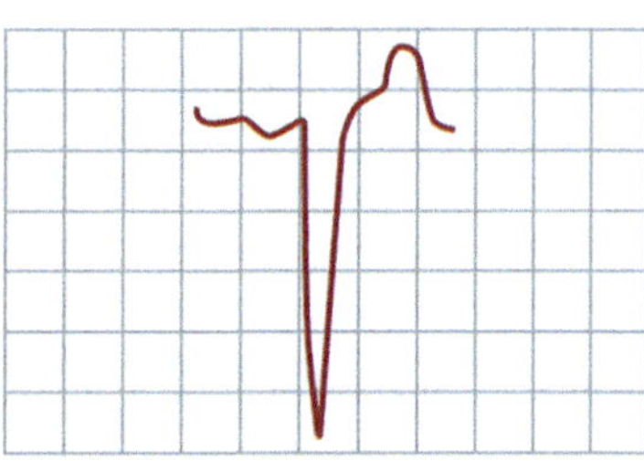

Posterior MI:

Take care not to miss a posterior MI. With chest pain and ST depression in V1-3 +/− dominant R wave in I consider posterior leads (V7-9) to assess for posterior ST elevation.

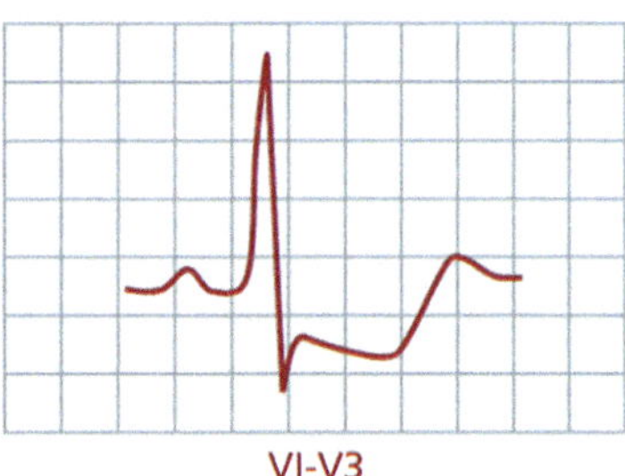

RV infarction:

RV infarction may accompany an inferior STEMI.
In inferior STEMI, additional ST elevation in V1 suggests RV infarction. If this is the case, place V4 in a reflected position on the right side of the chest (fifth right intercostal space, mid-clavicular line) to assess for ST elevation.
RV infarction is clinically significant since the use of nitrates can precipitate severe hypotension due to preload sensitivity.
Hypotension in RV infarction is treated with careful fluid resuscitation to ensure adequate filling pressure.

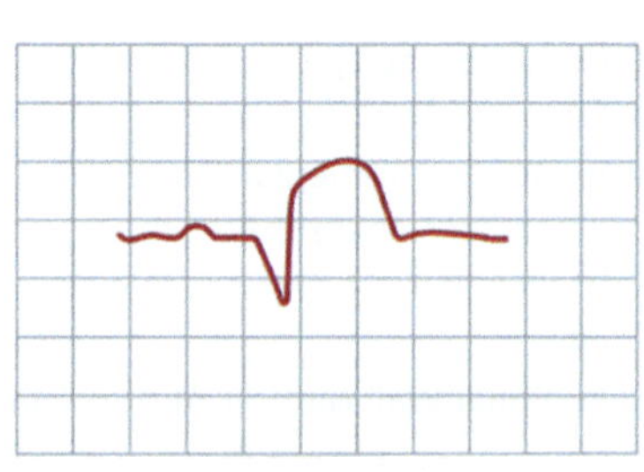

Changes in NSTEMI:

ST-segment depression:
Horizontal or down-sloping ST depression ≥0.5 mm in two or more contiguous leads.

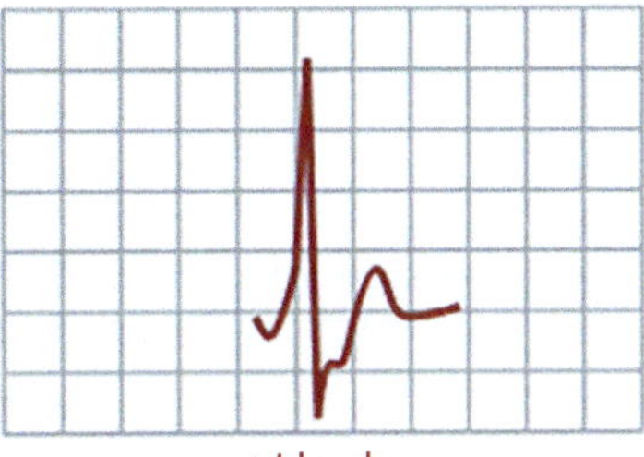

T-wave inversion:
Symmetrical T-wave inversion ≥1 mm in two contiguous leads with prominent R waves or R/S ratio > 1.

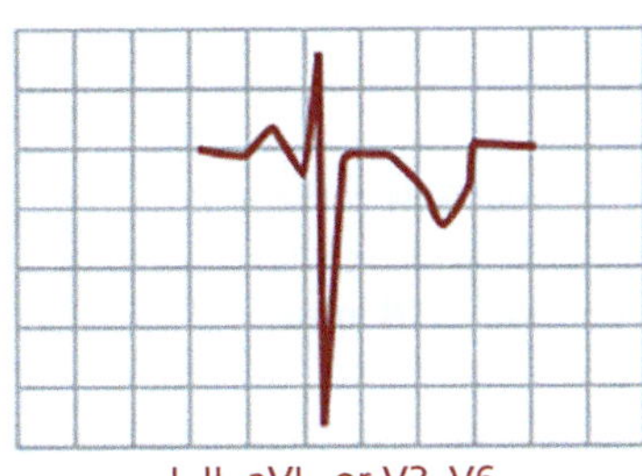

Wellen's syndrome:
Wellen's syndrome is characterised by biphasic (Type A) or deeply inverted (Type B) T waves in leads V2-V3. It is an indicator of significant stenosis of the proximal left anterior descending (LAD) artery and carries a high risk of anterior wall myocardial infarction. The ECGs often evolve quickly from V1-V6 so serial ECGs are vitally important.

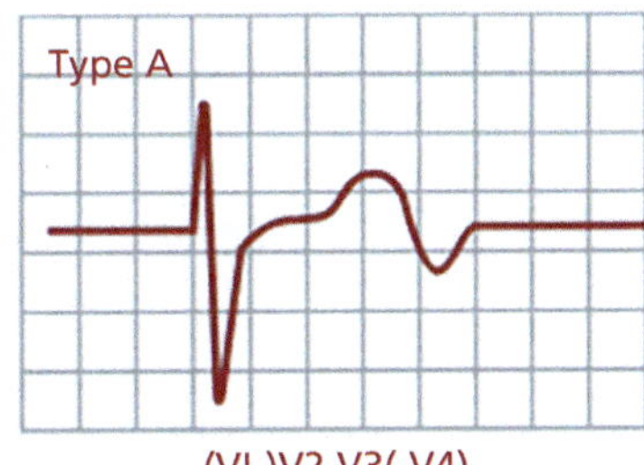

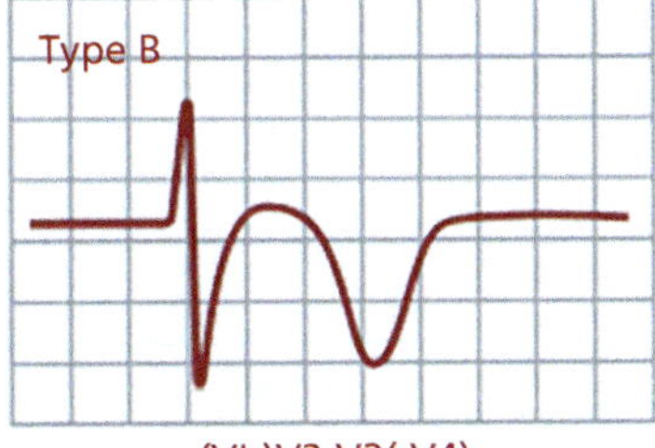

De Winter's sign:
De Winter's sign is an alternative presentation of anterior STEMI. It is characterised by upsloping ST depression >1 mm at the J-point in the precordial leads (V1-V6) along with tall, symmetrical T waves. This pattern signifies a critical occlusion of the LAD artery and requires immediate intervention.

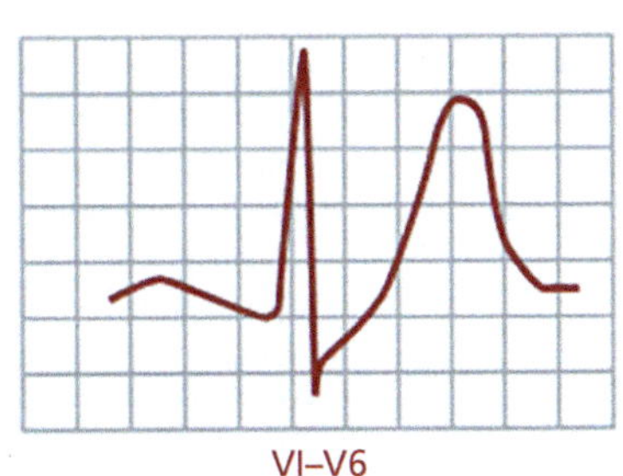

Source: Adapted from ESC Guidelines for the Management of Acute Coronary Syndromes (2023).

ECG leads	Location of MI
V1-3	Anteroseptal
V2-4	Anterior
I, aVL, V5-6	Lateral
II, III, aVF	Inferior
V1, V4R	Right Ventricle (RV)
V7-9 (with ST depression in V1-3)	Posterior

Initial Stabilisation:

- **Oxygen:** should be administered to patients with oxygen saturation below 90%. Routine use of oxygen in patients with normal oxygen saturation is no longer recommended as it has not been shown to improve outcomes.
- **Sublingual GTN:** for chest pain relief, unless contraindicated.
  - To be used with caution with evidence of RV infarction, hypotension or known severe aortic stenosis
  - **Consider GTN infusion** if ongoing chest pain, monitoring BP (local protocol will guide on BP but often aiming for systolic >90 mmHg)
  - Discuss with cardiology if ongoing chest pain requiring GTN infusion, as these patients may require urgent angiography
- **IV opioid:** titrate dose according to pain, with antiemetic if needed
- **In haemodynamic instability:** discuss with intensive care for consideration of inotropic support
  - There are multiple causes of cardiogenic shock in ACS, which can be identified with bedside echo
    - Acute LV or RV failure
    - Papillary muscle rupture with acute severe mitral regurgitation
    - LV wall rupture – either interventricular, or free wall rupture

Percutaneous coronary intervention

PCI is a cornerstone of ACS management, with the timing of PCI depending on the severity of the patient's condition (Table 12.1). Drug-eluting stents are recommended in all cases, and coronary artery bypass grafting (CABG) should be considered where PCI is not feasible or unsuccessful.

Table 12.1 Timing of PCI.

Risk level	Criteria	Timing of PCI
STEMI		Immediate or within 2 h of admission. *'Time is myocardium'*
Very high risk NSTEMI	• Haemodynamic instability or cardiogenic shock. • Recurrent or ongoing chest pain refractory to medical treatment. • Acute heart failure presumed secondary to ongoing myocardial ischaemia. • Life-threatening arrhythmias or cardiac arrest after presentation. • Mechanical complications of MI. • Recurrent dynamic ECG changes suggestive of ischaemia.	Immediate or within 2 h of admission.

Table 12.1 (*Continued*)

Risk level	Criteria	Timing of PCI
High risk NSTEMI	• Confirmed diagnosis of NSTEMI based on ESC troponin algorithms. • GRACE risk score > 140. • Transient ST-segment elevation. • Dynamic ST-segment or T wave changes.	Within 24 h of presentation.
No high or very high risk features	• Management based on degree of suspicion for ACS, for discussion with local cardiology team.	To discuss with cardiology team.

Source: Adapted from ESC Guidelines for the Management of Acute Coronary Syndromes (2023).

ST-segment elevation myocardial infarction
Primary PCI (PPCI)
The preferred method of reperfusion in STEMI is if it can be performed within 120 min of first medical contact. Cardiology should be contacted as soon as the diagnosis of STEMI is made.

Thrombolysis
Thrombolysis is indicated if anticipated time from diagnosis of STEMI to PCI exceeds 120 min – more likely in remote centres with a longer transfer time to the nearest PCI centre. Administer thrombolytic therapy as soon as possible, within 12 h of symptom onset. Follow local guidelines for thrombolysis protocol. If not easily accessible, the BNF has thrombolysis protocols for thrombolytics such as alteplase.

Post-thrombolysis care:
- All patients should be transferred to a PCI centre after initiation of thrombolysis
- Rescue PCI is indicated for failed thrombolysis:
  - ST-segment resolution <50% within 60–90 min of thrombolytic administration
  - Haemodynamic instability
  - Arrhythmias
  - Worsening ischaemia or persistent chest pain
- Otherwise, early routine PCI should be performed (within 2–24 h)

Follow local guidance or cardiology advice on antiplatelet therapy to be given in addition to thrombolysis – typically aspirin and clopidogrel.

NSTEMI
The management of NSTEMI involves risk stratification to guide the timing of PCI, and whether the patient should proceed to invasive angiography and PCI.

GRACE 3.0 score (predicts in-hospital, 6-month and 3-yearly mortality in ACS):

Age
Heart rate
Systolic BP
Creatinine
Sex
Cardiac arrest at admission
ST segment deviation
Raised troponin
Killip class

Source: Adapted from https://www.grace-3.com/about.

Myocardial infarction with non-obstructive coronary arteries

Myocardial infarction with non-obstructive coronary arteries (MINOCA) refers to a condition where patients exhibit symptoms suggestive of ACS, elevated troponin levels, but have less than 50% coronary artery stenosis in major coronary arteries during angiography. It is a broad term encompassing various coronary and non-coronary causes, and serves as a provisional diagnosis requiring further investigation to identify the underlying cause. Definitive diagnosis typically involves further investigations, including specialist invasive imaging and cardiac MRI, which can diagnose the cause of the majority of cases.

Anti-thrombotics

Antiplatelets

- Administer aspirin (300 mg loading dose) immediately to all patients with suspected ACS unless contraindicated.
- Consider second antiplatelet with a P2Y12 inhibitor (clopidogrel, ticagrelor or prasugrel), according to bleeding risk and local guidelines. The second antiplatelet should be given before or at the time of PCI.
- Bleeding risk can be assessed with scores such as the Academic Research Consortium on High Bleeding Risk (ARC-HBR) – presence of one major or two minor risk factors indicates high bleeding risk.
- If the patient is already on antiplatelet or anticoagulant therapy prior to admission, discuss with cardiology to determine the preferred treatment regimen going forward.

Anticoagulation

- Initiate anticoagulation with unfractionated heparin or low molecular weight heparin (LMWH) in patients with ACS.
- The choice of anticoagulant and duration of therapy depend on the clinical scenario and timing of invasive procedures, as well as local guidelines.

Gastric protection

For patients on dual antiplatelet therapy (DAPT), proton pump inhibitors (PPIs) should be considered in those with a high risk of gastrointestinal bleeding. ESC guidance suggests prescribing a PPI if one of the following is present:

- History of gastrointestinal bleeding or
- Concurrent use of anticoagulants, NSAIDs or steroids or
- Presence of two or more of the following factors:
    1 Age > 65 years
    2 Dyspepsia
    3 Gastroesophageal reflux disease (GORD)
    4 *Helicobacter pylori* infection
    5 Chronic alcohol use

Complications in ACS

Arrhythmias:
- **Tachyarrhythmias:**
    - Atrial Fibrillation (AF): Manage as usual with rate/rhythm control and anticoagulation. If unstable follow ALS guidance. If long-term anticoagulation is started this should be considered when deciding on antiplatelet therapy for ACS.

- Ventricular Fibrillation and Ventricular Tachycardia:
  - Treat as per ALS tachyarrhythmia guideline.
  - Incidence has significantly reduced with the advent of emergency reperfusion.
  - Consider secondary prevention with an Implantable Cardioverter Defibrillator (ICD), especially if the arrhythmia occurs >48 h post reperfusion.
- **Bradyarrhythmias:**
  - Treat as per ALS bradyarrhythmia guideline.
  - High-Degree AV Block: A permanent pacemaker (PPM) should be considered after at least five days post reperfusion. Occasionally a pacemaker is inserted before this with particularly unstable bradyarrhythmias.

Heart failure and cardiogenic shock:

- Heart failure and cardiogenic shock are severe complications of ACS that require urgent management. The main causes of this in ACS are LV or RV failure secondary to infarction, or mechanical complications (see below).
- Diuretics, vasodilators, inotropes +/− vasopressors may be required, as directed by the cardiology and intensive care teams.
- Mechanical circulatory support should be considered by the appropriate expert teams.
- Mechanical complications:
  - All mechanical complications are potentially life-threatening.
  - These include left ventricular free wall rupture (and subsequent pericardial effusion and tamponade), interventricular septal rupture with resulting left to right shunt, and acute severe mitral regurgitation secondary to papillary muscle rupture.
  - These typically present with sudden hypotension and cardiogenic shock, a recurrence of chest pain, and/or a new murmur.
  - They can either be a presenting feature of ACS (particularly in those who present late) or may develop during admission.
  - Immediate echocardiography is required to identify the complications, and emergency surgery/percutaneous structural intervention is often required. An MDT approach is paramount in managing such complications.

LV thrombus:

- More likely to develop with large anterior infarcts.
- All patients should have an ECHO during admission. If visualisation of the left ventricular apex is inconclusive then a contrast ECHO or cardiac MRI should be considered.
- Treatment is with anticoagulation for 3–6 months with possible reimaging to ensure resolution of thrombus, as guided by the cardiology team.

Pericarditis:

- Pericarditis can occur following myocardial infarction and should be managed with anti-inflammatory medications. Pericarditis typically presents with pleuritic chest pain, pericardial friction rub, and diffuse ST-segment elevation on ECG. Nonsteroidal anti-inflammatory drugs (NSAIDs) and colchicine are commonly used for treatment. Oral steroids can also be used as third line treatment.

Complications post PCI

1 Vascular complications:

  - Vascular complications at the site of access can occur in the minutes-to-days post procedure. These include bleeding and haematoma formation and are usually self-limiting.
  - Pseudoaneurysm presents as a pulsatile mass at/near the site of access and may require ultrasound-guided compression, thrombin injection or rarely vascular surgical repair (usually from femoral access).

2 Stent thrombosis
- Formation of thrombus within the stent, partially or fully obstructing blood flow.
- This typically occurs within the first 30 days following stent insertion, presenting with chest pain and ischaemic ECG changes.
- Patients who are non-compliant with antiplatelets are particularly at risk.

3 In-stent restenosis:
- Regrowth of the vessel around and within the stent causing narrowing of the lumen and reducing blood flow. This typically presents later than stent thrombosis, around 6–12 months after stent insertion. Treat as per ACS.

Long-term management

Cardiac rehabilitation

Participation in a structured cardiac rehabilitation program is essential for recovery and secondary prevention. These programs include exercise training, education on heart-healthy living, and counselling to reduce stress. Cardiac rehabilitation has been shown to improve functional capacity, quality of life and reduce the risk of recurrent cardiac events.

Lifestyle modifications (as per NICE guidelines)

Smoking cessation

Advise to stop smoking, and offer assistance from a smoking cessation service. If unable/unwilling to accept referral then offer pharmacotherapy in line with NICE guidance (including transdermal patches, gum, inhalation cartridges, tablets, lozenges, mouth spray and nasal spray).

Dietary recommendations

Emphasise a diet rich in fruits, vegetables, whole grains, lean proteins and low in saturated fats, trans fats, cholesterol, salt and added sugars. NICE and BHF guidance advocates a Mediterranean-style diet.

Physical exercise

Encourage regular aerobic exercise (e.g. walking, cycling and swimming) tailored to the patient's capacity and cardiovascular risk. About 30 min a day to the point of slight breathlessness is advised. People who are not active to this level should increase their activity in a gradual, step-by-step way, to increase their exercise capacity.

Weight management

Aim for a healthy BMI through diet and exercise. Offer advice to those who are overweight and obese.

Alcohol consumption

Advise moderation and adherence to recommended limits.

Medical therapy

1 Antiplatelets and anticoagulation:
- Continue DAPT for 6–12 months post-PCI, after which aspirin monotherapy should be continued lifelong.

- Strategies to reduce bleeding risk in high bleeding risk patients include reducing duration of DAPT to 3–6 months or de-escalation from prasugrel/ticagrelor to clopidogrel after 30 days; however, evidence is limited in higher-risk ACS patients.

2 **Secondary prevention lipid management:**
- Aggressive lipid-lowering therapy, typically with high-intensity statins, should be initiated to achieve target lipid levels and reduce the risk of recurrent events.
- Lipid management, including target cholesterol levels and emerging treatments, are changing frequently. Therefore, the most up-to-date guidelines should be consulted on secondary prevention lipid management.
- If a patient already on maximum statin dose has not achieved the target level, second-line medications such as ezetimibe can be added, with consideration of referral to lipid clinic.
- ESC (2023) guidance recommends:
  1 LDL < 1.4 mmol/L and achieve a ≥ 50% LDL reduction from baseline.
  2 If LDL goal is not achieved in 4–6 weeks, consider adding in ezetimibe.
  3 If LDL goal is still not achieved in a further 4–6 weeks, consider adding in PCSK9 inhibitor.

3 **Heart failure management – patients with LVEF < 40%**
- Patients with Heart Failure with reduced Ejection Fraction (HFrEF) should aim to be started on the four pillars of medical management of heart failure:
  1 ACE inhibitors or angiotensin II receptor blockers (ARBs) – also recommended in patients with diabetes, hypertension or CKD.
  2 Beta-blockers.
  3 Mineralocorticoid receptor antagonists (spironolactone and eplerenone).
  4 SGLT-2 inhibitors (empagliflozin and dapagliflozin).
- The patient should be referred to the local heart failure team, who can advise on initiation of medical therapy and titrate medications in the community following discharge.
- These patients should have repeat echocardiography in 6–12 weeks after revascularisation and on optimal medical therapy, to assess recovery.
- Consideration for ICD placement is based on persistent left ventricular dysfunction (LVEF < 35%) after 3 months of optimal medical therapy.

4 **Diabetes management**
- Aim for a target HbA1c of less than 53 mmol/mol (7.0%).
- The choice of anti-hyperglycaemic agents should be personalised based on the patient's comorbidities and preferences.

5 **Hypertension management**
- Aim for a target blood pressure (BP) of less than 130/80 mmHg if tolerated.
- For patients over 70 years old, aim for a target BP of less than 140/90 mmHg, but ideally 130/80 mmHg.

6 **Vaccination:**
- All ACS patients should be offered annual influenza vaccination.

Management of bystander disease

Complete revascularisation of bystander disease is now recommended either during the index PCI or within 45 days to reduce the risk of future cardiac events. This approach aims to ensure all significant coronary lesions are addressed, thereby improving long-term outcomes. The decision between staged PCI or CABG should be made by an MDT involving cardiologists and cardiac surgeons. DAPT is stopped pre-operatively and a single agent continued to undergo CABG. DAPT should be resumed following surgery and continued for at least 12 months.

Further reading

Byrne RA, Rossello X, Coughlan JJ, Barbato E, Berry C, Chieffo A, et al. 2023 ESC guidelines for the management of acute coronary syndromes: developed by the task force on the management of acute coronary syndromes of the European Society of Cardiology (ESC). Eur Heart J 2023;44(38):3720–3826. 10.1093/eurheartj/ehad191.

Driver and Vehicle Licensing Agency (DVLA) (2024) Assessing fitness to drive: a guide for medical professionals. Driver and Vehicle Licensing Agency (DVLA) Last updated: February 2024. https://www.gov.uk/government/collections/assessing-fitness-to-drive-guide-for-medical-professionals.

Maas AH, Rosano G, Cifkova R, Chieffo A, van Dijken D, Hamoda H, et al. Cardiovascular health after menopause transition, pregnancy disorders, and other gynaecologic conditions: a consensus document from European cardiologists, gynaecologists, and endocrinologists. Eur Heart J 2021;42(10):967–984. 10.1093/eurheartj/ehaa1044.

National Institute for Health and Care Excellence (NICE). Acute Coronary Syndromes: NICE Guideline [NG185]. London: NICE; 2020. Available from: https://www.nice.org.uk/guidance/ng185.

Soar J, Deakin CD, Nolan JP, et al. (2021) Adult advanced life support guidelines. Resuscitation Council UK. https://www.resus.org.uk/library/2021-resuscitation-guidelines/adult-advanced-life-support-guidelines.

Yndigegn T, Lindahl B, Mars K, Alfredsson J, Benatar J, Brandin L, et al. Beta-blockers after myocardial infarction and preserved ejection fraction. N Engl J Med 2024;390(15):1372–1381. 10.1056/NEJMoa2401479.

CHAPTER 13

Cardiac arrhythmia

David Sprigings and Basma A. A. Abdelsalam

Priorities

If there is imminent cardiac arrest, call the arrest team and manage along standard lines (see Chapter 1).

If there is a reduced level of consciousness, severe pulmonary oedema or the systolic BP is <90 mmHg:

- Record a 12-lead electrocardiogram (ECG) (if possible) for later analysis.
- If the heart rate is >150/min, call an anaesthetist in preparation for DC cardioversion (Chapter 106) and attach defibrillator pads.
- If the heart rate is <40/min, give atropine 0.6–1.2 mg IV, with further doses at 5-min intervals up to a total dose of 3 mg if the heart rate remains below 60/min. Consider an isoprenaline infusion 5 μg/min in severe bradycardia unresponsive to atropine; use with caution in patients with a history of ischaemic heart disease. If bradycardia is unresponsive or recurs, use an external cardiac pacing system or put in a temporary transvenous pacemaker (Chapter 107).

If the patient is haemodynamically stable, there is time to make a working diagnosis and plan management. Clinical assessment is summarized in Table 13.1 and urgent investigation in Table 13.2. Record a 12-lead electrocardiogram and a long rhythm strip. Further management is determined by the type of arrhythmia. Drugs used in the management of arrhythmias are summarized in Table 13.3.

Regular broad complex tachycardia:

- The diagnosis is usually ventricular tachycardia (VT). Haemodynamic stability does not exclude VT.
- If there is ischaemic heart disease or cardiomyopathy, the diagnosis is virtually always VT.
- Suspect diagnoses other than VT in younger patients (age<40 years), or with known Wolff–Parkinson–White syndrome or bundle branch block. If there is doubt, assess the effect of adenosine.

Irregular broad complex tachycardia:

- This is likely to be atrial fibrillation with bundle branch block or, less commonly, pre-excited atrial fibrillation (Figure 13.5). The difference between the maximum and minimum instantaneous heart rates calculated from the shortest and longest RR intervals is usually >30/min.
- The differential diagnosis is polymorphic ventricular tachycardia. This is usually due to therapy with antiarrhythmic and other drugs which prolong the QT interval (e.g. amiodarone and sotalol), especially in patients with hypokalaemia or hypomagnesaemia.

Acute Medicine: A Practical Guide to the Management of Medical Emergencies, Sixth Edition.
Edited by Mridula Rajwani, Leila Vaziri, and Ivie Gbinigie.

Table 13.1 Focused assessment of the patient with an acute arrhythmia.

Symptoms?
- Of arrhythmia (palpitations, presyncope and syncope).
- Of underlying cardiac disease (chest pain and breathlessness).

Haemodynamically stable? Signs of instability are:
- Pulmonary oedema.
- Heart rate <40/min or >150/min.
- Bradycardia with pauses >3 s.
- Systolic BP <90 mmHg or diastolic BP <60 mmHg.
- Chest pain.
- Reduced conscious level.

Known arrhythmia?
- Specific diagnosis? How was this established?
- Previous management (by DCCV, pharmacological therapyor ablation?).
- Current maintenance therapy.

Evidence of ischaemic or other structural heart disease (e.g. history of ACS, Q waves on ECG, known cardiomyopathy)?
- This makes ventricular tachycardia almost certainly the diagnosis if there is a regular broad complex tachycardia (BCT).
- Flecainide (class Ic antiarrhythmic medication) should be avoided for cardioversion or preventing atrial fibrillation because of the risk of precipitating ventricular arrhythmias.

Could LV systolic function be significantly impaired (e.g. exertional breathlessness, large cardiac silhouette on chest X-ray, LV ejection fraction <40% on previous echocardiography)?
- If so, avoid high-dose beta-blocker and flecainide in the acute decompensated phase.

Is there Wolff-Parkinson-White syndrome? This may cause:
- AV re-entrant or orthodromic tachycardia (narrow complex, regular): conduction forward through the AV node and back via the accessory pathway.
- Pre-excited atrial fibrillation (broad complex, irregular): fast conduction of atrial fibrillation down the accessory pathway.
- Antidromic tachycardia (broad complex, regular): conduction forward down the accessory pathway and back via the AV node.

Associated acute or chronic illness?
- Acute atrial fibrillation commonly complicates pneumonia and other infections.
- Electrolyte disorders (especially of potassium, calcium and magnesium) should be excluded/corrected.

Table 13.2 Urgent investigation of the patient with an acute arrhythmia.

12-lead ECG and long rhythm strip during the arrhythmia and after resolution (check heart rate and for delta wave, AV conduction abnormality, bundle branch block, Q waves, evidence of LV hypertrophy, QT interval, ST/T abnormalities)

Electrolytes (if on diuretic, include magnesium) and creatinine

Blood glucose

Thyroid function (for later analysis)

Plasma digoxin level if taking digoxin (at least 8 h after digoxin last taken)

Plasma troponin

Chest X-ray (heart size, evidence of raised left atrial pressure, coexistent pathology, for example pneumonia?)

Echocardiogram (for LV function, RV function, valve disease and pericardial effusion) if there is VT. Can be done the next day for other primary arrhythmias.

Table 13.3 Drugs used in the management of arrhythmias.

Drug	Class	Comment	Dose	Indications
Drugs used in tachyarrhythmias				
Lidocaine	Ib (Fast sodium channel blocker)	Converts ~30% Appropriate when VT is due to myocardial ischaemia or infarction. May cause hypotension and neurological side effects.	Loading: 1.5 mg/kg over 2 min Maintenance: 1–4 mg/min	Stable monomorphic VT
Flecainide	Ic (Slow sodium channel blocker)	May cause hypotension Avoid if known/possible structural or coronary heart disease	IV 2 mg/kg (to a maximum of 150 mg) over 10–30 min *or* PO 200–300 mg stat	Atrial flutter Atrial fibrillation Haemodynamically stable pre-excited atrial fibrillation
Verapamil	IV (Calcium channel blocker)	May cause hypotension Contraindicated in patients taking beta blockers or in heart failure.	5 mg IV over 5 min, to maximum dose of 15 mg *or* PO 40–80 mg 8-hourly	SVT (AVRT, AVNRT) Atrial tachycardia, Atrial flutter Atrial fibrillation
Esmolol	II (Beta blocker)	Short-acting (half-life 8 min) beta-1 selective beta-blocker	500 µgm/kg over 1 min, followed by 200µgm/kg over 4 min	SVT (AVRT, AVNRT) Atrial tachycardia, Atrial flutter Atrial fibrillation
Metoprolol	II (Beta blocker)	May cause hypotension	5 mg IV over 5 min, to maximum dose of 15 mg *or* PO 25–100 mg 12-hourly	SVT (AVRT, AVNRT) Atrial tachycardia, Atrial flutter Atrial fibrillation
Adenosine	V (AV Node blocker)	May cause facial flushing, chest pain, hypotension, bronchospasm May cause brief asystole, atrial fibrillation and non-sustained ventricular tachycardia Use with caution in patients with severe airway disease Contraindicated in patients with heart transplant	6 mg IV bolus through large bore cannula, followed by rapid saline flush. Repeat as necessary, if no response within 2 min, with 12, 18 and 24 mg boluses	SVT (AVRT, AVNRT) with or without bundle branch block
Digoxin	Cardiac glycoside	May cause hypotension Use if there is heart failure	Loading: 500–1000 µgm in 50 mL saline over 1 h PO maintenance dose: 62.5–250 µg daily, according to renal function/age	Atrial tachycardia Atrial flutter Atrial fibrillation

(continued)

Table 13.3 (*Continued*)

Drug	Class	Comment	Dose	Indications
Amiodarone	III (Potassium channel blocker)	May be combined with digoxin for rate control in haemodynamically unstable patients	Cardioversion: Loading: 300 mg, diluted in 5% glucose to a volume of 20–50 mL, infused over 20 min via a central vein Maintenance: 900–1200 mg over 24 h Rate control: PO dose 200 mg 8-hourly for one week, then 200 mg 12-hourly for one week, then 200 mg daily	SVT (AVRT, AVNRT) Atrial tachycardia Atrial flutter Atrial fibrillation Haemodynamically stable pre-excited atrial fibrillation Stable monomorphic/polymorphic ventricular tachycardia
Drugs used in bradyarrhythmias				
Atropine	Anticholinergic alkaloid	Inhibits vagal tone	Bolus of 500–1000 µgm, with further doses at 5 min intervals up to a total dose of 3 mg to achieve target heart rate	
Dobutamine	Beta-1 agonist	Cardiac beta-1 receptor stimulation. High doses may provoke ventricular arrhythmias	Start infusion at 10 µgm/kg/min. Adjust rate of infusion to achieve target heart rate	
Isoprenaline	Non-selective beta agonist	Positive inotrope and chronotrope Avoid in ischaemic heart disease, hyperthyroidism, diabetes	Bolus of 5-20 µgm IV Start infusion at a rate of 5 µg/min	
Glucagon		To reverse beta-blockade	Bolus of 2–10 mg followed by infusion of 50 µgm/kg/h	

Table 13.4 Differential diagnosis of bradycardia and AV block.

Diagnosis	ECG features
Sinus bradycardia	Constant PR interval < 200 ms QRS regular.
Junctional bradycardia	P wave absent or position constant either after, immediately before or hidden in the QRS complex.
First-degree AV block	Constant PR interval > 200 ms.
Second-degree AV block, Mobitz type 1	Progressively lengthening PR interval followed by dropped beat.
Second-degree AV block, Mobitz type 2	Constant PR interval with dropped beats.
Third-degree (complete) AV block	Relationship of P wave to QRS varies randomly.

Regular narrow complex tachycardia:

- The diagnosis in a younger patient is usually AV nodal re-entrant tachycardia and in an older patient, usually atrial flutter.
- Vagotonic manoeuvres increase AV block and may terminate the arrhythmia if it involves the AV node or reveal atrial activity. Ask the patient to perform a Valsalva manoeuvre, by attempting to blow the plunger from a 10 mL syringe, while semi-recumbent. Immediately following release, lay the patient flat and raise their legs passively for 15 s or try carotid sinus massage. If vagotonic manoeuvres do not restore sinus rhythm, give adenosine.
- Suspect atrial flutter with 2 : 1 AV conduction rather than sinus tachycardia if the rate is around 150/min.
- Suspect atrial tachycardia or junctional tachycardia in a younger patient with repaired congenital heart disease, in an older patient with structural heart disease, or if digoxin toxicity is possible. Digoxin toxicity is likely if plasma digoxin level is > 3.0 ng/mL (> 3.8 nmol/L), especially if there is hypokalaemia (< 3.5 mmol/L), hypomagnesaemia or hypercalcaemia. Systemic features include nausea, vomiting, diarrhoea and delirium.

Irregular narrow complex tachycardia:

- The diagnosis is usually atrial fibrillation (AF).
- Other possibilities are sinus rhythm with frequent supraventricular extrasystoles or multifocal atrial tachycardia (the rhythm looks half-way between sinus and AF).

Bradycardia (rate < 60/min):

- The differential diagnosis is given in Table 13.4. Look carefully at the PR interval and the relationship between the P wave and QRS complex.
- A regular ventricular rate < 50/min in a patient with atrial fibrillation indicates complete heart block (not 'slow AF'); always consider digoxin toxicity.

Regular broad complex tachycardia

(Figures 13.1 and 13.2, Table 13.5)

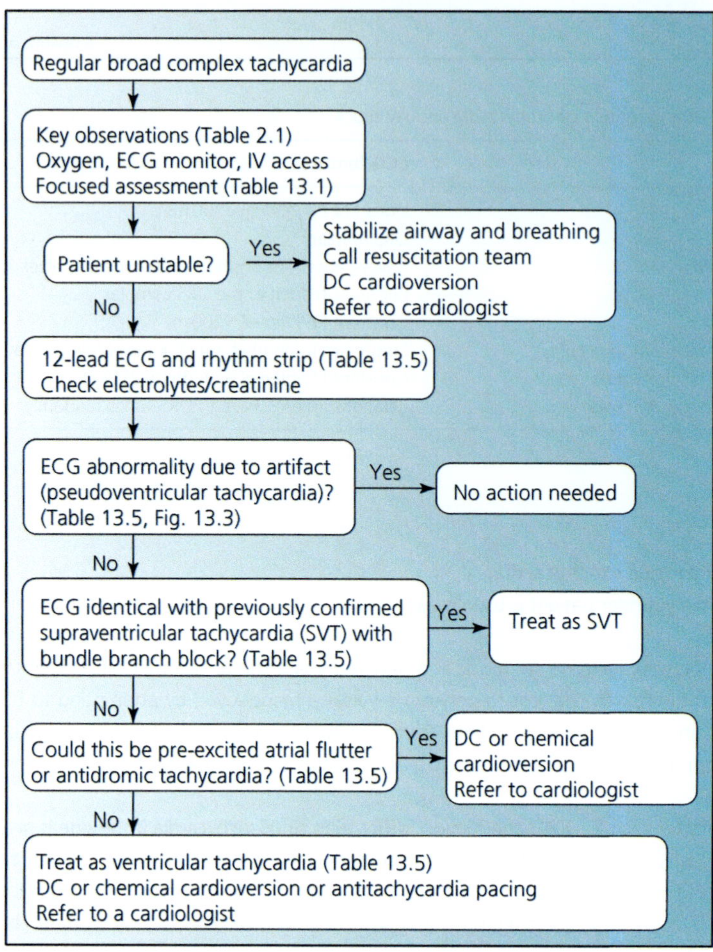

Figure 13.1 Approach to the patient with regular broad complex tachycardia (BCT). *In unstable patients, immediate resuscitation and arrhythmia control must always take precedence over rhythm analysis. Swift referral to a cardiologist is recommended.

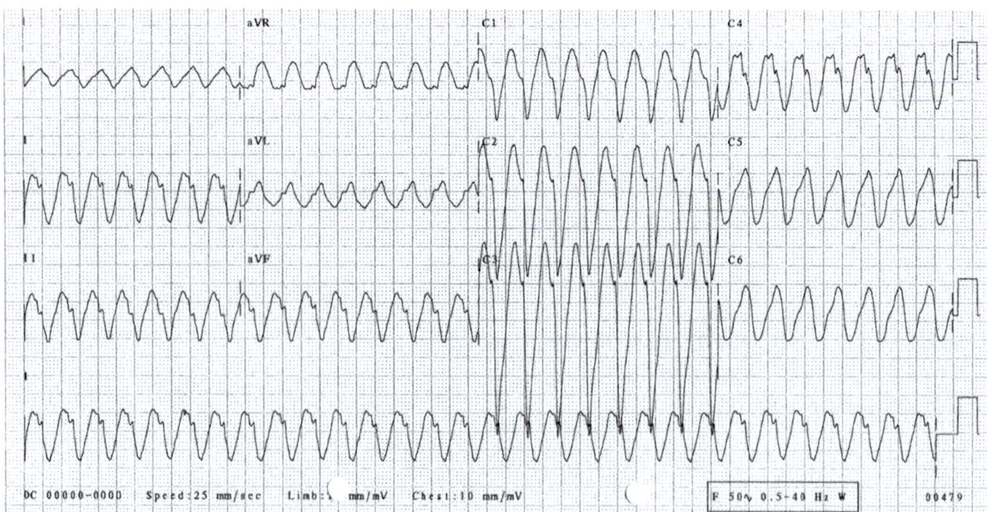

Figure 13.2 Monomorphic ventricular tachycardia (VT). VT is almost certain if there is a broad complex tachycardia with structural heart disease (e.g. myocardial infarction). Specific ECG features strongly suggestive of VT are the QRS width (approx. 200 ms) and the 'northwest axis' (positive QRS in lead aVR). Atrioventricular dissociation (see Table 13.6) is specific for VT, but often not seen, including in this trace.

Table 13.5 Regular BCT: differential diagnosis and management.

Arrhythmia	Comment	Management
Monomorphic ventricular tachycardia (Figure 13.2, Table 13.6)	The most common cause and should be the default diagnosis (especially if there is a history of previous myocardial infarction or other structural heart disease). Restore sinus rhythm as soon as possible, even in haemodynamically stable patients, as sudden deterioration may occur.	DC cardioversion (Chapter 106) if there is haemodynamic instability or other measures are ineffective. In stable patient, DC cardioversion, IV antiarrhythmic therapy or antitachycardia pacing. Refer to a cardiologist.
Supraventricular tachycardia (SVT) with bundle branch block	Confirm with adenosine test.	DC cardioversion if there is haemodynamic instability or other measures are ineffective. In stable patient IV adenosine, verapamil or beta-blocker. Record 12-lead ECG after sinus rhythm is restored to check for pre-excitation (WPW syndrome). Refer to a cardiologist if episodes are frequent or severe or if pre-excitation is found.
Antidromic tachycardia or atrial flutter in WPW syndrome	These are rarely seen but should be considered in a young patient with known WPW syndrome who does not have structural heart disease.	DC cardioversion. Refer to a cardiologist.
Pseudoventricular tachycardia	Caused by body movement and intermittent skin-electrode contact ('toothbrush tachycardia'). No haemodynamic change during apparent ventricular arrhythmia.	No action needed. It is important to avoid misdiagnosis as ventricular tachycardia.

Table 13.6 Regular BCT: ECG features that may help distinguish ventricular tachycardia (VT) from supraventricular tachycardia (SVT) with bundle branch block.

Feature	Comment
Atrioventricular dissociation	AV dissociation (with P waves interspersed between or within QRS complexes, and capture or fusion beats)is specific for VT, but is often not seen.
QRS complex morphology	QRS complex morphology incompatible with 'classical' left or right bundle branch blocks favours VT.
QRS duration	QRS >160 ms for BCT with left bundle branch block pattern and QRS >140 ms for BCT with right bundle branch block pattern favours VT.
Chest lead concordance	Chest lead concordance, with uniform QRS complexes across the chest leads (positive or negative), is specific for VT, but is often not seen.
QRS axis	'Northwest' axis (positive QRS in lead aVR) favours VT.

Irregular broad complex tachycardia

Figures 13.3, 13.4, 13.5; Table 13.7)

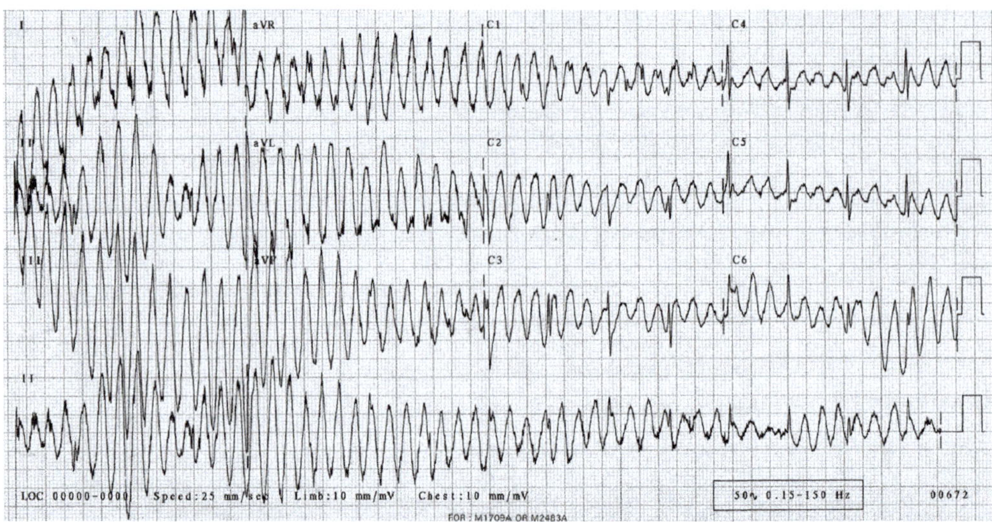

Figure 13.3 Pseudoventricular tachycardia. There are native QRS complexes at the cycle length of the baseline rhythm within the artifact, best seen in C4 and C5.

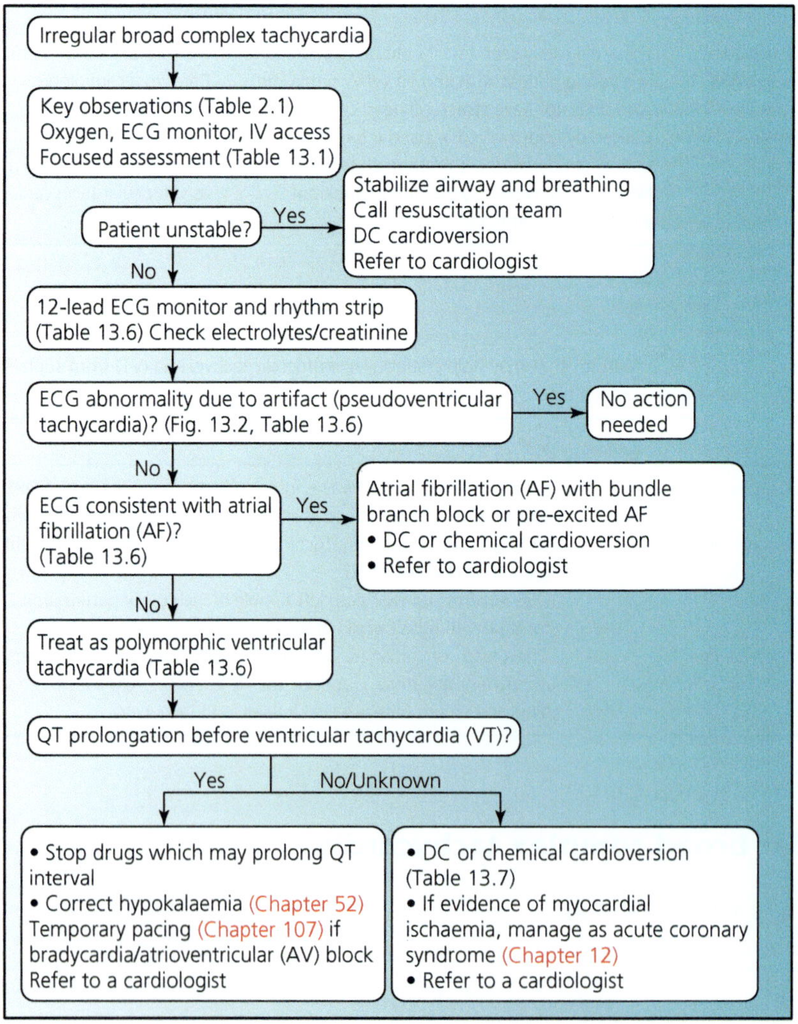

Figure 13.4 Approach to the patient with irregular broad complex tachycardia.

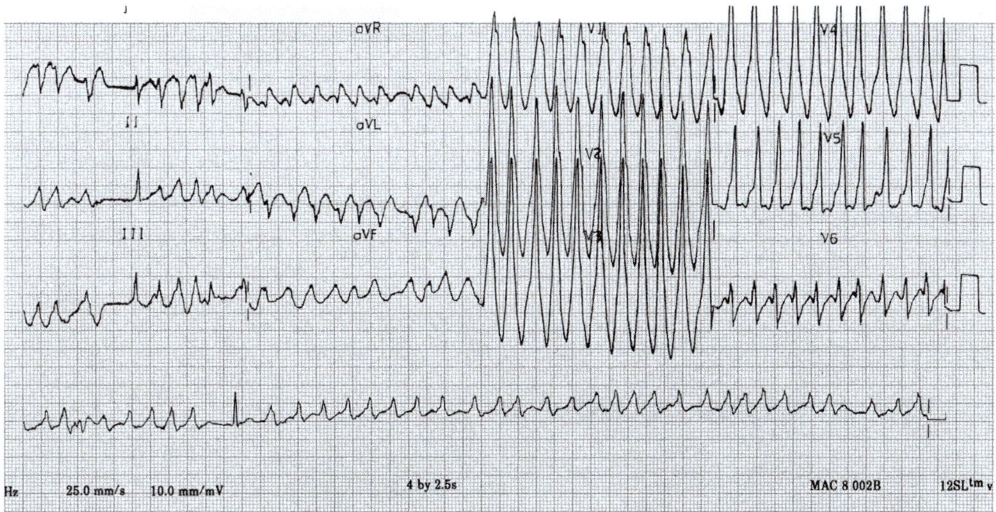

Figure 13.5 Pre-excited atrial fibrillation in Wolff–Parkinson–White syndrome. Despite the irregularity of the RR interval over the whole trace, some sections (e.g. V1–V6) look regular. By contrast, in atrial flutter the tachycardia is usually regular and in antidromic tachycardia, it is reproducibly regular.

Table 13.7 Irregular broad complex tachycardia: differential diagnosis and management.

Arrhythmia	Comment	Management
Atrial fibrillation with bundle branch block	Difference between maximum and minimum instantaneous heart rates, calculated from the shortest and longest RR intervals is usually >30/min, with QRS showing typical LBBB or RBBB morphology.	DC cardioversion if there is haemodynamic instability. In stable patient, aim for rate-control with AV node-blocking drugs.
Polymorphic ventricular tachycardia with preceding QT prolongation (torsade de pointes)	Usually due to therapy with antiarrhythmic and other drugs that prolong the QT interval (e.g. amiodarone, sotalol, erythromycin, psychotropic drugs), especially in patients with hypokalaemia and/or bradycardia Rarely congenital long QT syndrome (possible family history). Also advanced conduction system disease with block.	Stop drugs that may prolong QT interval. Correct hypokalaemia (target potassium 4.5–5 mmol/L). If there is bradycardia/AV block, use temporary pacing at 90/min (Chapter 107). If due to long QT syndrome, give magnesium sulphate 2 g IV bolus over 2–3 min, repeated if necessary, and followed by an infusion of 2–8 mg/min Refer to a cardiologist.
Polymorphic ventricular tachycardia without preceding QT prolongation	Usually due to myocardial ischaemia in the setting of acute coronary syndrome. Other causes include acute myocarditis, cardiomyopathies (e.g. arrhythmogenic right ventricular cardiomyopathy) and Brugada syndrome (VT/VF with RBBB and precordial ST elevation).	DC cardioversion (if there is haemodynamic instability or other measures are ineffective) or antiarrhythmic therapy with IV amiodarone or beta-blocker. Manage as acute coronary syndrome (Chapter 12) with urgent coronary angiography and revascularization if ischaemia is suspected or cannot be excluded. Refer to a cardiologist.

(*continued*)

Table 13.7 (*Continued*)

Arrhythmia	Comment	Management
Pre-excited atrial fibrillation (AF) in WPW syndrome (Figure 13.5)	AF conducted variably over accessory pathway. Ventricular rate typically 200–300/min. QRS morphology shows beat to beat variation in degree of pre-excitation.	DC cardioversion or antiarrhythmic therapy with flecainide or amiodarone. Refer to a cardiologist.
Pseudoventricular tachycardia (Figure 13.3)	Caused by skin-electrode contact ('toothbrush tachycardia'). No haemodynamic change during apparent ventricular arrhythmia.	No action needed. Important to recognize to prevent misdiagnosis as VT.

Narrow complex tachycardia

Figures 13.6-13.8, Tables 13.8 and 13.9.

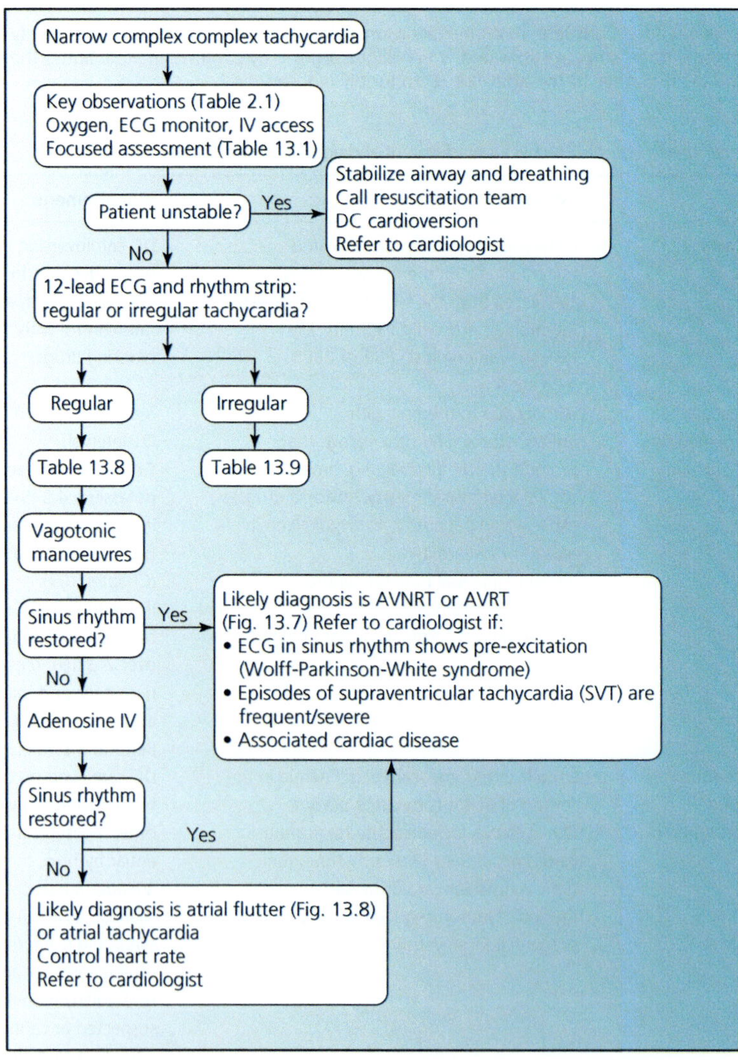

Figure 13.6 Approach to the patient with narrow complex tachycardia.

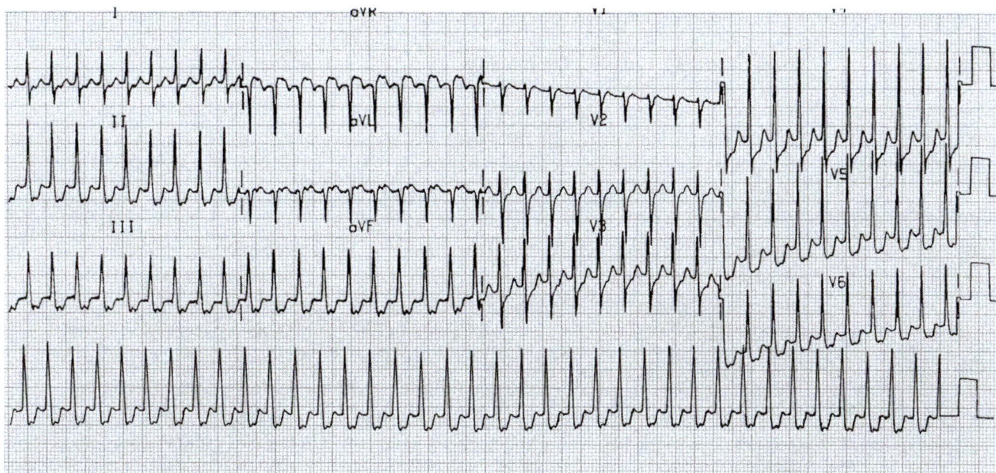

Figure 13.7 Paroxysmal supraventricular tachycardia, due to AV re-entrant tachycardia with retrograde P wave inscribed on ST segment.

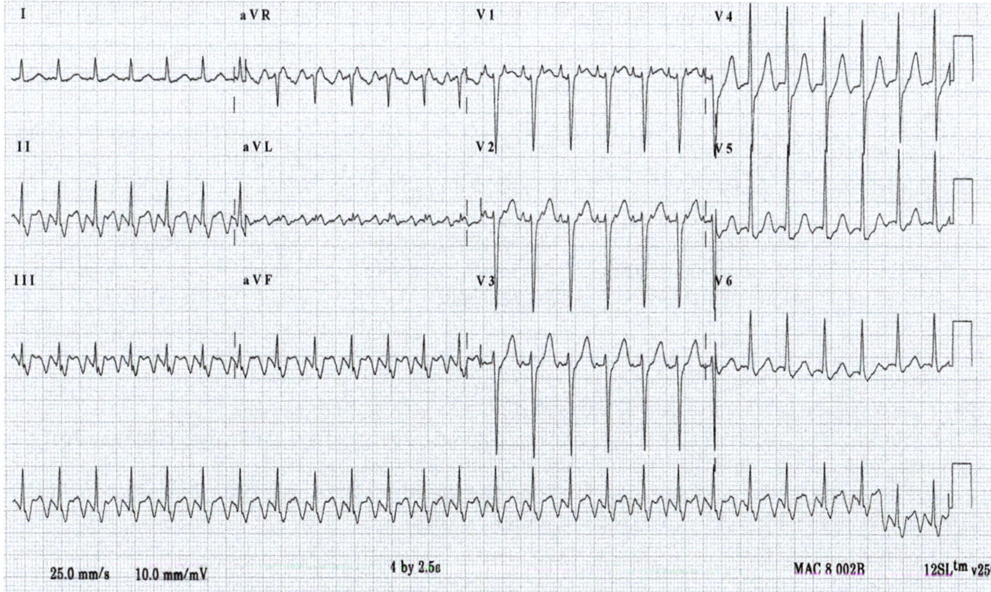

Figure 13.8 Atrial flutter with 2 : 1 conduction.

Table 13.8 Differential diagnosis and management of narrow complex regular tachycardia.

Arrhythmia	Characteristics	Comments	Management
Sinus tachycardia	Atrial rate 100–200 QRS rate 100–200 P wave precedes QRS	May sometimes be difficult to distinguish from other causes of tachycardia. Adenosine causes gradual deceleration of sinus rate followed by acceleration, with or without AV block.	Identify and treat the underlying cause. IV adenosine may be appropriate to exclude other causes of narrow-complex regular tachycardia if in doubt.

(continued)

Table 13.8 (*Continued*)

Arrhythmia	Characteristics	Comments	Management
AV nodal re-entrant tachycardia (AVNRT)	Heart rate usually 140–200/min. Retrograde P wave usually hidden within or inscribed at the end of the QRS complex (simulating S wave in inferior leads, partial RBBB in V1).	The commonest cause of paroxysmal SVT Typically presents in teenagers or young adults with no underlying cardiac disease, though may present at any age. Record 12-lead ECG after sinus rhythm restored to check for pre-excitation (WPW syndrome).	DC cardioversion if there is haemodynamic instability (uncommon) or other measures are ineffective. In stable patient try vagotonic manoeuvres. If these fail, use IV adenosine, or verapamil* if adenosine is not tolerated or is contraindicated. Record 12-lead ECG after sinus rhythm restored to check for pre-excitation (WPW syndrome).
AV re-entrant tachycardia involving accessory pathway (AVRT) (Figure 13.7)	Heart rate usually 140–230/min. Retrograde P wave may be seen inscribed in the ST segment or the ascending limb of the T wave.	Refer to a cardiologist if episodes are frequent or severe or if pre-excitation is found.	Refer to a cardiologist if episodes are frequent or severe or if pre-excitation is found.
Atrial flutter (Figure 13.8)	Suspect atrial flutter with 2 : 1 block when the rate is 150/min. 'Saw-tooth' in the inferior leads/V1.	Often associated with structural heart disease.	DC cardioversion if there is haemodynamic instability or other measures are ineffective. Vagotonic manoeuvres and adenosine slow the ventricular rate to reveal flutter waves. In stable patient, aim for rate control with AV node-blocking drugs. Discuss further management with a cardiologist.
Atrial tachycardia	P wave usually of abnormal morphology, at a rate 130–300/min, conducted with varying degree of AV block.	Caused by discrete focus of electrical activity. May be associated with structural heart disease in older patients.	DC cardioversion if there is haemodynamic instability or other measures are ineffective. In stable patient, aim for rate control with AV node-blocking drugs. Discuss further management with a cardiologist.

ALERT Atrial flutter and atrial tachycardia may be irregular if there is variable AV conduction.
NOTE: 1. In up to 50% of patients with AVRT the accessory pathway is concealed and a delta wave is never present in sinus rhythm. These patients do not have Wolff–Parkinson–White syndrome.
2. It may be impossible to distinguish AVRT from AVNRT on the surface ECG. Initial treatment is identical.
* Do not give verapamil if the patient is already taking an oral beta blocker.

Table 13.9 Differential diagnosis and management of narrow complex irregular tachycardia.

Arrhythmia	Comment	Management
Atrial fibrillation	Difference between maximum and minimum instantaneous heart rates, calculated from the shortest and longest RR intervals is usually >30/min. No organized atrial activity evident: fibrillation waves of varying amplitude may be seen.	DC cardioversion if there is haemodynamic instability. In stable patient, aim for rate control with AV node-blocking drugs.
Atrial flutter with variable AV conduction	Often associated with structural heart disease Vagotonic manoeuvres and adenosine slow the ventricular rate to reveal flutter waves ("saw-tooth" flutter waves in inferior limb leads).	DC cardioversion if there is haemodynamic instability. In stable patient, aim for rate control with AV node-blocking drugs.

Table 13.9 (*Continued*)

Arrhythmia	Comment	Management
Multifocal atrial tachycardia	Irregular tachycardia, typically 100–130/min, with P waves of three or more morphologies and irregular PP interval. Most commonly seen in COPD.	Treatment is directed at the underlying disorder and correction of hypoxia/hypercapnia. Consider verapamil if the heart rate is consistently over 110/min. DC cardioversion is ineffective.

Atrial fibrillation and flutter

Figures 13.9 and 13.10, Table 13.10.

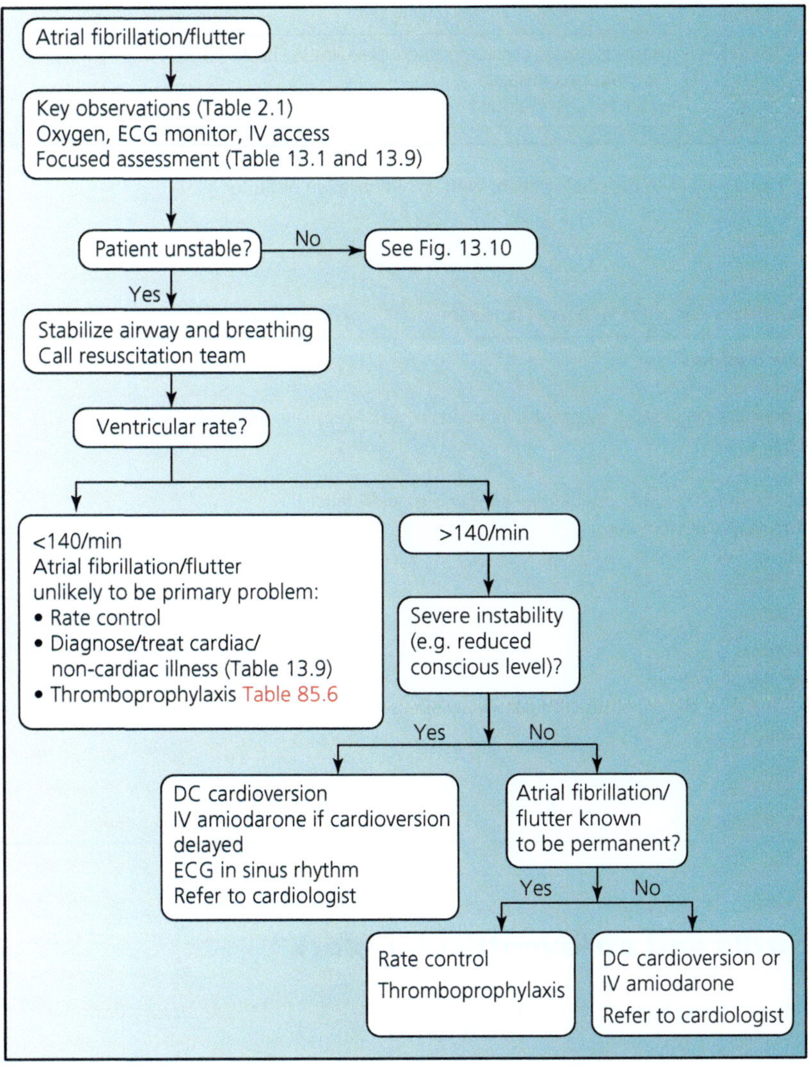

Figure 13.9 Approach to the patient with atrial fibrillation or flutter.

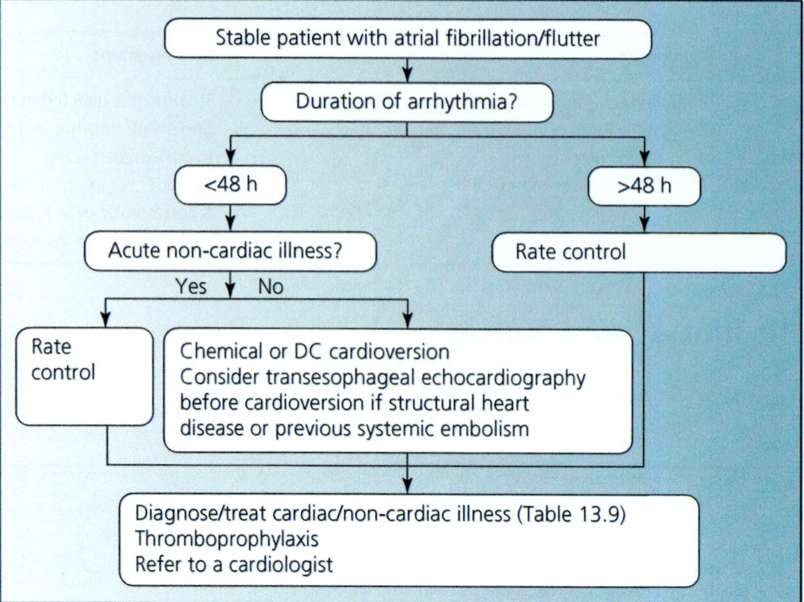

Figure 13.10 Management of the stable patient with atrial fibrillation or flutter.

Table 13.10 Disorders associated with atrial fibrillation.

Cardiovascular disorders
- Hypertension
- Coronary artery disease: previous myocardial infarction or acute coronary syndrome
- Cardiomyopathy
- Valve disease
- Any cause of heart failure (with resultant atrial hypertension/dilatation)
- Wolff–Parkinson–White syndrome
- Pulmonary embolism
- Acute pericarditis
- Cardiac surgery

Systemic disorders
- Sepsis, especially pneumonia
- Acute exacerbation of chronic obstructive pulmonary disease
- Alcohol binge
- Thyrotoxicosis
- Severe hypokalaemia
- Non-cardiac surgery

Bradycardia and atrioventricular block

Figures 13.11–13.16 and Tables 13.11.–13.14

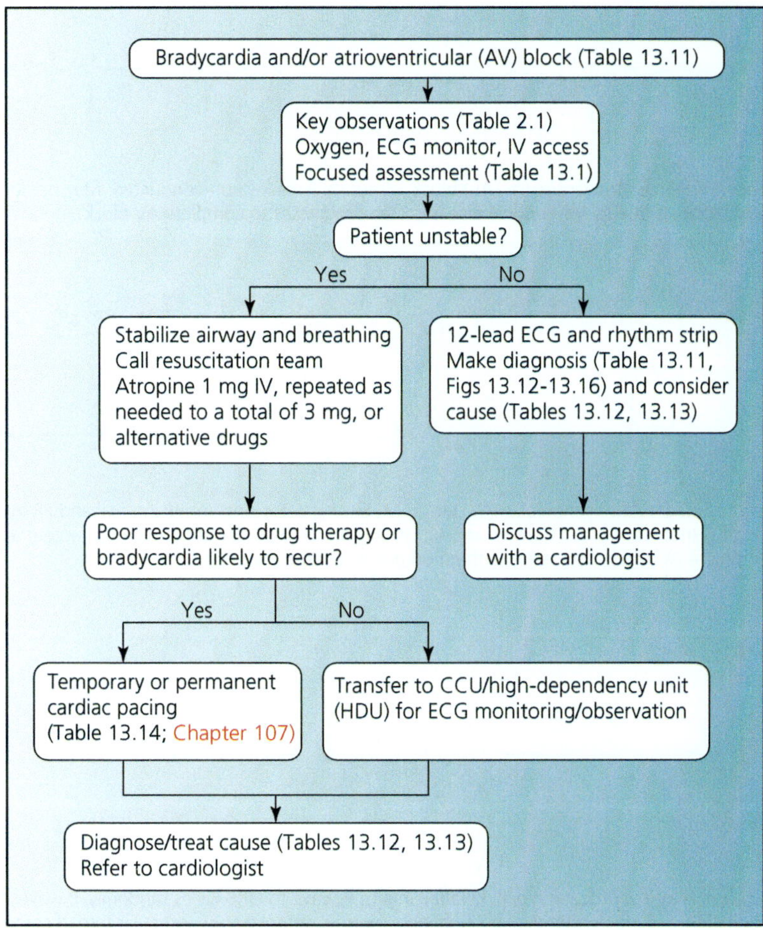

Figure 13.11 Approach to the patient with bradycardia and/or atrioventricular block.

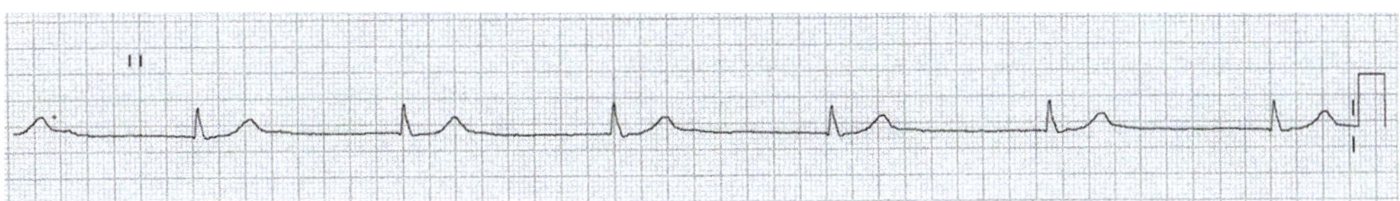

Figure 13.12 Junctional bradycardia secondary to sinus node disease. Heart rate 30–60/min with P wave absent or position constant either after, immediately before or hidden in QRS complex. Occurs when junctional pacemaker overtakes slow sinus node pacemaker or with complete sino-atrial exit block or sinus arrest.

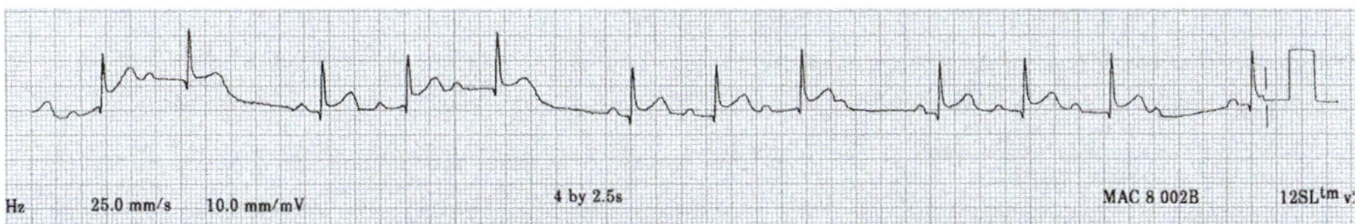

Figure 13.13 Second-degree atrioventricular block, Mobitz type 1 (Wenckebach). Progressively lengthening PR interval followed by dropped beat.

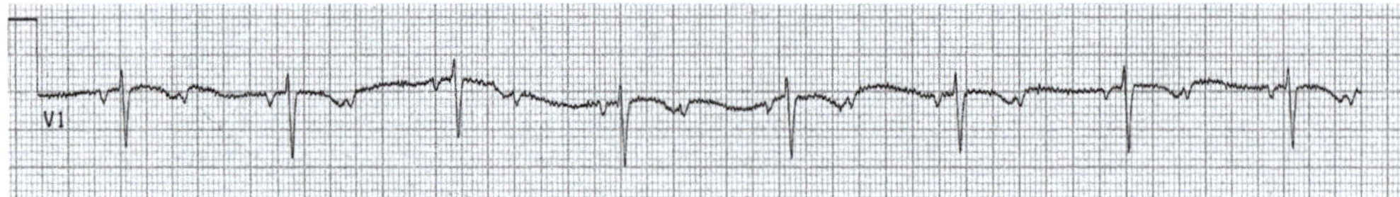

Figure 13.14 Second-degree atrioventricular (AV) block: alternate P waves non-conducted. May be due to disease in the AV node or below. If due to His-Purkinje disease often progresses to complete AV block.

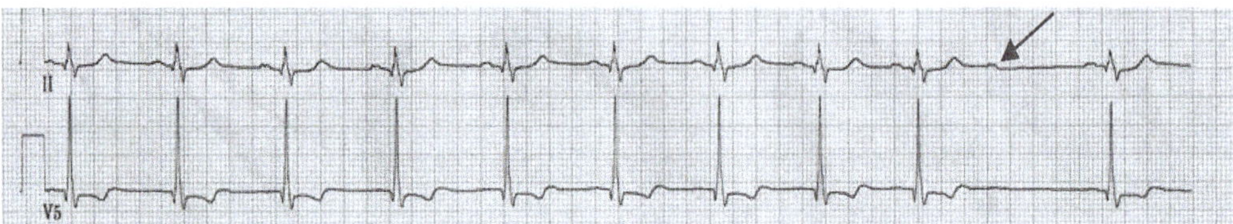

Figure 13.15 Second-degree atrioventricular (AV) block, Mobitz type 2. Constant PP interval and PR interval, with sudden dropped beat (non-conducted P wave, arrow). Usually due to disorder of His-Purkinje system and often progresses to complete AV block, frequently with an unreliable escape rhythm.

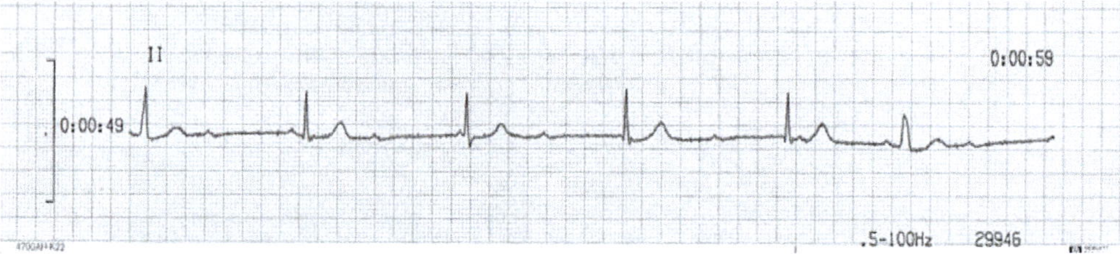

Figure 13.16 Complete atrioventricular block. Relationship of P wave to QRS varies randomly. P waves are absent if there is atrial fibrillation. Escape rhythm may be junctional (narrow complex) or ventricular (broad complex). Even in asymptomatic patients, this carries a risk of sudden death due to ventricular standstill or polymorphic ventricular tachycardia/ventricular fibrillation. The escape rhythm is usually slower and less reliable when it is ventricular.

Table 13.11 Classification of bradycardia and atrioventricular (AV) block.

Bradycardia (sinus node disease and atrioventricular block)
- Sinus bradycardia (see Table 13.12 for causes)
- Second-degree sino-atrial exit block
- Junctional escape secondary to profound sinus bradycardia or complete sino-atrial exit block or sinus arrest
- Atrial fibrillation with slow ventricular rate (distinguished from atrial fibrillation with complete AV block by irregular RR interval)
- Atrial flutter/atrial tachycardia with high-grade AV block
- Complete AV block with a junctional or ventricular escape rhythm

Atrioventricular block (see Table 13.13 for causes)
- First-degree AV block (constant PR interval >200 ms)
- Second-degree AV block, Mobitz type 1 (Wenckebach)
- 2 : 1 second-degree AV block
- Second-degree AV block, Mobitz type 2
- High-grade AV block (e.g. 4 : 1 or 5 : 1 AV block)
- Third-degree/complete AV block with junctional or ventricular escape rhythm

Table 13.12 Causes of sinus bradycardia.

Cardiovascular
- Chronic sinus node dysfunction (due to idiopathic degenerative/fibrotic change in sinus node).
- Acute sinus node dysfunction due to ischaemia (typically in inferior MI; sinus node artery arises from RCA in ~90%).
- Manoeuvres triggering high vagal tone, for example suctioning of airway.
- Vasovagal syncope
- Carotid sinus hypersensitivity

Systemic
- Drugs (beta-blockers, digoxin, diltiazem, verapamil and other antiarrhythmic drugs).
- Hypothermia
- Hypothyroidism
- Hypokalaemia and hyperkalaemia
- Raised intracranial pressure

Table 13.13 Causes of atrioventricular (AV) block.

Acute
- High vagal tone (may cause transient first-, second- and third-degree AV block)
- Myocardial ischaemia/infarction
- Drugs (beta-blockers, digoxin, diltiazem, verapamil and other antiarrhythmic drugs)
- Hyperkalaemia
- Infections: Lyme disease and others
- Myocarditis
- Infective endocarditis with aortic root abscess
- Transcatheter aortic valve implantation and surgical aortic valve replacement

Chronic
- Idiopathic conducting system fibrosis
- Congenital complete AV block
- Cardiomyopathies (e.g. in myotonic dystrophy)
- Cardiac sarcoidosis

Table 13.14 Temporary cardiac pacing: indications, contraindications and potential complications (for technique, see Chapter 107).*

Indications
- Bradycardia/asystole (sinus or junctional bradycardia or second/third-degree AV block) associated with haemodynamic compromise and unresponsive to atropine.
- After cardiac arrest due to bradycardia/asystole.
- To prevent perioperative bradycardia. Temporary pacing is indicated in:
- Second-degree Mobitz type 2 AV block or complete heart block *or*
- Sinus/junctional bradycardia or second-degree Mobitz type I (Wenckebach) AV block or bundle branch block (including bifascicular and trifascicular block) only if history of syncope or presyncope.
- Atrial or ventricular overdrive pacing to prevent recurrent monomorphic ventricular tachycardia or polymorphic ventricular tachycardia with preceding QT prolongation (torsade de pointes).

Contraindications
- Risks of temporary pacing outweigh benefits, for example rare symptomatic sinus pauses, or complete heart block with a stable escape rhythm and no haemodynamic compromise. Discuss management with a cardiologist. Consider using standby external pacing system instead of transvenous pacing.
- Prosthetic tricuspid valve.

(continued)

Table 13.14 (*Continued*)

Complications

- Complications of central vein cannulation, especially bleeding in patients with acute coronary syndromes treated with thrombolytic therapy (reduced with ultrasound-guided approach).
- Cardiac perforation by pacing lead (may rarely result in cardiac tamponade).
- Arrhythmias (including ventricular fibrillation) during placement of pacing lead.
- Infection of pacing lead.

* Always discuss first with a cardiologist. Where possible, temporary pacing should be avoided, because of the high risk of complications. When bradycardia is likely to be reversible or contraindications to early permanent pacing are present (e.g. sepsis), temporary cardiac pacing may be indicated.

Further reading

Acute arrhythmias: general principles of management

European Resuscitation Council (2021) ERC guidelines. https://cprguidelines.eu/.

Resuscitation Council (UK) (2021) Resuscitation guidelines. Resuscitation Council (UK). https://www.resus. org.uk/library/2021-resuscitation-guidelines

Broad complex tachycardia

Kashou A, Noseworthy P, DeSimone CV, *et al.* (2020) Wide complex tachycardia differentiation: a reappraisal of the state-of-the-art. *J Am Heart Assoc* 9, e016598.

Katritsis DG, Brugada J. (2020) Differential diagnosis of wide QRS tachycardias. *Arrhythmia Electrophysiol Rev* 9(3), 155–160. https://doi.org/10.15420/aer.2020.2.

Narrow complex tachycardia

Brugada J, Katritsis DG, Arbelo E, *et al.* (2020) 2019 ESC guidelines for the management of patients with supraventricular tachycardia. *Eur Heart J* 41(5), 655–720. https://doi.org/10.1093/eurheartj/ehz467.

Kotadia ID, Williams SE, O'Neill M. (2020) Supraventricular tachycardia: an overview of diagnosis and management. *Clin Med (Lond)* 20(1), 43–47. https://doi.org/10.7861/clinmed.cme.20.1.3. PMID: 31941731; PMCID: PMC6964177.

Peng G, Zei PC. (2024) Diagnosis and management of paroxysmal supraventricular tachycardia. *JAMA* 331(7), 601–610. https://doi.org/10.1001/jama.2024.0076.

Atrial fibrillation and flutter

2023 ACC/AHA/ACCP/HRS guideline for the diagnosis and management of atrial fibrillation: a report of the American College of Cardiology/American Heart Association Joint Committee on clinical practice guidelines. *Circulation* 149(1), e167.

Van Gelder IC, Rienstra M, Bunting KV, et al. 2024 ESC Guidelines for the management of atrial fibrillation developed in collaboration with the European Association for Cardio-Thoracic Surgery (EACTS). *Eur Heart J* 45, 3314–3414. https://doi.org/10.1093/eurheartj/ehae176.

Bradyarrhythmia and atrioventricular blocks

Glickson M, Nielsen JC, Kronborg MB, et al. ESC Guidelines on cardiac pacing and cardiac resynchronization therapy. *Eur Heart J* 42, 3427–3520. https://doi.org/10.1093/eurheartj/ehab364.

Sidhu S, Marine J. (2020) Evaluating and managing bradycardia. *Trends Cardiovasc Med* 30(5), 265–272.

CHAPTER 14

Heart failure

James Gamble and Sarah Fellows

Heart failure is defined as a clinical syndrome consisting of clinical signs and symptoms (Table 14.1) related to a structural or functional abnormality of the heart, resulting in inadequate cardiac output for current physiological requirements and/or elevated intracardiac pressures (congestion). Acute presentations are seen as both a 'de novo' first presentation of the underlying disease, or as decompensations of known pre-existing chronic heart failure.

Heart failure is highly treatable both in the acute and chronic phases. Despite this, hospital readmission rates and mortality remain high. In the acute context, the priorities are:

- To initially stabilise the patient and relieve severe pulmonary oedema.
- Undertake initial diagnostic tests to confirm the diagnosis and any provoking factor.
- To establish medications with a prognostic benefit before hospital discharge.

Probably the most common error seen in clinical practice is to discharge the patient without initiating prognostic medications and without adequate decongestion. This is strongly associated with readmission and poor outcomes for the patient.

Although the New York Heart Association (NYHA) classification of heart failure symptoms is widely used (Table 14.2), it has many practical limitations. The differences between class II and class III are very subtle. Many patients limit their activity such that they report no or minimal symptoms although would be very limited on significant exertion. Patients may also report no or minimal symptoms in the early stages of or in well-optimally treated heart failure.

Causes of heart failure

This is not an exhaustive list of the aetiology of heart failure but include some causes more likely to be seen in the acute setting or at hospital admission (Tables 14.3 and 14.4).

Table 14.1 Signs and symptoms of acute or decompensated heart failure.

Symptoms	Clinical signs
Fatigue	Peripheral oedema
Breathlessness	Elevated jugular venous pressure (JVP)
Orthopnoea/Paroxysmal Nocturnal Dyspnoea	Third heart sound
Peripheral oedema, e.g. ankle swelling, abdominal swelling	Coarse pulmonary crackles
Breathlessness on bending over ('bendopnoea')	Ascites
Poor appetite, weight loss	Cachexia

Acute Medicine: A Practical Guide to the Management of Medical Emergencies, Sixth Edition.
Edited by Mridula Rajwani, Leila Vaziri, and Ivie Gbinigie.
© 2026 John Wiley & Sons Ltd. Published 2026 by John Wiley & Sons Ltd.

Table 14.2 Classification of symptoms.

New York Heart Association (NYHA) functional classification
Class I Can manage ordinary physical activity without undue fatigue or breathlessness.
Class II Slight limitation of ordinary activity by fatigue or breathlessness.
Class III Marked limitation of ordinary activity by fatigue or breathlessness.
Class IV Cannot manage any activity without fatigue or breathlessness, and may have symptoms at rest.

Table 14.3 Causes of heart failure.

Myocardial ischaemia	Acute coronary syndromes Coronary artery dissection Coronary embolism
Dilated cardiomyopathy	'Idiopathic' Genetic predisposition Stress induced 'Takotsubo' Peripartum Toxins (alcohol, cocaine, iron)
Valvular disease	Aortic stenosis, aortic regurgitation Mitral regurgitation (including post ACS)
Mechanical or extrinsic cause	Ventricular septal defect, cardiac tamponade, pulmonary embolism or acute respiratory dysfunction, acute cerebrovascular insult or head injury
Hypertensive emergency	Renal artery stenosis, phaeochromocytoma, medication withdrawal/non-compliance
Arrhythmia	Persistent atrial or ventricular tachycardia
Drug induced	Anthracyclines, VEG-F inhibitors, Immune checkpoint inhibitors
Infective	Acute myocarditis, HIV, Lyme disease
Infiltrative	Cardiac amyloidosis
Metabolic	Thyroid disease, autoimmune disease

Table 14.4 Non-cardiac causes of acute pulmonary oedema.

Renal disease
- Acute kidney injury or advanced chronic kidney disease
- Renal artery stenosis

Iatrogenic fluid overload
Subarachnoid haemorrhage
Negative-pressure pulmonary oedema (e.g. post general anaesthetic)

Causes due to increased pulmonary capillary permeability
Acute lung injury/ARDS

Direct lung injury	**Indirect lung injury**
Pneumonia (viral or bacterial)	Sepsis
Aspiration of gastric contents	Cardiopulmonary by-pass
Pulmonary contusion	Drug overdose
Fat emboli	Acute pancreatitis
Drowning	Transfusions of blood products
Inhalational injury	
Reperfusion pulmonary oedema after lung transplantation or pulmonary embolectomy	

Focused assessment of the patient with acute heart failure

Acute heart failure

Acute heart failure occurs when there is a rapid deterioration in previously stable cardiac dysfunction or a new presentation of heart failure severe enough to require emergency medical assessment. Whilst patients can present acutely in pulmonary oedema or cardiogenic shock, more often they present sub-acutely, with fluid retention causing progressive breathlessness and oedema (Table 14.1). It is also important to consider other extrinsic factors that may be precipitating acute heart failure in stable valvular or left ventricular disease.

The typical presentations can be roughly divided into four categories:
- Acute decompensated heart failure: LV Dysfunction with or without RV failure. Usually gradual onset, often has another precipitating cause (Table 14.3).
- Acute pulmonary oedema: Elevated pressure in pulmonary capillaries leading to pulmonary congestion, often related to acute LV failure but can have a number of non-cardiac causes (Table 14.4).
- Isolated right ventricular (RV) failure: Increased RV and atrial pressures which can then impact LV filling and reduce systemic cardiac output. Caused by ACS with RV involvement, RV cardiomyopathy and pulmonary hypertension.
- Cardiogenic shock: acute cardiac dysfunction resulting in rapid loss of cardiac output and tissue hypoperfusion (cool peripheries, confusion and oliguria) but not always with hypotension if compensatory vasoconstriction has occurred. A high lactate, metabolic acidosis and rising creatinine are all demonstrating tissue hypoxia. This has a very high mortality and needs urgent assessment and treatment.

Management strategies

The approach to managing an acutely unwell patient with potential heart failure should follow the ABCDE approach (Tables 14.5 and 14.6). Table 14.7 below gives slight differences that might be applied in addition.

Table 14.5 Focused assessment of the patient with acute heart failure.

History
Total duration of symptoms and acute deterioration
Degree of exertional breathlessness (see NYHA functional classification)
Orthopnoea or paroxysmal nocturnal dyspnoea
Is heart failure or a cardiomyopathy known? What investigations have been done? Who normally manages care?
Is there a history of hypertension or coronary artery disease?
Drug history including any recent change and evidence for compliance?
Any aetiological factors: Alcohol, smoking, chemotherapy, family history of heart disease

Examination
General appearance
Body mass index (cachexia/obesity)
Heart rate and blood pressure
Jugular venous pressure, peripheral oedema, ascites
Respiratory rate, arterial oxygen saturation, inspiratory crackles, signs of pleural effusion
Murmurs, third heart sound, apex displacement
Poor peripheral perfusion, cold extremities, confusion, low urine output

Table 14.6 Urgent investigations.

ECG
- ST Elevation/features of acute ischaemia or myocarditis
- Abnormal rate and/or rhythm
- Evidence of LV hypertrophy (Aortic valve disease? Hypertrophic cardiomyopathy?)
- Low QRS voltage (Pericardial effusion? Cardiac amyloidosis?)

Chest X-ray
- Pulmonary oedema
- Cardiomegaly
- Pleural effusion (may contribute to breathlessness)
- Pulmonary consolidation

Arterial blood gases, pH and lactate
- High lactate and metabolic acidosis are markers of tissue hypoperfusion
- Hypoxia or respiratory failure as a marker of severity of pulmonary oedema

Blood tests
N-terminal pro-BNP (NT-pro-BNP)
- In the acute phase useful only as a rule-out; high negative predictive value but poor positive predictive value
- In acute setting, a normal value makes acute HF very unlikely (reasonable thresholds are BNP < 100 pg/mL, NT-proBNP < 300 pg/mL and MR-proANP < 120 pg/mL)
- NT-pro-BNP will be lower in obesity and younger patients
- BNP/NT-pro-BNP will also be raised in most acute illnesses including infection, pulmonary embolism, myocardial infarction, liver cirrhosis, kidney disease, COPD, advanced age

Other acute blood tests
Full blood count (exclude severe anaemia)
Sodium, potassium, urea and creatinine (including eGFR)
Albumin, liver function and INR (liver congestion)
Thyroid function
Troponin level (if history is suggestive of acute coronary syndrome)

Echocardiogram
- LV size/geometry, regional and global systolic function
- Ejection fraction and LV filling pressures
- RV size and systolic function
- Estimated pulmonary artery pressures/likelihood of pulmonary hypertension
- Valve disease
- Pericardial effusion

Table 14.7 The management of an acutely unwell patient with potential heart failure.

Acute decompensated HF (congestion/fluid overload)	Loop diuretics
	Initiate prognostic medications with diuretic effect (SGLT2i, aldosterone antagonist)
	Inotropic support when organ hypoperfusion is suspected
	Rarely, renal replacement therapy
Acute pulmonary oedema	Oxygen via nasal high flow or continuous positive pressure
	Loop diuretics
	Initiate prognostic medications with diuretic effect (SGLT2i, aldosterone antagonist)
	Vasodilators (if High BP) to reduce afterload
Isolated RV failure	Careful optimisation of fluid status
	Loop diuresis if congested
	Consider vasopressors

Inotropes and inodilators

- The choice of inotropic agents is complex and highly specialist. Please seek further advice and specialist input about this.
- Dopamine, dobutamine and milrinone are examples of inotropes used in acute heart failure.
- Used when the patient has low cardiac output and hypotension (SBP<90mmHG) and/or features of tissue hypoperfusion.
- Risk of sinus tachycardia, induced/worsened myocardial ischaemia, and arrhythmia; therefore, uptitrate from low doses with close monitoring.
- In a patient on beta-blockers, avoid dobutamine as they act on the same receptor with antagonistic actions.

Vasopressors: adrenaline/noradrenaline

- Used in severe hypotension to improve end-organ perfusion but often need to be used with an inotrope to combat the effect of increased afterload from the peripheral vasoconstriction.
- Only appropriate for use in an intensive care environment

Loop diuretics

- Furosemide IV at either twice the daily oral dose the patient was taking prior to admission or, if not taking previously, a starting dose of 40–80mg (see Table 14.8, for example, regimens).
- Bumetanide and torasemide can also be used. 1mg of bumetanide is equivalent to 40mg of furosemide. Bumetanide may be better absorbed from an oedematous gut. Torasemide is less widely available in some countries.
- Furosemide is usually given as bolus doses twice daily or as a continuous infusion (infusions need a loading dose first).

Table 14.8 Example regimens.

At initial presentation of heart failure, unknown ejection fraction, blood pressure not low 130/60, pulmonary and peripheral oedema, no comorbidity	Day 1: Furosemide 80mg IV, eplerenone 25mg once daily orally, dapagliflozin 10mg once daily orally Day 2: Clarify ejection fraction as soon as possible and consider specific treatment.
New presentation of heart failure with reduced ejection fraction, pulmonary and peripheral oedema, blood pressure 140/60, type 2 diabetes on metformin alone	Day 1: Furosemide 80mg IV, eplerenone 25mg once daily orally. Day 2: Start empagliflocin 10mg once daily if eating and drinking. Start candesartan 4mg once a day at night. Day 3: Stepdown to oral furosemide as oedema resolved. Start Bisoprolol 1.25mg once daily, switch candesartan to sacubitril/valsartan 24/26mg twice daily.
New presentation of heart failure with preserved ejection fraction and atrial fibrillation, pulmonary oedema. No diabetes.	Day 1: Furosemide 80mg IV, eplerenone 25mg once daily orally, dapagliflozin 10mg once daily orally, oral anti-coagulation with apixaban, initial rate control with digoxin. Day 2: Introduce bisoprolol for additional rate control as remains tachycardic.
New presentation of heart failure with reduced ejection fraction, hypertensive with blood pressure 90/50, pulmonary oedema, no diabetes	Day 1: Furosemide 80mg IV, eplerenone 25mg once daily. Specialist assessment for borderline shock. Day 2: Empagliflocin 10mg once daily, ramipril 1.25mg once a day at night.

- Response to diuresis should be measured in symptoms, weight change and urine output (>100 ml/h), and can also be assessed with urinary sodium levels 2 h after diuretics given.
- Re-assessment should be rapid and regular, ideally within 4–6 h, but as a minimum 24 hourly.
- Prognostic heart failure medications with a diuretic effect (aldosterone antagonist, SGLT2 inhibitor) should be initiated alongside loop diuretic in all patients with heart failure unless contraindicated.
- Inadequate response should trigger an increase in dosing, addition of adjunctive medications, or a switch to continuous infusion.
- Adjunctive treatments can be given alongside loop diuretics, e.g. thiazide diuretics or metolozone. Specialist input is recommended.

Specialist input

- Input from a heart failure specialist team is strongly associated with improved outcomes and should be sought as soon as possible for all patients admitted with heart failure.

When to seek advanced heart failure support/consider mechanical support:

- Early identification of cardiogenic shock is key. Untreated, this has an extremely high mortality.
- Early involvement of your local specialist heart failure team is vital to help assess those who would benefit from early referral for advanced heart failure assessment.
- Advanced heart failure centres assess patients for suitability for transplant and/or mechanical assist devices.
- These discussions and decisions can help guide the direction of care for a patient.
- The I NEED HELP pneumonic was developed to recognise signs that should prompt these discussions (Table 14.9).

Once stable and improving

- If not already done, seek advice from/refer to the local specialist heart failure team.
- Obtain an echocardiogram as soon as possible and clinically appropriate. Breathlessness should be controlled to the level that the patient can sit comfortably. If in atrial fibrillation, heart rate should ideally be controlled below 90 bpm before performing an echocardiogram.

Table 14.9 I NEED HELP.

I	Need for **Inotropes**
N	**New** York Heart Assoc stage IV
E	Worsening **end-organ** dysfunction
E	**Ejection fraction** <20%
D	**Defibrillator** shocks for ventricular arrhythmia
H	Recurrent **HF** admissions
E	**Escalating** diuretic dose
L	**Low** Blood Pressure
P	**Progressive** intolerance of heart failure medication

- 4–6 hourly obs (blood pressure [BP], heart rate [HR], oxygen saturations, respiratory rate [RR]).
- Monitor with a daily weight chart and check electrolyte and creatinine levels daily.
- Continue IV diuresis initially with aim for oral switch when fully diuresed. Premature cessation of diuretics and leaving the patient congested are strongly associated with poor outcomes.
- Optimise prognostic medical therapy for heart failure (Tables 14.10 and 14.11), aiming to start all indicated heart failure medications 48h prior to discharge with rapid uptitration both in hospital and in the weeks following discharge from hospital (aim for maximally tolerated doses within 6 weeks).

Table 14.10 Medications by subtype of heart failure.

	Empirical treatment	HF with reduced EF (HFrEF)	HF with mildly reduced EF (HFmrEF)	HF with preserved EF (HFpEF)
Left-ventricular ejection fraction	As yet unknown	Under 40%	40–49%	Over 50%
MRA	✓	✓	✓	✓
SGLT2i	✓	✓	✓	✓
ACEi/ARNI		✓	✓	
B Blocker		✓	✓	

Table 14.11 Prognostic medications in heart failure.

Mineralocorticoid receptor antagonist (MRA)	Eplerenone, spironolactone, finerenone	Mortality benefit in HFrEF, HFmrEF Symptom benefit in all HF Acute diuretic effort Increase potassium Minimal effect on blood pressure Renal protective effect	Caution with eGFR less than 30 ml/min/m², normally need to avoid if less than 20 Caution if potassium is greater than 5, avoid if potassium is greater than 5.5–6 mmol/L Spironolactone can cause gynaecomastia in males or breast enlargement in females
Sodium-glucose co-transporter 2 inhibitors	Dapagliflozin Empagliflozin	Mortality and symptom benefit in all HF Acute diuretic effort Slightly lowers potassium Minimal effect on blood pressure Renal protective effect	No evidence for benefit if eGFR less than 15 ml/min/m² Increased rate of genital fungal infection (thrush) Not licenced in type 1 diabetes Increased risk of ketoacidosis See safety notes below
ACE inhibitors, angiotensin receptor antagonists	Ramipril, lisinopril Candesartan, losartan	Mortality and symptom benefit in HFrEF, HFmrEF. No benefit in HFpEF Increases potassium Renal protective effect	Caution with eGFR less than 30 ml/min/m², normally need to avoid if less than 20 Caution if potassium greater than 5, avoid if potassium greater than 5.5–6 mmol/L Avoid in bilateral renal artery stenosis
Angiotensin receptor nephrolysin inhibitors	Sacubitril/ valsartan combination	Greater mortality benefit than ACEi in HFrEF, symptom benefit in HFmrEF, no benefit in HFpEF Increases potassium Renal protective effect	Cautions as per ACEi/ARB above Must have 48-h with no ACE inhibitor before starting (combination increases the risk of angioedema)
Beta-blockers	Bisoprolol, carvedilol, metoprolol XL, nebivolol	Mortality and symptom benefit in HFrEF, HFmrEF. Potentially harmful in HFpEF	Dangerous in acute heart failure, as a negative inotrope. Do not start until patient stabilised, i.e. no pulmonary oedema, oral diuretics, other agents started Caution if heart rate less than 60, significant conduction disease, severe asthma

Table 14.12 Subtypes of heart failure.

HF with preserved EF (HFpEF)	HF with mildly reduced EF (HFmrEF)	HF with reduced EF (HFrEF)
EF over 50%	EF 40–49%	EF under 40%

Although these divisions are widely used, clinicians should be aware that echocardiography is intrinsically inaccurate, and overreliance on an exact ejection fraction (EF) is unwise. Practically, heart failure is best divided into patients with reduced ejection fraction i.e. less than 50%, and those without this (Table 14.12). Heart failure (HF) due to left ventricular (LV) dysfunction is categorized by the LVEF.

In addition, be aware that in patients with severe valvular regurgitation, ejection fraction should be supranormal and normal range or reduced ejection fraction represents abnormal ventricular function.

Prognostic medications for treatment of heart failure

Safety of SGLT2 inhibitors

- The class is generally very safe, and can be used in acute heart failure.
- However, they are rarely associated with euglycaemic ketoacidosis in people with diabetes (higher risk in those with type 1 diabetes or mimics, patients on insulin or gliclazide, when acutely unwell).
- If a patient on an SGLT2 inhibitor becomes acutely unwell, ketones must be checked as well as glucose levels.
- Advise the patient of sick day rules: need to stop this medication when feeling unwell and unable to maintain adequate oral intake of fluid and food. It can be restarted once eating and drinking normally.

Other agents

- If ACE-inhibitor/ARB contra-indicated and in severe renal dysfunction, the combination of hydralazine (initially 25 mg 12-hourly PO) and isosorbide mononitrate (initially 10 mg 12-hourly PO) can be used. Weak evidence for mortality and symptom benefit in HFrEF.
- If the heart rate remains over 80 bpm on maximum tolerated dose of beta-blocker, Ivabradine (initially 2.5 mg BD, titrate to 7.5 mg BD) has evidence of symptom benefit and small mortality benefit in HFrEF. No effect in atrial fibrillation.
- Digoxin at low dose (62.5 mcg) probably provides a small additional mortality benefit in HFrEF. Digoxin is a useful agent for heart rate control in atrial fibrillation with heart failure as it is effective at rate control and is a weak positive inotrope.

Other considerations whilst in hospital
Heart rate and rhythm control in atrial fibrillation

- If haemodynamically unstable, consider cardioversion acutely.
- If hypotensive, in severe heart failure or with an unknown cause of heart failure, beta-blocker may be best avoided and digoxin is probably a safer option for heart rate control.
- If no signs of shock and well compensated, beta-blockers have a better heart rate control effect in the longer term.
- Increasing evidence suggests benefit from rhythm control of atrial fibrillation for patients with HFrEF, which should be reviewed by a specialist.

- In HFpEF, cardiac output may be dependent upon heart rate and a lax approach should be taken to rate control, aiming for resting heart rate 80–90 bpm.
- Anticoagulation should be initiated for all patients with atrial fibrillation and heart failure, unless contraindicated.

Heart failure and renal dysfunction

Two broad phenotypes need to be differentiated in the context of an acute deterioration in renal function and acute heart failure (type 1 cardiorenal syndrome)

1 In a low cardiac output state, renal dysfunction occurs due to renal hypoperfusion. The patient is likely to display signs of shock. This is seen less frequently, and is likely to be clinically evident from assessment. Treatment is likely to be with inotropic support.
2 In a congested state with high venous pressures, renal dysfunction occurs due to high renal venous pressures and renal capsular compression. The patient is likely to have raised JVP, ascites (although this may not always be clinically evident) and severe peripheral oedema. Treatment is to give higher dose diuretics to achieve fluid offloading and decongestion, which will result in improving renal function.

Chronic renal dysfunction will also occur commonly with advancing heart failure. This tends to develop over the years, and represents worsening cardiac dysfunction (type 2 cardiorenal syndrome; although concurrent renal damage due to comorbidities such as diabetes is also seen).

Thromboprophylaxis against systemic and venous thromboembolism

- Treatment-dose, low-molecular-weight heparin should be given whilst inpatient.

Ambulatory care for heart failure

This is often offered in current clinical practice. There are some specific considerations:

- Patient selection should be careful. Younger patients (who are more likely to have a rare cause of heart failure, and who would be potential candidate for advanced heart failure therapies) may be at higher risk to ambulate.
- Ambulatory care does not reduce the benefit of specialist input, and every attempt should still be made to include the specialist heart failure team.
- Generally, ambulatory patients are excellent candidates to start an SGLT2 inhibitor and aldosterone antagonist early as if they are well enough to be managed on an ambulatory basis, they are likely to be eating relatively normally and have a good blood pressure.
- Therapies may need to be modified for once daily administration of intravenous agents. This can be by bolus dosing of furosemide, for example 200 mg once daily rather than 100 mg twice daily, or by adding high-dose oral furosemide alongside once daily intravenous furosemide (e.g. furosemide 120 mg intravenously in the morning and bumetanide 1 mg orally in the afternoon).

Drugs to avoid

Avoid the following drugs which may cause harm:

- Calcium channel blockers (except dihydropyridine types e.g. amlodipine, felodipine), have a negative inotropic effect.
- Glitazones can exacerbate existing HF and increase the risk of new-onset HF
- NSAIDs and COX-2 inhibitors cause sodium and water retention.
- Angiotensin-receptor blocker, if already taking an ACE-inhibitor or ARNI and a mineralocorticoid antagonist, because of the risk of hyperkalaemia.

Special cases

New heart failure in pregnancy/peripartum cardiomyopathy
- The increased demands on the left ventricle during pregnancy, particularly into the third trimester, can unmask undiagnosed cardiac disease such as valvular heart disease or a susceptibility to cardiomyopathy.
- Peripartum cardiomyopathy (EF < 45%) occurs typically towards the end of the pregnancy or in the weeks following delivery.
- Usually, this presents with heart failure symptoms but, less often, can present as ventricular arrythmia and/or cardiac arrest.
- Seek urgent specialist/sub-specialist advise.

Acute myocarditis caused by Immune checkpoint inhibitors (ICI)
- Most commonly occurs in the first four cycles of ICI therapy.
- Poorly understood aetiology but known to cause acute myocarditis which requires immediate cessation of the ICI treatment and prompt treatment with high-dose IV steroids.
- Specialist input should be sought in all suspected cases from your local heart failure team.

Negative-pressure pulmonary oedema
- Seen in the early postoperative period.
- Due to forced inspiration in the presence of upper airway obstruction (e.g. from laryngospasm after extubation).
- After relief of laryngospasm, patients develop clinical and radiological features of pulmonary oedema.
- Typically resolves over the course of a few hours with supportive care.
- Cardiogenic pulmonary oedema should be excluded by clinical assessment, ECG and echocardiography.

Palliative care
Judging when palliative care (Chapter 97) is appropriate may be difficult. It should be considered for patients in whom transplantation, circulatory support or other definitive treatment including heart valve surgery has been ruled out and:
- In whom palliation has already been discussed and agreed as part of a chronic care plan.
- With severe recurrent and progressive heart failure despite maximally tolerated therapy.
- With multi-organ failure not responding to therapy.
- With a chronically poor quality of life and severe symptoms.

Opiates are useful in the symptomatic relief of dyspnoea and anxiety whilst also being sedating. Opiate choice will need to be selected depending on renal function. Advice should be sought from your local palliative care team.

Further reading

Harjola V-P, Mebazaa A, Celutkiene J, et al. (2016) Contemporary management of acute right ventricular failure: a statement from the Heart Failure Association and the Working Group on pulmonary circulation and right ventricular function of the European Society of Cardiology. *Eur J Heart Fail* 18, 226–241.

McDonagh TA, Metra M, Adamo M, et al. (2023) 2023 focused update of the 2021 ESC guidelines for the diagnosis and treatment of acute and chronic heart failure: developed by the task force for the diagnosis and treatment of acute and chronic heart failure of the European Society of Cardiology (ESC) With the special contribution of the Heart Failure Association (HFA) of the ESC. *Eur Heart J* 44(37), 3627–3639. doi: 10.1093/eurheartj/ehad195.

McDonagh TA, Metra M, Adamo M, *et al.* (2021) ESC guidelines for the diagnosis and treatment of acute and chronic heart failure. *Eur Heart J.* 2021 42(36), 3599–3726. doi: 10.1093/eurheartj/ehab368. Erratum in: Eur Heart J. 2021 Dec 21;42(48):4901. doi: 10.1093/eurheartj/ehab670.

National Institute for Health and Care Excellence 2021). Acute heart failure: diagnosis and management [NICE guideline No. 187] https://www.nice.org.uk/guidance/cg187

Page RL, O'Bryant CL, Cheng D, *et al.* (2016) Drugs that may cause or exacerbate heart failure. A scientific statement from the American Heart Association. *Circulation* 134, e32–e69. doi: 10.1161/CIR.0000000000000426.

CHAPTER 15

Infective endocarditis

JOHN CHAMBERS AND JOHN L. KLEIN

Infective endocarditis (IE) is uncommon but not rare and is still under-recognised. The incidence of IE in the general population is 14 per 100,000 per year but much higher in some clinical groups (Table 15.1). IV drug use greatly increases the risk of left as well as right-sided endocarditis.

IE has an average hospital mortality of 20%. Mortality is reduced by early detection, prompt initiation of appropriate antibiotics and timely surgery when indicated. About 40% of patients require surgery as an inpatient and a further 10% in the first two years after discharge.

Infection of the intra-cardiac leads of implanted cardiac devices causes a similar presentation to infection of heart valves. Removal of an infected device is almost always required to achieve a cure of infection.

Table 15.1 Conditions predisposing to infective endocarditis.

Condition	Relative risk*
High risk	
Previous episode of infective endocarditis	265.5
Ventricular assist device	124.2
Congenital disease corrected with a valved shunt	86.1
Replacement heart valve (or repair)	70.1 (76.7)
Cyanotic congenital heart disease	55.4
Moderate risk	
Bicuspid aortic valve	66.4
Acquired valve disease	41.4
Hypertrophic cardiomyopathy	32.8
Implanted electrical devices	9.7
Mitral valve prolapse with ≥ moderate regurgitation	5.4
Predisposing conditions	
Immunosuppression	
Indwelling lines, e.g. haemodialysis	
Intravenous drug use	

* Compared to the general population in England.

Priorities

1 Think of the diagnosis

Consider if there is fever or raised inflammatory markers and any of:

- High or moderate risk cardiac structural disease (Table 15.1)
- Stroke in a young patient
- Arterial embolism
- IV drug use ('pneumonia' can be caused by septic pulmonary emboli from tricuspid valve endocarditis)
- Tunnelled central venous catheter including Hickman line or haemodialysis catheter
- Multisystem illness
- Chronic malaise, sweating and weight loss, often for several weeks
- Acute aortic or mitral regurgitation (may present with acute pulmonary oedema)

2 Send blood cultures

- Before starting antibiotic therapy since prior antibiotic therapy is the most common cause of blood culture-negative endocarditis.
  - If the patient is stable, send three cultures taken at least 30 minutes apart.
  - If the patient is unstable because of sepsis or severe valve regurgitation take two cultures 30 minutes apart and then start antibiotics.
- IE is often first suspected when a typical organism is grown from the first blood culture (Table 15.2).

3 The clinical assessment is given in Table 15.3 and urgent investigation is in Tables 15.4 and 15.5. The diagnosis is aided by the modified Duke criteria (Table 15.6).

4 Emergency surgery may be indicated for heart failure caused by acute mitral or aortic regurgitation, and within 48 h if there are severe valve lesions associated with a stroke or with large residual vegetations. Seek an immediate cardiac opinion.

Table 15.2 Organisms and infective endocarditis.

Bloodstream isolates and their association with infective endocarditis

- Viridans group streptococci are the most common cause in non-IVDU without intracardiac prosthetic material (*Streptococcus mutans* bacteraemia is particularly associated with IE).
- *Streptococcus gallolyticus* (up to 40% are associated with colorectal tumours including carcinoma); around 40–50% risk of endocarditis in community-acquired infection.
- *Staphylococcus aureus* (the chance of having infective endocarditis is 20–30% with community-acquired infection and 5–10% in hospital-acquired infection).
- *Enterococcus faecalis* – risk of endocarditis is 20% in community-acquired infection; common in older age groups.
- The HACEK group (*Haemophilus* species, *Aggregatibacter* species, *Cardiobacterium hominis*, *Eikenella corrodens* and *Kingella* species) bacteraemia strongly associated with endocarditis.
- Coagulase-negative staphylococci are the most common cause of contaminated blood cultures but are common causes of endocarditis in patients with prosthetic valves or pacemakers.

Organisms that rarely cause infective endocarditis

The list is potentially almost endless, but common organisms isolated from blood triggering inappropriate requests for echocardiography are:

- *Pseudomonas aeruginosa* (usually associated with IV-line infections or pneumonia).
- *E. coli* and other coliforms (usually associated with urinary, biliary or intra-abdominal infections).
- *Streptococcus anginosus* group (commonly associated with hepatic and other intra-abdominal abscesses).

Table 15.3 Focused assessment in suspected infective endocarditis.

History
- Major symptoms and time course
- Symptoms of systemic embolism (transient ischaemic attack, stroke, abdominal pain, limb ischaemia) or pulmonary embolism (with right-sided valve endocarditis, typically seen with IV drug use)
- Previous endocarditis or other known high-risk cardiac lesion (Table 15.1)
- Antibiotic history *(prior antibiotic therapy may render blood cultures negative)*
- Dental history (regular dental surveillance? Dental extraction two to six weeks prior to symptom onset)
- IV drug use

Examination
- Physiological observations and systematic examination
- Careful examination of the skin, nails, conjunctival and oral mucosae and fundi, looking for stigmata of infective endocarditis (petechiae and splinter haemorrhages). Janeway lesions, Osler nodes, and Roth spots are rare
- Auscultation of the heart – in the right context, murmurs consistent with mitral or aortic regurgitation are strong pointers to a diagnosis of IE
- Search for alternative source of sepsis, e.g. inflamed venous cannula site, cellulitis and groin infection in IV drug-use
- Splenomegaly

Table 15.4 Urgent investigation in suspected infective endocarditis.

- Blood culture – *3 sets drawn at least 30 min apart unless critically ill in which case take two sets 30 min apart*
- Full blood count
- C-reactive protein
- Blood glucose
- Urea and electrolytes, liver function tests
- Urine dipstick, microscopy and culture
- ECG (lengthening of the PR interval is a sign of possible aortic root abscess)
- Chest radiograph
- Consider echocardiography (see Table 15.5)

Table 15.5 Indications for transthoracic echocardiography in suspected infective endocarditis.

Urgent
- Hypotension or pulmonary oedema
- Clinically severe aortic or mitral regurgitation (rapid deterioration may occur)
- Suspicion of an abscess (ill patient, long PR interval or *S. aureus* bacteraemia)

As soon as possible
- Positive blood culture with organism typically associated with endocarditis, e.g. viridans group streptococci, *Streptococcus gallolyticus*, *S. aureus*, *Enterococcus faecalis* or the HACEK group
- IV drug use
- Prosthetic heart valve (often needs TOE)
- Central venous catheter-related bloodstream infection persisting for >72 h after antimicrobial therapy
- New regurgitant murmur (endocarditis rarely causes new obstruction)

Not indicated
- Low clinical suspicion of endocarditis (e.g. fever with short ejection systolic flow murmur) (see Table 15.6)

Table 15.6 2023 Modified ESC criteria for the diagnosis of infective endocarditis.

Type of criterion	Description of criterion
Major	1 Blood culture positive • Typical microorganisms from two sets of blood cultures: viridans group streptococci, *S. gallolyticus*, HACEK group, *S. aureus* or *E. faecalis*. • Persistently positive with microorganisms consistent with IE (≥2 taken more than 12 h apart, or all of three or a majority of ≥4 drawn over a period of ≥1 h). • Single positive blood culture for *Coxiella burnetii* or phase I IgG antibody titre >1:800. 2 Imaging positive • Vegetations, local complication (abscess, fistula or pseudoaneurysm), new prosthetic valve dehiscence or metabolic lesion using echocardiography, cardiac computerised tomography (CT), [18F]-fluorodeoxyglucose-positron emission tomography/computerised tomography ([18F]-FDG-PET/CT) or white cell single-photon emission computed tomography (SPECT)
Minor	1 Known cardiac predisposition to endocarditis (including intravenous drug use) 2 Temperature >38 °C 3 Vascular phenomena (e.g. systemic or pulmonary embolus/infarct, intracranial haemorrhage/ischaemia, mycotic aneurysm, spondylodiscitis) including 'silent' cerebral or peripheral emboli on magnetic resonance imaging, conjunctival haemorrhages, Janeway lesions 4 Immunological features (e.g. glomerulonephritis, Osler's nodes, Roth spots or positive rheumatoid factor) 5 Positive blood culture but insufficient for major criteria or serological evidence of active infection with an organism consistent with IE

Definite IE: Two major criteria, *or* one major and three minor criteria *or* five minor criteria.
Possible IE: One major and one or two minor criteria, or three or four minor criteria.
IE Rejected: Firm alternative diagnosis; resolution with ≤four days of antibiotics; no evidence of IE at surgery/autopsy after ≤four days of antibiotics).

Further management

1 This must be done by an endocarditis team. At minimum, at a DGH, this is a cardiologist and infection specialist. The team must contact the local Heart Centre, usually within 12 h of the diagnosis if the patient is stable, to discuss whether care can continue at the DGH or transfer is needed (Table 15.7).
2 Discuss antibiotic therapy with an infection specialist (clinical microbiologist or infectious diseases physician). Current recommendations are given in Table 15.8.
3 Remove infected intravenous cannulae.
4 Consider the appropriate route for antimicrobial delivery (e.g. PICC line).

Table 15.7 Empirical antibiotic therapy in suspected infective endocarditis.

1 Patients with early (<one year) prosthetic valve IE or suspected MRSA:
• Vancomycin – 12-hourly (dose based on weight) IV plus
• Gentamicin 3 mg/kg od IV
2 Acute presentation (ill for <one week) in patients with native valves (including IVDUs)
• Flucloxacillin 2 g 4–6 hourly IV
3 Sub-acute presentation in patients with native or late (>one year) prosthetic valve IE
• Amoxicillin 2 g 4-hourly IV plus
• Gentamicin 3 mg/kg od IV

These are regimens for when antibiotic therapy must be started before blood culture results are available. Contact an Infection specialist for advice, particularly in patients with penicillin allergy.

Table 15.8 Indications for transfer to a cardiac surgical centre.

Prosthetic valve or implantable cardiac electronic device infection
Severe **valve** regurgitation even if currently stable haemodynamically
Abscess
Invasive organism, e.g. *S. aureus**
Organisms that are hard to manage medically, e.g. fungi
Failure to respond to antibiotics
Stroke (or other embolism) and large residual vegetation
Recurrent emboli
Renal failure**

* Some cases of *S. aureus* IE may respond to antibiotic therapy, but IE caused by this organism should trigger discussion with a surgical centre.
** Renal failure in IE has many and sometimes multiple origins including glomerulonephritis, renal emboli, aminoglycoside therapy and low cardiac output. It can contribute to the decision for early surgery when associated with severe valve destruction or failure to control sepsis and should therefore trigger a discussion with a surgical centre.

Table 15.9 Monitoring in infective endocarditis.

Clinical assessment daily, more frequently if there is a change
Regular monitoring of full blood count, urea and electrolytes and C reactive protein:
- Record blood results on a flow-chart if electronic systems are not in use, check creatinine and electrolytes initially daily then twice weekly as condition improves, check C-reactive protein and white cell count twice weekly.
- Check vancomycin/gentamicin levels as directed by Microbiology Dept.
- With aortic valve endocarditis, record an ECG daily while fever persists (prolongation of the PR interval is a sign of abscess formation: arrange transoesophageal echocardiography or cardiac CT).
- Only repeat transthoracic echocardiography if there is a change in clinical status or at the time of discharge (to provide a baseline against which to compare the grade of regurgitation and size of the left ventricle in outpatient studies).

5 Monitoring is given in Table 15.9.
6 Cardiac surgery is usually needed:
- As an emergency for critical valve destruction causing haemodynamic collapse.
- Within 48 h for severe valve regurgitation causing heart failure or a combination of a vegetation >10 mm long and other indications for surgery.
- At a time determined by the endocarditis team, usually at one to two weeks for: failure to control sepsis; organism unlikely to respond to antimicrobials; severe valve destruction; emboli despite treatment with the correct antibiotic at the correct dose.
7 Correct anaemia with transfusion if haemoglobin is <80 g/L.
8 If the creatinine rises:
- Consider the possible causes: pre-renal failure; glomerulonephritis related to IE; renal infarct/abscess; vancomycin- or gentamicin-nephrotoxicity; interstitial nephritis related to antibiotic; other causes, e.g. bladder outflow obstruction.
- Check urinalysis and urine microscopy and arrange ultrasound of the urinary tract.
- Reduce antibiotic doses as necessary.
- Discuss management with a cardiac surgeon if renal failure is due to severe valve regurgitation, uncontrolled sepsis or glomerulonephritis.
- Seek advice from a nephrologist if you suspect glomerulonephritis or interstitial nephritis (casts in urine, large kidneys on ultrasound scan).

9 Seek further opinions from a:
  - Maxillofacial surgeon if endocarditis is due to viridans group streptococci or other oral commensal;
  - Gastroenterologist if endocarditis is due to *Streptococcus gallolyticus* (up to 40% are associated with colorectal tumours including carcinoma);
  - Spinal surgeon if there is back pain with MRI evidence of spondylodiscitis.

Problems

Missed infective endocarditis

Some scenarios recur:
- Possible lymphoma in a patient with a prosthetic heart valve;
- Search for source of gastro-intestinal blood or malignancy in a patient with normochromic normocytic anaemia, weight loss and fever/sweats (often subtle and easily missed);
- IV drug use with a chest infection (lung cavitations).

Blood culture-negative endocarditis

Prior antibiotic therapy is the most common cause. Other causes to consider are given in Table 15.10. Ask advice from an infection specialist about:
- Stopping antibiotics and repeating blood cultures if the diagnosis is not secure.
- Sending blood for serology (especially for *Bartonella* and *Coxiella burnetii*).
- Sending blood for antinuclear antibodies and, in patients with a porcine valve, anti-pork antibodies.

IV drug use with cavitating lung lesions but normal tricuspid valve

Consider septic thrombophlebitis of the femoral veins and arrange an ultrasound scan of the leg veins.

Should echocardiography be done in all patients with *Staphylococcus aureus* bacteraemia?

All patients with community-acquired *S. aureus* bacteraemia should have echocardiography since the risk of endocarditis is high.

The need in patients with hospital-acquired (e.g. line-related) bacteraemia is less certain and you should be guided by local hospital protocols. Echocardiography is unequivocally indicated if:
- There are suggestive features, e.g. new regurgitant murmur or splinter haemorrhages.
- The fever fails to settle in 72 h.
- Persistent bacteraemia despite intravenous line removal and antibiotic therapy.

Table 15.10 Causes of blood culture-negative endocarditis

- Prior antibiotic therapy (at least 50%)
- Slow-growing organisms (some members of the HACEK group)
- Mould endocarditis, e.g. *Aspergillus* species
- *Coxiella burnetii* or *Bartonella* species
- Thrombotic, non-infected ('marantic') endocarditis, e.g. systemic lupus erythematosus or cancer

Mistakes to avoid

* Starting antibiotics without taking blood cultures
* Failing to involve the endocarditis team. Failing to keep in regular contact with the Heart Centre
* Requesting echocardiography as part of a fever screen (as well as wasting resources this introduces the possibility of false positive results from minor valve thickening and normal variants)

Further reading

Delgado V, Marsan NA, de Waha S, *et al*. (2023) 2023 ESC guidelines for the management of endocarditis. *Eur Heart J* 44(39), 3948–4042.

Katan D, Michelena HI, Avierinos JF, *et al*. (2016) Incidence and predictors of infective endocarditis in mitral valve prolapse: a population-based study. *Mayo Clin Proc* 91, 336–342.

Thornhill MH, Jones S, Prendergast B, *et al*. (2018) Quantifying infective endocarditis risk in patients with predisposing cardiac conditions. *Eur Heart J* 39, 586–595.

CHAPTER 16

Acute pericarditis

DAVID SPRIGINGS AND RUTH LITHGOW

- Consider acute pericarditis in the patient with pleuritic central chest pain. Pericarditis accounts for 5% of patients with acute severe chest pain.
- The typical patient is an otherwise healthy young adult, with a presumed viral ('idiopathic') aetiology (male: female ratio 2 : 1). Viral pericarditis may be preceded by a flu-like illness and is usually a self-limiting disorder lasting one to three weeks.
- Other causes are given in Table 16.1.
- There is a recurrence rate after a first episode of pericarditis of 15–30%, substantially reduced by treatment with colchicine.
- Patients with mild disease can be safely managed without hospitalisation.
- The management of the patient with suspected acute pericarditis is summarised in Figure 16.1.

Priorities

1 Review the observations and make a focused clinical assessment (Table 16.2). A pericardial friction rub is heard in less than one-third of cases, so its absence does not exclude the diagnosis.

2 If there are clinical signs of cardiac tamponade (breathlessness with distended neck veins or pulsus paradoxus; see Chapter 6) arrange urgent echocardiography and seek urgent advice from a cardiologist.

Table 16.1 Causes of acute pericarditis.

Infectious (80–85% of cases)

Viruses: e.g. enteroviruses, especially coxsackie and echoviruses; adenoviruses; parvovirus B19; herpes viruses (especially EBV and CMV); HIV; SARS-CoV-2

Pyogenic bacteria: e.g. *Streptococcus pneumoniae, S. pyogenes, S. aureus, Neisseria meningitidis*

Other bacteria: e.g. *Mycobacterium tuberculosis, Coxiella burnetii (Q fever agent), Borrelia burgdorferi (Lyme disease agent)*

Non-infectious (15–20% cases)

Post-cardiac injury syndrome: e.g. after cardiac surgery, cardiac device implantation, percutaneous cardiac procedure, chest trauma

Autoimmune: e.g. systemic lupus erythematosus, rheumatoid arthritis, systemic sclerosis

Neoplastic: e.g. breast or lung cancer, lymphoma

Metabolic: e.g. uraemia, hypothyroidism

Drug-related: e.g. chemotherapeutic agents, drugs causing lupus-like syndrome, vaccines including mRNA COVID vaccine

Acute Medicine: A Practical Guide to the Management of Medical Emergencies, Sixth Edition.
Edited by Mridula Rajwani, Leila Vaziri, and Ivie Gbinigie.
© 2026 John Wiley & Sons Ltd. Published 2026 by John Wiley & Sons Ltd.

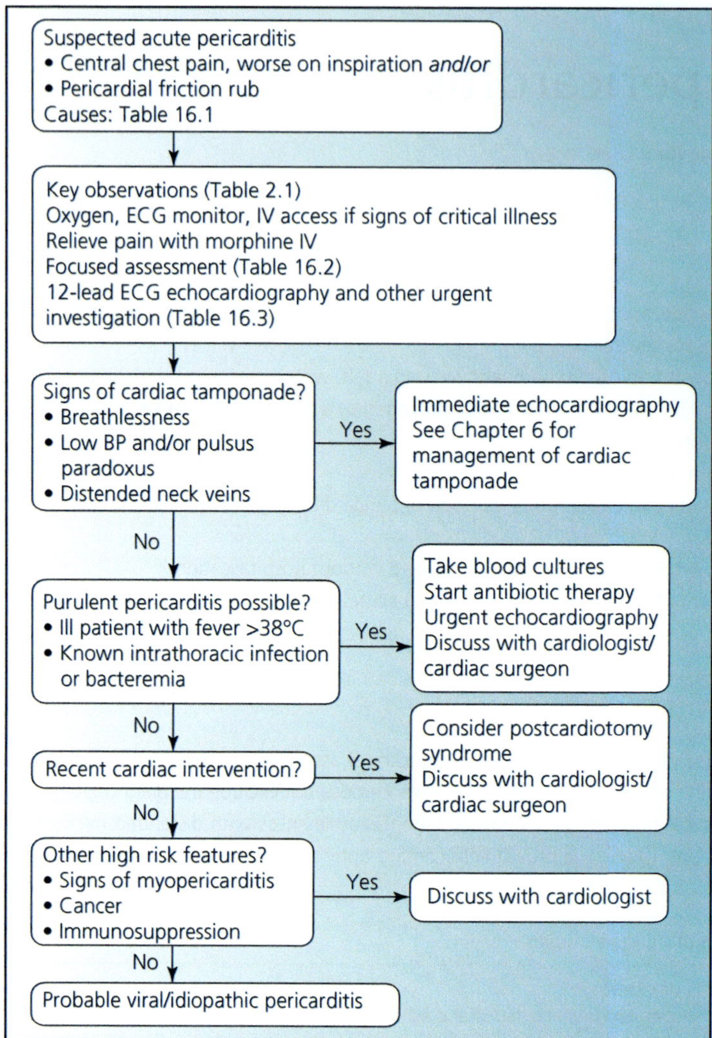

Figure 16.1 Management of the patient with suspected acute pericarditis.

Table 16.2 Focused clinical assessment in suspected acute pericarditis.

History

Quality of chest pain? The pain of acute pericarditis is typically worse on inspiration and in certain postures, for example lying back, and is relieved by sitting up or leaning forward.

Was there a viral prodrome (fever, malaise, sore throat, muscle aching)?

Are there any constitutional symptoms to suggest TB (weight loss, chronic cough) or underlying autoimmune disease?

History of predisposing conditions?

Risk for post-cardiac injury syndrome pericarditis: cardiac surgery, procedure or chest trauma, two to four weeks previously (range one week to three months)?

Examination

Patient ill or well?

Temperature

Signs of tamponade (breathlessness, distended neck veins, palpable pulsus paradoxus, hypotension)?

Signs of heart failure (basal lung crackles) to suggest myocarditis with ventricular dysfunction?

Pericardial friction rub?

Table 16.3 Investigation in suspected acute pericarditis.

ECG
Chest X-ray (usually normal unless a large pericardial effusion (>300 mL) is present)
Echocardiography (urgent if evidence of tamponade or myocarditis)
Plasma troponin
Renal function and electrolytes
Full blood count
C-reactive protein
ESR
Blood culture (if suspected bacterial infection)
Autoantibody screen
HIV serology
BNP or NT-proBNP

Table 16.4 High-risk features in acute pericarditis.

Ill patient
Fever >38 °C
Sub-acute course
Large pericardial effusion (>20 mm thick on echocardiography)
Clinical or echocardiographic features of cardiac tamponade (Chapter 6)
Immunosuppression
Evidence of myopericarditis (elevated plasma troponin/BNP, ventricular dysfunction on echocardiography)
Oral anticoagulation
Immunosuppression
Pericarditis in the context of chest trauma

3 Obtain an electrocardiogram (ECG) and other investigations (Table 16.3). The diagnosis of acute pericarditis is based on the clinical features supported by the ECG and requires at least two of the following four features:

- Pericarditic chest pain: central chest pain worse on inspiration and eased by sitting forward
- Pericardial friction rub
- New widespread ST-segment elevation and/or PR depression on ECG
- Pericardial effusion on echocardiography (new or worsening; present in 50–65% of patients).

The distinction between acute pericarditis, acute coronary syndrome with ST-segment elevation and non-specific chest pain with benign early repolarization can sometimes be difficult (Chapter 12).

4 Decide on the likely aetiology and risk-stratify the patient (Table 16.4).

Further management

1 In-patient or out-patient management?

Admit if there are high-risk features (Table 16.4) or a non-viral cause of pericarditis requiring specific treatment is suspected.

Patients with presumed viral ('idiopathic') or post-cardiac injury syndrome pericarditis, who have no high-risk features, can be managed without hospitalisation. Give an NSAID with gastroprotection, plus colchicine (Table 16.5). NSAID should be continued for one week after pain resolves, then tapered off, and colchicine given for three months. Arrange clinic review in one to two weeks and provide advice on how to obtain

Table 16.5 Treatment of acute pericarditis.

Drug	Comment/Dose/Duration
NSAID	Ibuprofen 600–800 mg 8-hourly PO or
	Aspirin 750–1000 mg 8-hourly PO
	(aspirin preferred in patients with coronary artery disease)
	Continue for one week after pain resolves, then taper off.
	Co-administer a proton-pump inhibitor for gastroprotection.
Prednisolone	If NSAID contraindicated or if there is evidence of auto-immune cause and infection has been excluded.
	Give prednisolone 0.2–0.5 mg/kg/day PO.
	Co-administer a proton-pump inhibitor for gastroprotection.
Colchicine	Co-administer with NSAID or prednisolone.
	Age <70 and weight >70 kg:
	Give colchicine 500 µgm twice daily PO
	Age >70 or weight <70 kg:
	Give colchicine 500 µgm once daily PO
	Continue for three months.

medical help if there is worsening pain or the development of breathlessness. Patients should avoid exercise until symptoms have fully resolved, and competitive sports for three months (six months if there is myopericarditis, with raised plasma troponin and/or ventricular dysfunction on echocardiography).

2 Purulent pericarditis

This is rare and is usually due to the spread of intrathoracic infection, for example following thoracic trauma or complicating bacterial pneumonia. Consider if the patient is ill with fever >38 °C or is known to have intrathoracic infection or bacteraemia.

Take blood cultures and start antibiotic therapy (e.g. IV vancomycin and ceftriaxone). Seek urgent advice from a microbiologist.

Perform pericardiocentesis if there is an effusion large enough to drain safely (thickness >20 mm) and send the fluid for Gram stain and culture. Consider tuberculosis or fungal infection if the effusion is purulent but no organisms are seen on Gram stain.

Discuss further management with a cardiologist or cardiothoracic surgeon.

3 Post-cardiac injury syndrome pericarditis

This is an acute self-limiting illness, with fever, pericarditis and pleuritis. Consider if the patient with acute pericarditis has had cardiac surgery, a cardiac procedure or chest trauma two to four weeks previously (range one week to three months). The ECG may show typical changes of acute pericarditis or only non-specific ST/T abnormalities. The chest X-ray may show an enlarged cardiac silhouette (due to pericardial effusion), bilateral pleural effusions and transient pulmonary infiltrates. The ESR is typically around 100 mm/h.

The differential diagnosis includes infectious or neoplastic pleuro-pericarditis, pulmonary embolism and oesophageal rupture.

Treat with NSAID plus colchicine as for acute viral pericarditis (Table 16.5).

Further reading

Chiabrando JG, Bonaventura A, Vecchie A, *et al.* (2020) Management of acute and recurrent pericarditis. *J Am Coll Cardiol* 75, 76–92.

Lazarou E, Tsioufis P, Vlachopoulos C, *et al.* (2022) Acute pericarditis: update. *Curr Cardiol Rep* 24, 905–913.

CHAPTER 17

Cardiomyopathies and congenital heart disease in adults

JONATHAN J. H. BRAY AND JULIAN O. M. ORMEROD

Priorities

- Cardiomyopathy is the underlying cause in approximately 15% of sudden cardiac deaths (SCDs) (1). Hypertrophic cardiomyopathy (HCM) is the most common type causing SCD in the United Kingdom. Arrhythmogenic cardiomyopathy (ACM) is also a frequent cause of SCD; serious arrhythmia can occur early in the course of disease, without major electrocardiographic (ECG) or echocardiographic changes.
- Shock in the context of hypertrophic obstructive cardiomyopathy (HOCM) is a medical emergency and should warrant urgent specialist input. If left ventricular (LV) obstruction is echocardiographically confirmed, treatment goals are to minimise outflow obstruction and avoid positive inotropes.
- Dilated cardiomyopathy (DCM) can present as acute heart failure or cardiogenic shock. It is the most common underlying reason for heart transplantation in the United Kingdom.
- Takotsubo cardiomyopathy is not a true cardiomyopathy (primary heart muscle disease); it can mimic the presentation of a myocardial infarction but, with supportive care through the initial event, the long-term prognosis can be very good and full recovery is common.
- Atrial arrhythmias are common in adult congenital heart disease (CHD) and should warrant urgent specialist input, rehydration as required and early cardioversion.

Cardiomyopathies are disorders of the myocardium in which the heart muscle is structurally and functionally abnormal, in the absence of other causes such as coronary artery disease, hypertension, valvular disease and CHD. In 2007, The European Society of Cardiology released a revised classification for cardiomyopathies (Figure 17.1) that is clinically oriented and is grouped according to ventricular morphology and function, followed by sub-division into familial and non-familial forms (2). Classification into familial and non-familial forms of cardiomyopathy is designed to support a framework for further investigations.

Familial forms occur in at least two family members (index case and a relative); whereas non-familial forms occur only in the index case and not within family members. Familial cardiomyopathies are often, but not always, monogenic in nature. It is useful to appreciate that LV dysfunction secondary to coronary ischaemia or myocardial infarction, sometimes termed 'ischaemic cardiomyopathy', is not considered a true cardiomyopathy as it is not a primary disorder of heart muscle. Channelopathies are primary electrical disorders and generally distinct from cardiomyopathies.

Hypertrophic cardiomyopathy

HCM is defined as the presence of increased ventricular wall thickness or mass in the absence of loading conditions (hypertension, valve disease) sufficient to cause the observed abnormality.

Acute Medicine: A Practical Guide to the Management of Medical Emergencies, Sixth Edition.
Edited by Mridula Rajwani, Leila Vaziri, and Ivie Gbinigie.
© 2026 John Wiley & Sons Ltd. Published 2026 by John Wiley & Sons Ltd.

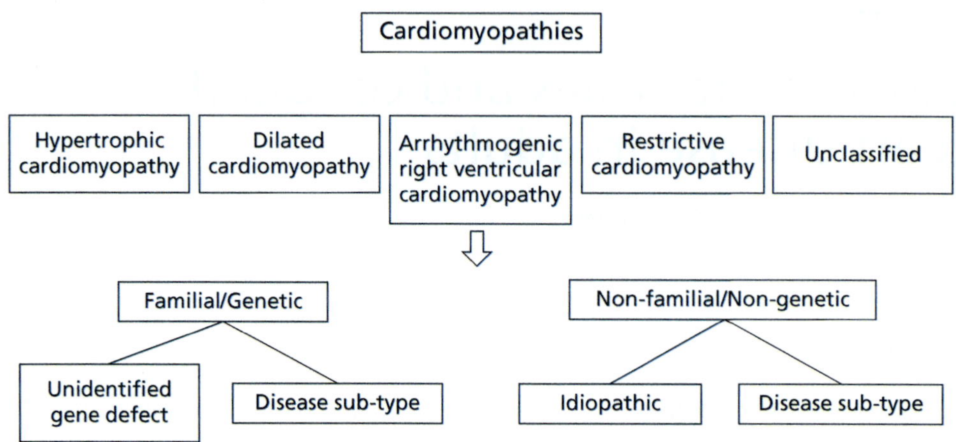

Figure 17.1 European society of cardiology classification of cardiomyopathy. Source: Adapted from Elliott and colleagues (2).

HCM is due to monogenic or polygenic gene changes, generally affecting proteins in the heart muscle units (the sarcomere). The polygenic ('sarcomere negative') form of disease tends to present later in life – 5th–7th decades – is associated with hypertension and obesity, and carries a more benign prognosis. The monogenic ('sarcomere positive') form typically presents before the age of 40; commonly in the late teens/twenties, but childhood presentation does occur and can be severe. The risk of SCD, atrial fibrillation (AF) and heart failure (HF) is higher in the monogenic form of HCM. Clinical context, specific phenotype and genetic testing can distinguish the two forms.

Similar phenotypes ('phenocopies') can be seen in metabolic disorders, mitochondrial disease or in association with congenital syndromes (e.g. Noonan or Williams syndromes). It is the most common cardiomyopathy and occurs in approximately 1:500 of the general population (3, 4). Athletic training can lead to physiological myocardial hypertrophy and can cause diagnostic uncertainty in some individuals. Careful phenotyping, genetic testing and sometimes detraining can be helpful.

Signs and symptoms

- Exertional dyspnoea
- Fatigue
- Chest pain (anginal or atypical) – with normal coronary angiography.
- Presyncope and syncope (particularly exertional) – up to a quarter of patients report at least one episode and almost half have presyncope.
- Palpitations

Symptoms of advanced heart failure are less common but can occur as part of 'burnt-out HCM'. This is progressive LV dysfunction and dilatation in HCM and has a poor prognosis. It more commonly occurs in monogenic ('sarcomere positive') disease. Symptoms include orthopnoea, paroxysmal nocturnal dyspnoea and oedema.

Symptoms are caused by numerous mechanisms, including left ventricular outflow tract (LVOT) obstruction, myocardial dysfunction, diastolic dysfunction, microvascular dysfunction or brady- or tachyarrhythmias. These mechanisms vary between individuals and at different stages of disease progression.

The presence of atrial fibrillation is four to six-fold higher than in the general population and is again more common in the monogenic form of the disease (5).

Table 17.1 Summary of the treatment of LVOT obstruction in HCM. *IV: intravenous.*

Minimise outflow obstruction	Increase preload	• Elevation of the legs • IV fluids/blood as necessary • Correction of anaemia
	Increase afterload	• Vasopressors (with minimal beta-1 agonist activity)
	Negative inotropes	• Beta-blockers (e.g. IV metoprolol) • IV disopyramide • Role for myosin ATPase inhibitors (e.g. mavacamten) in acute setting is unclear
	Mechanical circulatory support	• Extracorporeal membrane oxygenation can be considered
	Septal reduction	• In certain situations, urgent surgical myectomy or alcohol ablation
Treatments to avoid	• Positive inotropes, e.g. dobutamine, adrenaline	

Acute haemodynamic collapse can occur, manifesting with severe hypotension and symptoms of heart failure, and a thready, double-impulse peripheral pulse and a systolic murmur of LV obstruction ± mitral regurgitation on examination. Precipitating events include decreased preload (e.g. dehydration, diuretics and acute blood loss), decreased afterload (e.g. perioperative vasodilation), supraventricular tachyarrhythmia, or acute mitral regurgitation (e.g. endocarditis). LVOT obstruction should be confirmed by urgent echocardiography, and if present expert opinion should be sought. Treatment options are summarised in Table 17.1. Conventional treatment for heart failure with nitrates, diuretics and vasodilators may exacerbate hemodynamic impairment.

Investigations

- Blood tests: Troponin levels are often chronically raised in patients with established sarcomeric HCM and in mitochondrial disease; acute rises in troponin may be caused by decompensation and do not necessarily indicate ACS in this setting.
- Electrocardiogram: Most sensitive routine test.
  - T wave inversion in anterolateral leads (strain pattern) due to abnormal repolarisation (can be deeply inverted in apical HCM).
  - Prominent Q waves in inferior and lateral leads due to hypertrophied septal depolarisation.
  - P wave abnormalities from atrial enlargement.
  - Left axis deviation from LV hypertrophy.
- Echocardiography: Identification of LV hypertrophy.
  - ≥15 mm in any segment in an adult is considered pathological.
  - Systolic anterior motion of the mitral valve.
  - LVOT obstruction.
- Cardiac magnetic resonance (CMR) imaging can be useful, especially with suboptimal echocardiography; it also can demonstrate fibrosis and distinguish phenocopies.
- Ambulatory ECG monitoring: As part of SCD risk stratification and for evaluation of symptoms.
- Exercise testing: Risk stratification (especially in younger adults).
- Genetic testing: Wider panel testing in the affected patient (proband) when a genetic condition is suspected (diagnostic testing) or cascade family screening in at-risk individuals when a pathogenic (disease-causing) gene change is known in the family (predictive testing).
- Cardiac catheterisation: Can be useful to exclude coronary disease or assess pulmonary pressures in selected patients.

Management

LV outflow tract obstruction (LVOT gradient >50 mmHg at rest or on Valsalva) in HOCM may be managed conservatively if asymptomatic. If symptomatic, or in selected patients with high gradients (e.g. >100 mmHg at rest), initial therapy involves titration of a non-vasodilating beta-blockade (e.g. bisoprolol, nadolol or metoprolol) or a non-dihydropyridine calcium channel blocker (e.g. diltiazem or verapamil). Disopyramide is a negative inotrope and class I antiarrhythmic, and can be added to either of these, or used (with caution) as monotherapy. Cardiac myosin ATPase inhibitors (e.g. mavacamten) are relatively novel therapies that can be used with severe obstructive symptoms, but drug interactions and a narrow therapeutic window necessitate specialist prescribing and frequent monitoring. Short AV delay dual chamber pacing can be useful in selected individuals, especially with concomitant bradyarrhythmia or need for an implantable cardiovert defibrillator (ICD). Septal reduction therapy (either alcohol septal ablation or surgical myectomy) can be very effective for ongoing symptoms despite optimal medical therapy.

In patients with HCM without LV obstruction or coronary artery disease, chest pain is treated, as above, with a beta-blocker or a non-dihydropyridine calcium channel blocker. Treatment of arrhythmia and heart failure is similar to patients without HCM.

ICDs are recommended for secondary prevention of sustained ventricular tachycardia and for certain patients based on risk stratification for primary prevention. European guidelines recommend the use of a risk calculator (HCM-RISK) to assist with risk stratification and inform discussion.

Dilated cardiomyopathy

DCM is defined as the presence of LV dilatation and LV systolic dysfunction in the absence of abnormal loading conditions such as hypertension or valve disease, or coronary artery disease sufficient to cause global systolic impairment. The right ventricle (RV) is not required to be dilated for diagnosis but may also be affected. Chronic inflammatory cells may also be seen in histology or immunocytochemistry. Increasingly, it is recognised that patients may present with dilatation alone, or with non-dilated LV dysfunction. A variety of terminology is used (e.g. hypokinetic non-DCM).

Prevalence of DCM varies between populations (and with environmental factors such as alcohol use and obesity), but it is thought that approximately one quarter have a familial form such as caused by mutations in structural myocardial genes, including those associated with inherited muscular dystrophies (e.g. Becker and Duchenne) (Table 17.2) (7). Other causes of DCM include nutritional deficiencies, endocrine dysfunction and cardiomyopathy secondary to cardiotoxic drugs, though there are likely to be additional underlying genetic predisposing factors that are incompletely understood. Inflammatory disease such as sarcoidosis may mimic DCM and it can be challenging to distinguish DCM from chronic myocarditis.

Diagnosis of familial DCM

Familial DCM is diagnosed when idiopathic DCM is diagnosed in two or more family members; however, it is important to be mindful that adult-onset DCM has a variable age of onset ('age-related penetrance').

- It is recommended to obtain a comprehensive (three-generation) family history.
- DCM secondary to syndromic disease can be familial, and so when examining it is important to examine for subtle skeletal myopathy with proximal weakness of arms or legs.
- Certain genetic forms can present with early heart block.
- First-degree relatives of individuals with DCM should be considered for clinical screening.

Treatment

Treatment of DCM is similar to treatment of heart failure with reduced ejection fraction as is covered in Chapter 14.

Table 17.2 Examples of causes and disease modifiers of cardiomyopathies.

	Cause	Disease modifier	Phenotype
Genetic mutations			
Lamin A/C (LMNA)	x		DCM
Titin (TTN)	x	x	DCM, (HCM)
Ribonucleic acid binding motif 20 (RBM20)	x		DCM
Myosin heavy chain 7 (MYH7)	x		DCM, HCM
Myosin-binding protein C (MYPC)	x		DCM, HCM
Troponin-T	x		DCM, HCM
Phospholamban (PLN)	x		DCM, HCM, ACM
Desmoplakin (DSP)	x	x	ACM, DCM, myocarditis
Sodium channel alpha unit 5 (SCN5a)	x	x	ACM, (DCM)
Tropomyosin-1	x		DCM
Haemochromatosis (HFE gene, C282Y)	x		HCM, DCM
Galactosidase-A (Fabry disease)	x		HCM
Neuromuscular disorders			
Duchenne muscular dystrophy, Becker muscular dystrophy, myotonic dystrophy	x		DCM
Syndromic disorders			
Mitochondrial X-linked mutations	x		DCM
Acquired diseases			
Infection (viruses)	x	x	Myocarditis, DCM
Immuno-mediated diseases (rheumatoid arthritis, systemic lupus erythematosus, dermatomyositis)	x	x	Myocarditis, DCM
Toxic (alcohol, amphetamines, cocaine)	x	x	DCM, myocarditis
Drugs (anthracyclines, trastuzumab, immune checkpoint inhibitors)	x	x	DCM, myocarditis
Overload (hemochromatosis)	x	x	HCM, DCM
Peripartum (pregnancy)	x	x	DCM
Comorbidities with possible gene mutations interactions and effect on phenotype			
Tachy-arrhythmias	x	x	DCM
Diabetes mellitus	x	x	DCM, HCM
Hypertension	x	x	DCM, HCM
Hypo- and hyperthyroidism		x	DCM, HCM, myocarditis

Source: Adapted from McDonagh and colleagues (6).

Peripartum cardiomyopathy

Peripartum cardiomyopathy is diagnosed where signs of heart failure occur within the last month of pregnancy or within five months following delivery. It is more common in women over 30 and is strongly associated with gestational hypertension, pregnancy with twins and tocolytic therapy. Compared to the general DCM population, a similar proportion have an identifiable causative gene change.

Restrictive cardiomyopathy

Restrictive cardiomyopathy (RCM) is characterised by a large rise in ventricular pressure with a minimal increase in volume during ventricular diastole due to excess ventricular stiffness. European guidance has defined RCM as restrictive ventricular physiology in the presence of a) normal or reduced diastolic volumes (of one or both ventricles), b) normal or reduced systolic volumes and c) normal ventricular wall thickness. RCM is rare but occurs most frequently due to systemic disorders such as amyloidosis, sarcoidosis, scleroderma and carcinoid heart disease, and due to endomyocardial disorders causing fibrosis. Familial RCM can occur demonstrating autosomal dominant inheritance with mutations to structural myocardial genes such as troponin I or as autosomal recessive inheritance as part of metabolic disorders such as haemochromatosis or glycogen storage disease.

Clinical features

Symptoms

- Slowly progressive signs and symptoms of heart failure, often over months (e.g. exertional dyspnoea, oedema).
- Reduced exercise tolerance.
- Palpitations or syncope from arrhythmias.

Signs

- Findings of chronic or decompensated HF (left-sided e.g. pulmonary oedema, S3 or right-sided sided, e.g. raised jugular venous pressure (JVP), peripheral oedema, hepatomegaly.
- Pulses paradoxus: An exaggerated fall in blood pressure (>10 mmHg) upon inspiration.
- Kussmaul sign: A paradoxical rise in JVP on inspiration (more commonly seen in constrictive cardiomyopathy).

Investigations

- ECG: ECG abnormalities are common but non-specific. A reduced voltage ECG is common in *TTR* amyloidosis; there may alternatively be evidence of LV hypertrophy.
- Echocardiography.
- Blood tests: To assess severity of disease (e.g. end-organ dysfunction) and potential secondary causes.
- Chest radiograph: Cardiomegaly due to atrial enlargement, pulmonary venous congestion, pleural effusions, mediastinal lymphadenopathy in sarcoid, interstitial lung disease in scleroderma.

  If initial investigation does not identify a probable cause, then further diagnostics such as CMR, nuclear imaging, genetic testing and/or endomyocardial biopsy may be warranted.

Treatment

General principles of HF volume management apply including use of diuretics and treatment of arrhythmias such as AF.

However, there is little evidence to support to use of other commonly used agents including renin-angiotensin-aldosterone system inhibitors, neprilysin inhibitors, beta-blockers and nitrates in the context of decompensation. Sodium-glucose cotransporter-2 inhibitors (SGLT-2i) are often used but evidence specifically in RCM is lacking. Certain disease-specific therapies (e.g. tafamidis for TTR amyloidosis) may be available for specialist use.

Advanced heart failure therapies including transplantation can be considered in patients with refractory symptoms, depending on individual factors and overall prognosis.

Arrhythmogenic cardiomyopathy

In contrast to HCM, DCM and RCM, ACM is defined histologically with the presence of progressive replacement of right ventricular myocardium with adipose and fibrous tissue. This may be confined to the right ventricle, causing an ARVC phenotype, may be confined to the LV alone ('left-dominant ACM'), or may affect both ventricles. Ventricular arrhythmia can occur relatively early in the course of disease, and progressive heart failure can occur later. ACM is rare, with a prevalence of around 1:2500 in the United Kingdom, although there are areas of higher prevalence (e.g. northern Italy and The Netherlands) due to founder mutation effects. The majority of cases are caused by autosomal dominantly inherited mutations in intercalated disc proteins (the 'desmosome'). However, around 30% of cases are gene elusive (and may be oligogenic/polygenic in aetiology) and recessive disease is also seen (e.g. Naxos and Carvajal syndromes). This tends to cause a particularly severe phenotype with a high risk of sudden death and syndromic features such as woolly hair and palmo-plantar hyperkeratosis.

Endurance exercise appears to be a major modifiable risk factor for phenotypic expression, and affected individuals (and even unaffected gene carriers) should have specialist discussion regarding exercise intensity and duration.

Clinical presentation

- Most patients present with palpitations, syncope or atypical chest pain. However, approximately 40% of patients are diagnosed with ACM as part of cascade family screening.
- Palpitations may represent atrial arrhythmia but sustained monomorphic ventricular tachycardia (often self-terminating) is common in this condition.
- SCD, and appropriate ICD shocks, are more common in ACM than in other cardiomyopathies. Arrhythmia is frequently exercise-induced, though can occur at rest.
- Left-dominant ACM can also present as a DCM phenotype with features of heart failure (e.g. dyspnoea and signs of RV failure). Genetic testing and the presence of substantial fibrosis (ring-like, biventricular or involving the epicardium) on CMR may help distinguish the two.

Investigations

- 12-lead ECG: Anterior T wave inversion (V1-V3/4) +/− epsilon wave (Figure 17.2) is classical for ARVC phenotype but only present in around 40% of individuals and may be transient. This presentation is more common in ACM associated with *PKP2* mutations. Left-dominant ACM typically shows lateral T wave inversion but this is non-specific. ACM associated with desmoplakin (*DSP*) mutations show low voltages in the limb leads.
- Exercise ECG can reveal frequent ectopy, NSVT or sustained ventricular arrhythmia in high-risk individuals.
- Ambulatory ECG monitoring is helpful in diagnosis, risk stratification and to investigate symptoms.
- Transthoracic echocardiography.
- CMR imaging.
- Electrophysiologic testing if the diagnosis is not clear.
- Genetic testing of first-degree relatives when a diagnosis is confirmed.

Treatment

- Avoidance of vigorous exercise/competitive sports due to the risk of life-threatening arrhythmias.
- Avoidance of higher volumes of low-intensity exercise due to the risk worsening heart failure
- Beta-blockers: Cardioselective blockers such as metoprolol or bisoprolol.

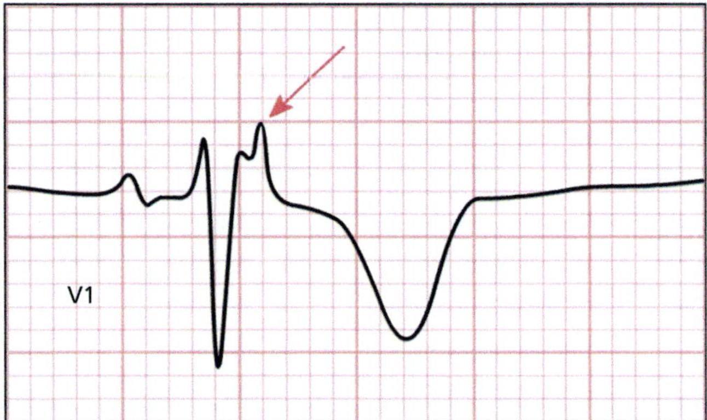

Figure 17.2 Epsilon wave seen in ACM.

- Medications as for DCM in LV dysfunction.
- Implantable cardioverter defibrillators in selected individuals (risk stratification tools are available).
- In severe cases, heart transplantation may be required for HF or intractable arrhythmias.

Unclassified cardiomyopathies

Excessive trabeculation/hypertrabeculation (previously known as LV non-compaction – LVNC) is characterised by prominent LV trabeculae and deep inter-trabecular recesses. It is an imaging finding that can be seen in normal individuals, athletes or in association with cardiomyopathy or CHD. It can also occur transiently with rapid LV dilatation and dysfunction in the context of critical illness, for example. True cardiomyopathy with excessive trabeculation in adults is rare and is generally associated with sarcomeric mutations when it occurs. In these families, it is not clear whether the presence of hypertrabeculation carries any additional risk of arrhythmia or thrombosis over and above that of the underlying cardiomyopathy. It is a common cause of diagnostic uncertainty and risks over-treatment in adults, but the finding may be of more significance in paediatric cohorts (8).

Takotsubo cardiomyopathy is not a true cardiomyopathy as it is not known to be an intrinsic disease of the heart muscle. However, it is listed as an unclassified cardiomyopathy and is commonly seen on the medical take. It is characterised by (usually transient) regional systolic dysfunction involving the LV apex and/or mid-ventricle without obstructive coronary disease on coronary angiography. Patients present similarly to myocardial infarction with subacute onset chest pain, diffuse T-wave inversion (sometimes preceded by ST-elevation) and a mild cardiac enzyme rise. Known colloquially as 'broken heart syndrome', onset of the condition is often preceded by emotional or physical stress. It is more frequent in post-menopausal women. Whilst the aetiology is not well understood, serum noradrenaline concentrations are transiently elevated in most patients. If the initial presentation is survived, prognosis is generally good, with LV dysfunction usually normalising within days to weeks. Recurrence occurs in around 10% and some individuals have persistent changes in the LV myocardium. This pattern of reversible myocardial dysfunction is also sometimes seen in patients sustaining cerebral injury such as intracranial haemorrhage.

Adult congenital heart disease

With >90% of individuals with CHD in the western world living through to adulthood, the prevalence of adults living with CHD or the sequelae of CHD is far greater than the number of children with CHD (9). It is therefore important that general physicians are aware of the common causes of CHD and potential complications.

CHD can be classified by its complexity and by whether it is cyanotic or acyanotic (Table 17.3).

Table 17.3 Example of complexity classification of adult CHD.

Mild	Moderate	Complex
Isolated congenital aortic valve disease/bicuspid aortic valve disease	Anomalous pulmonary venous connection	CHD pulmonary vascular disease (e.g. Eisenmenger syndrome)
Isolated congenital mitral valve disease	Aortic stenosis – subvalvular or supravalvular	Fontan circulation
Mild isolated pulmonary stenosis	ASD primum or secundum and VSD	Pulmonary atresia
Isolated small ASD, VSD or PDA	Coarctation of the aorta	Transposition of the great arteries
	Ebstein anomaly	Truncus arteriosus
	Tetralogy of Fallot – repaired	Univentricular heart
	Transposition of the great arteries after arterial switch operation	

Source: Adapted from Baumgartner and colleagues (10) *ventricular septal defect (VSD), atrial septal defect (ASD), patent ductus arteriosus (PDA)*.

Cyanotic heart disease

- Tetralogy of Fallot (TOF): Comprises four defects: a ventricular septal defect, pulmonary stenosis, overriding aorta and right ventricular hypertrophy. It is the most common cyanotic heart defect.
  - Most patients undergo primary intracardiac repair in infancy.
  - Patients require long-term follow-up and surveillance for complications.
  - Pulmonary valve replacement is often necessary before development of severe RV dysfunction.
- Transposition of the great arteries: The positions of the pulmonary artery and the aorta are reversed, resulting in two separate circulatory systems that require early surgical intervention with an arterial switch procedure.
- Truncus arteriosus: Involves a single large vessel arising from the heart, instead of pulmonary artery and aorta, and is often accompanied by a VSD.
- Tricuspid atresia: Characterised by the absence or abnormal development of the tricuspid valve, leading to inadequate blood flow from the right atrium to the right ventricle.
- Hypoplastic left heart syndrome (HLHS): HLHS involves underdevelopment of the left side of the heart, including the left ventricle, aorta and mitral valve. It is a severe condition requiring staged surgeries or heart transplantation.
- Ebstein's anomaly: Where the tricuspid valve is displaced downward into the right ventricle, leading to inadequate blood flow and cyanosis.

Acyanotic heart disease

- Atrial septal defect (ASD): A defect in the atrial septum allowing oxygenated blood from the left atrium to mix with deoxygenated blood in the right atrium. Corrected via transcatheter closure or open-heart surgery.
- Ventricular septal defect (VSD): A defect in the septum allowing oxygenated blood from the left ventricle to mix with deoxygenated blood in the right ventricle. Corrected via transcatheter closure or open-heart surgery.
- Patent ductus arteriosus (PDA): The ductus arteriosus enables the foetus' circulation to bypass the underdeveloped lungs, but remains open following birth causing abnormal blood flow between the aorta and pulmonary artery. Corrected through transcatheter closure or surgical ligation.
- Coarctation of the aorta: A narrowing of the aorta, usually near the former ductus arteriosus. Corrected with surgical resection with end-to-end anastomosis or balloon angioplasty with or without stent placement.
- ***Congenital aortic stenosis***
- ***Congenital pulmonary Stenosis***

Examples of surgical procedures

Fontan procedure

- A staged procedure that redirects deoxygenated blood directly to the pulmonary arteries without passing through the heart, resulting in a single functioning ventricle.
- It is performed for conditions such as tricuspid atresia and HLHS.

Norwood procedure

- Used to treat HLHS early in life with the aim of providing unobstructed blood flow from right ventricle to systemic circulation and establishing a controlled source of pulmonary blood flow.
- The procedure includes a) construction of a new aorta using pulmonary artery, b) inserting a shunt such as a modified Blalock-Taussig shunt and c) resecting the atrial septum.
- Patients may undergo further surgeries such as a Fontan surgery after this procedure.

Ross procedure

- This procedure is used to treat congenital aortic valve disease using a pulmonary autograft.
- It involves replacing the aortic valve with a pulmonic valve autograft and right-sided reconstruction with an aortic or pulmonary homograft.

Atrial arrhythmias in CHD

- Atrial arrhythmias are common in CHD, affecting approximately one-fifth of CHD patients and are a major cause of morbidity.
- They can lead to haemodynamic deterioration and so urgent specialist input should be sought, patients should be aggressively rehydrated where required and cardioversion should be considered early.

Pacemakers in CHD

- Generally, indications for pacing are similar in CHD to the general population.
- All symptomatic sinus or AV node diseases require pacemaker intervention.
- Lead access can pose a difficulty for these patients who require detailed surgical histories and cross-sectional imaging.
- Imaging of the heart and vessels using an echocardiogram with a bubble study or venography is required to exclude shunts that could lead to paradoxical thromboembolic strokes.

Implantable cardioverter defibrillators (ICD) in CHD

- As more individuals with CHD live into adulthood, SCD has become the most common cause of mortality due to the combination of surgical incisions and myocardial scarring creating a substrate for ventricular arrhythmias.
- The same indications to individuals without CHD apply, but in addition:
  1 Adults with CHD and presumed cardiogenic syncope with at least moderate ventricular dysfunction or inducible sustained monomorphic ventricular tachycardia.
  2 Individuals with a single ventricle or systemic RV dysfunction with an additional risk factor may be considered.
  3 Individuals with repaired TOF with arrhythmogenic symptoms, risk factors or before further interventions may be considered.

Anticoagulation in CHD

- Stroke is a major cause of morbidity in patients with adult CHD.
- It is recommended that individuals with moderate or complex defects and AF should be anticoagulated regardless of the CHA_2DS_2-VASc score.

References

1 Srinivasan NT, Schilling R. (2018) Sudden cardiac death and arrhythmias. *Arrhythmia Electrophysiol Rev* 7(2), 111–117.
2 Elliott P, Andersson B, Arbustini E, *et al.* (2008) Classification of the cardiomyopathies: a position statement from the European society of cardiology working group on myocardial and pericardial diseases. *Eur Heart J* 29(2), 270–276.
3 Elliott P, McKenna WJ. (2004) Hypertrophic cardiomyopathy. *Lancet* 363(9424), 1881–1891.
4 Maron BJ, McKenna WJ, Danielson GK, *et al.* (2003) American College of Cardiology/European Society of Cardiology clinical expert consensus document on hypertrophic cardiomyopathy. A report of the American College of Cardiology Foundation Task Force on Clinical Expert Consensus Documents and the European Society of Cardiology Committee for Practice Guidelines. *J Am Coll Cardiol* 42(9), 1687–1713.
5 Robinson K, Frenneaux MP, Stockins B, *et al.* (1990) Atrial fibrillation in hypertrophic cardiomyopathy: a longitudinal study. *J Am Coll Cardiol* 15(6), 1279–1285.
6 McDonagh TA, Metra M, Adamo M, *et al.* (2022) 2021 ESC Guidelines for the diagnosis and treatment of acute and chronic heart failure. *Eur J Heart Fail* 24(1), 4–131.

7 Petretta M, Pirozzi F, Sasso L, *et al.* (2011) Review and metaanalysis of the frequency of familial dilated cardiomyopathy. *Am J Cardiol* 108(8), 1171–1176.

8 Nugent AW, Daubeney PE, Chondros P, *et al.* (2005) Clinical features and outcomes of childhood hypertrophic cardiomyopathy: results from a national population-based study. *Circulation* 112(9), 1332–1338.

9 Moons P, Bovijn L, Budts W, *et al.* (2010) Temporal trends in survival to adulthood among patients born with congenital heart disease from 1970 to 1992 in Belgium. *Circulation* 122(22), 2264–2272.

10 Baumgartner H, De Backer J, Babu-Narayan SV, *et al.* (2021) 2020 ESC Guidelines for the management of adult congenital heart disease: The Task Force for the management of adult congenital heart disease of the European Society of Cardiology (ESC). Endorsed by: association for European Paediatric and Congenital Cardiology (AEPC), International Society for Adult Congenital Heart Disease (ISACHD). *Eur Heart J* 42(6), 563–645.

CHAPTER 18

Aortic dissection and other acute aortic syndromes

YANI PERERA AND PRIYADARSHINI MARATHE

Consider acute aortic syndrome in any patient with chest, back or upper-abdominal pain. Aortic dissection is the most common acute aortic syndrome and is classified as proximal (Type A; involving the ascending thoracic aorta) or distal (Type B; only involving the descending thoracic aorta) (Figure 18.1). The risk of death is high in the first few hours, so immediate discussion with an aortic surgical centre is vital. Management of suspected aortic dissection is summarized in Figure 18.2.

Priorities

- Insert an intravenous (IV) cannula and relieve pain with morphine 5–10 mg IV (2.5–5 mg in the small or elderly) with further doses every 15 min as required. Be mindful of potential haemodynamic instability in the patient.
- Obtain an electrocardiogram (ECG) to exclude acute myocardial infarction as an alternative cause for the pain. Very rarely, aortic dissection can involve the right coronary artery, causing inferior infarction.
- Complete your clinical assessment (Table 18.1) and urgent investigations (Table 18.2).

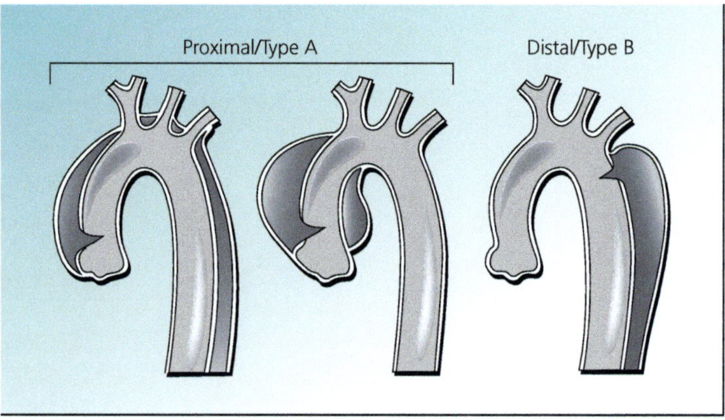

Figure 18.1 Classification of aortic dissection.

Acute Medicine: A Practical Guide to the Management of Medical Emergencies, Sixth Edition.
Edited by Mridula Rajwani, Leila Vaziri, and Ivie Gbinigie.
© 2026 John Wiley & Sons Ltd. Published 2026 by John Wiley & Sons Ltd.

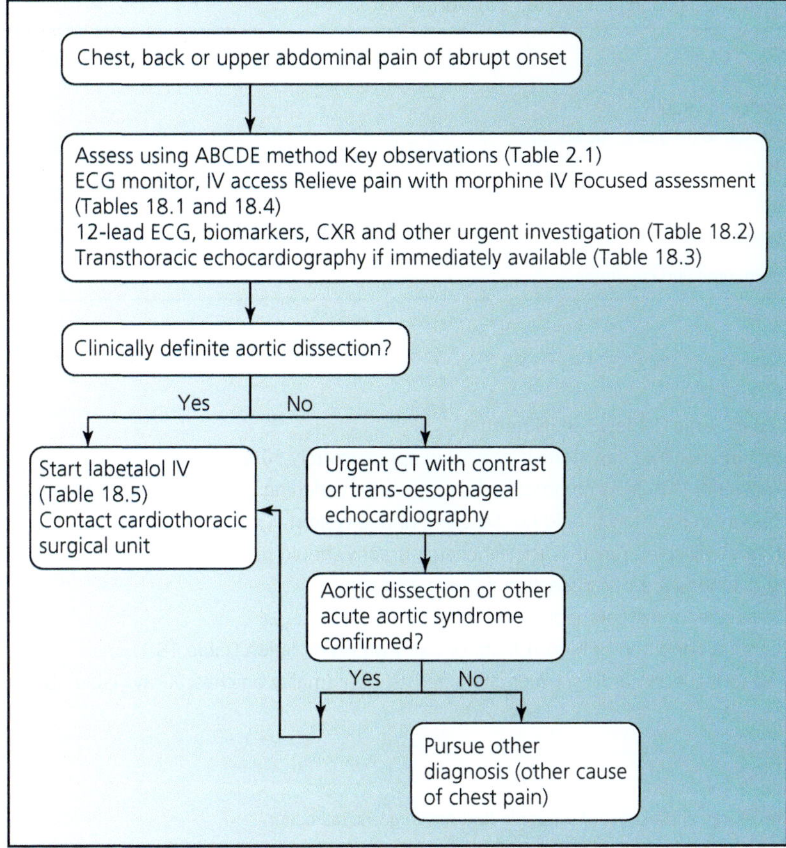

Figure 18.2 Management of suspected acute aortic dissection.

Table 18.1 Clinical assessment in suspected dissection.

History

Was the pain instantaneous in onset (like a hammer-blow or a light turning on)?

Did the pain radiate along the course of the aorta? Often, the pain is described as tearing.

Were there associated neurological symptoms (e.g. transient blurring of vision)? Symptoms are present in 15–40% of cases.

Was there syncope (present in 15% of dissections)?

Is the patient at increased risk of dissection because of:

- A congenital predisposition (Marfan, Ehlers–Danlos, Turner syndromes or bicuspid aortic valve)
- Pregnancy
- Dilated aorta
- Family history of dissection or sudden premature death?
- Recent cardiac surgery or cardiac catheterization?

Has there been cocaine use?

Examination

Blood pressure in both arms (the normal difference in systolic pressure is <20 mmHg).

Elevation of the jugular venous pressure (JVP) and arterial paradox as signs of tamponade.

Presence and symmetry of the peripheral pulses.

Early diastolic murmur of aortic regurgitation (due to distortion or dilatation of the aortic root).

Limb power and tendon reflexes.

Evidence of Marfan syndrome or other collagen abnormality.

Table 18.2 Urgent investigation in suspected aortic dissection.

ECG
Chest X-ray
Transthoracic echocardiography
Point-of-care ultrasound (to assess the aorta)
Full blood count
Plasma D-dimer level
Plasma troponin
Blood glucose
Sodium, potassium, urea and creatinine

- Review the chest X-ray (Table 18.3). Note that:
  - A posterior–anterior (PA) film alone is normal in approximately 50% of cases.
  - Anterior–posterior (AP) films commonly show apparent widening of the mediastinum in normal subjects and this feature in isolation should not be given undue weight.
  - If immediately available, transthoracic echocardiography should be done (Table 18.3).
  The working diagnosis is aortic dissection if (Table 18.4):
- The pain was severe, of instantaneous onset and;
- There is a high-risk condition or high-risk abnormality on examination (Table 18.1) or
- There is an abnormal echocardiogram or characteristic abnormality on chest X-ray (Table 18.3).

Table 18.3 Chest X-ray and echocardiographic findings in aortic dissection.

Chest X-ray
Widened mediastinum (caused by mediastinal haematoma)
Widened or double lumen to aortic knuckle
Irregular aortic contour
Small left pleural effusion (15–20% Type A or B dissections) resulting from inflammation
Large left pleural effusion as a sign of rupture

Transthoracic echocardiography
Dissection flap
Dilated aorta
Aortic regurgitation
Pericardial effusion

Transoesophageal echocardiography
As for transthoracic echocardiography but better definition of dissection flap with imaging of true and false lumen and entry tears

Intramural haematoma
- Aortic wall >5 mm thick.
- Echolucencies caused by blood in the aortic wall.
- Fascial planes in the aortic wall which 'shear' during systole.

Penetrating ulcer
- Usually descending thoracic aorta
- Crater-like outpouching through intima
- Extensive atheroma

Table 18.4 Clinical scoring in suspected acute aortic syndrome.

Aortic dissection is likely if there are >2 of
- Instantaneous onset chest or back pain
- One high-risk condition from:
  - A congenital predisposition (Marfan, Ehlers–Danlos, Turner's or Loeys–Dietz syndromes)
  - Pregnancy
  - Aortic valve disease or
  - Dilated aorta or
  - Recent cardiac surgery or cardiac catheterization
  - Family history of dissection or sudden premature death
- One high-risk sign from:
  - Asymmetric major pulses or blood pressure
  - Focal neurological deficit
  - Hypotension

Further management

1 **Working diagnosis of aortic dissection**
   - Make sure adequate analgesia has been given.
   - Start hypotensive treatment (Table 18.5).
     - Insert a bladder catheter to monitor urine output.
     - Aim to reduce systolic blood pressure to 100–120 mmHg, providing the urine output remains >30 mL/h.
   - Discuss further management with a cardiothoracic surgeon at your regional aortic centre.
   - Patients with clinically definite or a high suspicion of dissection should be transferred immediately for further investigation, unless they are not surgical candidates (e.g. due to advanced age or significant comorbidities)
     - Proximal dissections require urgent repair.
     - The early death rate is high and time should not be lost arranging investigations locally.
     - Distal dissections will usually be managed medically unless there are complications.
2 **Aortic dissection is the most likely clinical diagnosis but there is no dissection flap on transthoracic echocardiography**
   - Other causes of an acute aortic syndrome are:
     - Intramural haematoma (15–25% acute aortic syndromes)
     - Penetrating ulcer (occur in 2–7% acute aortic syndromes)

Table 18.5 Hypotensive therapy for acute aortic dissection.

The patient should be managed in a high dependency or intensive care unit.
- Make sure adequate analgesia has been given, as pain will contribute to hypertension.
- Consider placement of an arterial cannula to allow continuous BP monitoring. Insert a bladder catheter to monitor urine output.
- Start labetalol IV. Give a bolus of 20 mg over 2 min, followed by an infusion of 1–6 mg/min, increasing the infusion rate every 10 min as needed to achieve target systolic BP.
- Target systolic BP is 100–120 mmHg within 20–30 min, providing urine output remains >30 mL/h, and there is no other clinical evidence of organ ischaemia.
- If target BP is not achieved with labetalol 6 mg/min, add a nitrate infusion, for example isosorbide dinitrate 2–12 mg/h.
- Start or increase oral anti-hypertensive therapy.

- Aortic pseudoaneurysm
- Free or contained rupture
- Pseudoaneurysms and free or contained rupture should be suspected after deceleration injuries or cardiac catheterization or cardiac surgery.
- In the United Kingdom, Emergency and Acute Physicians are increasingly being trained in point-of-care ultrasound (POCUS). This includes assessing the aorta for acute aortic syndrome (i.e. aortic aneurysms and dissection flaps). If a trained practitioner is available, an early POCUS scan can be performed within minutes of the patient's arrival to aid in their diagnosis.
- The diagnosis is made with a computed tomography (CT) scan or transoesophageal echo (TOE). A scan without contrast shows an intramural haematoma and with contrast shows a dissection flap or leakage into a pseudoaneurysm or rupture. The CT must be ECG-gated and must have sufficiently frequent cuts. A CT pulmonary angiogram may not detect an abnormal aorta.
- The treatment for all acute aortic syndromes is surgery, except for intramural haematoma of the descending thoracic aorta which is initially treated medically.

3 **The diagnosis is clinically uncertain**
- If the clinical suspicion is low, a normal plasma D-dimer level (within 24 h of onset of symptoms) is a good rule-out for aortic dissection as well as pulmonary embolism. It may rarely be normal with intramural haematoma or localized dissections.
- Very high D-dimer level favours dissection over pulmonary embolism.
- If the chest X-ray is normal and expert emergency transthoracic echocardiography is not available, and if an acute aortic syndrome remains a clinical possibility with no alternative cause for pain (e.g. pleurisy, vertebral crush fracture), further investigation is needed: either CT or TOE (transoesophageal echocardiography) as available.
- Pitfalls of CT to be aware of are:
  - An intimal flap can be missed if the contrast is too dense.
  - Failure to gate to the ECG may cause artefacts resembling a dissection flap.
  - CT scans with a smaller number of cuts (as performed for detecting pulmonary emboli) may miss a localized dissection.
  - Views without contrast may be needed to show an intramural haematoma.
- TOE in trained hands detects aortic dissection and intramural haematoma (Table 18.3).
- If dissection remains highly likely clinically but the initial CT or TOE is normal, consider the alternative test or magnetic resonance imaging.

4 **Confirmed distal aortic dissection**
- If, after discussion, the decision is to manage locally, this means that the patient has a dissection unequivocally involving only the descending thoracic aorta. Emergency endovascular stent implantation for a stable Type B dissection is not routine and not definitely superior to medical therapy.
- Transfer the patient to the intensive care unit or coronary care unit, and continue IV hypotensive therapy. Start oral therapy, which should include a beta-blocker (with angiotensin-converting enzyme [ACE]-inhibitor/angiotensin receptor blocker added later) unless there are major contraindications.
- Maintain adequate pain relief (initially with a combination of opiate and non-steroidal anti-inflammatory drug).
- Monitor for evidence of complications (Table 18.6)
- Discuss with a cardiothoracic surgeon if the dissection becomes complicated as defined by one or more of:
  - Severe pain continues or recurs.
  - Signs of rupture (large pleural effusion, increasing para-aortic or mediastinal haematoma).
  - The urine output falls. If not due to excessive hypotensive therapy or hypovolaemia, this suggests involvement of the renal arteries and is an ominous sign.

Table 18.6 Monitoring in distal (Type B) dissection.

Pain score
Blood pressure
Heart rate and rhythm (continuous ECG monitoring)
Clinical assessment for evidence of:
- Brain or spinal cord ischaemia
- Myocardial ischaemia
- Renal ischaemia (creatinine, eGFR, urine output)
- Mesenteric ischaemia (abdominal pain, which is frequently non-specific, with bloody diarrhoea, rising lactate)
- Limb ischaemia (distal pulses)

- There is evidence of other branch artery involvement (e.g. abdominal pain with bloody diarrhoea due to ischaemic colitis).
- Refractory hypertension.
- Early aortic expansion.
- The preferred treatment for a complicated Type B dissection is with an endovascular stent, which has better outcomes than surgery (30-day mortality 8%, stroke 8% and spinal cord ischaemia 2%).

Problems

The patient is hypotensive

- Check for clinical evidence of a large left pleural effusion (as a sign of contained rupture).
- Review the CT scan for evidence of a contained rupture or extensive mediastinal or abdominal haematoma.
- On the transthoracic echocardiogram look for:
  - Pericardial tamponade
  - Impaired LV function either pre-existing or secondary to acute myocardial ischaemia
  - Severe aortic regurgitation
  - Evidence of hypovolaemia (flat IVC, small RV and LV cavities)
- If hypovolaemic, give a fluid challenge.
- If evidence of contained rupture, pericardial tamponade or severe aortic regurgitation discuss immediately with a cardiac surgeon.

Clinically dissection is possible but there is inferior ST elevation on ECG

- Coronary disease is the overwhelming cause of inferior infarction. Only about 3% of dissections involve the right coronary artery and acute dissection occurs at a frequency about 1% of an acute coronary syndrome (ACS).
- However, if the pain was of instantaneous onset and there are other reasons for concern (e.g. Marfan syndrome, widened mediastinum), investigate further for dissection before starting reperfusion therapy.
- The troponin level is raised in 25% of acute dissections and therefore will not be helpful in distinguishing between dissection and ACS.
- If a dissection flap is not definitely visible on transthoracic echocardiography arrange an urgent CT scan with contrast.
- If the diagnosis is confirmed the management is as for dissection. The coronary artery should not be treated as an ACS.

Box 18.1 Aortic dissection – alerts.

Both the chest X-ray and transthoracic echocardiogram may be normal in acute dissection.

Pulse abnormalities are found in <20% of patients with dissection and may also be caused by other conditions (e.g. arterial stenosis). Asymmetry of blood pressure <20 mmHg may be normal.

Further reading

Mussa FF, Horton JD, Moridzadeh R, *et al*. (2016) 2016 Acute aortic dissection and intramural hematoma: a systematic review. *JAMA* 316, 754–763.

The Task Force for the diagnosis and treatment of aortic diseases of the European Society of Cardiology (ESC). (2014) 2014 ESC Guidelines on the diagnosis and treatment of aortic diseases. *Eur Heart J* 35, 2873–2926. DOI: 10.1093/eurheartj/ehu28D1.

CHAPTER 19

Pulmonary hypertension

MUHAMMAD OWAIS MUSANI AND S. JOHN WORT

Overview

Pulmonary hypertension (PH) is estimated to affect up to 1% of the general population. The definition, recently updated, is described in Table 19.1, but requires a mean pulmonary artery pressure (mPAP) of greater than 20 mmHg. Accurate diagnosis requires right heart catheterisation: pre-capillary PH is defined by a pulmonary capillary wedge pressure (PCWP) of ≤15 mmHg, whereas a PCWP of >15 mmHg defines post-capillary PH. Clinical classification of PH is based on five groups, each with similar pathophysiology and anticipated response to treatments, and is described in Table 19.2. The most common causes are due to left heart disease (Group 2) and respiratory disease (Group 3), although the treatments are directed at the underlying causes and not specific treatment for underlying pulmonary vasculopathy. Pulmonary arterial hypertension (PAH; Group 1) and chronic thromboembolic PH (CTEPH; Group 4) are both very rare (prevalence around 50 and 25 cases per million population respectively) but have specific treatments aimed at the associated pulmonary vasculopathy.

Irrespective of the aetiology of PH, patients suffer increased morbidity and mortality. According to the REVEAL registry, the mortality of PAH remains remarkably high with one-, two- and three-year mortality rates of 10%, 19% and 25%, respectively. This is driven mainly by progressive right ventricular (RV) failure from increased pulmonary vascular afterload (measured as pulmonary vascular resistance; PVR). Impaired RV filling (diastolic dysfunction) and/or reduced RV output (systolic dysfunction) leads to systemic venous congestion and poor perfusion (reduced cardiac output; CO) which in turn leads to multiorgan dysfunction. The cause of

Table 19.1 Hemodynamic definitions and characteristics of pulmonary hypertension (PH).

Definition	Hemodynamic characteristics
Pulmonary hypertension (PH)	mPAP > 20 mmHg
Pre-capillary PH	mPAP > 20 mmHg
	PCWP ≤ 15 mmHg
	PVR > 2WU
Isolated post capillary PH (IpcPH)	mPAP > 20 mmHg
	PCWP > 15 mmHg
	PVR ≤ 2WU
Combined post- and pre-capillary PH (CpcPH)	mPAP > 20 mmHg
	PCWP > 15 mmHg
	PVR > 2WU
Exercise-induced PH	mPAP/CO slope between rest and exercise >3 mmHg/L/min

Acute Medicine: A Practical Guide to the Management of Medical Emergencies, Sixth Edition.
Edited by Mridula Rajwani, Leila Vaziri, and Ivie Gbinigie.
© 2026 John Wiley & Sons Ltd. Published 2026 by John Wiley & Sons Ltd.

Table 19.2 Clinical classification of pulmonary hypertension.

Clinical classification of pulmonary hypertension

Group I	Pulmonary arterial hypertension (PAH)
Group II	PH associated with left heart disease
Group III	PH associated with chronic respiratory diseases and/or hypoxia
Group IV	PH associated with pulmonary artery obstruction-mainly chronic thromboembolic PH (CTEPH)
Group V	PH associated with unclear/and or multifactorial mechanisms

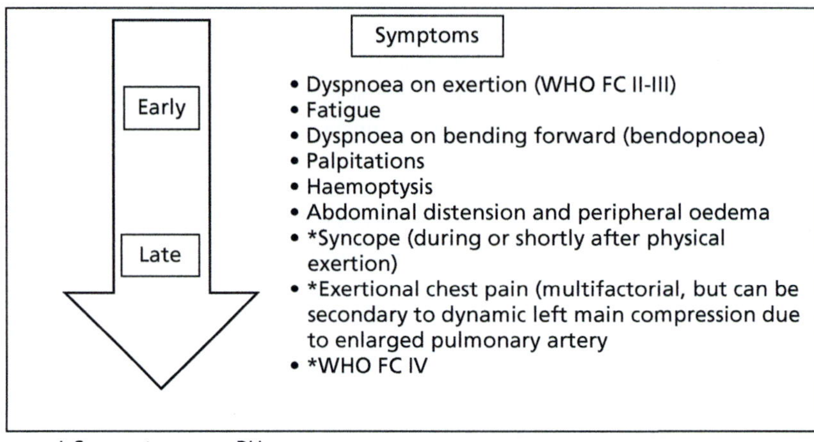

Figure 19.1 Symptoms and signs of a patient presenting with PH.

increased PVR will depend on the aetiology of PH but is primarily vascular remodelling of pulmonary arterioles in PAH and vascular obstruction and/or remodelling in CTEPH.

Significant PH in the acute clinical setting is rare but potentially life threatening. The probable scenarios are:

1 Decompensation of a patient with known PAH or CTEPH.
2 New presentation of PAH or CTEPH.
3 PH associated with acute exacerbation of chronic respiratory disease or chronic left heart disease (more common and likely to improve after treatment of the exacerbation).

It is rare to get significant PH in the setting of acute PE and if it is present should prompt thoughts of acute-on-chronic thromboembolic PH. Other signs suggestive of CTEPH in the context of a patient presenting with acute PE are discussed in Section Signs suggestive of acute-on-chronic PH.

For symptoms and signs of a patient presenting with PH see Figure 19.1 and Table 19.3. Warning signs of severe PH are WHO functional class 4, rapid progression of symptoms, signs of right heart failure, pre-syncope or syncope.

Priorities

1 Immediate echocardiography (echo), especially if severe PH is suspected. The probability of PH is defined by the ERS/ESC guidelines (see Figure 19.2). Echo signs of severe PH are explained in Figure 19.2 and Table 19.4.

Table 19.3 Signs of Pulmonary Hypertension.

Related to pulmonary hypertension
1. Central or peripheral cyanosis
2. Loud pulmonary component of second heart sound
3. RV third heart sound
4. Systolic murmur of tricuspid regurgitation and diastolic murmur of pulmonic regurgitation

Related to RV pump failure
1. Cool extremities with peripheral cyanosis (blue lips and fingertips)
2. Prolonged capillary refill
3. Distended and pulsatile jugular vein
4. Hepatomegaly
5. Ascites
6. Peripheral oedema

Signs suggesting underlying cause of PH
Clubbing: Cyanotic CHD, fibrotic lung disease, bronchiectasis or liver disease
Auscultation-murmurs, crepitations or wheeze: Lung or heart disease
Venous insufficiency or prior DVT sequelae: CTEPH
Telangiectasia: Hereditary haemorrhagic telangiectasis or systemic sclerosis (SSc)
Raynaud's phenomenon, sclerodactyly, digital ulceration: SSc

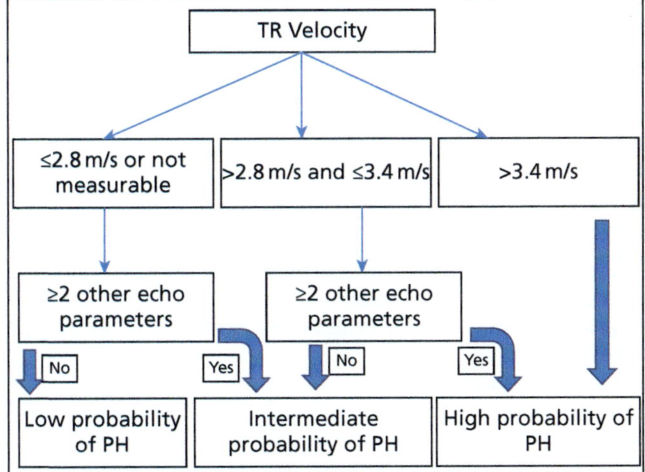

Figure 19.2 Echo features of pulmonary hypertension.

Table 19.4 Additional echocardiographic parameters associated with pulmonary hypertension.

Other echo parameters of PH

The ventricles	1. Right ventricle/left ventricle basal diameter ratio > 1.0 **
	2. Flattening of interventricular septum (LV eccentricity index >1.1 in systole, diastole, or both. **
	3. RV hypertrophy
The pulmonary artery	1. RV outflow Doppler acceleration time (ACT) <105 ms and/or mid systolic notching.
	2. Early diastolic PRV* > 2.2 m/s
	3. PA diameter >25 mm
Inferior vena cava and right atrium	1. IVC diameter >21 mm with <50% collapse on deep inspiration
	2. RA area (End systole) >18 cm²
Other	Presence of pericardial effusion**

*PRV, pulmonary regurgitation velocity; TRV, tricuspid regurgitation velocity (values suggestive of pulmonary hypertension severity, as per ESC/ERS Guidelines, 2022).
**Signs of severe pulmonary hypertension.

2 If the patient is known to a national specialist centre, look at any information the patient has with them and contact the centre for specialist advice. All centres usually have 24-hour on-call cover.

3 If a patient is not known to a specialist centre but has signs of severe PH, immediate referral to a specialist centre is recommended. All patients with a suspected new diagnosis of PAH or CTEPH should be referred to a specialist centre.

Management

Investigations

Investigation choice depends on the underlying cause and where possible should be coordinated with a specialist centre. Definitive diagnosis of PH requires right heart catheterisation, but this is best performed in a specialist centre where additional tests such as reversibility to nitric oxide and/or pulmonary angiography can be performed at the same time. However, immediate local tests should include specific tests, such as blood tests, imaging, or other diagnostic procedures, as outlined in Table 19.5, which provides associated findings for each test:

Signs suggestive of acute-on-chronic PH

It is unusual to develop significant PH in the context of acute PE. An RVSP >50 mmHg on echo plus the additional signs, usually seen on CT-PA, indicate acute-on-chronic thromboembolic PH:

- RV hypertrophy
- Flattening of interventricular septum

Table 19.5 Investigation findings suggestive of pulmonary hypertension.

Investigation findings suggestive of pulmonary hypertension	
ECG	• Normal ECG does not exclude pulmonary hypertension • Right axis deviation, RV hypertrophy, p-pulmonale, tall R wave in V1, RV strain pattern
Chest X ray	• Cardiomegaly • Elevated cardiac apex due to RVH • Enlarged right atrium • Prominent pulmonary trunk • Pruning of peripheral pulmonary vessels Associated findings related to underlying causes, i.e. kyphoscoliosis, valvular heart disease, emphysema and fibrosis.
Echo	Figure 19.2 and Table 19.4. Pericardial effusion is associated with, but not specific to, severe pulmonary hypertension
CT scan (HRCT)	Assessment of lung parenchyma can identify possible underlying causes, such as ILD, COPD etc; mosaic attenuation reflects areas of oligemia and is common in, but not specific to, CTEPH.
CT scan (CTPA)	• Enlarged pulmonary trunk. • RV hypertrophy • RV/LV >1 • Flattening of interventricular septum • Reflux of contrast into the IVC • Pericardial effusion
VQ scan	• Mismatched perfusion defects. A negative scan rules out CTEPH. VQ may be positive and CT-PA negative in distal CTEPH.
Bloods	• Basic blood tests as per clinical relevance in addition to brain natriuretic peptide (BNP) or NT-proBNP.

* CTPA, CT pulmonary angiogram; HRCT, High resolution CT scan; ILD, Interstitial lung disease (as defined in ESC/ERS Guidelines, 2022).

- Presence of organised filling defects including bands and webs
- Presence of bronchial artery collaterals

Treatment

Immediate treatment will depend on the severity of PH (and associated right heart failure), the underlying cause of PH and any other associated, exacerbating factors. In the emergency setting, the most common cause of suspected PH will be in association with exacerbations of left-heart disease and respiratory disease. The treatment is of the underlying cause in addition to the introduction/optimisation of diuretics and correction of hypoxaemia/hypercapnia (both causes of increased PVR). If PAH or CTEPH are suspected, then advice should be sought from a specialist centre as early as possible. As for any cause of PH, ensuring adequate oxygenation (always keep O_2 saturations above 90%) with correction of fluid balance (usually diuresis) is paramount. In patients who are unstable and/or not responding to supportive therapy, the following principles of management can be adopted and summarised in Figure 19.3. They are aimed at management of right heart failure: fluid optimisation, CO optimisation, improving RV afterload (PVR), treating exacerbating/pre-disposing factors and consideration of additional RV support.

Fluid optimisation

The aim is to reduce RV wall tension and move the RV to a more efficient part of the Starling curve. In most cases, this is with addition and/or optimisation of diuretics. This may include introduction of a loop diuretic to a diuretic naïve patient, conversion to intravenous loop diuretic in patients already on oral diuretics and consideration of the addition of an aldosterone receptor antagonist or thiazide diuretic in more resistant cases. In cases of patients with PH and co-existent sepsis cautious, small boluses of fluid may be necessary, but should be managed in a level 2/3 environment.

Cardiac output optimisation

In patients with preserved systemic pressure with signs of hypoperfusion, an inotrope should be considered. In patients with low systemic pressure and hypoperfusion, a vasopressor should be added. Systemic mean BP should be kept>70 mmHg. This is important to maintain aortic root pressure and coronary perfusion to the right ventricle (mainly supplied by the right coronary artery).

Inotropes

Dobutamine (β_1 receptor agonist): start at 2.5 µg/kg/min and progressively up titrate but not more than 10 µg/kg/min as high doses decrease the systemic vascular resistance with increasing risk of tachyarrhythmia.

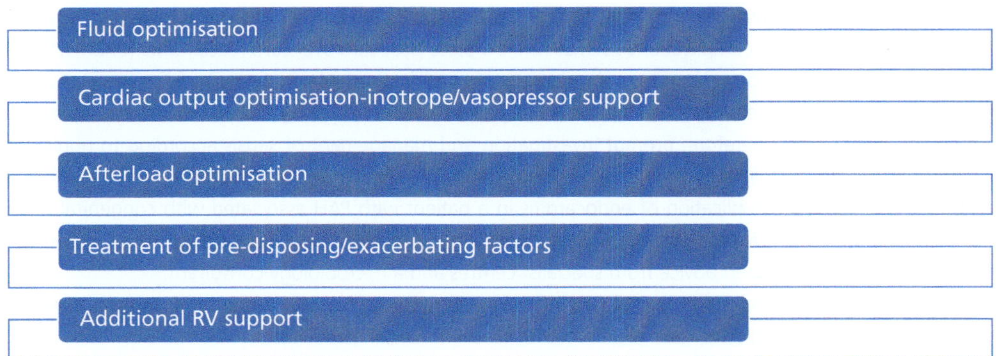

Figure 19.3 The principles of management of PH.

Dopamine: 2–5 µg/kg/min is useful when systemic vascular resistance is low, often in the context of co-existent sepsis.

Milrinone (phosphodiesterase -3 inhibitor): 50 µg/kg over 10 min then 0.375–0.75 µg/kg/min infusion.

Levosimendan (calcium sensitiser – stabilizes interaction of calcium and troponin C): initial infusion 0.05 then 0.1 µg/kg/min (without a bolus). Can increase to 0.2 µg/kg/min, for 24 h.

Vasopressors

Noradrenaline: 0.01–0.5 mcg/kg/min
Vasopressin: 0.02–0.04 units/min

As noradrenaline causes pulmonary vasoconstriction at higher doses the suggested regimen is to start with noradrenaline until 0.1 mcg/kg/min and then switch to vasopressin, which at the dose range stated is a pulmonary vasodilator.

Afterload optimisation

The use of pulmonary vasodilators will depend on what is available locally and how sick the patient is and is ideally initiated at a specialist centre. However, they may be started locally in a level 2/3 environment with advice. The most likely available medications are oral and IV sildenafil (a phosphodiesterase inhibitor) and intravenous epoprostenol (a prostanoid). Nebulised iloprost may be available. A patient already on pulmonary vasodilators should not have their therapy stopped unless they cannot absorb oral therapies (see also Section Advice on patients already known to a specialist centre on pulmonary vasodilator therapy).

Doses:

Oral sildenafil	12.5–50 mg TDS.
IV sildenafil	Half oral dose or as an infusion (1.25 mg/hr).
IV epoprostenol:	Start at 1 ng/kg/min and aim for 5–10 ng/kg/min in the first instance.
Nebulised iloprost:	2.5–5 µg, 6–9/day

Predisposing condition management

Supraventricular arrhythmia: Atrial flutter and atrial fibrillation are relatively common in patients with PH and are associated with deterioration and poor outcome. Cardioversion back to sinus rhythm should be attempted where possible. DC cardioversion and ablation techniques are preferred but should not be attempted outside a specialist centre or a centre with sufficient senior cardiac anaesthetic experience. Advice from a specialist centre should always be sought. Medical cardioversion with amiodarone can be attempted. In general, the use of beta-blockers and rate-limiting calcium channel blocker should be avoided especially in patients with more advanced right heart failure. Patients should always be observed in a level 2/3 environment as there is a risk of complications such as low CO state post cardioversion. Precipitants for arrhythmia such as sepsis and disturbed electrolytes should be sought and corrected.

Infection/sepsis: Sepsis is the most common cause of a patient with PH requiring ICU admission; the associated mortality is very high. Therefore, prompt investigation and management of sepsis according to published guidelines should be followed. Two special circumstances are worth mentioning: a) consideration of a cerebral abscess as a complication of endocarditis in a patient with PAH associated with congenital heart disease and b) catheter-related sepsis and/or tunnelitis in a patient on IV epoprostenol via an indwelling catheter. Both require expert advice from specialist centres and a microbiology consultant.

Thromboembolism: Apart from the special case of CTEPH, thromboembolism is a cause of deterioration in a patient with PH and should be managed according to international guidelines.

Noncompliance: Non-adherence with pulmonary hypertension medications is a cause of deterioration in patients already on therapy and should be considered.

Management of refractory heart failure

There are a number of bridging techniques available to potentially rescue a patient with medically resistant right heart failure and/or prepare a patient for lung transplantation. These include atrial septostomy and extra-corporal life support, including extra-corporal membrane oxygenation. These can only be done in an appropriate specialist centre.

Special circumstances

Advice on patients already known to a specialist centre on pulmonary vasodilator therapy

As a basic principle pulmonary vasodilator therapy should never be stopped as this may result in rebound rises in pulmonary pressure. However, if oral intake is not possible alternatives are intravenous sildenafil and epoprostenol or nebulised iloprost. Rarely a patient already on intravenous epoprostenol, via an indwelling catheter, may present with line or pump failure. Re-establishment of epoprostenol supply quickly is mandatory.

Possibilities include

- **If the patient is acutely unwell and the line is the issue**, connect the patient's pump to a large bore cannula.
- **Ideally, epoprostenol should be delivered by a hospital pump via a central cannula (central line or PICC line)**. A large bore cannula may suffice but side-effects are more common, and the rate of delivery should be reduced. A patient should have details of the rate of delivery and concentration of epoprostenol with them.
  - **In all cases, advice from the specialist centre should be sought.**
  - **Some patients will have other prostanoids such as trepostinil or iloprost delivered intravenously**.

The pregnant patient with PH

Although the principles of management described apply to a pregnant patient with PH, the associated mortality to mother and baby are much higher and can approach 50%. These patients should be managed in a specialist centre with obstetric sub-speciality.

Patients with PH requiring surgery or other invasive intervention

Sedation and anaesthesia are associated with increased risk in patients with PH and should be avoided if possible and, if necessary, discussed with a specialist service. Even procedures such as upper and lower GI endoscopy should be discussed in a specialist multidisciplinary team meeting (MDT) before proceeding. In the case of the need for emergency surgery or intervention, patients should be discussed with specialist centres for advice on anaesthetic, peri-procedural care and use of pulmonary vasodilators.

Further reading

Erythropoulou-Kaltsidou A, Alkagiet S, Tziomalos K. (2020) New guidelines for the diagnosis and management of pulmonary embolism: key changes. *World J Cardiol* 12(5), 161.

Humbert M, Kovacs G, Hoeper MM, *et al.* (2022, 2022) ESC/ERS Guidelines for the diagnosis and treatment of pulmonary hypertension: Developed by the task force for the diagnosis and treatment of pulmonary hypertension of the European Society of Cardiology (ESC) and the European Respiratory Society (ERS). Endorsed by the International Society for Heart and Lung Transplantation (ISHLT) and the European Reference Network on rare respiratory diseases (ERN-LUNG). *Eur Heart J* 43(38), 3618–3731.

Price LC, Dimopoulos K, Marino P, *et al.* (2017) The CRASH report: emergency management dilemmas facing acute physicians in patients with pulmonary arterial hypertension. *Thorax* 72, 1035–1045.

Price LC, Martinez G, Brame A, *et al.* (2021) Perioperative management of patients with pulmonary hypertension undergoing non-cardiothoracic, non-obstetric surgery: a systematic review and expert consensus statement. *Br J Anaesth* 126(4), 774e790.

CHAPTER 20

Heart valve disease: native, prosthetic and repaired valves

JOHN CHAMBERS

Significant valve disease occurs in 11% of people aged over 65 . It is undetected in over half and so may present acutely in a patient with no past history of valve disease. The main valve lesions in industrialised countries are calcific aortic stenosis and secondary mitral regurgitation as a result of left ventricular (LV) dysfunction.

Native valve disease may present to hospital:

- With infective endocarditis (see Chapter 15).
- With arrhythmia (usually atrial fibrillation), hypotension or pulmonary oedema.
- With syncope, breathlessness, or chest pain.
- Incidentally, when it increases the mortality in other acute illnesses including acute coronary syndrome, stroke or after road traffic collisions.
- Incidentally, when a murmur is detected peri-operatively (e.g. after hip fracture).

Priorities

- Correct arrhythmia. The haemodynamic effects of mitral stenosis are amplified by high heart rates. Slow the ventricular rate in atrial fibrillation using rate-control medication (see Chapter 13).
- Treat pulmonary oedema:
  - Start a loop diuretic.
  - If systolic BP is <100 mmHg, start dobutamine (Chapter 14).
  - Mechanical ventilation can be considered if the pO_2 is <92% despite 60% oxygen and the patient is tiring.
- Immediate echocardiography is indicated for unexplained hypotension or pulmonary oedema. A murmur may be inaudible in the presence of low flow even with severe valve disease.
- Consider the causes of acute valve disease or deterioration in previously stable valve disease (Table 20.1).
- If there is a significant newly detected murmur in a patient presenting with a clear non-valve problem, echocardiography is indicated with an urgency depending on the clinical circumstance. Echocardiography should be performed before moderate or high-risk non-cardiac surgery (see Table 20.2) unless this is an emergency.

Acute Medicine: A Practical Guide to the Management of Medical Emergencies, Sixth Edition.
Edited by Mridula Rajwani, Leila Vaziri, and Ivie Gbinigie.

Table 20.1 Causes of acute presentation in valve disease.

Acute new aortic or mitral regurgitation
Ruptured chord in mitral valve prolapse
Infective endocarditis
Deceleration injury (mitral > aortic)
Papillary muscle rupture after myocardial infarction (mitral)
Aortic dissection (aortic)

Acute decompensation of previously stable native, prosthetic or repaired valve disease
Infective endocarditis
Progression of native valve disease
Prosthetic valve dysfunction
Dehiscence causing a leak around the valve
Thrombosis
Structural degeneration
Failure of valve repair

Non-valvular
Decompensation of long-standing LV dysfunction
Acute myocardial infarction or myocardial ischaemia
Arrhythmia
Fluid-load
* Poor compliance with diuretic therapy
* Drugs causing fluid retention (e.g. NSAIDs and steroids)
* Iatrogenic fluid overload
Intercurrent illness, e.g. pneumonia and anaemia

Table 20.2 Management of asymptomatic severe disease during non-cardiac surgery.

Valve disease	Risk of non-cardiac surgery*
Aortic stenosis	High: MDT should consider aortic valve surgery or TAVI or strict intraoperative monitoring ideally with a cardiac anaesthetist Low/moderate: proceed with NCS
Aortic regurgitation	High/moderate/low: No increased risk if LV ejection fraction normal or mildly reduced
Mitral stenosis	High/moderate/low: Proceed if pulmonary artery systolic pressure <50 mmHg High: Consider balloon valvotomy if pulmonary artery systolic pressure >50 mmHg
Mitral regurgitation	High/moderate/low: No increased risk if LV ejection fraction normal

* **Low risk,** Breast, dental, thyroid, eye, minor gynaecological or urological, skin.
Moderate risk, Carotid endarterectomy, endovascular aortic, head and neck, intra-abdominal, intrathoracic non-major, orthopaedic, peripheral artery angioplasty, major gynaecological or urological.
High risk, Aortic and major vascular, duodenal and pancreatic surgery, liver resection, oesophagectomy, open lower limb revascularisation, pneumonectomy, lung or liver transplant, repair of perforated bowel, total cystectomy.

* Mistakes to avoid are given in Box 20.1.
* Refer for immediate advice from a cardiologist if there is:
  * Evidence of infective endocarditis (Chapter 15) *or*
  * Severe valve disease even in the absence of symptoms *or*
  * A repaired or prosthetic valve or apparently moderate native valve disease with hypotension, pulmonary oedema or LV impairment on the echocardiogram.

Box 20.1 Heart valve disease – mistakes to avoid.

In severe valve disease, a murmur may be absent if the cardiac output is low and/or breath-sounds loud.

In severe aortic stenosis with a low cardiac output, the transvalve gradient will fall and the aortic stenosis may be erroneously graded as moderate.

Severe aortic stenosis may be associated with systemic hypertension rather than a low blood pressure and narrow pulse pressure.

A low ejection fraction in severe aortic stenosis may recover and is not a contraindication to surgery.

If mitral regurgitation is reported as 'mild' or 'moderate' or it is associated with a hyperdynamic LV in a patient with shock, the likely diagnosis is severe regurgitation. An inexperienced echocardiographer can easily miss severe regurgitation since the jet area may be small as a result of the low pressure difference between the left ventricle and left atrium.

Management of problems in patients with repaired or prosthetic heart valves

Repaired valves

- Surgical mitral valve repair is the optimal treatment for mitral valve prolapse. Aortic valve repair is only performed at a few Heart Centres and transcatheter edge-to-edge repair for mitral regurgitation is still uncommon.
- Repairs can break down causing regurgitation which may be severe. Initial treatment is as for native valve disease until the patient can be transferred to the Heart Centre which performed the procedure.
- Infective endocarditis is more likely than in the general population so have a high index of suspicion in the presence of fever or valve failure.

Prosthetic heart valves

With hypotension or pulmonary oedema

- Emergency treatment with loop diuretics or inotropes is as for native valves.
- Because of the difficulty of assessing prosthetic valve failure, a cardiac referral should be made even if there is severe LV dysfunction sufficient to cause the presentation.
- Obstruction is recognised by reduced or absent opening of cusps or mechanical leaflets associated with a high pressure drop across the valve on echocardiography.
- Regurgitation is obvious if there is a large regurgitant colour jet but may be suspected if there is rocking of the prosthesis or the combination of highly active LV and low cardiac output.

Mechanical prosthetic valve and high or low international normalised ratio (INR)

- Involve a haematologist.
- **If there is active bleeding** that cannot be controlled by direct pressure (e.g. intracerebral or gastrointestinal):
  - Give vitamin K 5 mg IV slowly. Repeat as necessary after 12 h.
  - Consider IV prothrombin complex concentrate or, if not available, then fresh frozen plasma.
  - Recheck the INR in 30 min then 4–6 hourly until close to the therapeutic range.

Table 20.3 Target international normalized ratio (INR) for mechanical prostheses.

Prosthesis thrombogenicity	No patient risk factors*	>1 risk factor*
Low	2.5	3.0
Medium	3.0	3.5
High	3.5	4.0

Prosthesis thrombogenicity:
- **Low:** Carbomedics, Medtronic Hall, St Jude Medical, On-X
- **Medium:** other bileaflet valves
- **High:** Lillehei-Kaster, Omniscience, Starr-Edwards, Bjork-Shiley and other tilting-disc valves.

* Patient-related risk factors: mitral or tricuspid valve replacement; previous thromboembolism; atrial fibrillation; mitral stenosis of any degree; left ventricular ejection fraction <35%.

- **No active bleeding:**
  - If INR is >10, stop warfarin and give one dose of vitamin K orally 2.5–5.0 mg. Recheck INR daily.
  - If INR is 4.5–10, stop warfarin and consider a dose of vitamin K 1–2 mg orally.
  - If INR is < 4.5, omit one to two doses, check the INR daily and restart at a lower dose.
- **If INR is low or a surgical procedure is planned**

  Intravenous unfractionated heparin is the standard treatment but subcutaneous (SC) low molecular weight heparin (LMWH) is increasingly used off-licence.
  - If INR is below 1.5 in low-risk valves or 2.0 in all other risk valves (see Table 20.3), start IV heparin or SC LMWH. Increase daily dose of warfarin until INR is therapeutic.
  - If minor surgery is planned with little anticipated bleeding which can be easily controlled, do not interrupt anticoagulation.
  - If more major surgery is planned, stop warfarin and start IV heparin or SC LMWH when the INR falls to 1.5 in low-risk valves or 2.0 in all other risk valves (Table 20.3). Restart warfarin the day after the procedure unless the risk of bleeding remains high.

Thromboembolism

- The risk of thromboembolism is most closely related to non-prosthetic factors, e.g. atrial fibrillation, large left atrium or impaired left ventricle.
- Check that there are no signs of prosthetic dysfunction (breathlessness, abnormal murmur, muffled closure sound) or signs of infective endocarditis (Chapter 15).
- Look at the anticoagulation record and check INR, full blood count, C-reactive protein and blood cultures (three sets) if white cell count or C-reactive protein is raised.
- If INR is <2.0 for a mechanical valve and there is no evidence of infective endocarditis discuss with a haematologist an increase in warfarin dose. Target INR according to European Society of Cardiology (ESC) guidelines (Table 20.2). Arrange an early appointment with the anticoagulation clinic.
- Refer to a cardiologist to consider transoesophageal echocardiography looking for thrombus or pannus formation (endothelial overgrowth which can be a nidus for thrombus formation).
- Consider carotid ultrasonography looking for other common causes of TIA.

Fever

- The risk of infective endocarditis is higher than the general population. Have a low index of suspicion but do not forget non-cardiac causes.
- Send three sets of blood cultures before starting antibiotic therapy.
- Surgery is more likely to be necessary in prosthetic than native valve endocarditis.

Anaemia

- Investigate as for any anaemia, not forgetting the possibility of endocarditis.
- Virtually all mechanical valves produce minor haemolysis (disrupted cells on the blood film, high LDH (lactate dehydrogenase) and bilirubin and low haptoglobin) caused by normal transprosthetic regurgitation. Usually, the haemoglobin remains normal.
- Haemolytic anaemia suggests leakage usually around the valve (paraprosthetic regurgitation) which is often small and only detectable on transoesophageal echocardiography.
- Refer for advice from a cardiologist and haematologist.

Further reading

Otto CM, Nishimura RA, Bonow RO, *et al.* (2021) 2020 ACC/AHA guideline for the management of patients with valvular heart disease: a report of the American College of Cardiology/American Heart Association Joint Committee on Clinical Practice Guidelines. *Circulation* 143(5), e72–e227.

Vahanian A, Beyersdorf F, Praz F, *et al.* (2022) 2021 ESC/EACTS guidelines for the management of valvular heart disease. *Eur Heart J* 43(7), 561–632.

CHAPTER 21

Hypertensive emergencies

DAVID SPRIGINGS AND ZAINAB ZAFAR

Severe hypertension is characterised by a systolic blood pressure over 180 mmHg or a diastolic blood pressure over 120 mmHg. Acute management is determined by the clinical context and the presence and type of organ damage. Intravenous therapy, although warranted in certain situations, is potentially dangerous, as a sudden drop in blood pressure may lead to cerebral, myocardial or renal ischaemia.

The management of the patient with severe hypertension is summarised in Figure 21.1.

Priorities

Establish the context and comorbidities by focused clinical assessment and investigation (Tables 21.1 and 21.2). Management of severe hypertension in specific contexts is discussed below. If IV therapy is indicated, transfer the patient to an intensive therapy unit (ITU) or high-dependency unit (HDU) for arterial blood pressure monitoring and general care.

Acute aortic dissection and other acute aortic syndromes

- Make sure adequate analgesia with morphine has been given, as untreated pain and distress can exacerbate hypertension.
- Put in an arterial line to allow continuous BP monitoring and a bladder catheter to monitor urine output.
- Start labetalol IV (Table 21.3). Give a bolus of 20 mg over 2 min, followed by an infusion of 1–6 mg/min, increasing the infusion rate every 10 min as needed to achieve target systolic BP and heart rate.
- Target systolic BP is 120 mmHg within 20–30 min, and heart rate <60/min, providing urine output remains >30 mL/h, and there is no other clinical evidence of organ ischaemia.
- If target BP is not achieved with labetalol 6 mg/min, add a nitrate infusion (Table 21.3).
- Start or increase oral therapy.
- See Chapter 18 for further management of aortic dissection.

Acute ischaemic stroke

- See Chapter 56 for the assessment of the patient with ischaemic stroke.
- If the patient is a candidate for thrombolysis, start antihypertensive therapy if BP is >185/110 mmHg, aiming to reduce BP below this. If BP is not maintained at or below 185/110 mmHg, do not give thrombolysis.
- If the patient is not a candidate for thrombolysis, start therapy if BP is greater >220/120 mmHg. Aim to reduce mean arterial pressure (estimated by diastolic BP plus one-third of pulse pressure) by no more than 15% in the first 24 h.

Acute Medicine: A Practical Guide to the Management of Medical Emergencies, Sixth Edition.
Edited by Mridula Rajwani, Leila Vaziri, and Ivie Gbinigie.
© 2026 John Wiley & Sons Ltd. Published 2026 by John Wiley & Sons Ltd.

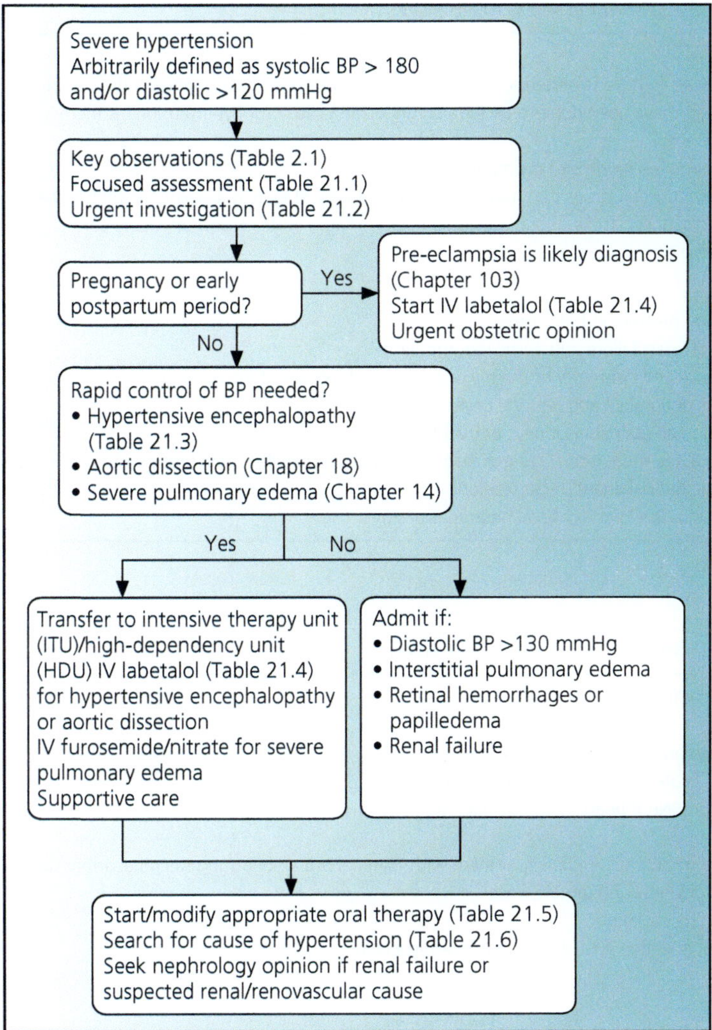

Figure 21.1 Management of the patient with severe hypertension.

- Give labetalol 10 mg IV bolus over 1 min, followed by an infusion of 1–8 mg/min, increasing the infusion rate every 10 min as needed to achieve target BP.
- If target BP is not achieved with labetalol 8 mg/min, add a nicardipine infusion (Table 21.3) at 5 mg/h, and increase the infusion rate by 2.5 mg/h every 10 min to a maximum of 15 mg/h.

Intracerebral haemorrhage

- If the patient presents within 6 h of the onset of intracerebral haemorrhage, with systolic BP >150 mmHg, start antihypertensive therapy.
- Target systolic BP is 140 mmHg within 6 h and maintained for at least 7 days. Ensure that the drop in BP does not exceed more than 60 mmHg within the first hour.
- Give labetalol or nicardipine by infusion (as for acute ischaemic stroke).
- Start or increase oral therapy.

Table 21.1 Focused assessment in severe hypertension.

History
- Is the patient known to have hypertension? What treatment has been given? What is the compliance with treatment? What investigations have been done to exclude an underlying cause for hypertension? Is there associated cardiac or renal disease?
- Pregnant or within three months of giving birth?
- Drug history? Recent use of drugs that may give hyperadrenergic state (e.g. cocaine, amphetamines and phencyclidine)?
- Any symptoms to suggest stroke or subarachnoid haemorrhage, aortic dissection, acute coronary syndrome and pulmonary oedema?

Examination
- Measure the blood pressure in both arms.
- Check for signs of heart failure and aortic regurgitation.
- Check the presence and symmetry of the major pulses, and for radio-femoral delay.
- Listen for carotid, abdominal and femoral bruits.
- Examine the abdomen (palpable kidneys or bladder?)
- Examine the fundi: are there retinal haemorrhages, exudates or papilloedema (not due to other causes), which define accelerated-phase or 'malignant' hypertension?
- Assess the conscious level and for focal neurological signs.

Table 21.2 Urgent investigation in severe hypertension.

Electrolytes and renal function (check daily)
Blood glucose
Plasma renin/aldosterone (for later analysis)
Plasma troponin, if acute coronary syndrome suspected
Plasma BNP or NT-proBNP, if heart failure suspected
Full blood count
Urine stick test and microscopy (renal impairment with minimal proteinuria suggests renal artery stenosis)
Ultrasonography of kidneys and urinary tract
Urinary catecholamine excretion
Urinary free cortisol excretion if Cushing syndrome suspected
Chest X-ray
ECG
Echocardiography, if heart failure suspected
Computed tomography (CT) or magnetic resonance imaging (MRI) of the brain, if there are neurological symptoms, headache, nausea and vomiting, or retinal haemorrhages, exudates or papilloedema
Contrast-enhanced CT of the chest, if aortic dissection is suspected.

Table 21.3 Intravenous therapy for severe hypertension with organ damage.

Drug	Properties	Administration
Labetalol	Beta- and alpha-adrenergic blocker	IV bolus: 10–20 mg over 1–2 min IV infusion: 1–8 mg/min (see text)
Esmolol	Short-acting beta-adrenergic blocker	IV bolus: 1 mg/kg over 30 s IV infusion: 150–300 μgm/kg/min (see text)
Isosorbide dinitrate	Nitric-oxide-mediated vasodilatation	IV infusion: 2–12 mg/h (see text)
Nicardipine	Dihydropyridine calcium-channel blocker	IV infusion: 5–15 mg/h (see text)
Phentolamine	Short-acting non-selective alpha-adrenergic blocker	IV bolus: 1 mg (response is maximal in 2–3 min and lasts 10–15 min) IV infusion: 1 mg/h

Subarachnoid haemorrhage

- Make sure adequate analgesia has been given.
- If systolic BP is >160 mmHg, start antihypertensive therapy.
- Target systolic BP is <160 mmHg.
- Give labetalol or nicardipine by infusion (as for acute ischaemic stroke).
- See Chapter 53 for further management of subarachnoid haemorrhage.

Hypertensive encephalopathy

- This is rare. Hypertensive encephalopathy is due to cerebral oedema resulting from hyperperfusion, as a consequence of severe hypertension, with failure of autoregulation of cerebral blood flow. Clinical features are summarized in Table 21.3.
- It may be difficult to distinguish clinically between hypertensive encephalopathy, subarachnoid haemorrhage and stroke. Hypertensive encephalopathy is favoured by the gradual onset of symptoms and the absence (or late appearance) of focal neurological signs. CT should be done to exclude other diagnoses. In hypertensive encephalopathy, neurological status improves with lowering of blood pressure.
- Target BP is 10–20% lower than initial BP after 1 h of therapy, and 25% lower after 24 h.
- Give labetalol or nicardipine by infusion, as for ischaemic stroke.
- Start or increase oral therapy.

Acute heart failure

- Treat with a nitrate infusion plus a loop diuretic IV (e.g. furosemide 40 mg initially).
- See Chapter 14 for further management of acute pulmonary oedema and acute heart failure.

Acute coronary syndrome

- Make sure adequate analgesia has been given.
- Treat with a nitrate infusion plus esmolol IV (Table 21.3).
- See Chapter 12 for further management of acute coronary syndromes. Revascularisation is the priority in acute coronary syndrome with ST-segment elevation.

Phaeochromocytoma hypertensive crisis

- See Chapter 17 for the diagnosis and management of phaeochromocytoma.
- Treat with phentolamine IV (Table 21.3). Seek expert advice from an endocrinologist.

Table 21.4 Hypertensive encephalopathy

Early features
- Headache
- Nausea and vomiting
- Delirium
- Retinal haemorrhages, exudates or papilloedema

Late features
- Focal neurological signs
- Fits
- Coma

Suspected pre-eclampsia/eclampsia: pregnant or within three months of giving birth

- The diagnosis of pre-eclampsia/eclampsia is discussed in Chapter 103.
- Seek urgent advice from an obstetrician.
- Target BP is 130–150/80–100 mmHg.
- Give labetalol 20 mg IV bolus over 2 min, followed by an infusion of 1–2 mg/min.
- If there is pulmonary oedema, add nitrate IV.

Cocaine-induced hypertension

- Sedation with a benzodiazepine is the preferred initial treatment for cocaine-induced hypertension.
- Target diastolic BP is 100–105 mmHg within 2–6 h.
- Blood pressure will fall as cocaine is metabolized. If treatment in addition to benzodiazepine is needed, use phentolamine IV.

Other patients with BP > 180/110 mmHg

1 Recheck the blood pressure after the patient has rested for 30 min in a quiet room. Admit for investigation and management if there are any of the following features:
   - Retinal haemorrhages, exudates or papilloedema.
   - Acute kidney injury.
   - Interstitial pulmonary oedema.
   - Diastolic pressure > 130 mmHg.
2 Start or increase oral therapy. Aim to reduce BP to 160/100 mmHg over the first 24 h:
   - Initial therapy for the patient who is not already receiving anti-hypertensive therapy is given in Table 21.5.
   - Nifedipine MR should be co-administered with amlodipine for the first three days of treatment with amlodipine (as amlodipine has a large volume of distribution and is therefore of limited efficacy during this period).
   - For patients already on treatment, check compliance, prescribe usual treatment at increased dose if appropriate, or add an agent from another class. If the patient is already taking triple therapy with an ACE-inhibitor or angiotensin-receptor blocker, a calcium-channel blocker and a thiazide, consider adding spironolactone 25–50 mg daily.

Table 21.5 Initial oral therapy for severe hypertension in a patient not already receiving anti-hypertensive therapy.

Clinical setting	Drug therapy
Phaeochromocytoma suspected (see Table 21.6)	Labetalol 100–200 mg 12-hourly PO
Renal artery stenosis suspected (see Table 21.6)	Amlodipine* 5–10 mg daily PO plus Bisoprolol 2.5–5 mg daily PO
Heart failure (see Chapter 14)	Amlodipine* 5–10 mg daily PO plus Furosemide 20–40 mg daily PO
Other patients, either with type 2 diabetes (of any age or family origin) or aged < 55 but not of Black African or African–Caribbean heritage	ACE-inhibitor (ACEi) or angiotensin-receptor blocker (ARB) ARB should be given in preference to ACEi to patients of Black African or African–Caribbean family origin
Other patients without type 2 diabetes, aged > 55 or of Black African or African–Caribbean heritage	Calcium-channel blocker or thiazide (if fluid retention present)

* Nifedipine MR should be co-administered with amlodipine for the first three days of treatment with amlodipine (as amlodipine has a large volume of distribution, and is therefore of limited efficacy during this period).

Table 21.6 Causes of secondary hypertension.

Cause	Clues/investigation
Intrinsic renal disease	May have family history of heritable renal disease (e.g. polycystic kidney disease)
	Abnormal urine stick test and microscopy
	Raised creatinine
	Abnormal kidneys on ultrasound
	Discuss further investigation with nephrologist if intrinsic renal disease suspected
Primary	Low plasma potassium
hyperaldosteronism	High plasma aldosterone with suppressed plasma renin
	Typically due to aldosterone-producing adenoma or bilateral adrenal hyperplasia
Cushing syndrome	Truncal obesity, thin skin with purple abdominal striae, proximal myopathy
	Increased urinary-free cortisol excretion
	Due to pituitary or adrenal disease, or exogenous corticosteroid
Phaeochromocytoma	Paroxysmal headache, sweating or palpitation
	Hypertensive crisis following anaesthesia or administration of contrast
	May have family history of pheochromocytoma
	Increased urinary catecholamine excretion
Coarctation of aorta	Radiofemoral delay
	Coarctation demonstrated by echocardiography, CT or MRI
Renal artery stenosis	May be due to fibromuscular dysplasia (age < 50 with no family history of hypertension) or, more commonly, to atherosclerosis (age > 50 with other atherosclerotic arterial disease)
	Refractory hypertension
	Deteriorating blood pressure control in compliant, long-standing hypertensive patients
	Rise in creatinine on treatment with ACE-inhibitor
	Renal impairment with minimal proteinuria
	Low plasma potassium due to secondary hyperaldosteronism
	Difference in kidney size >1.5 cm on ultrasound
Other causes	Many causes including drugs, obstructive sleep apnoea, acromegaly

3 What is causing severe hypertension?

Causes of secondary hypertension, and clues to specific diagnoses, are summarized in Table 21.6.

4 Seek advice from a nephrologist if there is

- Acute kidney injury or chronic kidney disease.
- Evidence of acute glomerulonephritis or vasculitis (2+ or more proteinuria and/or red cell casts in the urine).
- Suspected renal artery stenosis (see Table 21.6).
- Suspected scleroderma renal crisis (a complication of systemic sclerosis characterised by hypertension with acute kidney injury, microangiopathic haemolytic anaemia and thrombocytopenia and hypertensive retinopathy; hypertensive encephalopathy, acute heart failure and acute pericarditis may also be present).

Further reading

Kulkarni S, Glover G, Kapil V, *et al.* (2023) Management of hypertensive crisis: British and Irish Hypertension Society position document. *J Hum Hypertens* 37, 863–879.

Miller JB, Hrabec D, Krishnamoorthy V, *et al.* (2024) Evaluation and management of hypertensive emergency. *BMJ* 386, e077205.

Respiratory Medicine

CHAPTER 22

Acute asthma

SWAPNA MANDAL

Asthma (Box 22.1) is one of the most common causes of breathlessness and wheeze, but other causes should be considered, especially if the response to initial treatment is slow (Table 22.1).

The severity of an attack is easily underestimated (Table 22.2).

It is important to establish the severity of the exacerbation to monitor progress and determine if early involvement of the intensive care team is required.

Priorities

Is this acute asthma? If so, how severe?

Many other diseases can mimic acute asthma (Table 22.1). Important diagnoses to consider include:

An **exacerbation of chronic obstructive pulmonary disease** (Chapter 23). The patient tends to be older, with a smoking history.

Upper airway obstruction (Chapter 105). PEF is disproportionately lower than the FEV_1.

Vocal cord dysfunction. Symptoms can be similar to asthma, but usually the periods of breathlessness are short, with difficulty in inspiration (as opposed to expiration in asthma).

Anaphylaxis may also present with wheeze and breathlessness, but typically there are additional features such as urticarial rash and hypotension (Chapter 4).

The severity of acute asthma can be judged by the clinical features and PEF (Table 22.2).

Box 22.1 Asthma.

- Asthma is characterized by variable airway obstruction and defined by the presence of one or more of the following symptoms: breathlessness, wheeze, chest tightness or cough, with reversible airway obstruction shown by diurnal variation in peak expiratory flow >25%.
- The National Review of Asthma Deaths has shown that the United Kingdom has one of the highest death rates for asthma in Europe, with 195 deaths attributable to an acute exacerbation between 2012 and 2013.
- Acute asthma is diagnosed by worsening symptoms with associated signs and a reduction in the patient's usual peak expiratory flow (PEF).

Acute Medicine: A Practical Guide to the Management of Medical Emergencies, Sixth Edition.
Edited by Mridula Rajwani, Leila Vaziri, and Ivie Gbinigie.
© 2026 John Wiley & Sons Ltd. Published 2026 by John Wiley & Sons Ltd.

Table 22.1 Differential diagnosis of acute asthma.

Disorder	Comment
Acute exacerbation of chronic obstructive pulmonary disease	A relevant smoking history will assist in differentiating between an exacerbation of asthma and an exacerbation of Chronic Obstructive Pulmonary Disease (COPD).
Upper airway obstruction	These individuals may have a more chronic course; however, they may present acutely, for example inhalation of a foreign body or acute anaphylaxis. The key in determining the differences will be in the history. In a more chronic setting, flow-volume loops are very helpful.
Vocal cord dysfunction	Acutely Vocal Cord Dysfunction (VCD) can present in a similar manner to acute asthma. It can be difficult to differentiate VCD from asthma as some patients with VCD may also have asthma and respond to acute treatment. Arterial blood gases will be normal in VCD and often patients with VCD find inspiration more difficult than expiration.
Anaphylaxis	Individuals with anaphylaxis can have wheeze and allergy is common in those with asthma. The key to determining the difference will be the history, that is, an acute trigger in those with anaphylaxis and other signs such as an urticarial rash and angioedema. Treatment for both will include bronchodilators and steroids. Individuals with anaphylaxis will also require adrenaline.
In atypical histories, signs or symptoms, other important diagnoses to consider:	
Gastro-oesophageal reflux	This often presents more chronically as a cough; however, gastro-oesophageal reflux can exacerbate symptoms of asthma.
Cystic fibrosis	This is an inherited disorder resulting in deficiency of the cystic fibrosis transmembrane receptor. These individuals often have bronchiectasis and can also develop cystic fibrosis-related asthma and can therefore present with wheeze and cough. Often these patients will also have thick sputum that can be difficult to expectorate, this would be an unusual finding in those with asthma that is not related to CF.
Heart failure	Heart failure can also present with breathlessness and wheeze. The history is key, the symptoms are often progressive over a period of time, heart failure tends to occur in the older population and those with a significant history of cardiac disease. These individuals will respond well to diuresis.
Foreign body aspiration	There will often be a very acute history involving a feeling of 'choking' whilst having eaten something. If the foreign body is lodged within the upper airway and there is complete obstruction, respiratory arrest may occur. Partial obstruction of the upper airway may cause stridor. If the foreign body passes below the carina a more chronic course of symptoms will occur, such as cough, wheeze and recurrent infection.
Eosinophilic lung disease	Eosinophilic pneumonias are a group of disorders characterized by peripheral blood eosinophilia and evidence of eosinophilia within the airways. Causes of eosinophilic pneumonia include: helminth and tropical infections; medication such as non-steroidal anti-inflammatory drugs (NSAIDs) and antibiotics; Churg–Strauss syndrome (eosinophilic granulomatosis with polyangiitis); ABPA and idiopathic eosinophilic pneumonias. The history and searching for a trigger, for example medication or travel to endemic areas will assist in the diagnosis. These individuals tend to present with a chronic course of symptoms and blood tests, and often bronchoscopy/lung biopsy may be necessary to clinch the diagnosis. Many of these conditions will respond to steroid treatment.

Immediate management

All patients presenting with an acute exacerbation of asthma should receive **oxygen** therapy to maintain an arterial oxygen saturation between 94 and 98% (Figure 22.1).

High-dose nebulized **β-agonists** (5 mg **salbutamol**) should be given as quickly as possible (the nebulizer should preferably be driven by oxygen); doses can be repeated every 15–30 min.

Ipratropium bromide (500 mcg 6-hourly) can be given to those with acute severe or life-threatening asthma, or in those who have a poor initial response to salbutamol.

Table 22.2 Assessment of severity of acute asthma.

	Moderate exacerbation of asthma	Acute severe asthma	Life-threatening asthma
Symptoms	Worsening chest tightness, breathlessness, wheeze, cough	Worsening chest tightness, breathlessness, wheeze, cough	
PEF Physiological variables	50–75% of best/predicted	33–50% of best/predicted RR > 25 breaths/min HR > 110 breaths/min	<33% of best/predicted $SaO_2 < 92\%$ $PaO_2 < 8\,kPa$ $PaCO_2$ 4.6–6.0 kPa
Other signs		Unable to complete sentences in one breath	Reduced GCS Exhaustion Silent chest Cyanosis Poor respiratory effort Arrhythmia Hypotension

Source: Adapted from BTS/SIGN/NICE guidelines.

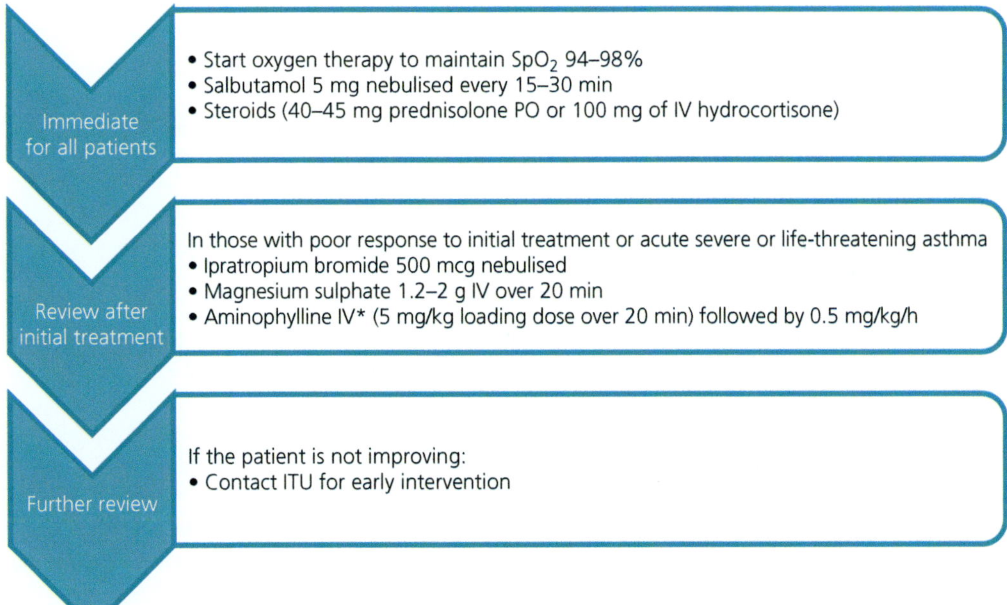

Figure 22.1 Management of acute asthma. Source: Adapted from BTS/SIGN/NICE guidelines.

Corticosteroids should be administered immediately. Either 40–50 mg of oral prednisolone daily or hydro-cortisone 100 mg 6-hourly IV or IM should be given. Corticosteroids should be given for a minimum of 5 days.

In those with acute severe asthma with poor response to initial therapy or life-threatening asthma, a single dose of **magnesium sulphate** (1.2–2 g IV over 20 min) can be given.

Aminophylline may be considered in those with life-threatening asthma where there has been poor response to treatment and discussion with senior medical staff has taken place. A loading dose of 5 mg/kg should be given parenterally over 20 min (omit if the patient is on oral aminophylline) followed by an infusion of 0.5 mg/kg/h.

Consider referral to ITU if: hypoxia worsens, hypercapnia or acidaemia is evident, the patient is exhausting, GCS is deteriorating or PEF is deteriorating.

Non-invasive ventilation (NIV) is **not** recommended for asthma and should not be given outside the intensive care environment.

Other treatments

- Antibiotics may be considered in those with signs of infection but should not be routinely used in the management of acute asthma.
- Patients who are dehydrated may require IV fluids.

Investigations and monitoring

Whilst treating these patients, investigations can be initiated, these include (Table 22.3):
- PEF (once the patient is stabilized PEF should continue to be monitored).
- Arterial blood gas (ABG).
- Serum electrolytes (as patients will be receiving salbutamol, they may become hypokalaemic).
- Chest X-ray to rule out exacerbating factors including pneumothorax or pneumonia.

Further management

All patients with life-threatening asthma must be admitted. Those with moderate or acute severe asthma may be considered for discharge home (Figure 22.2). Pitfalls to avoid are summarised in Box 22.2.

Asthma in pregnancy

Asthma control can deteriorate in pregnancy. Pregnant women with acute asthma should be treated in exactly the same manner as those who are not pregnant. In addition, there should be continuous foetal monitoring and involvement of the obstetric team.

Table 22.3 Monitoring of the patient with acute asthma.

Regular monitoring	To be monitored as required
Peak expiratory flow rate	ABG (initially if SpO_2 <92% and repeat after treatment)
SaO_2	Serum theophylline concentrations
Respiratory rate	Serum electrolytes
Heart rate	

<table>
<tr><td>Moderate asthma</td><td>Acute severe asthma</td><td>Life threatening asthma</td></tr>
<tr><td>↓</td><td>↓</td><td>↓</td></tr>
<tr><td>If after initial treatment:
Patient is clinically stable
AND
PEF >75%</td><td>Patient will require initial inpatient admission for observation and monitoring and continued treatment.
If patient stabilises AND PEF >50%
OR
Patient stable after initial treatment AND PEFR >75%</td><td>All patients with life threatening asthma will require **ADMISSION** with early ICU involvement</td></tr>
<tr><td>↓</td><td>↓</td><td></td></tr>
<tr><td>Consider discharge home with prednisolone 40–50 mg for 5 days and early GP follow up (2 days) and referral to chest clinic
If above criteria not met **ADMIT** patient</td><td>Consider discharge home with prednisolone 40–50 mg for 5 days and early GP follow up (2 days) and referral to chest clinic
If above criteria not met or ongoing signs of severe or life threatening asthma **ADMIT**</td><td></td></tr>
</table>

Figure 22.2 Discharge planning of the patient with acute asthma. Source: Adapted from BTS/SIGN guidelines.

Box 22.2 Pitfalls in the management of acute asthma.

- Be vigilant for pneumothoraces; small ones may be difficult to detect.
- Beware of the tiring patient. Escalate treatment and involve the ICU team if:
  - Wheeze disappears: this is a silent chest not an improvement in symptoms.
  - $PaCO_2$ normalizes.
- If you are giving a one-off stat dose of IV hydrocortisone, ensure you give a dose of oral prednisolone also.
- Ensure at discharge that:
  - Inhaled corticosteroid is started in addition to a course of oral steroids.
  - Inhaler technique is checked.
  - Smoking cessation advice given if necessary.
  - A peak flow meter is given to continue monitoring.
  - Specialist follow-up is arranged (urgently for those with an acute, severe or life-threatening episode).

Further reading

British Thoracic Society and Scottish Intercollegiate Guidelines Network (2016) British guideline on the management of asthma: a national clinical guideline. Available from https://www.brit-thoracic.org.uk/document-library/clinical-information/asthma/btssign-asthma-guideline-2016/.

CHAPTER 23

Exacerbation of chronic obstructive pulmonary disease (COPD)

Jo Riley

An exacerbation of chronic obstructive pulmonary disease (COPD) is defined as an event characterised by dyspnoea and/or cough and sputum that worsen over <14 days. These are often associated with increased inflammation locally in the lungs and systemically, caused by airway infection (in approx. 60–70% of cases), pollution or other insults to the lungs.

Patients will present with increased dyspnoea which is a key symptom, and increased mucus production – often purulent, together with cough and wheezing.

For patients admitted to hospital with an exacerbation of COPD, mortality at 30 days is 6.1%, increasing to 11.9% at 90 days post admission, with 43% of patients being readmitted within 90 days (NACAP Clinical Outcomes Report 2023).

COPD exacerbations are associated with a decline in lung function, worsening quality of life and therefore increased burden on patients and their carers.

COPD often exists alongside other co-morbidities particularly cardiac disease which can make diagnosis more complex. When assessing patients, it is important to look for other causes of the patients' symptoms including pneumonia, PE, decompensated heart failure, and less often, pneumothorax, pleural effusion or myocardial infarction.

Priorities

The working diagnosis is made in patients with a known or suspected diagnosis of COPD with symptoms that are acute within days and worse than normal day-to-day variation in symptoms. Alternate diagnosis should be addressed especially when symptoms are less typical.

Obtain history

Known COPD? Post bronchodilator FEV1/VC <70% (or below lower limit of normal).

- FEV1 >80% predicted = Mild (or stage 1);
- FEV1 50–79% predicted = Moderate (or stage 2);
- FEV1 30–49% predicted = Severe (or stage 3);
- FEV1 <30% predicted = Very Severe (or stage 4).

Features suggestive of an acute exacerbation include:

- Worsening breathlessness.
- Increased sputum volume and purulence.
- Cough.

- Wheeze.
- Fever without an obvious source.
- Upper respiratory tract infection in the past 5 days.
- Respiratory rate or heart rate increased more than 20% above baseline.

A severe exacerbation may be suggested by:
- Marked breathlessness and tachypnoea.
- Pursed-lip breathing and/or use of accessory muscles at rest.
- New-onset cyanosis or peripheral oedema.
- Acute confusion or drowsiness.
- Marked reduction in activities of daily living.

Carry out a thorough clinical assessment:
- Check vital signs (including temperature, oxygen saturations [using pulse oximetry], blood pressure and heart rate).
- Assess for confusion or impaired consciousness.
- Examine the chest. Accessory muscle use, hyperinflated chest, added lung sounds and reduced breath sounds
- Evidence of cor pulmonale – oedema
- Evidence of hypercapnia – asterixis (flapping tremor), bounding pulse and excessively flushed.

Further information
- Check ability to cope at home.
- Consider pre-hospital treatment – antibiotics and/or oral corticosteroids.
- Usual inhaler usage – increased use of short-acting bronchodilator or decreased efficacy.
- Co-morbidities.
- Exacerbation frequency.
- Home oxygen therapy and/or home non-invasive ventilation (NIV).
- Previous NIV or mechanical ventilation.

Investigations
In all patients assessed in hospital with an acute exacerbation of COPD (1)
- Obtain a chest X-ray.
- Measure arterial blood gas tensions and record the inspired oxygen concentration.
- Record an electrocardiogram (ECG) (to exclude co-morbidities).
- Perform a full blood count and measure urea and electrolyte concentrations.
- Measure a theophylline level on admission in patients taking regular theophylline therapy.
- Send a sputum sample for microscopy, culture and sensitivities if the sputum is purulent.
- Take blood cultures if the patient has pyrexia.
- Refer patient for respiratory review within first 24 h of admission (evidence for shorter length of stay, reduced mortality and reduced risk of readmission).

Management
Oxygen
- Administer controlled oxygen – starting with 28% oxygen via venturi mask.
- Aim for peripheral oxygen saturations whilst breathing supplemental oxygen to be 88–92% until arterial blood gas is available to guide treatment (if the first blood gas is a venous sample, arterial sample must be obtained if acidosis is present [pH < 7.35]).

- Monitor for signs of oxygen-induced hypercapnic encephalopathy, particularly decreases in respiratory rate and conscious level – repeat arterial blood gas (ABG) if this occurs and consider reducing FiO_2 if hypercapnic and pO_2 >8 kPa.
- If PaO_2 <8 kPa and the patient has respiratory acidosis, consider NIV if no improvement within 1 h of optimal medical treatment (bronchodilators and corticosteroids) (Figure 23.1 and Chapter 113).

Bronchodilators

- Give nebulised salbutamol 2.5 mg 4 hourly, and initially back-to-back for severe breathlessness and wheeze.
- Consider increasing the usual dose of short-acting bronchodilator (salbutamol usually) to up to 10 doses via spacer 4 hourly for patients with moderate breathlessness.

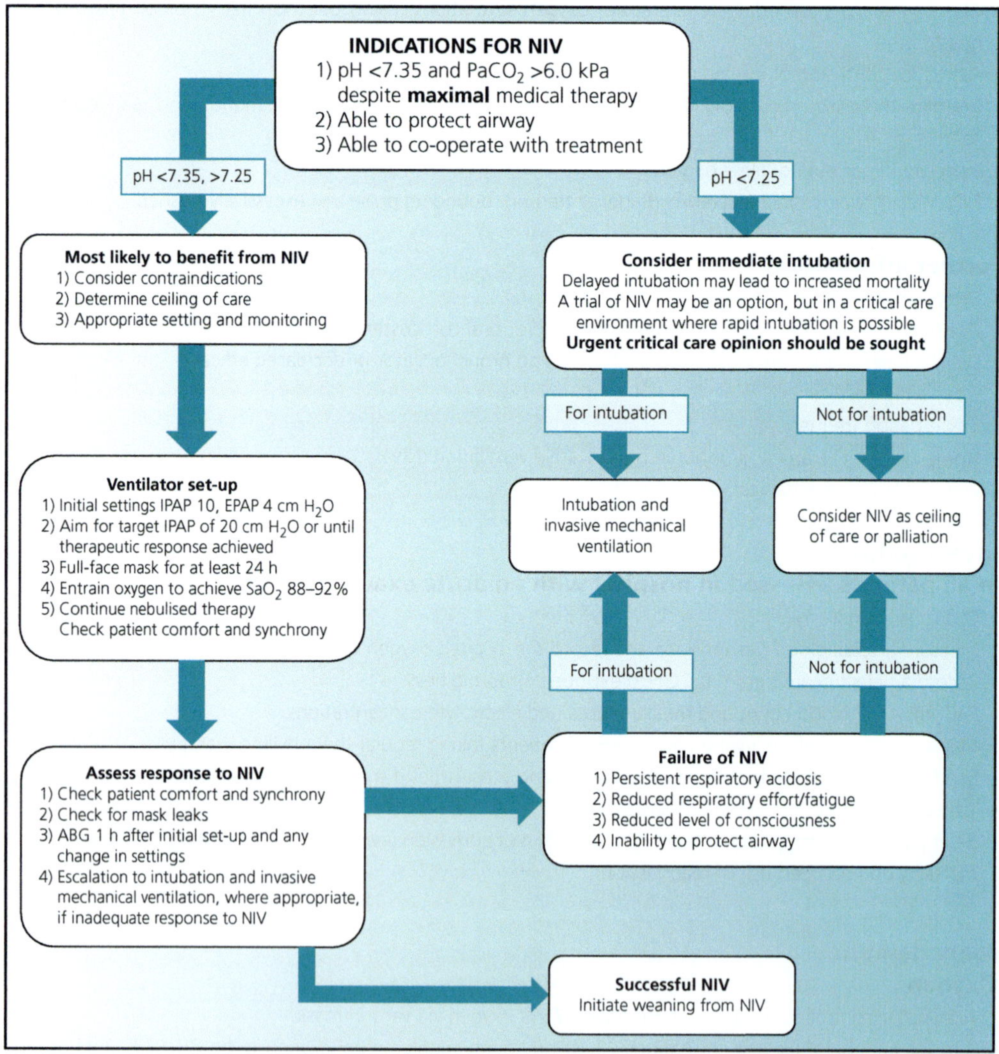

Figure 23.1 Algorithm for the use of NIV in acute exacerbations of COPD. IPAP, inspiratory positive airway pressure; EPAP, expiratory positive airway pressure.

- Add nebulised ipratropium 500 mcg 4 times/day for severely breathless patients – If continuing for more than 24 h, stop patient's usual long-acting antimuscarinic inhaler for the duration of Ipratropium therapy – Consider switching triple therapy inhaler to Inhaled Corticosteroid (ICS)/Long acting Beta 2 agonist (LABA) for the duration of ipratropium.
- If a person with COPD is hypercapnic or acidotic the nebuliser should be driven by compressed air rather than oxygen (to avoid worsening hypercapnia). If oxygen therapy is needed, administer it simultaneously by nasal cannulae (ensure this is prescribed).
- Change patient back to inhaled therapy at the earliest opportunity to expedite discharge.

Corticosteroids

- Give prednisolone 30 mg daily for 5 days (discuss longer courses with respiratory specialists for patients with blood eosinophil count >0.3 × 10^9/L and persistent wheeze/breathlessness).
- Hydrocortisone (100 – 200 mcg IV 6 hourly) would only be considered for patients unable to swallow tablets.
- In the presence of radiographic consolidation, patient should be treated as having pneumonia. Data to support the use of oral corticosteroids in patients with pneumonia suggests that this may prevent the need for mechanical ventilation but requires more study regarding potential adverse effects (2).

Antibiotic therapy

- Indicated in patients where there is an increase in sputum purulence above their usual status, radiological evidence of pneumonia or CRP > 20 mg/L if no evidence of pneumonia.
- Amoxycillin, doxycycline or macrolides would be first-line treatment choice (or according to local policy).
- Consider intravenous antibiotics in severely unwell patients.
- Review sputum and blood culture results when available – only change antibiotic if bacteria are resistant and no indication of clinical improvement.
- Previous recent sputum results can be used to guide antibiotic choice in patients with frequent infective exacerbations.

Aminophylline

- Use under expert guidance – only use intravenous theophylline as an adjunct to exacerbation management if there is an inadequate response to nebulised bronchodilators.
- Take care when using intravenous theophylline, because of its interactions with other drugs and potential toxicity if patient has been taking oral theophylline.
- For patients who are not taking theophylline orally, provide loading dose 250 – 500 mg IV (5 mg/kg) over 20 min.
- Continue 0.5 mg/kg/h IV infusion until clinical improvement.
- Check theophylline levels within 24 h of commencing therapy and then as often as clinically indicated.

Non-invasive ventilation

- In acute hypercapnic respiratory failure complicating an exacerbation of COPD, NIV improves survival, reduces intubation rates and reduces the length of ITU stay. The highest survival rates are achieved with onset of NIV within 1 h of failure to improve using conventional therapy for acute exacerbation of COPD.
- Use NIV as the treatment of choice for persistent hypercapnic ventilatory failure during exacerbations despite optimal medical therapy.
- The use of NIV should not delay escalation to Invasive Mechanical Ventilation (IMV) where this is more appropriate.
- It is recommended that NIV should be delivered in a dedicated setting, with staff who have been trained in its application, who are experienced in its use and who are aware of its limitations.

- When people are started on NIV there should be a clear plan covering what to do in the event of deterioration, and ceilings of therapy should be agreed.
- Time on NIV should be maximised in the first 24h depending on patient tolerance and/or complications.
- Improved survival is seen in those whose respiratory rate and pH are seen to improve within 4h of therapy.

Establishing ceiling of care

Predicting survival in COPD patients who require admission to the ICU is difficult: clinicians' estimates of mortality are variable, inaccurate and generally pessimistic.

Any decision to limit the escalation of care should be made by a senior physician, taking into account the patient's wishes expressed during or before hospital admission. A ruling by the Court of Appeal in England and Wales in 2014 now places a legal obligation on physicians to consult with patients before making do-not-attempt-resuscitation orders.

Age, arterial blood pH and reduced conscious level are predictive of mortality. Functional status, body mass index, requirement for supplemental oxygen when stable, co-morbidities and previous admissions to the ICU should also be considered when assessing whether IMV is appropriate.

Further management

Supportive care

- Ensure a fluid intake of 2–3 L/day.
- Check electrolytes the day after admission. Salbutamol and steroids may result in significant hypokalaemia. Give potassium supplement if the plasma level is <3.5 mmol/L.
- Refer for chest physiotherapy to aid with airway clearance, particularly if there is mucus plugging with lobar atelectasis.
- DVT prophylaxis with stockings/LMW heparin. Assess/treat co-morbidities, for example atrial fibrillation and congestive heart failure.
- Encourage early mobilisation to reduce the risk of deconditioning.

If the patient is not improving, consider:

- Wrong diagnosis: reconsider pneumonia, heart failure and pulmonary embolism. Other causes of respiratory failure with raised $PaCO_2$ are given in Table 23.1. Echocardiography is indicated to exclude left ventricular dysfunction.

Table 23.1 Alternate diagnosis to consider in patients with suspected COPD exacerbation.

Most Frequent	**Pneumonia**
	Chest X-ray
	Pulmonary Embolism
	Assess for risk factors (surgery, immobility, fracture, history of cancer and DVT)
	D-dimer
	CT pulmonary angiography
	Heart Failure
	Chest X-ray
	NT pro-brain natriuretic peptide (ProBNP) and BNP
	Echocardiography
Less frequent	**Pneumothorax, Pleural effusion**
	Chest X-ray
	Thoracic ultrasound
	Atrial Fibrillation, Myocardial infarction
	Electrocardiography ECG
	Troponin

- Missed pneumothorax.
- Inadequately treated infection. Consider changing to cefuroxime or cefotaxime IV and adding a macrolide.
- Inadequate bronchodilator therapy. Check that nebulisers are being run at the correct flow rate. Nebulised salbutamol can be given 2-hourly if necessary, or salbutamol can be given by IV infusion 5–30 mg/min.
- Cor pulmonale. Fluid retention with peripheral oedema may occur in patients with COPD complicated by acute or chronic respiratory failure even without right ventricular dysfunction. The diagnosis of cor pulmonale is made from a raised JVP, enlarged cardiac silhouette on the chest X-ray, and ECG evidence of right ventricular hypertrophy (not an invariable feature). Obtain an echocardiogram to confirm right ventricular dysfunction, estimate pulmonary artery pressures and exclude left ventricular or aortic/mitral valve disease. Treat fluid retention with a diuretic. There is no definite evidence for the use of digoxin (unless indicated for rate control in atrial fibrillation) or ACE inhibitors in cor pulmonale. Resistant cor pulmonale raises the suspicion of obstructive sleep apnoea.

Arrhythmias

- Supraventricular arrhythmias are common in acute exacerbations of COPD. Check plasma potassium: salbutamol and steroids may result in significant hypokalaemia. Give potassium replacement if plasma potassium is <3.5 mmol/L.
- Treat atrial fibrillation/flutter with digoxin, combined if needed with verapamil or diltiazem. Treat multifocal atrial tachycardia with verapamil if the ventricular rate is >110/min. DC cardioversion is ineffective.

Chest pain

- Chest pain from coronary disease occurs in acute exacerbations of COPD and may be caused by hypoxia, sepsis or tachycardia. A rise and fall in troponin T may also occur without chest pain or acute ECG changes.
- Ask for advice from a cardiologist. There is evidence that a beta blocker, aspirin and a statin improve outcome.
- Further cardiac investigation with a functional test may be indicated in individual cases.

Ensuring safe discharge

- Patients should be off intravenous therapy for >24h before discharge and established on discharge medication.
- COPD discharge bundle should be completed following every COPD admission – This includes:
  - Referral for early post-exacerbation pulmonary rehabilitation.
  - Optimising therapy.
  - Checking inhaler technique and changing devices when indicated.
  - Addressing ongoing smoking and providing support.
  - Arranging respiratory review and support in the community following discharge where community services exist.
  - Prescribing rescue packs of antibiotics and oral corticosteroids for patients with frequent exacerbations.
  - Providing self-management education.
  - Counselling regarding vaccination for Flu, pneumonia and COVID-19.
- Check functional status in the context of the patients' home circumstances.
- Arrange social support where indicated
- Arrange primary care review within 1 week and refer for Chest Clinic review, ideally within 4–6 weeks.

References

1 NICE Scenario: acute exacerbation of chronic obstructive pulmonary disease revised May 2024 scenario: acute exacerbation|Management|Chronic obstructive pulmonary disease|CKS|NICE. Available from https://www.nice.org.uk/cks-uk-only. [Accessed 29 August 2024].

2 CHEST (2023) Effect of corticosteroids on mortality and clinical cure in community-acquired pneumonia. CHEST. chestnet.org. [Accessed 1 September 2024].

Further reading

Davidson AC, Banham S, Elliott M, *et al.* (2016) BTS/ICS guideline for the ventilatory management of acute hypercapnic respiratory failure in adults. *Thorax* 71(Supplement 2), ii1–ii35.

Global Initiative for Chronic obstructive Lung Disease Global strategy for prevention, diagnosis and management of COPF 2024 report 2024 GOLD report – global initiative for chronic obstructive lung disease – GOLD. Available from https://www.goldcopd.org. [Accessed 18 August 2024].

NACAP National Asthma and Chronic Obstructive lung Disease Audit Programme, clinical outcomes report 2018–2020. Published: 2023 – (NACAP_Outcomes_Summary_Report_2023_03.pdf). Available from https://www.nrap.org.uk. [Accessed 28 August 2024].

NICE COPD (acute exacerbation) antimicrobial prescribing 2018 overview | Chronic obstructive pulmonary disease (acute exacerbation): antimicrobial prescribing | Guidance | NICE. Available from https://www.nice.org.uk/guidance/ng114. [Accessed 1 September 2024].

NICE Quality standard chronic obstructive pulmonary disease in adults. Overview | Chronic obstructive pulmonary disease in adults | Quality standards | NICE. Published: 28 July 2011 Last updated: 19 September 2023. Available from https://www.nice.org.uk/guidance/qs10. [Accessed 24 August 2024].

CHAPTER 24

Haemoptysis

AHMED YOUSUF

Haemoptysis

Haemoptysis, deriving its name from the Greek words 'haima' (blood) and 'ptysis' (spitting), is the presence of blood within sputum and ranges from blood-streaking of sputum to gross blood in the absence of any accompanying sputum. The causes of haemoptysis are shown in Table 24.1.

The term life-threatening haemoptysis (formerly massive haemoptysis) was previously used to describe the expectoration of a large amount of blood within a particular period of time. However, criteria based solely on the volume of blood cannot be used precisely since quantifying the amount of blood that a patient has expectorated is challenging and small amounts in patients with underlying cardiorespiratory disease may be enough to endanger life. Therefore, in clinical practice the term 'life-threatening haemoptysis' is more useful. It pertains to cases that lead to airway obstruction, significant disruptions in gas exchange, or haemodynamic

Table 24.1 Causes of haemoptysis.

Cause	Comment
Bronchogenic carcinoma*	Frank haemoptysis or blood-stained sputum, weight loss, cough, risk factors for lung cancer
Tuberculosis (TB)*	Cough, fever, night sweat, weight loss, risk factors for TB (e.g. homeless, from high prevalent countries)
Bronchiectasis*	Chronic cough with purulent sputum, known history of bronchiectasis, previous episodes of haemoptysis
Pneumonia*	'Rusty' sputum, fever, cough, consolidation on chest X-ray (CXR)
Pulmonary embolism (PE)	Pleuritic chest pain, breathlessness, risk factors for PE
Pulmonary oedema	Frothy 'pink' sputum, breathlessness, ↑JVP, bilateral pitting oedema of legs, raised NT-pro-BNP, pulmonary oedema on CXR
Vasculitides**	Granulomatosis with polyangiitis (formerly known as Wegner's), Goodpasture's syndrome, SLE
Mycetoma**	Fungal ball on CXR, previous TB
Arteriovenous malformation**	Recurrent haemoptysis, Osler–Weber–Rendu syndrome (telangiectasia)
Iatrogenic**	Post-lung biopsy or bronchoscopy

* Common.
** Rare.

Acute Medicine: A Practical Guide to the Management of Medical Emergencies, Sixth Edition.
Edited by Mridula Rajwani, Leila Vaziri, and Ivie Gbinigie.
© 2026 John Wiley & Sons Ltd. Published 2026 by John Wiley & Sons Ltd.

compromise. One limitation of this definition is that it excludes those patients with a good physiological reserve who can expectorate large volumes of blood without significant clinical deterioration during the early stages of life-threatening haemoptysis.

Assessment

The primary objectives of the initial assessment are to ascertain the extent and intensity of bleeding, pinpoint the origin of the bleeding and establish a list of potential diagnoses (Table 24.1).

History

A focused history is essential. This should evaluate the severity of haemoptysis and the clues pointing towards the underlying aetiology, including smoking history, existing medical conditions, medications (e.g. anti-coagulant) and family history.

Physical examination

A targeted physical examination should aim to gauge the extent of respiratory impairment, and identify clues of diseases beyond the respiratory system (e.g. telangiectasia indicating Osler–Weber–Rendu syndrome, skin rash may suggest underlying vasculitis).

Management

- Management is summarized in Figure 24.1. Haemoptysis can be distinguished from haematemesis by its colour and pH: haemoptysis is bright red and alkaline, haematemesis is brown ('coffee ground') and acidic. Bleeding from the nasopharynx may be mistaken for haemoptysis: if in doubt, ask the advice of ear, nose and throat (ENT) surgeon.

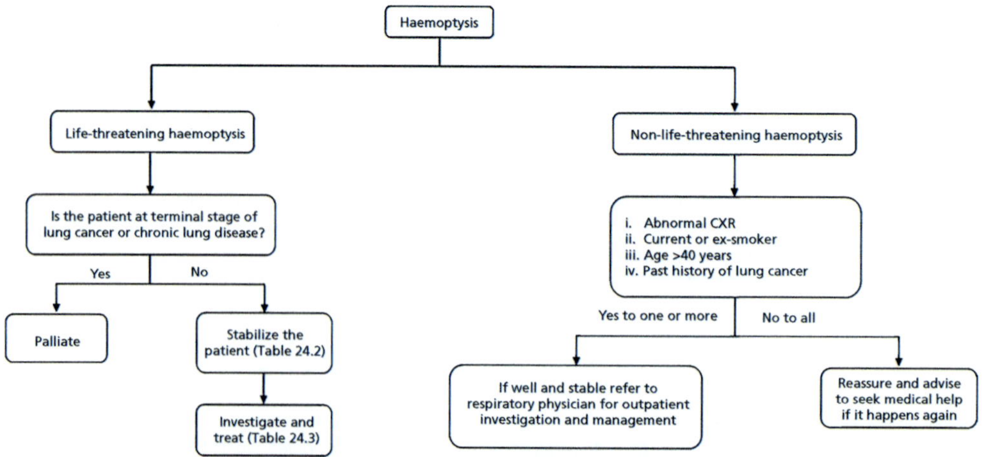

Figure 24.1 Management of haemoptysis.

Table 24.2 Management of life-threatening haemoptysis.

1. Airway protection and improving ventilation: this could be achieved by sitting up the patient, or lying the patient on the bleeding side (if known) to avoid spillage of blood to the unaffected lung. Give oxygen to maintain oxygen saturation above 94% (unless the patient is known to have chronic type 2 respiratory failure).
2. Cardiovascular support:
   - Insert two large bore (at least 16 gauge) cannulas.
   - Send blood for FBC/cross match/clotting screen/renal function.
   - Fluid resuscitation.
   - Blood transfusion (if Hb < 70 g/L).
   - Arterial +/− CVP line (in HDU/ICU setting).
3. Assess patient's GCS, if <8 or unable to protect airway, ask for anaesthetist's help.
4. Correct any clotting disorders as per hospital protocol.
5. Give IV tranexamic acid (1 g TDS, avoid if known renal failure).
6. Consider giving nebulized adrenaline (1 mL of 1 : 1000 with 4 mL of NaCl 0.9%).
7. Consider giving intravenous terlipressin (2 mg IV stat, then 1 mg IV every 4–6 h).

Once patient is stabilized arrange:

8. Bronchoscopy (flexible or rigid): diagnostic (biopsy, bronchial wash) and therapeutic interventions (e.g. injecting cold saline or 1 : 20,000 adrenaline, cryocautery and diathermy) can be undertaken.
9. Endovascular embolization: most effective and minimally invasive procedure in managing haemoptysis.
10. Surgery: resection of the bleeding lobe (if all other measures have failed).

Table 24.3 Investigation of haemoptysis.

Full blood count
Clotting screen
Renal function
ECG
Auto-antibodies (ANA, ANCA, anti-GBM), urine dip and microscopy for red cells casts (if vasculitides are suspected)
Arterial blood gases if O_2 saturation < 92%
CXR can help with lateralizing bleeding and may reveal a focal or diffuse lung involvement. It has 35–50% positive diagnostic yield. A quarter of patients presenting with haemoptysis due to malignancy will have normal CXR.
Sputum Ziehl–Neelsen stains and culture, if there is suspicion of TB.
CT scan – CT bronchial arteriography if bleeding is thought to be originating from bronchial circulation. If it does not identify the source of bleeding, and there is a high suspicion of the pulmonary artery source of bleeding, then CT pulmonary angiogram should be performed. Performing CT scan before bronchoscopy will improve diagnostic yield.
Bronchoscopy (flexible or rigid): it helps to visualize the airways and localize the site of bleeding.

- In the majority of cases, haemoptysis originates from the bronchial circulation. Bronchial arteries usually arise directly from the aorta and carry blood at systemic blood pressure. Therefore, bleeding that originates from bronchial circulation causes life-threatening haemoptysis; if left untreated it has a mortality rate of up to 80%. Management of life-threatening haemoptysis is summarized in Table 24.2.
- Investigation of haemoptysis is given in Table 24.3.

Management of life-threatening haemoptysis

The priority is to stabilize the patient, identify the bleeding site and stop the bleeding (Table 24.2). Active intervention is not appropriate for all patients and in some cases (e.g. metastatic lung cancer, end-stage chronic pulmonary or cardiac disease) a palliative approach might be the best option.

Further reading

Kathuria H, Hollingsworth HM, Vilvendhan R, Reardon C. (2020) Management of life-threatening hemoptysis. *J Intensive Care* 8, 23.

Larici AR, Franchi P, Occhipinti M. (2014) Diagnosis and management of hemoptysis. *Diagn Interv Radiol* 20, 299–309.

Radchenko C, Alraiyes AH, Shojaee S. (2017) A systemic approach to the management of massive hemoptysis. *J Thorac Dis* 9(Supplement 10), S1069–S1086.

CHAPTER 25

Respiratory infection: CAP, HAP and TB

AHMED YOUSUF

Community-acquired pneumonia

Community-acquired pneumonia (CAP) is a very common respiratory infectious disease. Incidence of CAP ranges between 1 and 25 cases per 1000 head of population per year. CAP (see Box 25.1 for definition) usually presents with acute respiratory symptoms, but should always be considered in patients with unexplained sepsis or delirium. Examination of the chest may be normal and, if you suspect pneumonia, a chest X-ray (CXR) is needed to make the diagnosis. Approximately 40% of patients with CAP will require hospitalisation, and 5% of these patients will be admitted to the intensive care unit (ICU). See Figure 25.1 for management of CAP.

A broad range of pathogens can cause CAP. *Streptococcus pneumoniae* (pneumococcus) is the main pathogen that causes CAP worldwide, independent of age. Other common pathogens are *Staphylococcus aureus*, *Haemophilus influenza* and the so-called atypical bacteria (*Mycoplasma pneumoniae*, *Chlamydia pneumoniae*, *Chlamydia psittaci* and *Coxiella burnetii*).

In recent years, the availability of molecular microbiological tests has increased isolation of respiratory viruses in CAP. In adults, viruses, particularly *influenza, rhinovirus and coronaviruses*, cause a third of cases of pneumonia.

Box 25.1 Definitions.

Community-acquired pneumonia (CAP): pneumonia acquired outside hospital, or which appears within 48 h of admission to hospital.

Hospital-acquired pneumonia (HAP): pneumonia that develops 48 h or longer after hospital admission, and was not subclinical on admission.

Lower respiratory tract infection: an acute illness with cough and at least one other lower respiratory tract symptom, presumed to be due to infection. The definition includes pneumonia, acute bronchitis and infective exacerbation of chronic obstructive pulmonary disease.

Acute Medicine: A Practical Guide to the Management of Medical Emergencies, Sixth Edition.
Edited by Mridula Rajwani, Leila Vaziri, and Ivie Gbinigie.
© 2026 John Wiley & Sons Ltd. Published 2026 by John Wiley & Sons Ltd.

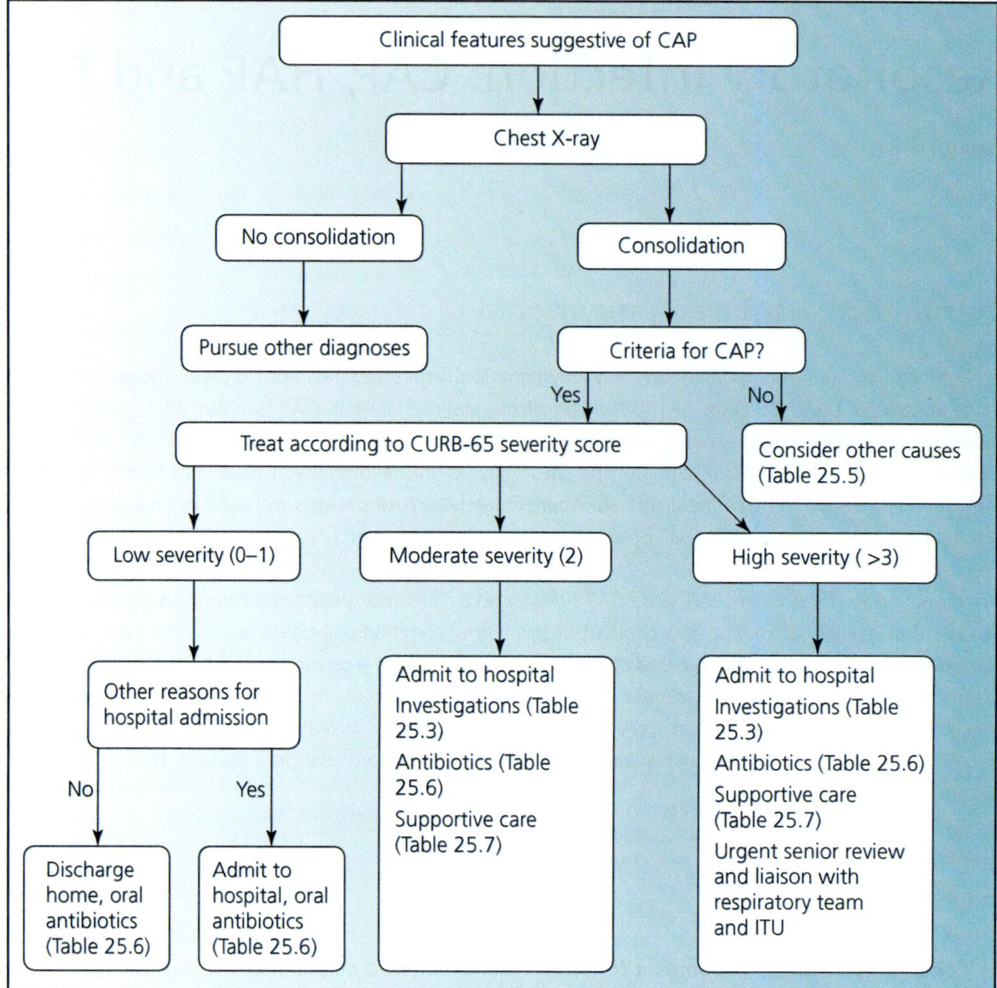

Figure 25.1 Management of suspected community-acquired pneumonia (CAP).

Priorities
Is this pneumonia? How severe is it?
- Suspect pneumonia in the presence of one or more of the following clinical features:
  - Fever
  - Cough
  - Purulent sputum
  - Dyspnoea
  - Pleuritic chest pain
  - Focal lung crackles or bronchial breathing
- Consider the differential diagnosis (Table 25.1). A CXR showing new focal shadowing is essential for the diagnosis (Table 25.2). Other investigations needed are given in Table 25.3.
- The severity of CAP can be assessed by the CURB-65 score (Table 25.4).

Table 25.1 Differential diagnosis of suspected pneumonia.

Disorder	Comment
Cardiovascular disorders	
Pulmonary embolism	Risk factor(s) for venous thromboembolism Sudden-onset shortness of breath See Chapter 31.
Tricuspid valve endocarditis	IVDU (intravenous drug user) or indwelling venous cannula e.g. for haemodialysis in blood cultures.
Neoplastic disorders	
Bronchial carcinoma	Weight loss, chronic cough, abnormal CXR (nodule or mass, mediastinal lymphadenopathy).
Alveolar cell carcinoma	Similar CXR appearance to pneumonia. If there is no leucocytosis or fever or if the patient doesn't respond to antibiotics.
Immune-mediated disorders	
Wegener granulomatosis	Haematuria, haemoptysis, epistaxis, scleritis, uveitis.
Diffuse alveolar haemorrhage	Haematuria, haemoptysis, positive anti-GBM (anti glomerular basement membrane antibodies), ANCA (antineutrophil cytoplasmic antibodies) antibodies.
Systemic lupus erythematosus	Skin rash, sensitivity to sunlight, positive ANA (antinuclear antibodies).
Acute interstitial pneumonia	Ground glass changes and traction bronchiectasis on HRCT (high resolution CT).
Eosinophilic pneumonia	Peripheral blood eosinophilia, peripheral infiltrate within the outer two-thirds of the lung fields on CXR, responds to steroids.
Organizing pneumonia	Acute to subacute onset of symptoms, migratory patchy infiltrates on CXR, responds to steroids.
Other disorders	
Drug toxicity (e.g. amiodarone pneumonitis)	Restrictive spirometry, decreased gas transfer, responds to steroids and stopping offending drug(s).
Radiation pneumonitis	History of recent radiotherapy, responds to steroids.

Table 25.2 Chest X-ray (CXR) findings in pneumonia.

Element	Comment
Focal shadowing	Required to make the diagnosis of pneumonia. Lobar pneumonia is the result of disease that starts in the periphery and spreads from one alveolus to another. As the disease reaches a fissure, this will result in a sharp delineation, since consolidation will not cross a fissure. The alveoli that surround the bronchi become denser and the bronchi become more visible, resulting in an air-bronchogram. Bronchopneumonia starts in the airways as acute bronchitis. It will lead to multifocal ill-defined densities. When it progresses it can produce diffuse consolidation.
Pleural effusion	If present, and high suspicion of pleural infection, arrange for ultrasound-guided aspiration of effusion and send samples for Gram stain and culture, pH and biochemistry (lactate dehydrogenase [LDH], protein, glucose).
Cavitation	Associated with tuberculosis and *Staphylococcus aureus* infection, but may also occur in Gram-negative and anaerobic infections.
Lung abscess	CXR typically demonstrates an air-fluid level, but chest CT is more sensitive and can confirm the diagnosis in difficult cases. Most patients with lung abscess do well with conservative management and a prolonged course of antibiotics.
Pneumothorax	May occur in cavitating pneumonia and is particularly associated with *Pneumocystis jirovecii* pneumonia (Chapter 28).

Table 25.3 Urgent investigations in suspected community-acquired pneumonia.

Test	Comment
CXR	See Table 25.2.
Full blood count	Leucocytosis or leucocytopenia are markers of sepsis and severe infection.
Urea &electrolytes	To assess renal function and disease severity (urea >7.0).
C-reactive protein	As biomarker of treatment response.
Liver function tests	The identification of underlying or associated hepatic disease.
Arterial blood gas (ABG)	If oxygen saturations <92% on air, or in patients with Chronic Obstructive Pulmonary Disease COPD to assess for type 2 respiratory failure.
Urine for Legionella antigen	In those with severe CAP or during an outbreak.
Blood culture	Identification of pathogens and antibiotic sensitivity patterns allows selection of optimal antibiotic regimens. Blood for culture must be taken prior to starting antibiotics.
'Atypical' serology	For patients with severe CAP or unresponsive to beta-lactam antibiotics. 'Atypical' pathogens that cause pneumonia are *Mycoplasma pneumoniae*, *Chlamydia pneumoniae*, *Chlamydia psittaci* and *Coxiella burnetii*.
Sputum culture	For patients with CAP who are able to expectorate sputum. Sputum samples should be sent for Gram stain, culture and sensitivity tests.
HIV test	CAP is considered a HIV indicator condition. Therefore, HIV testing should be offered to all adults age 65 years or younger with CAP.

Table 25.4 CURB-65 score.

Score 1 point each for:
- New **C**onfusion (abbreviated mental test score 8 or less, or new disorientation in person, place or time).
- Blood **U**rea > 7.0 mmol/L.
- **R**espiratory rate ≥ 30 breaths/min.
- Low **B**lood pressure (systolic BP < 90 mmHg or diastolic BP ≤ 60 mmHg).
- Age ≥ 65 years.

Choice of initial antibiotic therapy for CAP

Antibiotic treatment is typically chosen empirically because of the absence of microbiological results upon diagnosis. The choice of the empirical antibiotic depends on the most likely pathogen, individual risk factors, comorbidities, allergies and local antimicrobial policy (Table 25.5).
- Start antibiotic therapy as soon as diagnosis of CAP is suspected. Antibiotics should not be withheld if there is a delay in taking blood for culture.

Further management
Oxygen

Humidified O_2 should be continued to keep arterial $PaO_2 > 8.0$ kPa (oxygen saturation 88–92% in patients with chronic obstructive pulmonary disease and risk of CO_2 retention).

Fluid balance

- Insensible losses are greater than normal due to fever (allow 500 mL/day/°C fever) and tachypnoea.
- Patients with severe pneumonia should receive IV fluids (2–3 L/day), with daily assessment of fluid status and measurement of renal function. Adequate hydration also helps with expectoration of sputum.

Table 25.5 Initial empirical treatment regimens for CAP in adults (this is only intended as a guide. You should prescribe antibiotics according to your local antimicrobial policy).

Severity	Site	Preferred treatment	Penicillin allergy
Low (CURB-65 = 0–1, mortality <3%)	Home	Amoxicillin 500 mg TDS orally for 5 days.	Doxycycline 200 mg loading dose then 100 mg orally *or* clarithromycin 500 mg bd orally for 5 days.
Low severity (CURB-65 = 0–1, mortality <3%) but admission indicated for reasons other than pneumonia severity (e.g. social reasons)	Hospital	Amoxicillin 500 mg TDS orally. If oral administration not possible: amoxicillin 500 mg TDS IV for 5 days.	Doxycycline 200 mg loading dose then 100 mg od orally *or* clarithromycin 500 mg bd orally for 5 days.
Moderate severity (CURB-65 = 2, 3–15% mortality)	Hospital	Amoxicillin 500 mg–1.0 g TDS orally *plus* clarithromycin 500 mg bd orally. If oral administration not possible: amoxicillin 500 mg TDS IV *plus* clarithromycin 500 mg bd IV.	Doxycycline 200 mg loading dose then 100 mg orally *or* levofloxacin 500 mg od orally *or* moxifloxacin 400 mg od orally.
High severity (CURB-65 ≥ 3, 15–40% mortality)	Hospital	Co-amoxiclav 1.2 g TDS IV *plus* clarithromycin 500 mg bd IV.	Vancomycin 1 g bd IV plus clarithromycin 500 mg bd IV *or* levofloxacin 500 mg bd IV *or* Cefuroxime 1.5 g TDS IV or cefotaxime 1 g TDS IV *or* ceftriaxone 2 g od IV, *plus* clarithromycin 500 mg bd IV.

Antibiotic therapy

- Review this after 48 h. If there has been clinical improvement, with a fall in C-reactive protein level, switch to oral therapy in those patients initially given IV therapy.
- Management of patients who fail to improve after 48 h antibiotic therapy is discussed below (see Problems).

Venous thromboembolism prophylaxis

Give prophylaxis with anti-embolism stockings and low-molecular-weight heparin.

Pain relief

Relieve pleuritic chest pain with paracetamol and/or NSAIDs, to facilitate sputum expectoration.

Chest physiotherapy

- Chest physiotherapy is helpful if the patient is producing sputum but having difficulty expectorating it, and in bronchiectasis.
- Nebulized hypertonic saline may be helpful when sputum is thick and difficult to expectorate, but tends to cause a greater degree of bronchoconstriction than normal saline. Give bronchodilator therapy before nebulized hypertonic saline.

Bronchodilator therapy

Nebulized salbutamol or ipratropium should be prescribed to patients with asthma or COPD if there is wheeze on auscultation.

Checklist before discharge

Clinically stable for >24h:

- Normal mental state (or at baseline).
- Temperature < 37.5 °C.
- Respiratory rate < 24/min.
- Arterial oxygen saturation breathing air >92% (>88% if COPD).
- Heart rate < 100/min.
- Systolic BP >90 mmHg.
- Advice on smoking cessation given if needed.
- General practitioner follow-up arranged within one week.
- Follow-up CXR at six weeks' time.

Prevention

The main preventable risk for pneumonia is tobacco smoking. In those with comorbidities and elderly, influenza and pneumococcal vaccinations reduce the risk of developing pneumonia.

Problems
Failure to improve after 48h antibiotic therapy

Address the following points:

- Review the clinical, microbiological and radiological findings.
  - Are you confident the diagnosis is pneumonia (consider the diagnoses in Table 25.1), and that the patient's current antibiotic therapy is appropriate for the possible pathogens?
  - Consider broadening your antibiotic therapy, in case the organism is unusual or resistant: ask advice from a microbiologist.
- Re-examine the patient, and check for signs of metastatic infection, such as septic arthritis or infective endocarditis.
- Repeat the CXR. Are there any new findings such as cavitation or pleural effusion? If there is sufficient pleural effusion for safe pleural aspiration, this should be aspirated and sent for Gram stain and culture. If the fluid is cloudy rather than mildly turbid, and/or the pleural fluid pH <7.20, liaise with chest physicians to arrange for urgent chest drain insertion. In an IV drug user or a patient with an indwelling venous cannula consider tricuspid valve endocarditis with septic pulmonary emboli.
- Consider underlying airways or lung disease, such as chronic obstructive pulmonary disease, bronchiectasis, bronchial carcinoma and inhaled foreign body.
- Consider pulmonary tuberculosis in patients with risk factors for TB. Send sputum for Ziehl–Neelsen stain and liaise with chest physicians for advice. Consider HIV/AIDS. Test for HIV if this has not already been done.
- CT or fibreoptic bronchoscopy may be indicated to clarify the diagnosis. Therefore, close liaison with chest physicians is strongly recommended.

Hospital-acquired pneumonia

Hospital-acquired pneumonia (HAP) (Box 25.2) is defined as a lower respiratory tract infection occurring 48h or more after admission which was not present at the time of admission OR infection present on admission but patient is within 10 days of previous in-patient stay. HAP (which includes ventilator-associated pneumonia) is the second most common cause of infection among hospital inpatients and is the leading cause of death due to infection, with mortality rates ranging from 20% to 70%.

Consider HAP in a patient with:

- New cough productive of purulent sputum or purulent tracheal secretions.
- Acute breathlessness.

Box 25.2 Hospital-acquired pneumonia.

HAP affects 0.5–1.0% of inpatients and is one of the most common nosocomial infections contributing to death.

The mortality rate of HAP is between 20 and 70%. It increases hospital stay by 7–9 days.

In immunocompetent patients, HAP is typically caused by bacteria (e.g. *Pseudomonas aeruginosa*, *Escherichia coli*, *Klebsiella pneumoniae* and *Staphylococcus aureus*) and rarely by viral or fungal pathogens.

Risk factors for HAP are:
- Age > 70
- Chronic lung disease
- Diabetes
- Reduced level of consciousness
- Recent chest or abdominal surgery
- Mechanical ventilation
- Nasogastric feeding
- Immunosuppression (e.g. long-term corticosteroid use and chemotherapy).

- Increased oxygen requirement/respiratory failure (Chapter 30).
- New delirium.
- Core temperature >38 or <36 °C.

Severe HAP is defined as one or more of the following features:
- Admission to ICU.
- New confusion.
- Bilateral or multi-lobar consolidation on CXR.
- Respiratory rate > 30.
- New hypoxia (PO_2 <8 kPa or SaO_2 <92% on any FiO_2).
- FiO_2 >35% to maintain O_2 saturation.
- Need for ventilator support (non-invasive or invasive ventilation).
- Haemodynamic compromise (systolic BP < 90 mmHg or diastolic BP < 60 mmHg).

Priorities

Make a rapid but systematic assessment using the ABCDE approach (Chapter 2).

Airway: ensure a clear airway (Chapters 1 and 105). If the airway is compromised, seek urgent help from an anaesthetist.

Breathing: maintain adequate oxygenation. Give supplemental oxygen as needed to maintain oxygen saturation at 94–96% (88–92% if at risk of CO_2 retention).

Circulation: maintain adequate cardiac output/systemic blood pressure:
- Volume replacement with IV crystalloid if dehydrated.
  - Correct major arrhythmia (Chapter 13). Rate-control if in atrial fibrillation with fast ventricular rate (Chapter 13).
  - While doing this, collect information about the patient, the current problem, the context and comorbidities. Establish what has been decided regarding the ceiling of care and resuscitation status of the patient.

Check arterial blood gases, arrange a CXR and record an ECG

See Chapter 30 for the management of respiratory failure. Compare the CXR with the previous CXR, if available. Focal shadowing (Table 25.2) is required to make the diagnosis of pneumonia. Consider the differential diagnosis (Table 25.1). CT chest may be needed in patients with abnormal CXR.

If the working diagnosis is hospital-acquired pneumonia, start antibiotic therapy.

The choice of antibiotic therapy is governed by local hospital policy (which takes into account knowledge of local microbial pathogens). Seek advice from a microbiologist on antibiotic therapy for patients with severe HAP (Table 25.6).

- Aspiration is the misdirection of oropharyngeal or gastric contents into the larynx and lower respiratory tract. Around 45% of healthy people aspirate during sleep. Aspiration is more common in hospital patients, particularly after a stroke or with a reduced conscious level, when the upper airway becomes colonized with Gram-negative bacteria. See Table 25.7 for management of aspiration pneumonia

Table 25.6 Initial antibiotic therapy of hospital-acquired pneumonia (HAP).

Severity of HAP	Initial antibiotic therapy*	
	No penicillin allergy	**Penicillin allergy**
Non-severe	Oral Co.-amoxiclav 625 mg 8-hourly for 5 days	Doxycycline 200 mg on 1st day, then 100 mg once a day for 4 days OR Cefalexin 500 mg twice or three times a day for 5 days OR Levofloxacin (off-label use) 500 mg once or twice a day for 5 days
Severe	Tazocin 4.5 g 8-hourly IV Ceftazidime 2 g 8-hourly IV (+ vancomycin if MRSA is suspected) Ceftriaxone 2 g IV once a day	Meropenem 0.5–1 g 8-hourly IV Levofloxacin 500 mg 12-hourly IV or oral

*This is only intended as a guide. You should prescribe antibiotics according to your local antimicrobial policy

Aspiration pneumonia.

Table 25.7 Aspiration pneumonia management.

Inoculum	Effects on airway and lungs	Clinical features	Management
Acid	Chemical pneumonitis	Acute dyspnoea, tachypnoea, possible cyanosis, bronchospasm, fever, pink frothy sputum, infiltrates in one or both lower lobes, hypoxaemia	Positive-pressure breathing, IV fluids, tracheal suction
Oropharyngeal bacteria	Bacterial infection	Usually insidious onset; cough, fever, purulent sputum, infiltrate involving dependent pulmonary segment or lobe, with or without cavitation	Antibiotic therapy (Table 25.6)
Inert fluids	Mechanical obstruction, reflex airway closure	Acute dyspnoea, cyanosis, pulmonary oedema	Tracheal suction, intermittent positive-pressure breathing with oxygen, bronchodilator
Particulate matter	Mechanical obstruction	Dependent on level of obstruction, ranging from acute apnoea to chronic cough with or without recurrent infections	Extraction of particulate matter, antibiotic therapy

- Conditions that predispose to aspiration pneumonia include:
  - Reduced consciousness, resulting in a compromise of the cough reflex and glottic closure
  - Dysphagia from neurologic deficits
  - Disorders of the upper gastrointestinal tract including oesophageal disease, surgery involving the upper airways or oesophagus and gastric reflux
  - Mechanical disruption of the glottic closure due to tracheostomy, endotracheal intubation, bronchoscopy, upper GI endoscopy and nasogastric feeding
  - Protracted vomiting
  - Large-volume NG tube feedings
  - Feeding gastrostomy

Pulmonary tuberculosis

Tuberculosis (TB) is a preventable and curable disease. According to World Health Organization's 'Global TB Report 2023', TB was the world's second leading cause of death from a single infectious agent, after COVID-19, with the reported global number of people newly diagnosed with TB of 7.5 million and an estimated 1.30 million deaths globally in 2022. More than 90% of people who develop the disease are adults and there are more cases among men than women. There were 4425 cases of TB in United Kingdom in 2021, with males accounting for 60% of the cases. More than half (52.8%) of the notified cases had pulmonary TB. For signs and symptoms of TB please see Table 25.8

Pathophysiology

It is caused by infection with *Mycobacterium tuberculosis* (MTB). MTB bacteria can spread through air droplets from infectious individuals while coughing, sneezing or even speaking. Close contacts (*i.e.* those with prolonged [>8h] contact with contagious case) are at the highest risk of becoming infected. For risk factors and investigations of TB see Tables 25.9 and 25.10, respectively.

Table 25.8 Clinical presentations of pulmonary TB.

- Chronic cough
- Pyrexia of unknown origin
- Haemoptysis (more common with cavitation on CXR, and most will be smear positive)
- Systemic symptoms- weight loss, night sweats, lethargy
- Unresolved pneumonia
- Pleural effusion, usually exudative and lymphocytic
- Breathlessness
- Asymptomatic

Table 25.9 Risk factors for developing active TB in the United Kingdom.

- Alcohol misuse (4.5%)
- Drug misuse (5.3%)
- Caucasian (30%)
- Afro-Caribbean immigrants (10%)
- Close contacts of smear positive TB
- Indian-subcontinent immigrants (35%)
- Homelessness (4.9%)
- Overcrowding (e.g. prison, 4.1%)
- Cigarette smoking, cannabis
- Certain medical factors: chronic renal disease (3.1%), chronic liver disease (1.6%), immunosuppression (6.7%), diabetes mellitus (11.9%), silicosis, vitamin D deficiency and haematological malignancy (e.g. lymphoma and leukaemia)

Table 25.10 Investigations of suspected pulmonary TB.

CXR	The most useful investigation for the diagnosis of TB. There is a strong predilection for the upper zones. The CXR findings vary from paratracheal or hilar lymph node enlargement, to cavitating pneumonia and pleural effusion.
Sputum staining, microscopy and culture	Required for definitive diagnosis. At least three sputum samples (including at least one obtained in the early morning) from a spontaneously produced deep cough. Induced sputum may be used in those unable to expectorate.
Baseline blood tests–FBC, renal and liver function tests.	Liver function tests at baseline are helpful before treatment is started as Anti-Tuberculosis Treatment (ATT) tends to cause hepatotoxicity.
Bronchoscopy	To obtain bronchoalveolar lavage in those with dry cough and high index of clinical suspicion.
Endobronchial ultrasound (EBUS)	To obtain lymph node samples in those with dry cough or inconclusive sputum sample and high index of clinical suspicion.
Nucleic acid amplification tests (e.g. GeneXpert)	These provide rapid identification of MTB and rifampicin resistance. The sensitivity of the tests varies depending on the specimen. Testing sputum is more accurate than other specimens such as pleural fluid or urine.
Interferon gamma release assays (IGRAs)	Due to their high sensitivity and low specificity, a negative result rules out active or latent TB, but a positive result cannot distinguish between active and latent TB.
HIV test	Due to close links between HIV and TB and high mortality rate in HIV-positive TB patients, all patients with TB should be tested for HIV infection.
CT scan	It may show cavitating disease, it also helps to distinguish active from non-active disease, guide site of BAL and identify any mediastinal lymphadenopathy.

Treatment

The treatment objectives are to cure the patient, minimizing the risk of morbidity and mortality associated with the disease, reduce risk of transmission to others and avert the development of clinically significant drug resistance. The therapeutic approach to tuberculosis (TB) adheres to a fundamental strategy, comprising an initial intensive phase (phase I) aimed at killing actively growing MTB, followed by a continuation phase (phase II) focused on the eradication of any residual bacteria. The latest WHO guidelines recommend a 6-month regimen of isoniazid (H), rifampicin (R), ethambutol (E) and pyrazinamide (Z) for people with drug-susceptible TB, with all four drugs for the first two months (phase I), followed by H and R for the remaining four months (phase II). Treatment should be started promptly in any patient who is smear-positive, and in those who are smear-negative but with typical CXR changes and no response to standard antibiotics. It is strongly advised to promptly consult local TB specialists regarding any suspected TB cases before starting ATT.

It is important to consider the following points when starting someone on ATT:

- Never treat with a single drug.
- Never add a single drug to failing regime.
- Most patients can be managed as outpatients.
- All patients should be discussed at local TB MDT. The treatment of all cases of TB must be supervised by a consultant with appropriate experience.
- TB is a notifiable disease under the Public Health Regulations of 1988. All new cases must be notified and reported to local public health.
- All multi-drug-resistant patients should be managed by TB specialists.
- Advise patients to stop drugs and contact the TB team if they have persistent vomiting.
- All patients should be warned about orange-coloured bodily fluids (urine, tears, saliva) due to rifampicin.
- All patients should have their visual acuity and colour vision checked before starting ATT. If they develop visual disturbance, they should immediately stop ATT and contact the TB team.

- For women of childbearing age, give them contraception advice as the efficacy of oral contraceptive pills will be reduced by rifampicin.
- A patient who is infectious and presents risk to others in the community can be admitted to hospital under court order, but cannot be compulsorily treated.

Complications
Pulmonary TB

- Fibrosis
- Pneumothorax
- Haemoptysis
- Aspergilloma

Extra-pulmonary TB

- Spinal cord damage
- Constrictive pericarditis
- Cranial nerve palsy

Common terminologies used in TB

Smear positive TB: indicates the detection of acid-fast bacilli (AFB) on a sputum smear using the Ziehl-Neelsen stain. These patients are highly infectious, and if a patient is admitted to hospital, isolation is necessary.

Culture-positive TB: refers to cases where AFB are not observed on the smear (smear-negative), but tuberculosis is confirmed through culture, which may take up to nine weeks. While less contagious than smear-positive disease, there is still a risk of transmission in culture-positive cases.

Multidrug-resistant Tb (MDR-TB): MTB resistant to two or more first-line agents, usually isoniazid and rifampicin.

Extensively drug-resistant TB (XDR-TB): MDR-TB with added resistance to all fluoroquinolones and one of three injectable anti-TB drugs (e.g. capreomycin and amikacin).

Interferon Gamma Release Assay (IGRA): two blood tests (T-SPOT.TB and QuantiFERON-TB Gold). These tests detect IFN-γ released by T-cells in response to MTB-specific antigens. Both tests are very sensitive for the diagnosis of latent TB than the tuberculin skin test. IGRA should not be used to diagnose active TB as it cannot distinguish between active and latent TB.

Latent TB: A positive skin test or IGRA, showing MTB infection but with no signs, symptoms or CXR changes of active TB. Treatment with chemoprophylaxis reduces the risk of active disease by 90%.

Further reading

Further reading for CAP

National Institute for Health and Care Excellence (2014) Pneumonia in adults: diagnosis and management. Clinical guideline (CG191) Last updated: October 2023. https://www.nice.org.uk/guidance/cg191.

National Institute for Health and Care Excellence (2019) Pneumonia (community acquired): antimicrobial prescribing. Available from www.nice.org.uk/guidance/ng138.

Prina E, Ranzani OT, Torres A. (2015) Community-acquired pneumonia. *Lancet* 386, 1097–1108.

Further reading for HAP

Clinical practice guidelines by the infectious diseases Society of America and the American Thoracic Society. *Clin Infect Dis* 63, e61–e111. http://cid.oxfordjournals.org/content/63/5/e61.long.

National Institute for Health and Care Excellence Guideline (2019) Pneumonia (hospital acquired): antimicrobial prescribing. Available from ww.nice.org.uk/guidance/ng139.

Further reading TB

WHO The World Health Organization routinely offers updated information on the latest advancements in tuberculosis. Available from https://www.who.int/health-topics/tuberculosis.

CHAPTER 26

Bronchiectasis

WILLIAM FLOWERS

Radiologically, bronchiectasis is defined by the irreversible dilation of the bronchi, while clinically it is characterised by a chronic cough with sputum production and a history of exacerbations.

There are several aetiologies and conditions associated with bronchiectasis but in a substantial proportion of patients, the disease is idiopathic.

The pathophysiology of bronchiectasis is believed to involve a 'vicious vortex' of complex interacting processes of mucus obstruction and impaired muco-ciliary clearance, chronic neutrophilic inflammation, persistent airway infection and airway damage.

Retained purulent secretions and the associated inflammatory cells and mediators significantly contribute to persistent airway injury and exacerbations in bronchiectasis.

In 2012, it was estimated that over 210,000 individuals in the United Kingdom were living with bronchiectasis.

Exacerbations of bronchiectasis are significant events for those affected by the disease. Patients experiencing three or more exacerbations annually have double the mortality rate of those who do not, and exacerbations necessitating hospitalisation more than double the subsequent mortality risk.

Although most acute exacerbations are followed by a return to baseline health, frequent exacerbations indicate a poor prognosis. The median duration of symptoms for a bronchiectasis exacerbation is 16 days; however, approximately 16% of patients do not return to baseline for at least one month.

A history of frequent exacerbations is the strongest predictor of future exacerbation rate and is linked to increased hospitalisations, reduced quality of life and higher mortality rates.

Presentation

The diagnosis of an exacerbation of bronchiectasis is based largely on the clinical history, plus the appropriate exclusion of alternative diagnoses (Table 26.1).

A bronchiectasis exacerbation is defined as a *deterioration in 3 or more of the following* for more than 48 h:

- Cough
- Sputum volume and/or consistency
- Sputum purulence
- Breathlessness
- Fatigue
- Haemoptysis

Acute Medicine: A Practical Guide to the Management of Medical Emergencies, Sixth Edition.
Edited by Mridula Rajwani, Leila Vaziri, and Ivie Gbinigie.
© 2026 John Wiley & Sons Ltd. Published 2026 by John Wiley & Sons Ltd.

Table 26.1 Assessing for alternative acute diagnoses.

Acute lower respiratory tract infection	Typically no significant prior history of chronic productive cough or recurrent exacerbations. Usually viral in origin.
Pneumonia	Fever, chills/rigors may be more suggestive of pneumonia, often with significantly raised CRP >70. Focal consolidation on chest X-ray.
Heart failure/pulmonary oedema	May present with acute cough, breathlessness and bibasal crackles on examination. Usually other features of cardiac failure such as raised JVP or oedema. Abnormal ECG or NTproBNP.
Asthma exacerbation	Chest tightness, wheeze, atopic features, may be mildly productive cough. Blood eosinophilia >0.3. May co-exist with bronchiectasis.
COPD exacerbation	Patients will have a significant history of smoking. Typically, mucus production may be a less-prominent symptom in between exacerbations. May co-exist with bronchiectasis.
Interstitial lung disease	Cough (usually dry) and fine lung crepitations that do not alter on coughing.
Pulmonary tuberculosis	Clinical features include persistent productive cough, which may be associated with breathlessness and haemoptysis or weight loss. Associated with typical pulmonary radiological changes. Consider in patients from high-prevalence countries or with a history of immunosuppression.
NTM pulmonary disease	Associated with bronchiectasis and clinical presentation can overlap.
Immunodeficiency	Possible risk factor for bronchiectasis. May be primary or secondary. Consider if there is a history of severe, persistent, unusual pathogens or recurrent infections.

Fever is relatively uncommon, and its presence may be more suggestive of another diagnosis such as viral respiratory tract infection or community-acquired pneumonia.

Patients may present acutely in one of two ways; an exacerbation of known bronchiectasis or as a first presentation of undiagnosed bronchiectasis. Most patients with a pre-existing diagnosis of bronchiectasis will have a recognisable change in symptoms that they can attribute to an exacerbation.

→ *In patients with an existing diagnosis of bronchiectasis – assess the following:*

Is there a history of frequent exacerbations?

Is there a known chronic airway infection with positive sputum cultures?

Is there a documented response to previous treatments?

What recent antibiotic therapies have been taken?

Any long-term antibiotic therapy?

What is the usual airway clearance regimen and inhaled treatments?

→ *In patients with no prior diagnosis of bronchiectasis:*

Consider whether a patient presenting with clinical features of lower respiratory tract infection may have an underlying diagnosis of bronchiectasis if they have features of the following:

- Patients with a history of chronic mucopurulent or purulent sputum and frequent lower respiratory tract infections.
- Chronic obstructive pulmonary disease (COPD) with >3 exacerbations and a previous positive sputum culture for *Pseudomonas aeruginosa* whilst stable.
- Patients with inflammatory bowel disease or rheumatoid arthritis with a history of chronic productive cough.

- In patients with asthma with severe or poorly controlled disease, especially with frequent productive cough and/or poor response to steroid therapy.
- Patients with a history of HIV infection, solid organ and bone marrow transplant, and history of immunosuppressive therapy for lymphoma and vasculitis with symptoms of chronic productive cough or recurrent chest infections.

Pitfalls

- Avoid making a diagnosis of bronchiectasis on a computed tomography (CT) scan of the thorax in an acute setting, as acute infection may cause reversible airway dilatation that can be misdiagnosed as bronchiectasis.
- Consider CT imaging when the patient has recovered or is in a stable state, typically 6–8 weeks after treatment.
- Radiological bronchiectasis may be evident in healthy, asymptomatic individuals, particularly those over 75 years, so ask about a history of chronic productive cough and exacerbations before considering further investigation.

→ *Review previous imaging for signs of bronchiectasis:*

CT signs of bronchiectasis

- Broncho-arterial ratio > 1 (internal airway lumen vs adjacent pulmonary artery).
- Lack of tapering of the bronchi.
- Airway visibility within 1 cm of costal pleural surface or touching mediastinal pleura.
- Other associated features may include bronchial wall thickening, mucoid impaction and mosaic attenuation (air trapping) on expiratory phase CT.

Examination

- May be normal.
- Inspect sputum – dark yellow or green sputum present, often viscous.
- Audible airway sputum may be heard on coughing.
- Focal crackles or squawks, especially basal, represent sputum retention (may alter on coughing).
- Wheezing may be present, especially if co-existing COPD/asthma.
- Fever, tachypnoea, tachycardia, hypotension etc. may suggest pneumonia.

Investigations

- Send sputum for routine culture and sensitivity testing.
- Viral swabs for specific viruses (e.g. Influenza A & B, RSV and SARS-CoV-2) during appropriate viral season.
- FBC
- U&E – may assist in CURB65 scoring if pneumonia.
- CRP – does not form part of the diagnostic criteria for an exacerbation, although a significantly elevated CRP may suggest pneumonia. Patients can have a significant exacerbation with relatively normal CRP values.
- CXR – not necessary for all exacerbations, especially in mild exacerbations in patients with a typical exacerbation but in patients requiring admission, with more severe features, haemoptysis or an unclear diagnosis it is essential to evaluate for alternative causes.
- Arterial blood gas analysis if significant hypoxia or at risk of hypercapnic respiratory failure.

Determine the location of treatment

Most patients can be managed in an ambulatory fashion, with either oral antibiotic therapy or outpatient intravenous antibiotic therapy.

→ *Criteria for admission*
- Severe illness or signs suggesting the patient is at risk of sepsis.
  - altered mental status, SpO_2 <93%, tachypnoea, hypotension, tachycardia.
- High sputum burden that cannot be managed without inpatient physiotherapy intervention.
- Have any comorbidities or other factors that make ambulatory management impractical such as poor oral intake, reduced mobility or significant frailty.
- Where oral antibiotics have failed and there are no outpatient intravenous antibiotics options (as may be the case in patients with chronic *P. aeruginosa* infection).
- Have clinically significant haemoptysis.

Management
- Treatment aims to remove abnormal secretions through airway clearance techniques (ACT or chest physiotherapy) and to reduce the microbial load through selective antibiotic use.

Airways clearance
- Encourage the patient to regularly perform and/or increase the frequency of their ACT.
- For patients managed in an ambulatory setting, consider an outpatient referral to a respiratory specialist and/or a specialist respiratory physiotherapist if the patient has not already been taught ACT.
- In the inpatient setting, refer patients to a respiratory physiotherapist.
- If sputum is viscous or difficult to expectorate, prescribe nebulised 0.9% sodium chloride 5–10 mL BD – QDS and/or carbocisteine 750 mg TDS.
- If there is wheeze, prescribe nebulised salbutamol 2.5 mg QDS.
- Respiratory physiotherapists may recommend standard techniques such as autogenic drainage (AD), active cycle of breathing technique (ACBT) with or without oscillatory positive expiratory pressure (OPEP) devices.
- Intermittent positive pressure breathing (IPPB) or non-invasive ventilation (NIV) may be required during a severe exacerbation to help offload the work of breathing so patients can perform longer ACT sessions.

Antibiotics
- Ensure sputum samples are submitted for culture and sensitivity testing before initiating antibiotic therapy but do not delay antibiotic treatment while awaiting the culture results.

Antibiotic selection
- Prescribe antibiotics based on previous sputum culture results, considering past antibiotic susceptibility profiles and local prescribing guidelines.
- The British Thoracic Society (BTS) guidelines for bronchiectasis 2019 provides a suggested table of antibiotics, Table 26.2.
- In the absence of prior positive sputum cultures, amoxicillin 500 mg tds or doxycycline 100 mg bd are suitable initial options.
- Fluoroquinolones (e.g. ciprofloxacin and levofloxacin) should only be prescribed if no other suitable alternatives exist. Patients must be informed about the risks of tendon rupture, muscle pain, muscle weakness, joint pain, joint swelling, peripheral neuropathy and central nervous system effects. They should also be updated on the latest MHRA advice regarding fluoroquinolones.

Antibiotic duration
- Prescribe a 14-day course of antibiotics for patients:
  - Who require admission

Table 26.2 Antibiotic selection based on BTS guideline for bronchiectasis.

Organism	Recommended first-line treatment	Recommended second-line treatment
Streptococcus pneumoniae	Amoxicillin 500 mg three times a day	Doxycycline 100 mg twice a day
Haemophilus influenzae beta-lactamase negative	Amoxicillin 500 mg three times a day OR Amoxicillin 1 g three times a day OR Amoxicillin 3 g twice a day	Doxycycline 100 mg twice a day OR Ciprofloxacin 500 mg OR 750 mg twice a day OR IV Ceftriaxone 2 g once a day
H. influenzae beta lactamase positive	Co-amoxiclav 625 mg three times a day	Doxycycline 100 mg twice a day OR Ciprofloxacin 500 mg or 750 mg twice a day OR IV Ceftriaxone 2 g once a day
Moraxella catarrhalis	Co-amoxiclav 625 mg three times a day	Doxycycline 100 mg twice a day OR Ciprofloxacin 500 mg or 750 mg twice a day OR Clarithromycin 500 mg twice daily
Staphylococcus aureus (MSSA)	Flucloxacillin 500 mg four times a day	Clarithromycin 500 mg twice daily OR Doxycycline 100 mg twice a day OR Co-amoxiclav 625 mg three times a day
S. aureus (MRSA) – seek specialist advice	Doxycycline 100 mg twice a day OR Rifampicin (<50 kg) 450 mg once a day OR Rifampicin (>50 kg) 600 mg once a day OR Trimethoprim 200 mg twice a day	Linezolid 600 mg twice a day OR OR IV Vancomycin (monitor serum levels and adjust dose accordingly) OR OR Teicoplanin 400 mg once a day
Coliforms	Ciprofloxacin 500 or 750 mg twice a day	
Pseudomonas aeruginosa	Ciprofloxacin 750 mg twice a day	IV monotherapy Ceftazidime 2 g three times a day OR Tazocin 4.5 g three to four times a day OR Aztreonam 2 g three times a day or Meropenem 2 g three times a day Combination therapy The above can be combined with iv tobramycin or iv colomycin

Source: Adapted from Hill AT, Sullivan AL, Chalmers JD *et al*. British Thoracic Society guideline for bronchiectasis in adults. *Thorax*. 2019;74(Supplement 1):1–69.

- - With more severe disease
  - Chronic *P. aeruginosa* infection
  - Whose symptoms have responded inadequately to community treatment
  - Who have experienced a rapid relapse in symptoms despite antibiotics
- Milder cases may be treated with a 7–10 day course, provided an effective clinical response is observed.
- Note that patients with a long history of bronchiectasis often have preferences regarding antibiotic selection and duration.
- Improvement should typically be seen within 5–7 days. If no clinical improvement is evident, consider altering the antibiotic regimen based on culture results and consider alternative diagnoses as above.
- If the sputum culture identifies a pathogen resistant to the current antibiotic, there is no need to change antibiotics if the patient is responding adequately.

Other medications

Do not routinely prescribe oral or inhaled corticosteroids outside their usual indications in asthma or COPD.

Haemoptysis in bronchiectasis

Haemoptysis in bronchiectasis is associated with acute infection during exacerbations and arises from inflammatory injury to neovascularisation of airway mucosa.

Estimating haemoptysis volume can be challenging and there are no agreed universal definitions. One suggested classification is listed below.

Ask patients to cough all their sputum into a standard universal container (usual volume 30–50 mL) to help quantification.

Define the severity of haemoptysis

- Mild – Haemoptysis where blood is 'streaky', i.e. streaks of blood mixed in with recognisable sputum.
- Moderate – More than a teaspoon (5 mL) of blood more than two or three times a day with episodes continuing for more than a few hours.
- Life-threatening – Any haemoptysis causing severe difficulty breathing, airway obstruction, hypoxaemia or haemodynamic instability. One suggested definition defines life-threatening haemoptysis as more than 100 mL in 24 h.

Management of haemoptysis

Mild haemoptysis

1 Send sputum for culture and treat exacerbation with antibiotics.
2 Chest X-ray to assess for pneumonia or new focal changes suggestive of alternative diagnosis.
3 Consider CT chest if worsening symptoms, failure to improve on treatment.

Moderate haemoptysis

1 Strongly consider admission.
2 Send sputum for culture and treat exacerbation with antibiotics.
3 Correct any abnormal bleeding tendency.
4 Involve respiratory physiotherapist for modified airways clearance.
5 Oral or iv tranexamic acid 500 mg–1 g three times a day (caution with risk of thromboembolism).
6 Emerging evidence that nebulised tranexamic acid 500 mg in 5 ml 0.9% sodium chloride TDS may be useful.
7 Chest CT with bronchial arterial contrast to assess lung parenchyma and any targets for bronchial artery embolisation.
8 Early discussion with respiratory and interventional radiology teams.

Life-threatening haemoptysis

1 Involve intensive care medicine early with senior respiratory medicine and thoracic surgical teams.
2 Initial measures should focus on securing the airway, maintaining adequate ventilation, ensuring hemodynamic stability and correcting any abnormal bleeding tendency.
3 If known, place the patient with the bleeding side down to prevent aspiration of blood into the non-bleeding lung.
4 Other measures as above.
5 Early bronchoscopy (possibly rigid bronchoscopy in intensive care unit (ICU) or theatres) to identify the site of bleeding is helpful.
6 Chest CT with arterial contrast as for moderate haemoptysis.

Further reading

Gopinath B, Mishra PR, Aggarwal P, *et al.* (2023) Nebulized versus IV tranexamic acid for hemoptysis: a pilot randomized controlled trial. *Chest* 163(5), 1176–1184.

Hill AT, Sullivan AL, Chalmers JD, *et al.* (2019) British Thoracic Society guideline for bronchiectasis in adults. *Thorax* 74(Supplement 1), 1–69.

Ibrahim WH. (2008) Massive haemoptysis: the definition should be revised. *Eur Respir J* 32(4), 1131–1132.

National Institute for Health and Care Excellence (2024) Bronchiectasis [Internet]. London: NICE Last updated: March 2024. Available from: https://cks.nice.org.uk/topics/bronchiectasis/.

CHAPTER 27

Interstitial lung disease

VISHAL NATHWANI, SABRINA ZULFIKAR, AND PETER SAUNDERS

Interstitial lung diseases (ILDs) represent a broad group of lung diseases with variable outcomes clinically.

Some diseases may be expected to improve or stabilise with treatment whereas others may progress despite treatment.

These diseases may be inflammatory or fibrotic or a combination of both.

Most ILD diagnoses are made on the basis of imaging patterns and multidisciplinary team (MDT) discussion with the role of biopsy and histology being usually reserved for more complex cases because of the risk of morbidity associated with sampling.

ILDs are often classified by their causes (Figure 27.1).

One of the most common of these diseases is idiopathic pulmonary fibrosis (IPF).

Idiopathic pulmonary fibrosis

Introduction

IPF is the most common ILD. Prevalence increases with age (over 50 with a mean age of 79) (1).

Prognosis remains poor with a median survival of three to five years and five-year survival rates 45% – lower than most cancers (2).

IPF is a progressive fibrotic lung disease with a gradual decline in lung function that presents with worsening exertional breathlessness and functional impairment. Symptoms develop insidiously, on average nine months prior to presentation. The clinical course is variable, and a subset of patients can suffer acute exacerbations with a sudden deterioration in respiratory symptoms and accelerated decline (Figure 27.2) (3).

Whilst patients are generally managed in specialist respiratory outpatient clinics they may be encountered in acute or ambulatory care settings as:

i. A new presentation of unexplained progressive breathlessness or hypoxia or identified incidentally after presenting with a separate complaint.
ii. In a patient with an established diagnosis of IPF with a sudden deterioration of respiratory symptoms suggestive of an acute exacerbation.
iii. A combination of (i) and (ii) presenting with acute on chronic unexplained breathlessness.

Acute Medicine: A Practical Guide to the Management of Medical Emergencies, Sixth Edition.
Edited by Mridula Rajwani, Leila Vaziri, and Ivie Gbinigie.

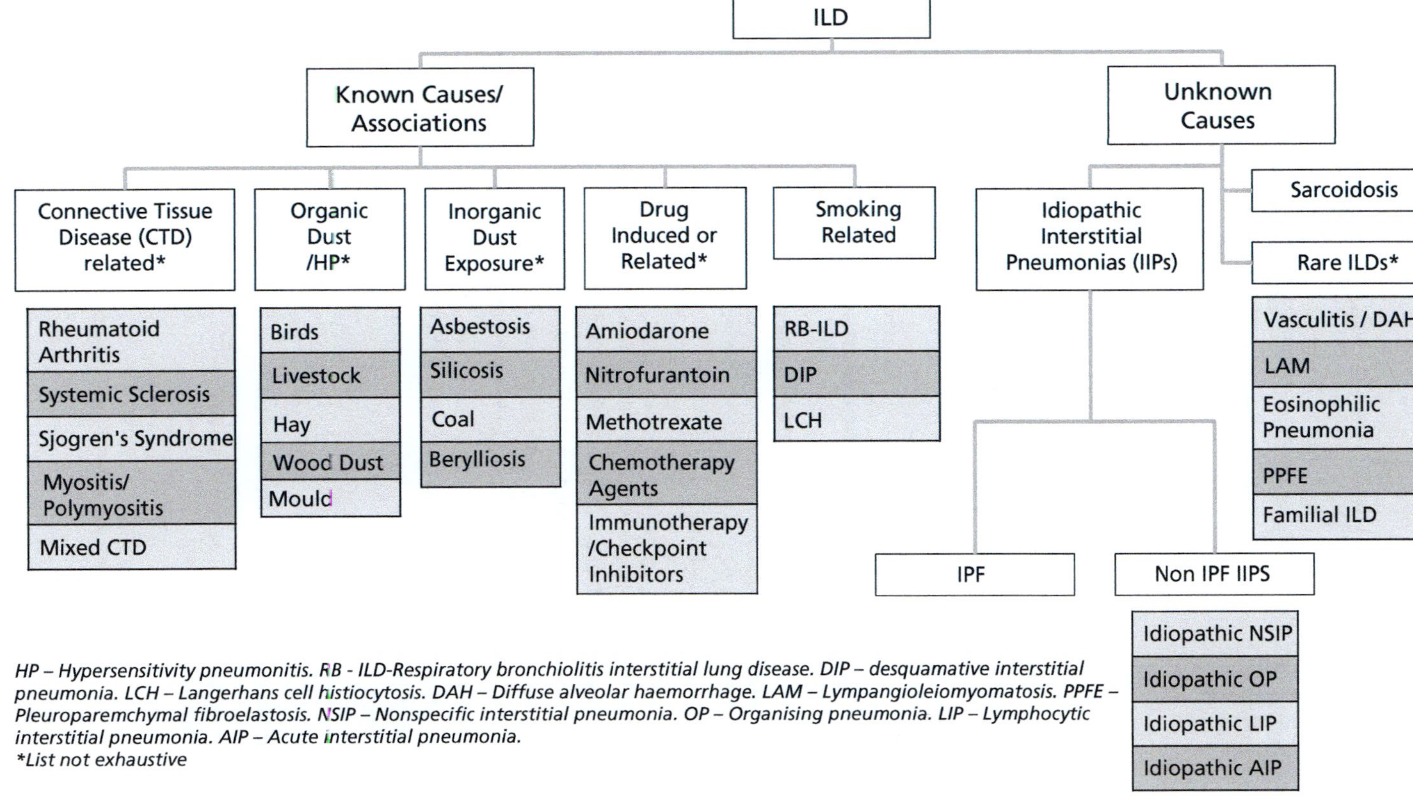

HP – Hypersensitivity pneumonitis. RB - ILD-Respiratory bronchiolitis interstitial lung disease. DIP – desquamative interstitial pneumonia. LCH – Langerhans cell histiocytosis. DAH – Diffuse alveolar haemorrhage. LAM – Lympangioleiomyomatosis. PPFE – Pleuroparemchymal fibroelastosis. NSIP – Nonspecific interstitial pneumonia. OP – Organising pneumonia. LIP – Lymphocytic interstitial pneumonia. AIP – Acute interstitial pneumonia.
*List not exhaustive

Figure 27.1 ILD classification.

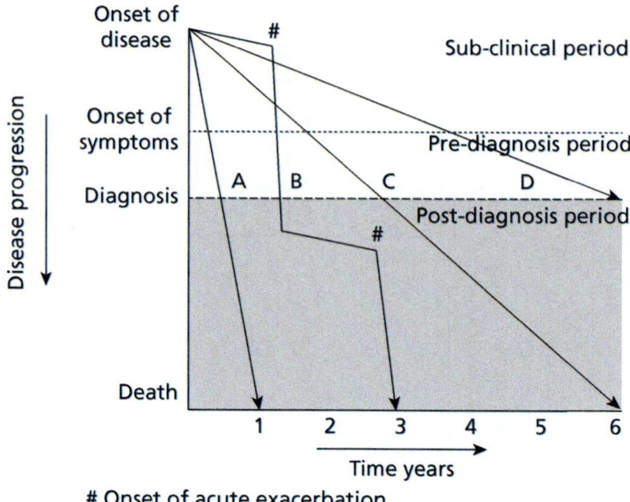

Figure 27.2 Clinical course of IPF.

Diagnostic evaluation in suspected/new presentation of IPF
Clinical features

IPF presents insidiously and non-specifically with gradually progressive breathlessness and a dry cough often resulting in delays in presentation (Figure 27.2) and correct diagnosis with reports of a median time to diagnosis of 2.2 years (4).

Clinicians should consider ILDs including IPF in the differential diagnosis of chronic breathlessness (Table 27.1) particularly in patients >50.

Patients with IPF often have multiple co-morbidities including emphysema, ischaemic heart disease, anaemia, and gastro-oesophageal reflux that symptoms of IPF can be incorrectly attributed to.

Features that should raise suspicion of a diagnosis of IPF in elderly patients presenting with breathlessness.

1 Slowly progressive (over months) exertional breathlessness with minimal day-to-day or diurnal variability.
2 Typically, a dry/minimally productive cough, if productive then sputum often clear unless coexistent infection or coexistent respiratory airway disease.
3 Wheeze/chest tightness are unusual in IPF. However, up to 40% of patients have coexistent chronic obstructive pulmonary disease (COPD).
4 Weight loss is common.

Table 27.1 The differential diagnosis of chronic breathlessness.

Differential diagnosis in (acute on) chronic breathlessness in adults >50
Chronic obstructive pulmonary disease (COPD)
Asthma
ILD's (including IPF)
Hypoventilation (neuromuscular disease, chest wall deformity and obesity)
Ischaemic heart disease (IHD)
Heart failure and pulmonary oedema
Unexplained anaemia
Pulmonary vascular disease

5 Peripheral oedema is an unusual feature unless advanced disease with secondary (group 3) pulmonary hypertension.

6 A family history of an ILD or IPF.

7 Finger clubbing may be present but is often absent.

8 Bibasal fine, end-inspiratory crackles.

Chest radiograph features suggestive of an ILD (including IPF):

1 Fine linear/reticular opacities in a lower zone and peripheral distribution, which may mimic features of pulmonary oedema (although additional features of oedema including prominent fissures, upper lobe diversion, costophrenic blunting and cardiomegaly will be absent).

2 Coarse reticulation suggestive of honeycombing and volume loss in advanced disease.

3 Whilst the radiograph is often abnormal, findings may be subtle and non-specific. If there is uncertainty cross-sectional imaging is recommended.

High resolution CT features of IPF - usual interstitial pneumonia (UIP) pattern

Subpleural reticulation (fine lines) associated with traction bronchiectasis.

Basal dominant distribution.

May have dendriform calcification.

May have honeycomb cyst formation (definite usual interstitial pneumonia pattern [UIP]) or not (probable UIP).

The diagnosis of IPF is made based on typical radiological features on high-resolution chest computed tomography (HRCT) *after* exclusion of known causes of ILD (Figure 27.1) including domestic and occupational environmental exposure, connective tissue disease and drug toxicity (ATS 2018) (Figure 27.3).

Distinguishing IPF from other ILDs

The UIP pattern of pulmonary fibrosis on CT is seen in other diseases and a careful history for occupational exposure to substances such as asbestos should be taken.

Connective tissue diseases such as rheumatoid arthritis and Sjogren's disease can also be associated with the UIP pattern of ILD.

Other fibrotic ILDs may have a similar course to IPF despite initial imaging and features reflecting an non-IPF ILD.

Non IPF ILDs should be carefully considered in patients aged <70 and in women.

Whilst most ILDs including IPF present with a gradual onset of symptoms, it is also important to consider certain cases of ILD may have a more rapid (days to weeks) onset of symptoms including acute interstitial pneumonia, acute eosinophilic pneumonia, acute hypersensitivity pneumonitis, diffuse alveolar damage/pulmonary vasculitis, organising pneumonia, drug reactions and myositis related ILDs.

Acute exacerbations of ILDs including IPF may also present with a rapid deterioration of symptoms (discussed below).

The following should be explored during clinical assessment.

1 A previous diagnosis or features of a connective tissue disease including; arthralgia, myalgia, proximal muscle weakness, skin rashes, skin thickening, sclerodactyly, Raynaud's, calcinosis, digital ulceration, dysphagia, microstomia and recurrent miscarriage.

2 Environmental and occupational exposures specifically asbestos, metal dusts (iron, tin, beryllium and tungsten), silica, wood dust, mouldy environments, farm work or bird exposure.

3 A thorough review of medication including current/previous exposure to nitrofurantoin, amiodarone, DMARDs including methotrexate, sulfasalazine, penicillamine, etanercept, non-steroidals, chemotherapy agents including bleomycin, cyclophosphamide, newer immune checkpoint inhibitors and previous radiotherapy.

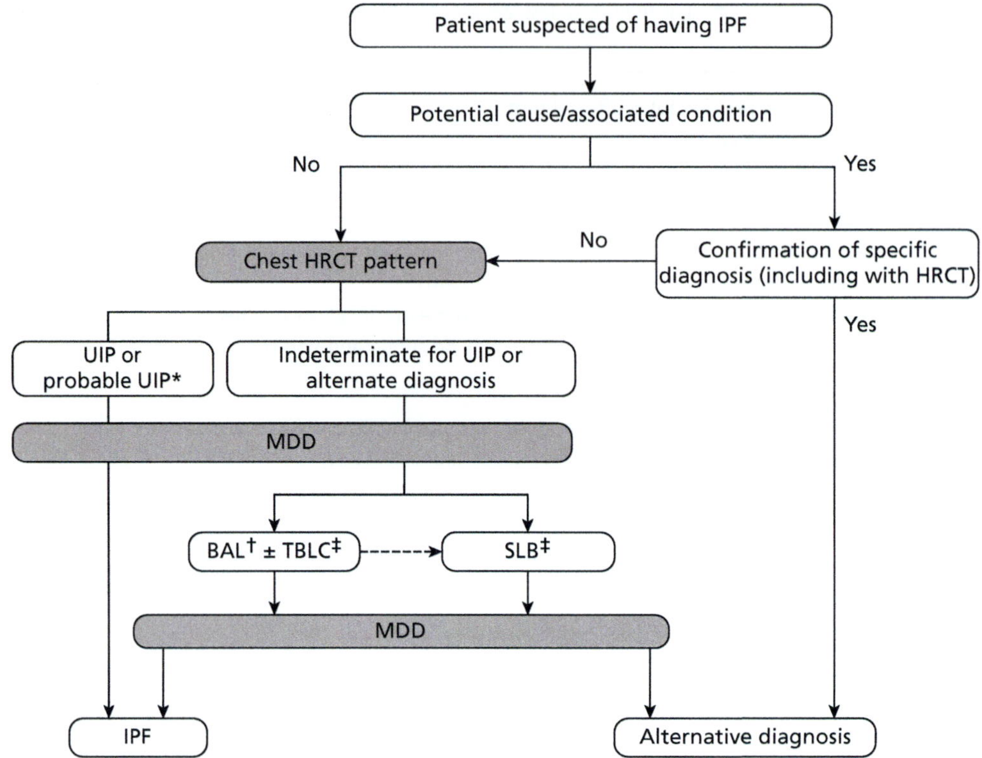

Figure 27.3 3 IPF diagnostic workflow. *Patients with a radiological pattern of probable usual interstitial pneumonia (UIP) can receive a diagnosis of IPF after multidisciplinary discussion (MDD) without confirmation by lung biopsy in the appropriate clinical setting (e.g. 60yr old, male, smoker). BAL may be appropriate in some patients with a probable UIP pattern. †BAL may be performed before MDD in some patients evaluated in experienced centers. ‡Transbronchial lung cryobiopsy (TBLC) may be preferred to surgical lung biopsy (SLB) in centers with appropriate expertise and/or in some patient populations.

Investigations in suspected ILD/IPF

All cases where an ILD including IPF are suspected require further investigations to classify the radiological pattern, rule out causative factors, assess lung physiology and functional impact of the lung disease. Whilst there is regional variability in arranging these tests if requested alongside a referral for respiratory review will facilitate the diagnostic journey and potentially expedite initiating specific treatments.

1 Serological analysis for a connective tissue disorder or alternative cause should include, full blood count, erythrocyte sedimentation rate (ESR), c-reactive protein (CRP), renal function, liver function tests, rheumatoid factor, anti-cyclic citrullinated peptide antibody and anti-nuclear antibody titre and pattern. Additional autoantibodies can be included dependent on the clinical suspicion and a positive ANA (Table 27.2).

2 Lung function testing including spirometry and gas transfer assessment. Forced vital capacity (FVC) remains the standard measurement to classify the severity of disease at baseline, whilst changes in FVC over time are used to define progressive disease, determine eligibility for treatment and useful predictor of mortality (5).

Haemoglobin corrected transfer factor for carbon monoxide (TLCOc) often correlates well with functional ability (<40% severe disease) but may be confounded by emphysema and pulmonary hypertension.

Table 27.2 Extended serological testing.

Connective tissue disease or exposure history	Additional tests and auto-antibodies
Systemic sclerosis	anti-Scl-70/topoisomerase-1, anti-centromere, anti-RNA polymerase III antibodies
Sjogren's	anti-SSA/Ro and anti-SSB/La antibodies
mCTD	anti-U1 RNP antibody
Myositis (polymyositis/dermatomyositis)	Serum creatinine kinase anti-Jo-1, anti PL-7, anti PL-12, anti-MDA5, anti-Mi2, anti-NXP2, anti-TIG1-g, anti-SRP, anti-SAE, anti U1RNP, anti-PM/Scl75, Anti-PM/Scl100 and anti-Ku antibodies
Vasculitis	ANCA, anti-PR3, anti-MPO, anti-GBM antibodies
Occupational/environmental exposures	IgG antibodies against avian proteins (bird exposure), aspergillus (mould and farm exposure), *Micropolyspora faeni* (farm and livestock exposure)

Table 27.3 Specifications when requesting a high-resolution CT to investigate a suspected ILD.

Condition	Rationale
Type	A 'non-contrast high-resolution CT' (HRCT) will include thinner (1 mm) sections with greater detail to visualise subtle abnormalities in the lung parenchyma and reduce artefact related to contrast
Position	A prone CT will reduce any dependent change or atelectasis that may obscure parenchymal change at the lung bases or periphery
Additional images	Expiratory (in addition to inspiratory) phase images to evaluate for large or small airway involvement
Contrast	If an additional contrast CT is required (i.e. for additional investigating pulmonary embolism or lung cancer) the non-contrast HRCT should be performed prior to the use of contrast
Timing	If suspicion of an active acute lung pathology (infection, oedema or haemorrhage) that will potentially obscure the underlying lung abnormality the diagnostic HRCT should be deferred for a minimum six to eight weeks

3 Lung functional assessments including pulse oximetry and a 6-minute walk test, the latter being a reliable, inexpensive measure of a patient's functional status and may guide treatment decisions regarding supplementary oxygen.

4 Cross-sectional Imaging. Accurate diagnosis of ILDs including IPF is highly dependent on cross-sectional imaging specifically a 'high-resolution chest CT'. Specific requirements are necessary when requesting a chest CT for investigation of an ILD which are detailed in Table 27.3.

5 The diagnostic value of the cellular composition of broncho-alveolar lavage and tissue histology (by transbronchial lung biopsy, transbronchial cryobiopsy and video-assisted surgical lung biopsy) has been extensively investigated (6, 7) and at present are not routinely recommended. Whilst they have a role in specific cases, these tests should be considered on a case-by-case basis in specialist clinics or following mutidisciplinary team review.

6 Additional tests including a serum beta natriuretic peptide (BNP) level and Echocardiography may be useful to assess for the presence of coexistent left heart disease and assess for secondary pulmonary hypertension in advanced disease.

Management

Patients with suspected ILD including IPF should be referred to specialist respiratory clinics for assessment, establishing a definitive diagnosis and consideration of specific treatments. Supportive treatments should be considered from the outset and may include the following.

General measures

1 Pulmonary rehab: Should be offered to all patients with a Medical Research Council score of 2 or more (breathlessness on hurrying or walking up a slight incline).
2 Smoking cessation: IPF is an independent risk factor for lung cancer. Amongst IPF patients, current smokers are five times more likely to develop lung cancer than ex-smokers (8).
3 Vaccine immunisation: IPF patients are at risk of poor outcomes following infections and should be routinely offered vaccines including annual influenza and pneumococcal vaccines.

Supportive therapies

1 Oxygen therapy: IPF patients often present with exertional desaturation and then chronic hypoxia in advanced disease or following an exacerbation. Chronic hypercapnic respiratory failure and CO_2 retention are unusual unless coexistent COPD or hypoventilation is present. Ambulatory oxygen is the more commonly prescribed oxygen therapy.
2 Symptom-specific treatments (often delivered in conjunction with palliative care).
   a Breathlessness – a handheld fan is often overlooked but may relieve symptoms of dyspnoea (9) if required oral morphine 1.25 mg four times daily (QDS) as required (PRN) or lorazepam 0.5 mg tds PRN are often beneficial.
   b Cough – if evidence of coexistent gastro-oesophogeal reflux disease (GORD) a protein pump inhibitor can be trialled. If productive cough with tenacious sections mucolytics can be considered. MST 5 mg BD is effective in reducing cough.

Specific therapies in IPF

Targeted IPF therapies may slow progression but at the risk of side effects and therefore may not be suitable in frailer patients with more co-morbidity.

Nintedanib

Oral tyrosine kinase inhibitor taken twice a day.
Common side effects include diarrhoea, abdominal pain and weight loss.
Potentially slows wound healing/increases bleeding risk so should be stopped perioperatively.
Reduces disease progression by around 50%.

Pirfenidone

Oral small molecule with multiple mechanisms of action taken thrice daily with food.
Common side effects include nausea, indigestion, anorexia, photosensitivity and weight loss.
Some evidence may have a role in exacerbation prevention/treatment.
Reduces disease progression by around 50%.

There is no role for steroids or immune suppression in the long-term management of IPF which are associated with an increase in serious adverse events and death (10).

Exacerbation of idiopathic pulmonary fibrosis
Epidemiology

Around 5–10% of IPF patients develop exacerbations annually. It is also one of the biggest killers in IPF, with up to 46% of deaths in IPF being preceded by an acute exacerbation (11).

Diagnosis

The 2016 International Working Group (11) has proposed the following criteria to make a diagnosis of acute exacerbation of IPF (Figure 27.4):

1 Acute respiratory deterioration of less than one month in a patient with a known or concurrent diagnosis of IPF.

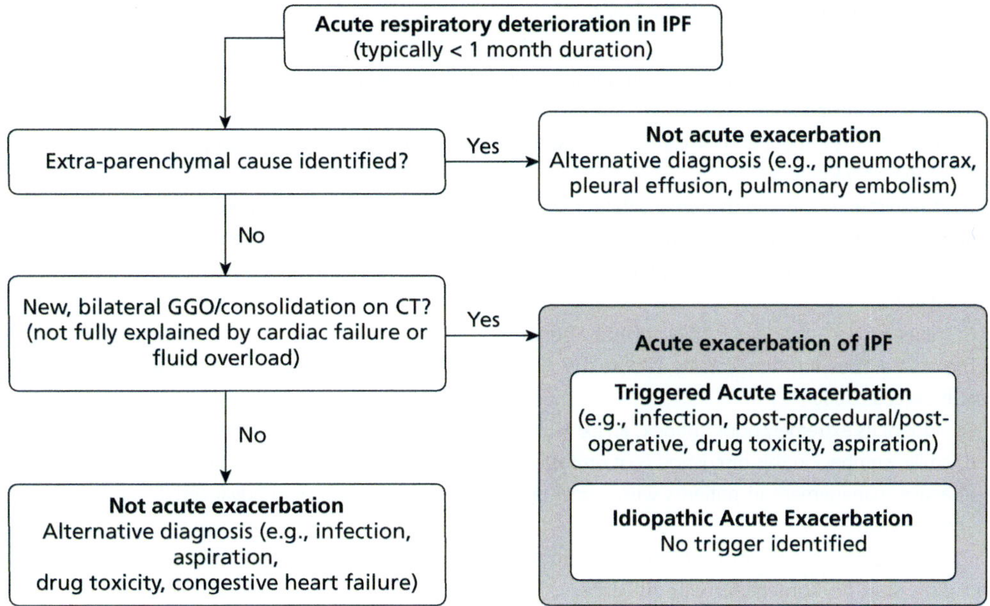

Figure 27.4 Diagnostic criteria for acute exacerbation of IPF by 2016 International Working Group.

2 Computed tomography (CT) of chest showing new bilateral ground-glass opacities and consolidation which cannot be explained by heart failure or fluid overload.

Assessment when suspecting acute exacerbation of IPF:

1 Assess clinically and perform chest X-ray to rule out other causes of breathlessness such as pneumothorax, pleural effusion and fluid overload, and CT pulmonary angiogram to rule out pulmonary embolism.

2 If chest imaging shows new bilateral opacities and this cannot be explained by heart failure or fluid overload, a high-resolution CT is recommended.

3 Presence of new bilateral ground-glass opacities and consolidation on HRCT confirms a diagnosis of acute exacerbation of IPF.

4 In patients without a known diagnosis of IPF and without a previous CT, presence of probable or definite usual interstitial pneumonia pattern on the new CT can be used to make a diagnosis of IPF.

Common triggers for acute exacerbation include:

1 infection

2 recent lung procedure or surgery

3 drug toxicity

4 aspiration

If no cause is identified, it is labelled as idiopathic acute exacerbation.

Management

1 Alert usual IPF care provider.

2 Send viral PCR – influenza/COVID, BNP, CRP and ANCA. Anti-neutrophil cytoplasmic antibodies (ANCA) are autoantibodies against neutrophil that are often present in certain autoimmune diseases such as GPA (Granulomatous polyangiitis), EGPA (Eosinophilic granulomatosis with polyangiitis) and MPA (Microscopic polyangitis).

3 Consider starting broad-spectrum antibiotics.

4 Steroids should be discussed – in most patients, there is a benefit to treating infection in the first instance. There is probably no role for other immunosuppressants and indeed a recent trial suggested harm from the use of cyclophosphamide (12).

5 Discuss with the patient and IPF care provider sensible ceilings of care – usually, these patients do not do well with invasive ventilation.

6 Treat respiratory failure with oxygen; there may be a role for nasal high-flow oxygen although this can be difficult to wean. Extracorporeal membrane oxygenation (ECMO), a method of oxygenating blood outside the body in the event of severe respiratory failure, is only ever used as a bridge to transplant in those already listed (13).

7 Consider early involvement of palliative care support.

The overall three-month mortality is more than 50% and in patients who have required mechanical ventilation, it exceeds 90% (12).

Because of its extremely poor outlook, an early plan for treatment escalation and the involvement of patients and family members in this discussion is of utmost importance. Often palliative care is included in conjunction with active management in patients with worse prognoses such as those with advanced IPF and significant co-morbidities.

There is increasing support for preventative strategies such as anti-fibrotic treatment, anti-acid treatment, and protection from infection with Influenza, COVID-19 and Pneumococcal vaccines; however, this is still without robust evidence from randomised clinical trials.

References

1 Raghu G, Chen SY, Yeh WS, *et al.* (2014) Idiopathic pulmonary fibrosis in US Medicare beneficiaries aged 65 years and older: incidence, prevalence, and survival, 2001-11. *Lancet Respir Med* 2(7), 566–572.

2 Tran T, Sterclova M, Mogulkoc N, *et al.* (2020) The European MultiPartner IPF registry (EMPIRE): validating long-term prognostic factors in idiopathic pulmonary fibrosis. *Respir Res* 21(1), 11.

3 Maher TM. (2013) PROFILEing idiopathic pulmonary fibrosis: rethinking biomarker discovery. *Eur Respir Rev* 22(128), 148–152.

4 Lamas DJ, Kawut SM, Bagiella E, *et al.* (2011) Delayed access and survival in idiopathic pulmonary fibrosis: a cohort study. *Am J Respir Crit Care Med* 184(7), 842–847.

5 Neely ML, Hellkamp AS, Bender S, *et al.* (2023) Lung function trajectories in patients with idiopathic pulmonary fibrosis. *Respir Res* 24(1), 209.

6 Raghu G, Remy-Jardin M, Myers JL, *et al.* (2018) Diagnosis of idiopathic pulmonary fibrosis. An official ATS/ERS/JRS/ALAT clinical practice guideline. *Am J Respir Crit Care Med* 198(5), e44–e68.

7 Raghu G, Remy-Jardin M, Richeldi L, *et al.* (2022) Idiopathic pulmonary fibrosis (an update) and progressive pulmonary fibrosis in adults: an official ATS/ERS/JRS/ALAT clinical practice guideline. *Am J Respir Crit Care Med.* 205(9), e18–e47.

8 Karkkainen M, Kettunen HP, Nurmi H, *et al.* (2017) Effect of smoking and comorbidities on survival in idiopathic pulmonary fibrosis. *Respir Res* 18(1), 160.

9 Khor YH, Saravanan K, Holland AE, *et al.* (2021) A mixed-methods pilot study of handheld fan for breathlessness in interstitial lung disease. *Sci Rep* 11(1), 6874.

10 Raghu G, Anstrom K, King TE Jr, *et al.* (2012) Prednisone, azathioprine, and N-acetylcysteine for pulmonary fibrosis. *NEJM* 366, 1968–1977.

11 Collard HR, Ryerson CJ, Corte TJ, *et al.* (2016) Acute exacerbation of idiopathic pulmonary fibrosis. An International Working Group Report. *Am J Respir Crit Care Med* 194(3), 265–275.

12 Naccache JM, Jouneau S, Didier M, *et al.* (2022) Cyclophosphamide added to glucocorticoids in acute exacerbation of idiopathic pulmonary fibrosis (EXAFIP): a randomised, double-blind, placebo-controlled, phase 3 trial. *Lancet Respir Med* 10(1), 26–34.

13 Trudzinski FC, Kaestner F, Schafers HJ, *et al.* (2016) Outcome of patients with interstitial lung disease treated with extracorporeal membrane oxygenation for acute respiratory failure. *Am J Respir Crit Care Med* 193(5), 527–533.

CHAPTER 28

Pleural disease

ALGUILI ELSHEIKH AND ROB HALLIFAX

Pleural effusion

Pleural effusions are a common and significant clinical problem and are often a feature of underlying diseases.

Evaluation requires clinical assessment, imaging by chest X-ray (CXR), thoracic ultrasonography (TUS) and pleural phase contract CT chest and examination of pleural fluid. Assessment and management of pleural effusions are summarised in Figure 28.1. Transudative and exudative effusions (Tables 28.1 and 28.2) are caused by distinctive pathogenic mechanisms, and Light's criteria should be used for their differentiation (1, 2).

Clinical assessment and imaging

The clinical assessment is summarised in Table 28.3.

- Review the history, with a focus on occupational exposures, drugs, risk factors for pulmonary embolism or tuberculosis, extrapleural sources (e.g. ascites) and comorbid conditions, e.g. heart failure, connective tissue diseases, etc.
- Review the CXR. Pleural effusion results in basal shadowing obscuring the hemidiaphragm with a concave upper border. Massive effusion demonstrates a complete 'white-out' of the hemithorax with mediastinal displacement away from the effusion. If a mediastinal shift is not present with massive effusion, consider the possibility of a co-existing bronchial obstruction with the effusion (e.g. lung cancer).
- TUS is the standard of care in the diagnosis and management of pleural effusions (1, 3). TUS is more sensitive than CXR in detecting pleural effusion and provides additional diagnostic information on the cause of the effusion (exudative, empyema and malignant pleural effusion), and is essential in guiding intervention.
- Chest CT scan with pleural phase contrast (late venous phase) is useful in distinguishing nodular, mediastinal or circumferential pleural thickening (features present in around 80% of cases of malignant pleural disease).

Thoracentesis

- Thoracentesis (drainage of pleural fluid) is not necessarily required if the patient has a clear cause of pleural effusion (e.g. small bilateral pleural effusions and a history of heart failure or known hypothyroidism) as this cause should be treated first (1).
- Thoracentesis may be diagnostic (50–60 mL of fluid) and/or therapeutic (target: symptomatic relief, removal of 1–1.5 L of pleural fluid).
- In most cases, 1–1.5 L of pleural fluid can be aspirated with careful attention to the development of chest symptoms; re-expansion pulmonary oedema is a recognised but rare consequence of large-volume aspiration. Pleural aspiration should be stopped, if the patient develops chest tightness, chest pain or severe coughing.

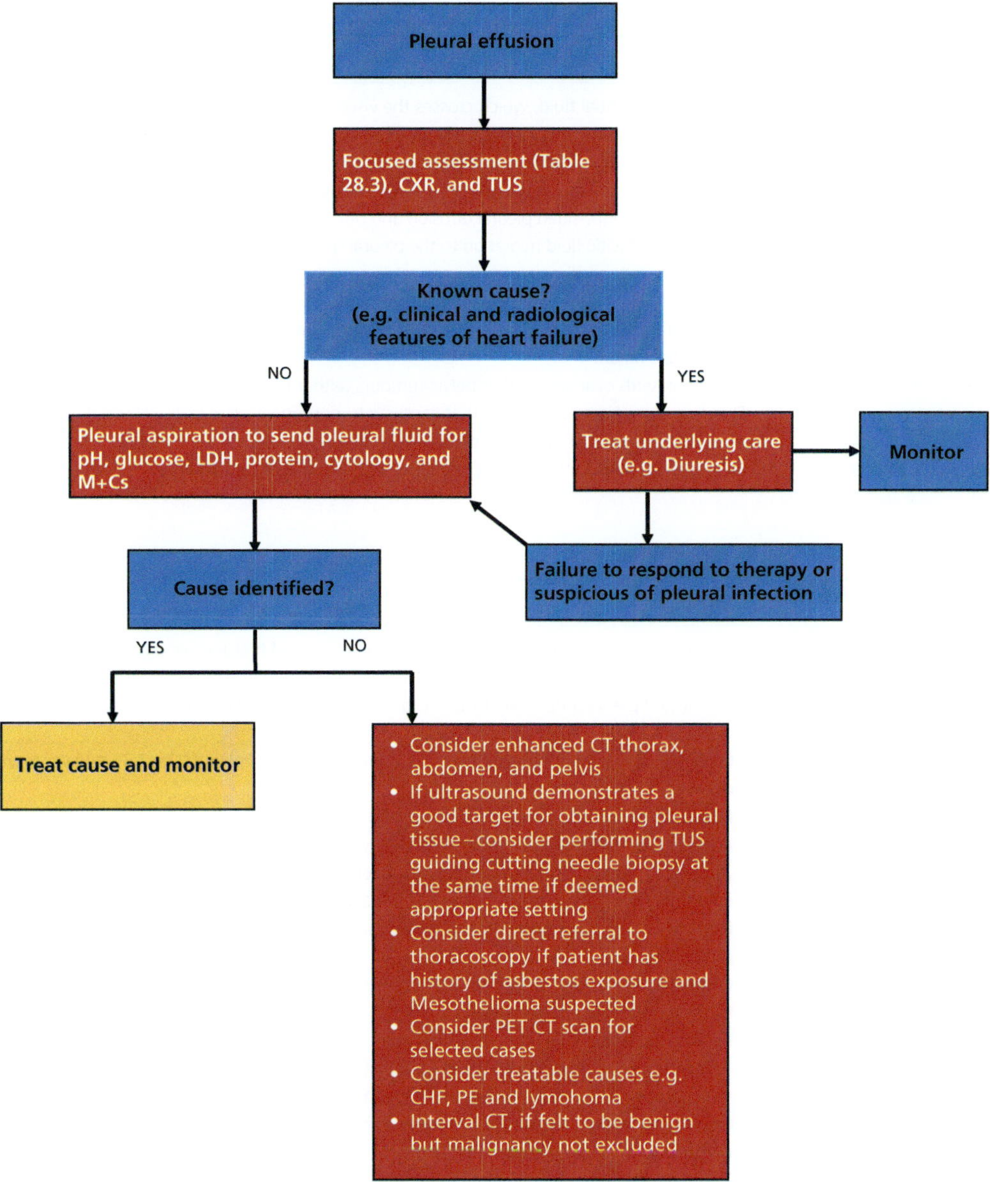

Figure 28.1 Investigation of pleural effusion. CXR chest X-ray; TUS thoracic ultrasound; LDH lactate dehydrogenase; PET CT positron émission tomography; PE pulmonary embolism; CHF chronic heart failure.

Pleural fluid should be sent for testing (summarised in Table 28.4).

- If pleural infection is suspected, inoculate pleural fluid into blood culture bottles in addition to white top containers and pleural fluid pH should be measured using a blood gas analyser: but do not analyse a purulent sample (frank pus), as this is unnecessary and may damage the machine.
- Cytology (approximately 40–50 mL should be sent for malignant cell identification and cell differential diagnosis). The sensitivity of the technique for detecting malignant pleural effusion is around 60%

Table 28.1 Causes of transudative pleural effusion.

Cause	Comment
Heart failure	Increased interstitial fluid, which crosses the visceral pleura and enters the pleural space. Investigate further if atypical features are present (unilateral effusion or failure to response to medical therapy, fever and chest pain)
Nephrotic syndrome	Usually bilateral effusions, decreased oncotic pressure causing transudate effusion
Cirrhosis with ascites	Predominantly right-sided pleural effusion and often ascites are present. Features of chronic liver disease. Ascitic fluid migration to the pleural space through diaphragmatic defects
Hypoalbuminaemia (serum albumin <25 g/L)	Associated with oedema
Hypothyroidism	May be transudate or exudate, commonly in combination with ascites, pericardial effusion and cardiac failure
Meigs' syndrome	In women with ovarian or other pelvic tumours (either bilateral or unilateral)
Urinothorax	Due to urinary tract obstruction that causes retroperitoneal urine leak. pH usually low, pleural fluid smells of urine and pleural fluid creatinine > serum creatinine is diagnostic
Constrictive pericarditis	Increases intravenous hydrostatic pressure, associated with oedema

Table 28.2 Causes of exudative pleural effusion.

Cause	Comment
Pleural infection (complicated parapneumonic effusion and empyema)	Commonly among young patients with infective clinical features; empyema is defined as pus in the pleural cavity. Confirmed pleural infection; if there is purulent pleural fluid (positive Gram stains or cultures (pleural fluid or pleural biopsy). High risk of pleural infection if pH ≤ 7.2 intermediate risk if pH > 7.21 < 7.39 and very low risk if pH ≥ 7.4.
Malignancy	Most common cause in older patients and a frequent cause of recurrent massive effusions, blood stained or straw coloured, lymphocytic predominance, positive cytology.
Tuberculosis	Delayed hypersensitivity reaction to mycobacteria released into the pleural space. Straw coloured, lymphocytic predominance, acid-fast bacillus smear or cultures often negative from fluid, caseating granuloma of pleural biopsy, ADA > 50 U/L based on the pre-test probability.
Chylothorax	Often milky effusions, diagnosis with presence of chylomicrons or pleural fluid triglyceride level >1.24 mmol/L.
Oesophageal rupture	Food particles, pH < 7.20, increased levels of salivary amylase.
Pulmonary embolism	Almost always exudative; bloody in <50%; it should be suspected when dyspnoea is disproportionate to size of effusion, or when patient is hypoxic.
After coronary artery bypass surgery (CABG)	Commonly left-sided pleural effusions and most resolve spontaneously. If <30 days of surgery, blood stained due to post-operative bleeding. If >30 days of surgery: clear fluid due to immune reaction.
Acute pancreatitis	Pleural fluid pancreatic amylase may be raised.
Rheumatoid arthritis	Typical low pleural fluid glucose (<1.6 mmol/L).
Yellow nail syndrome	Triad of nail discolouration, lymphoedema and pleural effusion.

ADA, adenosine deaminase.

(i.e. false-negative rate 40%) and the additional yield from sending more than two specimens of pleural fluid taken on different occasions is low.

- Additional tests may be indicated, depending on the clinical settings, e.g. chylomicrons, cholesterol, triglycerides, tuberculosis fluid markers (adenosine deaminase or interferon-gamma based on pre-test probability), amylase and antinuclear antibody.

Table 28.3 Focused assessment of the patient with pleural effusion.

History
Dyspnoea
Pleuritic chest pain, chest discomfort or 'heaviness', pain referred to the shoulder or abdomen but usually localised to the site of inflammation
Dry cough
Symptoms of malignancy: loss of appetite and weight, lack of energy
Symptoms of infection: fever, sputum, night sweats
May also be asymptomatic

Examination
Reduced chest expansion
Reduced tactile vocal fremitus
Dull percussion
Reduced breath sounds
Pleural friction rub may be heard in patient with pleural inflammation

Table 28.4 Pleural fluid analysis: (1) in all patients and (2) additional tests for exudative effusions.

Pleural fluid analysis (1): In all patients

Test	Comment
Visual inspection	Blood-stained effusion (pleural fluid haematocrit 1–20% of peripheral haematocrit) is likely to be due to malignancy, pulmonary embolism or trauma. Purulent fluid signifies empyema. Milky coloured caused by chylothorax or pseudochylothorax
Protein and lactate dehydrogenase (LDH)	Pleural fluid LDH correlates with the degree of pleural inflammation. Exudative pleural effusions have a protein concentration >30 g/L. If the pleural fluid protein is around 30 g/L, Light's criteria are helpful in distinguishing between a transudate and exudate. An exudate is identified by one or more of the following: • Pleural fluid protein to serum protein ratio >0.5 • Pleural fluid LDH to serum LDH ratio >0.6 • Pleural fluid LDH more than two-thirds the upper limit of normal for serum LDH

Pleural fluid analysis (2): Additional tests for exudative pleural effusion

Test	Comment
Pleural fluid pH and glucose (check these if parapneumonic or malignant pleural effusion is suspected. Send sample in heparinized syringe for measurement of pH in blood gas analyser)	Low pH (<7.2)/low glucose (<3.3 mmol/L) pleural fluid may be seen in: • Complicated parapneumonic effusion and empyema • Malignancy • Rheumatoid or lupus pleuritis • Tuberculosis • Oesophageal rupture
Cytology (total and differential cell count; malignant cells)	Neutrophilia (>50% cells) indicate acute pleural disease. Lymphocytosis is seen in malignancy, tuberculous pleuritis and in pleural effusions after CABG. The yield of cytology is influenced by the histological type of malignancy: >70% positive in adenocarcinoma, 25–50% in lymphoma, 10% in mesothelioma.
Microbiology (Gram stain culture; markers of tuberculosis [TB])	Send fluid for markers of TB, e.g. ADA if TB is suspected or there is a pleural fluid. lymphocytosis.
Other tests depending on clinical setting (e.g. amylase, triglyceride, ANA, ADA)	Elevated pleural fluid amylase is seen in the acute pancreatitis and oesophageal rupture. Check triglyceride level if chylothorax is suspected (opaque white effusion); chylothorax (triglyceride >1.1 g/L) is due to disruption of the thoracic duct by trauma or lymphoma.

ADA, adenosine deaminase; ANA, antinuclear antibody; CABG, coronary artery bypass graft; TB, tuberculosis.

To answer this important question, Light's criteria should be employed. The effusion is an exudate if it meets one of the following criteria:

- Pleural fluid protein/serum protein ratio >0.5.
- Pleural fluid LDH/serum LDH ratio >0.6.
- Pleural fluid LDH greater than two-thirds of the upper limit of normal serum LDH.

Light's criteria correctly identify almost all exudates, but mis-classifies about 20% of transudates as exudates. If a transudative effusion is suspected (e.g. due to heart failure or liver cirrhosis) and none of the biochemical measurements are >15% above the cut-off levels for Light's criteria, the difference between serum and the pleural fluid protein is measured. If the difference is >31 g/L, the effusion is probably a transudate.

Further management

Treatment of symptoms and underlying disorder

- The effusion itself generally does not require treatment if the patient is asymptomatic.
- Many effusions resorb spontaneously when the underlying disorder is treated, especially effusions due to heart failure, pulmonary embolism, hypothyroidism or after coronary artery bypass surgery (CABG).
- Pleuritic pain can usually be managed with non-steroidal anti-inflammatory drugs (NSAIDs) or other oral analgesics including opioids.

Drainage of a symptomatic effusion

- Therapeutic aspiration is a sufficient treatment for many symptomatic effusions and can be repeated for effusions that re-accumulate. Seek advice from a chest physician or pleural specialist.

Specific management for complicated parapneumonic effusions and empyema

- Seek advice from a chest physician or pleural specialist. For indications for chest drain insertion see Table 28.5.
- Consider using a risk stratification tool to predict mortality and morbidity (such as the RAPID score) but these have not validated to guide patient management.
- All patients with pleural infection should be treated with antibiotics (refer to local hospital prescribing guidelines) and chest drain insertion, should this fail (a persistent feature of systemic inflammatory syndrome and significant residual fluid collection on radiology (TUS, CT or CXR) in 48–72 hours then consider intrapleural fibrinolytic enzyme therapy or referral to surgeons if deemed appropriate (1).
- Antibiotic options ought to be rationalised with culture and sensitivity results of the pleural fluid or blood cultures (note that anaerobes are frequently difficult to culture and may coexist with other organisms).

Table 28.5 Indications for chest tube insertion for parapneumonic effusions/empyema (1, 3).

Purulent pleural fluid
High-risk CPPE or pleural infection (pH ≤ 7.20)
Moderate risk CPPE or pleural infection diagnosed when pH between 7.2 and 7.39 plus LDH ≥ 900 with any of the following:

- Large effusion
- Septation on thoracic ultrasound
- Pleural contrast enhancement on CT chest (if performed)
- Pleural fluid glucose ≤ 4 mmol/L or 72 mg/dL (non-diabetic)

Pleural fluid pH > 7.4 plus septation on radiology (thoracic ultrasound or CT chest)
Pleural fluid positive culture or Gram stain

NB: The ideal chest drain size is subject to debate but small (≤ 14 F) drains may be as effective as larger ones (>14 F) in the management of empyema, and cause less pain and discomfort. Regular flushes with normal saline (0.9%) are needed (20 mL four times per day).

Specific management for malignant pleural effusions
- Seek advice from a chest physician or pleural specialist.
- Asymptomatic effusions and those causing dyspnoea unrelieved by thoracentesis do not require additional procedures.
- If dyspnoea caused by malignant pleural effusion is relieved by thoracentesis but fluid and dyspnoea redevelop, definitive treatment is required (talc pleurodesis or placement of an indwelling pleural catheter [IPC]) based on patient choice.
- Pleurodesis is performed by instilling a sclerosing agent into the pleural space in order to seal the visceral and parietal pleura and hence to stop fluid recurrence. The most effective and commonly used sclerosing agent is talc. Talc pleurodesis can be performed either by the insertion of a chest tube (14–18F) as a slurry or by medical thoracoscopy as a poudrage.
- IPC drainage is the preferred approach for ambulatory patients because hospitalisation is not necessary for catheter insertion and the pleural fluid can be drained intermittently into vacuum bottles. IPC is the preferred option for patients with significant trapped lung (when the tumour encases the visceral pleura and prevents lung re-expansion).
- A thoracoscopic or image-guided pleural biopsy may be used depending on the clinical indication and local availability of techniques however blind biopsies should not be conducted.
- Image-guided biopsies or thoracoscopic techniques have significantly better results compared to closed pleural biopsies. Thoracoscopy also offers diagnostic and therapeutic approaches to patients with pleural effusion (e.g. talc poudrage pleurodesis).
- Even after extensive investigations, 25% of pleural effusions remain undiagnosed. These are often due to occult pulmonary embolism, TB, viral infection or cancer.

Pneumothorax

Pneumothorax is a common pathology. Spontaneous pneumothorax (SP) is conventionally defined as the accumulation of air in the pleural space in the absence of trauma or causative medical intervention. The incidence of SP has increased from 9.1 to 14.1 per 100,000 population over the last 50 years in the United Kingdom (4). It is associated with a significant symptom burden and healthcare utilisation (4, 5). The disease is more common in men than women (4, 6). Data from the United Kingdom suggest that the annual admission rate for pneumothorax of 16.7 per 100,000 for men and 5.8 per 100,000 for women, with a corresponding mortality rate of 1.26 per million and 0.62 per million per year, respectively (6). An annual pneumothorax rate of 22.7 per 100,000 population in national data from France (6).

Spontaneous pneumothorax can be subdivided into primary spontaneous pneumothorax (PSP) in the absence of suspected lung disease, or secondary spontaneous pneumothorax (SSP) in patients with an established underlying lung disease. However, although it is still widely used, the utility of making such a distinction is being challenged in many articles. The peak incidence for PSP occurs at 35 years of age, whereas SSP occurs later in life at 53 years, reflecting a parallel increase in chronic lung disease as age increases (6).

The risk of PSP is thought to be increased by smoking, being of tall stature and having a low body mass index (BMI). Importantly, Cigarette smoking increases the risk of pneumothorax ninefold in women and 22-fold in men (7). The most common causes of SP are listed in Table 28.6. When the accumulation of air around the lung compromises cardiac and respiratory function, this is called tension pneumothorax. This is a life-threatening condition that requires urgent intervention. Signs of tension pneumothorax and needle decompression are shown in Tables 28.7 and 28.8.

The assessment and management of pneumothorax is summarised in Figure 28.2.

Table 28.6 Classification and causes of pneumothorax.

1. **Spontaneous pneumothorax**
   Primary (PSP)
   - No underlying lung disease
   - Typically occurs in tall thin males aged 15–30 years
   - Association with tobacco and cannabis smoking
   - Rare in patients over 40
   Secondary (SSP)
   - Airways disease (COPD, cystic fibrosis, acute severe asthma)
   - Infectious lung disease (*Pneumocystis carinii* (*jirovecii*) pneumonia; necrotizing pneumonia caused by anaerobic, Gram-negative bacteria or Staphylococcus aureus and tuberculosis)
   - Interstitial lung disease (e.g. sarcoidosis)
   - Connective tissue disease (e.g. rheumatoid arthritis and Marfan syndrome)
   - Genetic syndrome (e.g. Birt–Hogg–Dube syndrome, Tuberous sclerosis and pulmonary LAM)
   - Malignancy (bronchial carcinoma or sarcoma)
   - Other (e.g. thoracic endometriosis 'catamenial pneumothorax')
2. **Traumatic pneumothorax** (due to penetrating or blunt chest trauma)
   Should be managed by surgical team
3. **Iatrogenic pneumothorax**
   - Transthoracic needle aspiration
   - Transbronchial needle aspiration or biopsy
   - Subclavian vein puncture
   - Thoracentesis and lung biopsy
   - Pericardiocentesis
   - Barotrauma related to mechanical ventilation

COPD, chronic obstructive airway disease.

Table 28.7 Signs of tension pneumothorax.

1. Pleuritic chest pain
2. Respiratory distress (dyspnoea, tachypnoea, ability to speak only in short sentences or single words, agitation and sweating)
3. Falling arterial oxygen saturation
4. Ipsilateral hyperexpansion, hypomobility and hyperresonance with decreased breath sounds
5. Tachycardia
6. Hypotension (late sign)
7. Tracheal deviation (inconsistent sign)
8. Elevated jugular venous pressure (inconsistent sign)

Table 28.8 Needle aspiration of pneumothorax.

1. With the patient semi-recumbent, identify the second or third intercostal space in the mid-clavicular line
2. Infiltrate with lidocaine 1% to the skin and down to and around the pleura
3. Connect a 21 G (green) needle to a three-way tap and a 60 mL syringe
4. Withdraw air and expel it via the three-way tap
5. Aspirate up to a maximum of 2.5 L of air
6. Obtain a chest X-ray to assess the resolution of the pneumothorax
7. If aspiration fails to sufficiently re-inflate the lung, insert a small bore (<14 F) chest drain

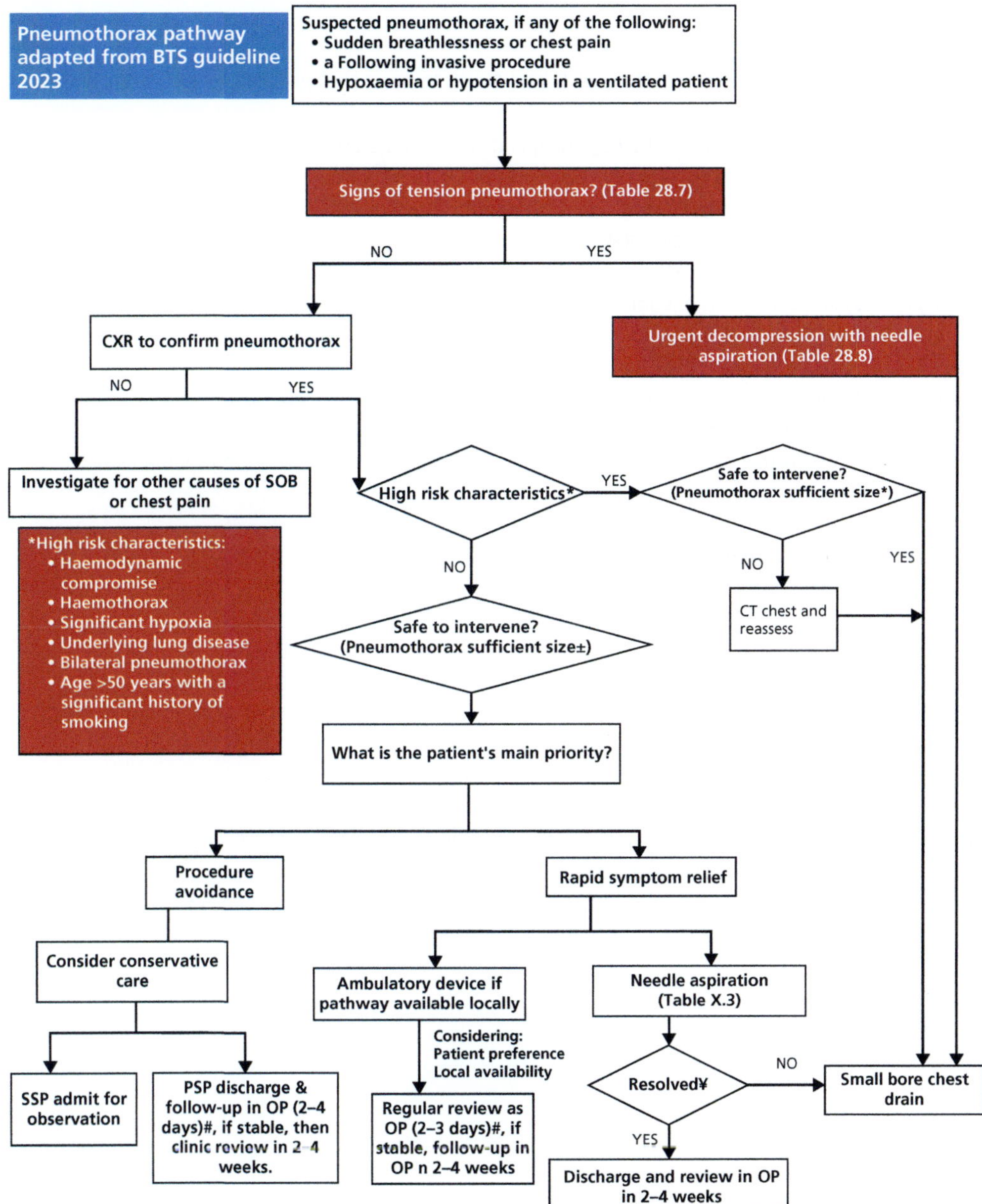

Figure 28.2 ± Pneumothorax of sufficient size to intervene depends on the clinical context but, in general, usually ≥2cm laterally or apically on CXR, or any size on CT scan which can be safely accessed with radiologist support. # At review, consider chest drain insertion and admission if enlarging pneumothorax or worsening symptoms. ¥ Resolution: improvement in symptoms and sustained improvement on CXR. CXR: chest x-ray; CT: computed tomography scan SSP: secondary spontaneous pneumothorax; PSP: primary spontaneous pneumothorax; OP: outpatient.

References

1 Roberts ME, Rahman NM, Maskell NA, *et al*. (2023) British Thoracic Society Guideline for pleural disease. *Thorax* 78(Suppl 3), s1–s42.
2 Light RW. (2013) The light criteria: the beginning and why they are useful 40 years later. *Clin Chest Med* [cited 2024 Sep 4] 34(1), 21–26. https://www.sciencedirect.com/science/article/pii/S0272523112001244.
3 Asciak R, Bedawi EO, Bhatnagar R, *et al*. (2023) British thoracic Society Clinical Statement on pleural procedures. *Thorax* 78(Suppl 3), s43–s68.
4 Hallifax RJ, Goldacre R, Landray MJ, *et al*. (2018) Trends in the incidence and recurrence of inpatient-treated spontaneous pneumothorax, 1968-2016. *JAMA* 320(14), 1471–1480.
5 Gupta D, Hansell A, Nichols T, *et al*. (2000) Epidemiology of pneumothorax in England. *Thorax* 55(8), 666–671.
6 Bobbio A, Dechartres A, Bouam S, *et al*. (2015) Epidemiology of spontaneous pneumothorax: gender-related differences. *Thorax* 70(7), 653–658.
7 Bense L, Eklund G, Wiman LG. (1987) Smoking and the increased risk of contracting spontaneous pneumothorax. *Chest* 92(6), 1009–1012.

Further reading

Corcoran JP, Psallidas I, Gerry S, *et al*. (2020) Prospective validation of the RAPID clinical risk prediction score in adult patients with pleural infection: the PILOT study. *Eur Respir J* 56(5), 2000130. doi: 10.1183/13993003.00130-2020. Erratum in: *Eur Respir J*. 2020 Dec 17;56(6):2050130. doi: 10.1183/13993003.50130-2020. PMID: 32675200.
Elsheikh A, Bhatnagar M, Rahman NM. (2023) Diagnosis and management of pleural infection. *Breathe* 19(4).
Porcel JM. (2013) Identifying transudates misclassified by Light's criteria. *Curr Opin Pulm Med.* 19(4), 362–367. doi: 10.1097/MCP.0b013e32836022dc. PMID: 23508114.
Psallidas I, Kalomenidis I, Porcel JM, *et al*. (2016) Malignant pleural effusion: from bench to bedside. *Eur Respir Rev* 25, 189–198. doi: 10.1183/16000617.0019-2016.

CHAPTER 29

Sleep-disordered breathing

Su Latt Phyu and Christopher Turnbull

Sleep-disordered breathing (SDB) refers to a range of conditions that result in abnormal breathing during sleep. They can be broadly categorised into two main types: obstructive sleep apnoea (OSA), and central breathing disorders including central sleep apnoea (CSA) and hypoventilation syndromes.

Obstructive sleep apnoea (OSA)

OSA is the most prevalent SDB. It is one end of a spectrum that includes snoring, snoring-induced arousals and upper airway resistance syndrome. OSA is caused by recurrent partial or complete upper airway obstruction during sleep resulting in recurrent oxygen desaturations. It is a common cause of nocturnal desaturations in hospitalised patients.

Epidemiology

It is estimated that OSA affects approximately 1 billion people worldwide (1) and around 80% of people with OSA remain undiagnosed (2). Untreated OSA is associated with higher cardiovascular risks including hypertension, ischaemic heart diseases and atrial fibrillation (3).

Clinical features

The most common risk factor for OSA is obesity. Other risk factors include anatomical factors such as retrognathia, enlarged tonsils, hormonal causes such as hypothyroidism and neuromuscular causes such as muscular dystrophies.

NICE guidelines state that individuals with ≥2 of the following symptoms should be assessed for OSA:
- loud snoring
- witnessed apnoeas
- unrefreshing sleep
- waking headaches
- unexplained excessive sleepiness, tiredness or fatigue
- nocturia
- choking during sleep
- sleep fragmentation or insomnia
- cognitive dysfunction or memory impairment

Acute Medicine: A Practical Guide to the Management of Medical Emergencies, Sixth Edition.
Edited by Mridula Rajwani, Leila Vaziri, and Ivie Gbinigie.
© 2026 John Wiley & Sons Ltd. Published 2026 by John Wiley & Sons Ltd.

Other less common symptoms include enuresis, reduced libido and nocturnal sweating. Symptomatic reflux and/or nocturnal cough is reported in <10% of sufferers.

Referral

Anyone with suspected OSA should be referred to a sleep service for further assessment. It is important to include the following: the results of the person's assessment scores, for example Epworth Sleepiness Scale (ESS), symptoms and their effects on daily activities, co-morbidities, occupational risk and if available, oxygen saturations and blood gas results.

Priority factors for rapid assessment include:

- vocational driving or vigilance critical job
- unstable cardiovascular disease
- pregnancy
- preoperative assessment for major surgery
- non-arteritic anterior ischaemic optic neuropathy

Investigations

- The key investigation to diagnose OSA and determine severity is home respiratory polygraphy which includes oximetry recording, noise recording, nasal cannulae measuring airflow, and abdominal and thoracic bands measuring respiratory effort.
- Hospital respiratory polygraphy can be considered if home respiratory polygraphy is impractical or additional monitoring is needed.
- Overnight oximetry alone is not usually recommended unless other tests are unavailable as it cannot differentiate between OSA and CSA.
- Full polysomnography can be considered if respiratory polygraphy results are negative, but symptoms continue. This is rarely needed for diagnosis of OSA and is more useful in diagnosis of narcolepsy and some parasomnias.

Treatment

Lifestyle modification such as losing weight, reducing alcohol intake and maintaining a good sleep hygiene is the first step approach in management of individuals with OSA. In those with moderate to severe OSA or mild OSA with significant symptom burden, treatment with continuous positive airway pressure (CPAP) should also be offered.

CPAP is a mechanical treatment that delivers pressurised air to splint the upper airway open during sleep. It has been shown to improve symptoms, reduce arousals and improve quality of life for patients with OSA. CPAP can deliver either a fixed continuous pressure or pressure that is constantly self-adjusting according to the airflow resistance called auto-titrating positive airway pressure (APAP). Common problems while on CPAP treatment and troubleshooting are detailed in Table 29.1.

Admissions in patients on CPAP treatment

When admitted with unrelated problems, patients should continue using their own CPAP machines in hospital unless there is any contraindication, e.g. recurrent vomiting, craniofacial trauma. If there are any concerns with CPAP machine or mask, consider contacting the team responsible for their CPAP.

Table 29.1 Problems encountered with CPAP treatment.

Problem	Solution
Air leak around the mask	Adjust the mask size and head straps, ensure mask is cleaned regularly
Nasal blockage	Occasionally, a heated humidifier needs to be added to the circuit
Aerophagy – uncomfortable/ bloating sensation	Reduce CPAP pressure if possible
Continued snoring	Consider increasing CPAP pressure
Continued sleepiness	Review the CPAP compliance. Consider if there is a mask leak making the treatment less effective. May need repeating the sleep study on CPAP to ensure hypopnoeas/ apnoeas are well controlled. Consider other additional issues, e.g. lack of sleep opportunities, shift work or other sleep disorder like periodic limb movement disorder

Perioperative management of patients with OSA

OSA is an established risk factor for a difficult airway during intubation. Patients with moderate to severe OSA have a higher risk of respiratory complications, including respiratory failure, hypoxaemic episodes, and reintubation (4). The anaesthetic team should be informed of the patient's diagnosis and treatment. Sedatives and opioids should be used to a minimum and with close monitoring for respiratory depression. Many pre-operative clinics now screen for sleep apnoea routinely and if surgery can be deferred, anaesthetics teams will sometimes request surgery is deferred to establish CPAP in people with confirmed moderate to severe OSA.

Other treatment options

Jaw advancement devices (JADs)

These devices hold the bottom jaw in protrusion relative to the upper jaw overnight. This pulls the tongue base forward off the posterior pharyngeal wall, reducing apnoeas. JADs are most suitable for patients with retrognathia, a slim neck, age over 18 years and optimal dental and periodontal health. They can come as customised or semi-customised mandibular advancement splints. They can be considered in patients with all severities of OSA who do not tolerate or decline CPAP. They are inappropriate in people with active dental problems, who have no or few teeth or in those with generalised tonic-clonic seizures.

Positional therapies

Positional OSA relates to those who have an apnoea-hypopnoea index (AHI) at least twice as high when lying supine compared with non-supine. Techniques to encourage patients not to sleep on their back can help, these include sleeping with a tennis ball sown onto the back of a T-shirt, lumbar or abdominal binders or sleeping alongside a full-length pillow. Newer vibro-tactile devices, which vibrate when patients lie supine have been shown to be effective in reducing AHI, but further research is needed. If other treatments are not suitable or not tolerated, positional modifiers can be used in people with mild or moderate positional OSA. They are unlikely to work in severe OSA.

Surgery

Tonsillectomy: NICE guidelines recommend considering tonsillectomy for people with OSA who have large obstructive tonsils and a BMI < 35 kg/m^2. Individuals with a higher BMI are more likely to have multi-level upper airway obstruction and are therefore less likely to benefit from tonsillectomy.

Modified uvulo-palatopharyngoplasty and tongue reduction: Patients with severe OSA who have not been able to tolerate CPAP and a customised mandibular advancement device can be referred for oropharyngeal surgery. The aim of surgery is to widen and stabilise the upper airway; this has been shown to improve outcomes in individuals who have not been able to tolerate other treatment options (5).

Hypoglossal nerve stimulation

This is a novel treatment for OSA. It involves an implantation device under the skin in the chest with leads running up under the chin to stimulate the hypoglossal nerve to activate muscles in the tongue and reduce upper airway collapsibility. This can be considered in individuals who failed CPAP therapy and who have a BMI$<35\,kg/m^2$ and suitability is assessed on a case-by-case basis.

Driving

The Driver and Vehicle Licensing Agency (DVLA) includes sleep disorders as part of its guidance on driving for individuals with medical conditions in the UK (Table 29.2). The rules for car and motorcycle drivers (group 1 driving licence holders) differ slightly from those for bus and lorry drivers (group 2 driving licence holders) (Table 29.2). The DVLA defines excessive sleepiness as having, or being likely to have, an adverse effect on driving. Asking about recent road traffic collisions, episodes of falling or nearly falling asleep behind the wheel, and use of alerting strategies (e.g. winding down the windows, turning up the radio) can help to identify high-risk drivers. The ESS should not be used alone to identify driving risk.

Table 29.2 DVLA guidance on excessive sleepiness for group 1 and 2 driving licence holders.

	Group 1 Car and motorcycle	Group 2 Bus and lorry
Excessive sleepiness due to a medical condition including mild obstructive sleep apnoea syndrome (AHI below 15) or medication.	• Must not drive. Driving may resume only after satisfactory symptom control. If symptom control cannot be achieved in three months DVLA must be notified.	• Must not drive. Driving may resume only after satisfactory symptom control. If symptom control cannot be achieved in three months DVLA must be notified.
Excessive sleepiness due to obstructive sleep apnoea syndrome – moderate and severe: • AH1 15–29 (moderate) • AHI 30 or more (severe) on the apnoea-hypopnoea index or equivalent sleep study measure	• Must not drive and must notify DVLA. Subsequent licensing will require: • control of condition • improved sleepiness • treatment adherence DVLA will need medical confirmation of the above, and the driver must confirm review to be undertaken every three years at the minimum.	• Must not drive and must notify DVLA. Subsequent licensing will require: • control of condition • improved sleepiness • treatment adherence DVLA will need medical confirmation of the above, and the driver must confirm review to be undertaken annually at the minimum.
Excessive sleepiness due to suspected obstructive sleep apnoea syndrome.	• Must not drive. Driving may resume only after satisfactory symptom control. If symptom control cannot be achieved in three months DVLA must be notified. See 'Excessive sleepiness due to obstructive sleep apnoea syndrome' above when diagnosis is confirmed.	• Must not drive. Driving may resume only after satisfactory symptom control. If symptom control cannot be achieved in three months DVLA must be notified. See 'Excessive sleepiness due to obstructive sleep apnoea syndrome' above when diagnosis is confirmed.

Individuals with OSA but no excessive sleepiness can continue to drive and do not need to inform the DVLA. Both group 1 and group 2 drivers who are diagnosed with moderate to severe OSA causing excessive sleepiness must stop driving and inform the DVLA in writing. The DVLA's Medical Group then sends a questionnaire to the driver and treating physician to assess symptom control, treatment compliance and response. Driving can usually resume once the OSA has been fully controlled. Although the treating physician has an obligation to advise patients that they must inform the DVLA of their diagnosis, it is the patient's responsibility to do this. Following treatment initiation, the DVLA requires a medical review every three years for group 1 drivers and annually for group 2 drivers.

Individuals with mild OSA or other sleep conditions causing excessive sleepiness sufficient to impair driving must stop driving until the symptoms satisfactorily resolve but should notify the DVLA only if symptom control cannot be achieved in three months. This rule is the same for drivers with excessive sleepiness who are suspected to have OSA but no formal diagnosis has yet been made. Regardless of the cause of excessive sleepiness, drivers should be advised not to drive but they need not notify the DVLA unless symptom control cannot be achieved in three months. Patients required to notify the DVLA should also notify their insurer.

Central sleep apnoea

CSA is a disorder where there are recurrent pauses in breathing due to a lack of respiratory drive during sleep. CSA may present with similar symptoms of daytime sleepiness, witnessed apnoeas but snoring is less common. It can be either primary (idiopathic) or secondary. In practice, it is commonly associated with underlying medical conditions such as heart failure and neurological conditions. Treatment of underlying medical conditions is the cornerstone of management of CSA. In certain cases, supplemental oxygen therapy, acetazolamide, sedatives, CPAP, and/ or adaptive servo ventilation may be indicated.

Hypoventilation syndromes

This is the term used to refer to a group of disorders associated with alveolar hypoventilation (indicated by arterial CO_2 ($PaCO_2$) > 6 kPa, usually with renal compensation and a high serum bicarbonate level). Hypoxia is also present in most cases, especially during sleep in early stages. Common causes include obesity hypoventilation syndrome (OHS), underlying lung diseases such as COPD, chest wall disorders such as kyphoscoliosis, and neuromuscular conditions (e.g. motor neurone disease). Symptoms of hypoventilation include those seen in OSA such as daytime sleepiness and waking headaches. In addition, there can be peripheral oedema suggesting the presence of cor pulmonale and unexplained polycythaemia which are not commonly seen in OSA alone. Orthopnoea is a common symptom of neuromuscular conditions such as motor neurone disease.

Obesity hypoventilation syndrome

OHS is defined as the combination of obesity (body mass index [BMI] of 30 kg/m² or more), raised arterial or arterialised capillary carbon dioxide (CO_2) level when awake, and breathing abnormalities during sleep, which may consist of obstructive apnoeas and hypopnoeas or hypoventilation or a combination of both. 70% of OHS overlaps with severe OSA and is adequately treated by CPAP in most cases unless there is the presence of acute ventilatory failure in which case non-invasive bi-level ventilation (NIV) should be offered. NIV is also indicated if symptoms do not improve, hypercapnia persists, AHI or oxygen desaturation index (ODI) are not sufficiently reduced, or CPAP is poorly tolerated.

COPD overlap with OSA

COPD can cause hypoventilation by complex mechanisms not fully understood. It is commonly associated with OSA, and the overlap increases the risk of COPD exacerbations, cardiovascular risks and carries a poorer prognosis than each condition alone. CPAP is the first-line treatment for people with COPD–OSA overlap syndrome if they do not have severe hypercapnia ($PaCO_2$ of 7.0 kPa or less). NIV should be offered if $PaCO_2 > 7$ kPa, as in these cases, NIV has been shown to improve admission-free survival.

References

1 Benjafield AV, Ayas NT, Eastwood PR, *et al.* (2019) Estimation of the global prevalence and burden of obstructive sleep apnoea: a literature-based analysis. *Lancet Respir Med* 7, 687–698.

2 Hidden Health Crisis Costing America Billions. https://aasm.org/resources/pdf/sleep-apnea-economic-crisis.pdf.

3 Yeghiazarians Y, Jneid H, Tietjens JR, *et al.* (2021) Obstructive sleep apnoea and cardiovascular disease: a scientific statement from the American Heart Association. *Circulation* 144, e56–e67.

4 Cozowicz C, Memtsoudis SG. (2021) Perioperative management of the patient with obstructive sleep apnea: a narrative review. *Anesth Analg* 132, 1231–1243.

5 MacKay S, Carney AS, Catcheside PG, *et al.* (2020) Effect of multilevel upper airway surgery vs medical management on the apnea-hypopnea index and patient-reported daytime sleepiness among patients with moderate or severe obstructive sleep apnoea: the SAMS randomized clinical trial. *JAMA* 324, 1168–1179.

CHAPTER 30

Respiratory failure: oxygenation and ventilatory support

Mia Cokljat and Nayia Petousi

Definition of respiratory failure

Respiratory failure is defined as inadequate gas exchange resulting in hypoxaemia.

- Acute respiratory failure develops over a time course of minutes (hyperacute), hours or days (sub-acute), whereas chronic respiratory failure develops over weeks, months or years.
- Respiratory failure is subdivided into:
- **Type 1**: PaO_2 <8 kPa and normal or low $PaCO_2$
- **Type 2**: PaO_2 <8 kPa with a raised $PaCO_2$ >6 kPa
- Type 1 respiratory failure is caused primarily by ventilation/perfusion ($\dot{V}/\dot{Q}$) mismatch and usually relates to diseases within the respiratory system. Type 2 respiratory failure is caused by alveolar hypoventilation, with or without V/Q mismatch and can thus be caused by diseases both intrinsic and extrinsic to the respiratory system.

Assessment of oxygenation and arterial blood gas analysis

Arterial oxygen tension and its determinants

Arterial oxygen tension refers to the partial pressure of oxygen in the arterial blood (PaO_2). In a person breathing air (fraction of oxygen in the inspired air (FiO_2) 21%), typically a normal PaO_2 is >10.7 kPa. Normal arterial carbon dioxide tension ($PaCO_2$) is 4.7–6.0 kPa. PaO_2 and $PaCO_2$ can be measured using arterial blood gas sampling and analysis.

Gas exchange occurs at the level of the alveolar capillaries. The relationship of alveolar partial pressure of oxygen (PAO_2) to inspired partial pressure of oxygen (PiO_2) and alveolar (or arterial) partial pressure of carbon dioxide ($PaCO_2$) is $PAO_2 = PiO_2 - PaCO_2/R$, where R is the respiratory quotient and normally has a value of 0.8. The difference between alveolar and arterial oxygen partial pressures is given as the A-a gradient = $PAO_2 - PaO_2$.

Factors that influence gas exchange, and therefore arterial oxygen tension are:

- The inspired oxygen concentration (FiO_2), which determines the inspired partial pressure of oxygen (PiO_2)
- Alveolar ventilation, which is determined by tidal volume, dead space and respiratory rate
- Diffusion of oxygen from alveoli to pulmonary capillaries
- Distribution and matching of lung ventilation and pulmonary blood flow (V/Q matching).

Thus, an increased A-a gradient indicates V/Q mismatching which may reflect a range of pulmonary and pulmonary vascular disorders.

Acute Medicine: A Practical Guide to the Management of Medical Emergencies, Sixth Edition.
Edited by Mridula Rajwani, Leila Vaziri, and Ivie Gbinigie.

Oxygen content of blood and peripheral oxygen saturation

Oxygen is carried in blood in two forms: dissolved (very small amount) and combined with Haemoglobin (Hb). The oxygen saturation of blood is the percentage of Hb-binding sites that have O_2 attached. Arterial oxygen saturation depends on arterial oxygen tension, and this relationship is governed by the oxyhaemoglobin dissociation curve. Arterial oxygen saturation can be measured either directly via arterial blood sampling or indirectly with pulse oximetry. Pulse oximetry is more readily available and less invasive for the patient, but can be subject to inaccurate readings (Table 30.1).

Acid-base balance

In addition to PCO_2 and PO_2, blood gas analysis will also give pH and bicarbonate readings, where normal is 7.35–7.45 and 23–29 mmol/L, respectively. The relationship between PCO_2, pH and HCO_3 is given by the Henderson–Hasselbalch equation: $pH = pK_a + log([HCO_3^-]/0.03PCO_2)$.

In type 2 respiratory failure, a low pH but normal bicarbonate level implies acute ventilatory failure with respiratory acidosis where there has not been time for metabolic compensation. Conversely, a bicarbonate level >29 mmol/L demonstrates a degree of chronicity to the ventilatory failure. A low pH superimposed on top of high carbon dioxide and high bicarbonate levels implies acute on chronic decompensated ventilatory failure; pH will be normal in chronic respiratory failure due to metabolic compensation (Table 30.2).

Management of acute respiratory failure

The management of the patient with suspected acute respiratory failure is summarized in Figures 30.1 and 30.2, according to the below priorities:

1 Is urgent intubation and/or ventilation required?

Assess if there is severe upper airway obstruction (Chapter 105), inability to protect airway due to decreased consciousness (Chapter 3), impending respiratory or cardiac arrest, severe hypoxia despite oxygen treatment or severe acidosis/hypercapnia.

Table 30.1 Pulse oximetry: causes of inaccurate reading.

- Probe not properly on finger
- Motion artefact
- Poor perfusion of finger
- Venous congestion
- Hypothermia
- Intense ambient light
- Abnormal haemoglobin (carboxyhaemoglobin, methaemoglobin and sickle haemoglobin)
- Severe anaemia (Hb < 50 g/L)

Table 30.2 Demonstrating primary (causal) changes in acid–base disturbance and secondary (compensatory) response.

Acid–base disturbance	pH	PCO_2	Bicarbonate
Respiratory acidosis	↓	↑ (1°)	↑ (2°)
Respiratory alkalosis	↑	↓ (1°)	=
Metabolic acidosis	↓	=/↓ (2°)	↓ (1°)
Metabolic alkalosis	↑	=	↓ (1°)

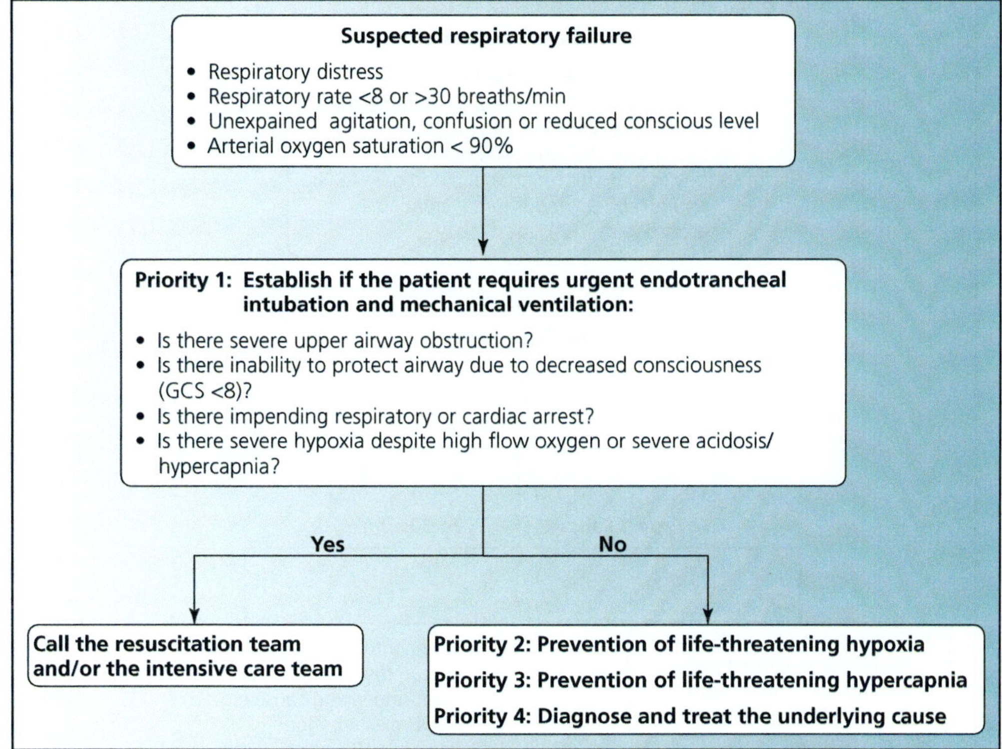

Figure 30.1 Management of the patient with suspected acute respiratory failure: priorities.

2 Prevent life-threatening hypoxia

Oxygen therapy is key in preventing life-threatening hypoxia, but caution should be taken. Patients known to suffer from chronic obstructive pulmonary disease (COPD) may have chronic respiratory failure with hypercapnia; in these patients, hypoxia acts as a stimulus to ventilatory drive and abolishing it completely may make respiratory failure worse. These patients need controlled oxygen therapy. Establish early, with the means of an arterial blood gas, whether the patient has type 1 or type 2 respiratory failure and instigate appropriate oxygen therapy (Figure 30.2). Methods of oxygen delivery are given in Table 30.3.

3 Prevent life-threatening hypercapnia

Patients with type 2 respiratory failure will require controlled oxygen therapy via a Venturi mask, aiming for SaO_2 of 88–92% (Figure 30.2). If high $PaCO_2$ or acidosis persists after treatment of the underlying cause, assisted ventilation will be required.

4 Diagnose and manage the underlying cause (Table 30.4)

Careful history, examination and appropriate investigations are paramount. Management will be determined by the working diagnosis and the response to initial treatment. For example:

- Inhaled bronchodilator therapy (e.g. salbutamol 2.5–5 mg) and steroids (e.g. prednisolone 30–40 mg) in acute exacerbation of asthma or COPD (Chapters 22 and 23).
- Intravenous diuretic (e.g. furosemide 40–80 mg) in acute pulmonary oedema (Chapter 14).
- Antibiotic therapy in pneumonia (Chapter 25).
- Anticoagulation (e.g. low-molecular-weight heparin) in pulmonary embolism (Chapter 31).
- Chest physiotherapy in the presence of copious respiratory secretions

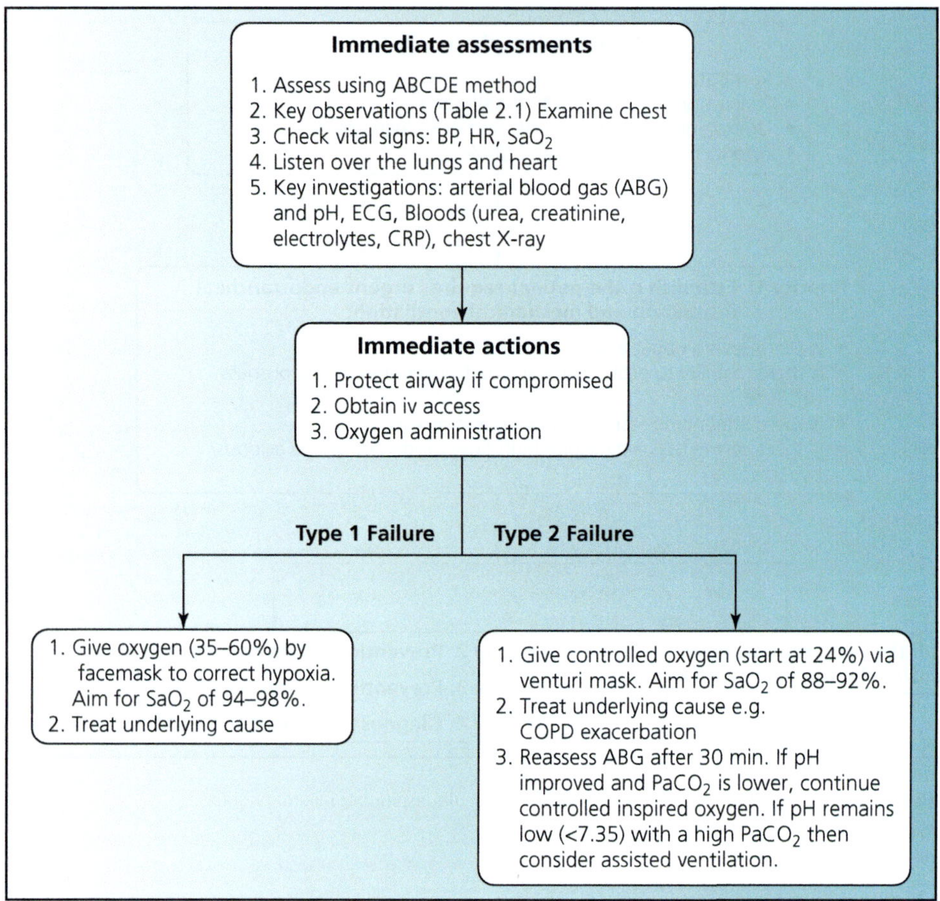

Figure 30.2 Management of the patient with suspected acute respiratory failure: assessment and actions.

Table 30.3 Oxygen delivery devices.

Device	Indication	Concentration of O_2 delivered	Advantages	Disadvantages
Facemask with reservoir bag (O_2 flow rate 10–15 L/min)	Cardiorespiratory arrest or peri-arrest	>80%	Highest O_2 concentration delivered	Some rebreathing of CO_2, risk of CO_2 retention in type 2 failure
Low-flow mask (e.g. Hudson)	Type 1 respiratory failure	28–60% depending on O_2 flow rate, leakage, and ventilatory minute volume	Simple and cheap No need to change mask if FiO_2 has to be changed	Unreliable $FiO2$ deliver and rebreathing may occur as above
High-flow mask (Venturi principle)	Type 2 respiratory failure, and when accurate FiO_2 is needed	24%, 28%, 35%, 40% and 60%, determined by the Venturi valve (colour coded) used and the O_2 flow rate	Delivers an accurate FiO_2 Reduces the risk of CO_2 retention in type 2 rate respiratory failure; 60% mask is useful in type 1 respiratory failure when hypoxaemia persists despite 10 L/min O_2 flow rate via low-flow mask	Uncomfortable to wear for long periods New valve needed if FiO_2 has to be changed

Table 30.3 (*Continued*)

Device	Indication	Concentration of O_2 delivered	Advantages	Disadvantages
Nasal cannulae	Patients with stable COPD or recovering from other causes of respiratory failure	Depends on the O_2 flow rate and ventilatory minute volume; 2 L/min gives an FiO_2 of roughly 25–30%	Prevents rebreathing Comfortable to wear for long periods	Nasal irritation with flow rates >3 L/min

Table 30.4 Causes of acute respiratory failure.

Type 1 respiratory failure	Type 2 respiratory failure
Pneumonia	**Reduced central respiratory drive**
Viral pneumonitis	Sedative drugs, for example opiates/opioids, benzodiazepines, alcohol
Pulmonary embolism	Head trauma
Acute exacerbation of COPD	Space-occupying CNS lesion
Acute exacerbation of asthma	Cerebrovascular accident
Pulmonary fibrotic lung disease	**Neuromuscular and thoracic wall disease**
Pulmonary oedema (heart failure)	Cervical cord lesion
Acute Respiratory Distress Syndrome (ARDS)	Guillain–Barré syndrome
Pneumothorax	Myasthenia gravis
	Poliomyelitis
	Diaphragmatic paralysis
	Flail chest
	Chest wall deformity (acute on chronic)
	Respiratory disease
	Acute upper airway obstruction (foreign body or reduced conscious level)
	Acute exacerbation of COPD
	Severe life-threatening asthma
	Pneumothorax
	Factors that can worsen respiratory failure of any cause
	Sedative drugs: benzodiazepines, opioids
	Aspiration of secretions or gastric contents
	Respiratory muscle fatigue
	Low cardiac output
	Severe obesity
	Chest wall abnormality, for example kyphoscoliosis
	Large pleural effusion
	Pneumothorax

Remember there may often be a combination of disease processes, for example pneumonia on a background of pulmonary fibrosis or heart failure. There may also be an acute-on-chronic presentation, for example decompensated chronic respiratory failure in a patient with an exacerbation of chronic obstructive pulmonary disease.

- Drainage of a large pleural effusion or pneumothorax (Chapter 28).
- Reversal of the effects of narcotic drugs (e.g. naloxone in opiate overdose and flumazenil in benzodiazepine overdose) (Chapter 8).

5 Institute assisted ventilation if indicated (Tables 30.5 and 30.6)

If, following treatment of the underlying problem, oxygen requirements remain high (e.g. >60%) or there is persistent acidosis with hypercapnia, assisted ventilation (invasive or non-invasive) should be considered. See Tables 30.5 and 30.6, and Chapter 113.

Table 30.5 Non-invasive ventilation in acute respiratory failure.

	Continuous positive airway pressure (CPAP)	**Bilevel positive airway pressure (BiPAP)**
Indications	Cardiogenic pulmonary oedema	Acidotic type 2 respiratory failure in acute exacerbation of COPD
	COVID-19 pneumonitis	Acidotic type 2 respiratory failure in patient with chest wall deformity
		Acidotic type 2 respiratory failure in pulmonary oedema
Contraindications	Vomiting or bowel obstruction	
	Unconscious or uncooperative patient	
	Copious secretions (relative)	
	Haemodynamic instability	
	Undrained pneumothorax	
	Recent facial, upper airway, or upper gastrointestinal surgery	
Disadvantages and complications	Patient must be conscious and cooperative	
	Discomfort from mask	
	Mask must seal well	
	Bloating due to aerophagia	
	May fail	

Table 30.6 Invasive ventilation in acute respiratory failure.

Endotracheal intubation and mechanical ventilation	
Indications	Upper airway obstruction
	Impending respiratory arrest
	Airway at risk due to reduced conscious level (GCS < 8)
	Oxygenation failure: $PaO_2 < 7.5\text{-}8kPa$, despite supplemental O_2/NIV
	Ventilatory failure: respiratory acidosis with pH < 7.25
Contraindications	Patient has expressed a wish not to be ventilated
	Chronic respiratory disease with severely impaired functional capacity and/or severe comorbidity
	Irreversible extensive neurological damage
Disadvantages and complications	Need for sedation and paralysis
	Pharyngeal, laryngeal and tracheal injury
	Ventilator-associated pneumonia
	Ventilator-induced lung injury (e.g. barotrauma)
	Weaning may pose ethical difficulties

Further reading

British Thoracic Society Emergency Oxygen Guideline Group (2015) BTS Guidelines for oxygen use in adults in healthcare and emergency settings. https://www.brit-thoracic.org.uk/standards-of-care/guidelines/bts-guideline-foremergency-oxygen-use-in-adult-patients/ [Accessed: 5 August 2024].

Chapman S, Robinson G, Stradling J, *et al.* (2014) *Oxford Handbook of Respiratory Medicine*, 3rd edition. OUP.

Davidson AC, Banham S, Elliott M, *et al.* (2016) British thoracic society/intensive care society acute hypercapnic respiratory failure guideline development group. BTS/ICS Guidelines for the ventilatory management of acute hypercapnic respiratory failure in adults. *Thorax* 71, ii1–ii35. https://www.brit-thoracic.org.uk/document-library/clinical-information/acute-hypercapnic-respiratory-failure/bts-guidelines-for-ventilatory-management-of-ahrf/.

Goligher EC, Ferguson ND, Brochard LJ. (2016) Clinical challenges in mechanical ventilation. *Lancet* 387, 1856–1866.

O'Driscoll R, Howard L, Earis J, Mak V, on behalf of the BTS Emergency Oxygen Guideline Group (2015) BTS Guidelines for oxygen use in adults in healthcare and emergency settings. https://www.brit-thoracic. org.uk/document-library/clinical-information/oxygen/emergency-oxygen-guideline-2015/bts-full-guideline-for-oxygen-use-in-adults-in-healthcare-and-emergency-settings-2015/ [Accessed: 5 August 2024].

Pepin JL, Timsit JF, Tamisier R, *et al.* (2016) Prevention and care of respiratory failure in obese patients. *Lancet Respir Med* 4, 407–418.

Schwartzstein RM, Parker MJ. (2006) *Respiratory Physiology: A Clinical Approach*, 1st edition. Lippincott Williams and Wilkins.

CHAPTER 31

Venous thromboembolism

EILISH DONNELLY, SANNA KHAWAJA, AND ROSHAN NAVIN

Risk factors

(see Table 31.1)

Table 31.1 Risk factors for VTE.

Intrinsic	Extrinsic
History of DVT/PE	Recent major surgery
Active cancer (known or undiagnosed)	Recent hospitalisation
Increasing age	Recent trauma
Obesity	Significant immobility
Male sex	Prolonged travel > 4 h
Inherited thrombophilia,	Pregnancy/postpartum period
e.g. Factor V Leiden, antiphospholipid syndrome	
Acquired thrombophilia,	Hormonal treatment,
e.g. Behcet's, nephrotic syndrome	e.g. HRT/COCP
Myeloproliferative disorders	Chemotherapy
Inflammatory disorders,	Smoker
e.g. IBD, autoimmune disease	
Varicose veins	Dehydration

Deep vein thrombosis (DVT)

History

Consider the diagnosis in any patient presenting with new onset of:

- Unilateral calf or leg swelling
  - Measure the circumference of each leg 10 cm below the tibial tuberosity – a difference of >3 cm increases the likelihood of a DVT
- Calf tenderness
- Erythema or warmth of the affected leg
- Distended veins

Acute Medicine: A Practical Guide to the Management of Medical Emergencies, Sixth Edition.
Edited by Mridula Rajwani, Leila Vaziri, and Ivie Gbinigie.
© 2026 John Wiley & Sons Ltd. Published 2026 by John Wiley & Sons Ltd.

Table 31.2 Wells' score for DVT.

Clinical feature	Points
Active cancer (treatment ongoing, within six months, or palliative)	1
Paralysis, paresis or recent plaster immobilisation of the lower extremities	1
Recently bedridden for 3 days or more or major surgery within 12 weeks requiring general or regional anaesthesia	1
Localised tenderness along the distribution of the deep venous system	1
Entire leg swollen	1
Calf swelling at least 3 cm larger than asymptomatic side	1
Pitting oedema confined to the symptomatic leg	1
Collateral superficial veins (non-varicose)	1
Previously documented DVT	1
An alternative diagnosis is at least as likely as DVT	−2
Clinical probability simplified score	
DVT likely	**2 points or more**
DVT unlikely	**1 point or less**

* Wells *et al.* (2003)/with permission of Elsevier.

Assessment

If deep vein thrombosis (DVT) is suspected, calculate a two-level DVT Wells' Score (Table 31.2) to assess the probability.

Wells' score ≤1

Check plasma D-dimer.

- If D-dimer is negative, DVT is effectively excluded.
  Pursue other diagnoses (Table 31.3).
- If D-dimer is positive, request a duplex scan of the proximal leg veins (if this is not possible within 4 h, begin interim therapeutic anticoagulation, pending the result of the scan).

Wells' score ≥2

Go straight to requesting a duplex scan of the proximal leg veins (if this is not possible within 4 h, begin interim therapeutic anticoagulation, pending the result of the scan).

- If the scan is positive for DVT, start anticoagulation.
- If the scan is negative for DVT:
  - If D-dimer negative, DVT is effectively excluded. Pursue other diagnoses (Table 31.3).
  - If D-dimer positive, stop interim therapeutic anticoagulation and repeat the duplex scan six to eight days later in patients to confirm no DVT.

For a confirmed venous thromboembolism (VTE), patients will require anticoagulation for at least three months.

For detailed pharmacological treatment of confirmed VTE please refer to Chapter 85.

Consider catheter-directed thrombolytic therapy for DVT patients with symptomatic iliofemoral DVT who have symptoms <14 days, good functional status, life expectancy >1 year and a low risk of bleeding.

Refer as an outpatient for thrombosis follow-up for investigation of secondary causes and sequelae, as well as appropriate two-week wait pathway if cancer is suspected.

Table 31.3 Causes of leg swelling.

Venous/Lymphatic	Skin
Deep vein thrombosis	Cellulitis (often presents with tenderness, erythema and
Superficial thrombophlebitis	induration of the skin)
IVC obstruction (e.g. by a tumour)	**SYSTEMIC (oedema is bilateral, but may be asymmetric)**
Varicose veins with chronic venous hypertension	Heart failure
Post-phlebitic syndrome	Liver failure
Congenital lymphoedema	Acute kidney injury/chronic kidney disease
After vein harvesting for coronary bypass grafting	Nephrotic syndrome
Dependent oedema (e.g. in a paralysed limb)	Hypoalbuminaemia
Severe obesity with compression of ilio-femoral veins	Chronic respiratory failure
Musculoskeletal	Pregnancy
Calf haematoma	Idiopathic oedema of women
Ruptured Baker's cyst	Dihydropyridine calcium antagonists
Muscle tear	Drugs causing salt/water retention

Pulmonary embolism (PE)

History

Consider the diagnosis in any patient presenting with:

- Acute breathlessness, or worsening of chronic breathlessness (e.g. in COPD/CCF)
- Chest pain (which may be non-pleuritic or pleuritic)
- Haemoptysis
- Pre-syncope or syncope (especially in combination with breathlessness, or with risk factors for venous thromboembolism)
- Shock or hypotension

  40% of patients with a PE have no identified predisposing factors.

  <25% of patients with a symptomatic PE have clinical evidence of a DVT.

Assessment

Review the physiological observations, make a focused clinical assessment and perform blood tests as indicated. Obtain an electrocardiogram (ECG) and chest X-ray. These can also help reveal or exclude alternative diagnoses (e.g. myocardial infarction, pneumonia and pneumothorax).

In PE, the ECG may be normal, or show sinus tachycardia. It may also show changes associated with right ventricular strain (right axis deviation, partial or complete right bundle branch block, t-wave inversion in V1–4 or S1Q3T3 pattern).

The chest X-ray may be normal or show non-specific abnormalities.

If PE is suspected, a pre-test prediction of PE probability should be performed using the Wells' score (see Table 31.4 and Figure 31.1).

If Wells' score ≤4

Request a D-dimer. If the D-dimer is negative, PE is effectively excluded and no further investigation for PE is required. If D-dimer is positive, proceed to specific imaging (see below).

If Wells' score >4

Proceed straight to specific imaging. Do not request a D-dimer as a normal result does not exclude a PE.

If imaging cannot be obtained within 4h, then offer interim therapeutic anticoagulation.

Table 31.4 Modified Wells' score for PE.

Variable	Points
Clinical signs and symptoms of DVT	3
An alternate diagnosis is less likely than PE	3
Heart rate >100	1.5
Immobilisation or surgery in the previous four weeks	1.5
Previous DVT/PE	1.5
Haemoptysis	1
Malignancy (treatment currently, in the previous six months or palliative)	1

Risk group	Points required	Risk of PE
Low	0–4	5.1%
High	>4	39.1%

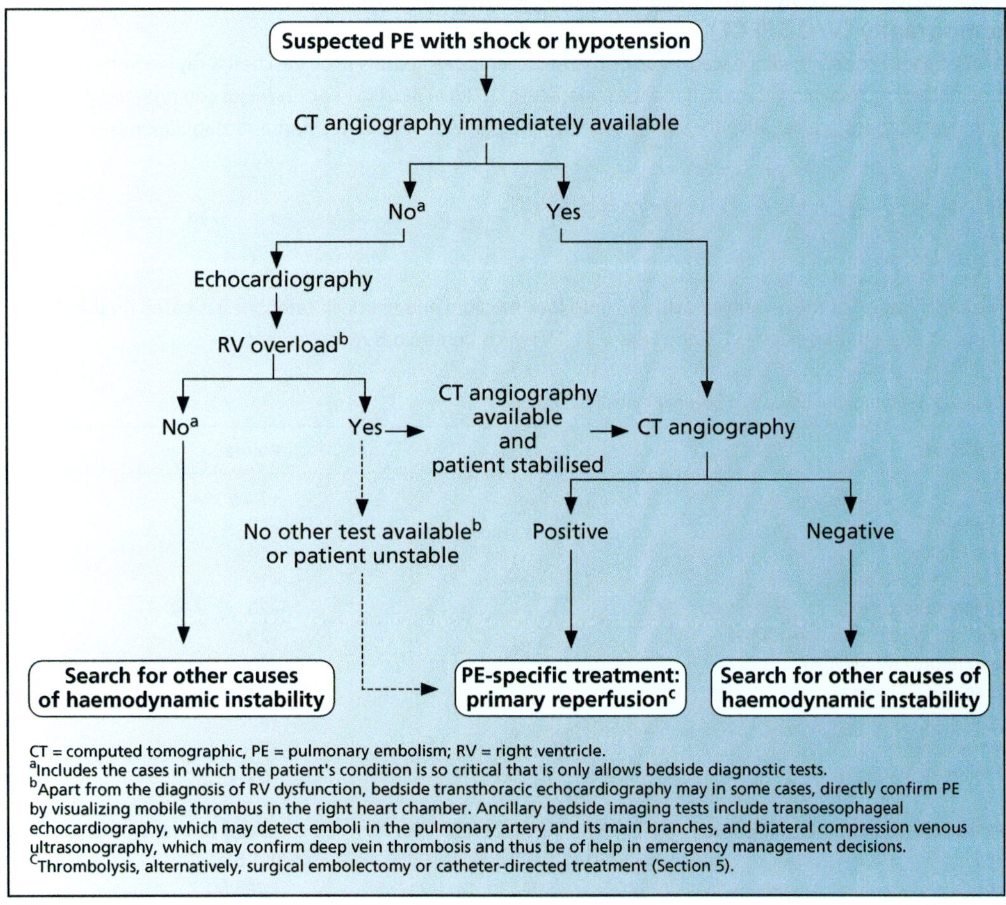

Figure 31.1 Suspected pulmonary embolism without shock or hypotension. Source: Konstantinides SV, Torbicki A, Agnelli G *et al.* (2014) 2014 ESC Guidelines on the diagnosis and management of acute pulmonary embolism. *Eur Heart J* 35, 3033–3080. Reproduced with permission of Oxford University Press.

D-dimer testing

The commonly used D-dimer assays have high sensitivity (95%) but only low specificity (50%) for VTE. Other causes of a raised plasma D-dimer include renal failure, aortic dissection, infection and malignancy.

Plasma D-dimer levels increase with age. The 2019 European Society of Cardiology (ESC) guidelines recommend using age-adjusted cut-off values (follow local guidance).

A negative D-dimer test in a patient with a Wells' score of ≤4 makes PE highly unlikely (0.14–0.5% probability); the negative predictive value of this combination is at least 99.5% and comparable to CT pulmonary angiography. Pursue other diagnoses.

Imaging

CT pulmonary angiography (CTPA)

CTPA has the advantage of providing valuable additional information on lung parenchyma, aorta, mediastinum, pleural spaces, bones and chest wall, and can reveal alternative diagnoses if PE is excluded. However, it carries higher radiation exposure than a V/Q scan (below).

Ventilation-perfusion imaging with single photon emission computed tomography (V/Q SPECT)

A V/Q scan is a nuclear medicine scan. It can be used in patients deemed low risk if the chest X-ray is normal and there is no underlying respiratory disease. It may be preferable to CTPA in renal failure or previous contrast reaction.

If investigations are negative for VTE, pursue other diagnoses. If positive, start anticoagulation (see below).

Management of confirmed VTE

Risk stratification

The classification of the severity of acute PE (into low, medium and high-risk categories) is based on the clinical status at presentation (Table 31.5 and Figure 31.1), which determines management.

Table 31.5 Pulmonary Embolism Severity Index (PESI) score.

Predictors	Points
Age	+1 per year
Male sex	+10
Heart failure	+10
Chronic lung disease	+10
Temperature <36 °C	+20
Arterial oxygen saturation <90%	+20
Respiratory rate >30/min	+20
Pulse rate >110/min	+20
Systolic BP <100 mmHg	+30
Active cancer	+30
Altered mental status	+60

PESI score (total number of points)	Risk class	30-day mortality rate (%)
<65	I	0–1.6
66–85	II	1.7–3.5
86–105	III	3.2–7.1
106–125	IV	4.0–11.4
>125	V	10.0–24.5

The Pulmonary Embolism Severity Index (PESI) score is commonly used as a validated clinical risk score to calculate overall mortality risk.

Low risk

PESI class I/II patients are deemed low risk if there are no known radiological or biochemical features of right heart dysfunction (Table 31.6). These patients may be considered for discharge and management in an ambulatory setting depending on local protocol.

The treatment of low-risk PE and DVT is with anticoagulation. Similar regimes are usually followed for both. Refer to local guidance for choice of agent.

Direct oral anticoagulants (e.g. rivaroxaban and apixaban) are direct Factor Xa inhibitors, and are first-line treatment unless contraindicated.

Table 31.6 2019 ESC Guidelines for the diagnosis and management of acute pulmonary embolism developed in collaboration with the European Respiratory Society (ERS) / Oxford University Press.

Early mortality risk		Indicators of risk			
		Haemodynamic instability[a]	Clinical parameters of PE severity and/or comorbidity:PESI class III–V or sPESI ≥1	RV dysfunction on TTE or CTPA[b]	Elevated cardiac troponin levels[c]
High		+	(+)[d]	+	(+)
Intermediate	Intermediate–high	–	+[e]	+	+
Intermediate	Intermediate–low	–	+[e]	One (or none) positive	
Low		–	–	–	Assessment optional; if assessed, negative

BP = blood pressure; CTPA = computed tomography pulmonary angiography; H-FABP = heart-type fatty acid-binding protein; NT-proBNP = N-terminal pro B-type natriuretic peptide; PE = pulmonary embolism; PESI = Pulmonary Embolism Severity Index; RV = right ventricular; sPESI = simplified Pulmonary Embolism Severity Index; TTE = transthoracic echocardiogram.

[a] One of the following clinical presentations (Table 4): cardiac arrest, obstructive shock (systolic BP <90 mmHg or vasopressors required to achieve a BP ≥90 mmHg despite an adequate filling status, in combination with end-organ hypoperfusion), or persistent hypotension (systolic BP <90 mmHg or a systolic BP drop ≥40 mmHg for >15 min, not caused by new-onset arrhythmia, hypovolemia, or sepsis).

[b] Prognostically relevant imaging (TTE or CTPA) findings in patients with acute PE, and the corresponding cut-off levels, are graphically presented in Figure 3, and their prognostic value is summarized in Supplementary Data Table 3.

[c] Elevation of further laboratory biomarkers, such as NT-proBNP ≥600 ng/L, H-FABP ≥6 ng/mL, or copeptin ≥24 pmol/L, may provide additional prognostic information. These markers have been validated in cohort studies but they have not yet been used to guide treatment decisions in randomized controlled trials.

[d] Haemodynamic instability, combined with PE confirmation on CTPA and/or evidence of RV dysfunction on TTE, is sufficient to classify a patient into the high-risk PE category. In these cases, neither calculation of the PESI nor measurement of troponins or other cardiac biomarkers is necessary.

[e] Signs of RV dysfunction on TTE (or CTPA) or elevated cardiac biomarker levels may be present, despite a calculated PESI of I–II or an sPESI of 0. Until the implications of such discrepancies for the management of PE are fully understood, these patients should be classified into the intermediate-risk category.

Alternatives can include low-molecular weight heparin (LMWH), unfractionated heparin (UFH) or warfarin (e.g. in pro-thrombotic conditions such as antiphospholipid syndrome).

The indications/contraindications of anticoagulation are discussed in detail in Chapter 85.

Refer to outpatient thrombosis clinic for investigation of secondary causes if appropriate, determination of treatment duration and long-term management.

Intermediate risk

Intermediate-risk patients should be admitted for observation and further work-up.

Subcutaneous LMWH is the treatment of choice (unless contraindicated) while ongoing risk is being determined.

Troponin, B-type natriuretic peptide (BNP), and inpatient echocardiography help further risk stratification as per ESC guidelines (Table 31.6).

If the patient falls into the intermediate-*low* risk category, and/or their monitored condition remains stable, the patient may be considered suitable for switch to oral agent if appropriate and discharge for ongoing ambulatory/outpatient management as above, following senior review.

If the patient's clinical condition deteriorates or fails to stabilise, they may fulfil criteria for escalation of treatment as a high-risk patient (see below).

High risk (haemodynamically unstable)

High-risk PE is defined by the presence of shock or refractory hypotension.

If a patient is haemodynamically unstable (systolic BP<90) and PE suspected, bedside echocardiography or emergency CTPA (depending on availability) is recommended to confirm diagnosis.

Right ventricular failure due to acute pressure overload is thought to be the primary cause of death in severe PE.

Systemic thrombolysis should be considered in:

- Refractory hypotension (systolic BP<90 mmHg for >30–60 min, or a drop of ≥40 mmHg for >15 min), not due to other causes, e.g. hypovolaemia, sepsis or new arrhythmia.
- Selected normotensive patients with clinical evidence of ongoing/worsening instability (intermediate-*high* risk) characterized by:
  - Significant right ventricular (RV) dysfunction (RV dilatation on echo, raised plasma BNP/raised troponin)
  - Worsening hypoxaemia and respiratory insufficiency
  - Extreme tachycardia
  - High clot burden
  - Deterioration or failure to improve on anticoagulation

A specialist multidisciplinary team approach to decision-making, on a case-by-case basis, in the intermediate-high risk cohort of patients is recommended.

Contraindications to thrombolysis are listed in Table 31.7.

It is important to consider that some 'absolute' contraindications to thrombolysis can become 'relative' in the context of an immediately life-threatening PE.

Thrombolytic agents

Systemic thrombolysis with tissue plasminogen activator (tPA) is most effective if initiated within 48 h of onset of symptoms.

Alteplase is the tPA approved for systemic thrombolysis in acute PE in the United Kingdom (Table 31.8).

Other agents are available. Follow local guidance.

These patients will usually be managed in a high dependency unit (HDU) or intensive care unit (ICU) environment.

Table 31.7 Thrombolytic therapy: contraindications.

Absolute
Active internal bleeding
Suspected aortic dissection
Prolonged or traumatic cardiopulmonary resuscitation
Recent head trauma or known intracranial neoplasm
Trauma or surgery within the previous two weeks, which could be a source of rebleeding
Diabetic haemorrhagic retinopathy or other haemorrhagic ophthalmic condition
Pregnancy
Recorded blood pressure >200/120 mmHg
History of cerebrovascular accident known to be haemorrhagic

Relative
Recent trauma or surgery (>2 weeks)
History of chronic severe hypertension with or without drug therapy
Active peptic ulcer
History of cerebrovascular accident
Known bleeding diathesis or current use of anticoagulants
Significant liver dysfunction
If there are one or more relative contraindications to thrombolytic therapy, you must weigh the risks and benefits of
therapy for the individual before deciding whether or not it should be given

Table 31.8 Thrombolysis regimen using alteplase.

Drug	Regimen
rtPA (alteplase)	10 mg of IV alteplase as a bolus over two minutes Then give 1.5 mg/kg over two hours (to a maximum of 90 mg)
Followed by unfractionated heparin infusion	

Consider ECMO (extracorporeal membrane oxygenation), where available, in patients with persistent shock, or severe respiratory failure despite optimal mechanical ventilation.

Endovascular interventions

- Catheter-directed thrombolysis /thrombus fragmentation, mechanical or surgical thrombectomy can all be considered for patients in whom thrombolysis is contraindicated, or who are at high risk of deterioration.
- UFH infusion can be used as a bridging measure whilst awaiting endovascular intervention.

PE management in cardiac arrest

PE is a differential diagnosis for a cardiac arrest with a non-shockable rhythm.

If the diagnosis is not confirmed, consider the following surrogates to help make the decision (Figure 31.2):

- History suggestive of PE
- VTE risk factors
- Bedside echocardiogram confirming RV enlargement or strain

Management

- Continue as per Advanced Life Support (ALS) algorithm
- Perform bedside echocardiography if immediately available
- The decision to treat for acute PE must be taken early to be most effective
- Administer systemic thrombolysis as detailed above

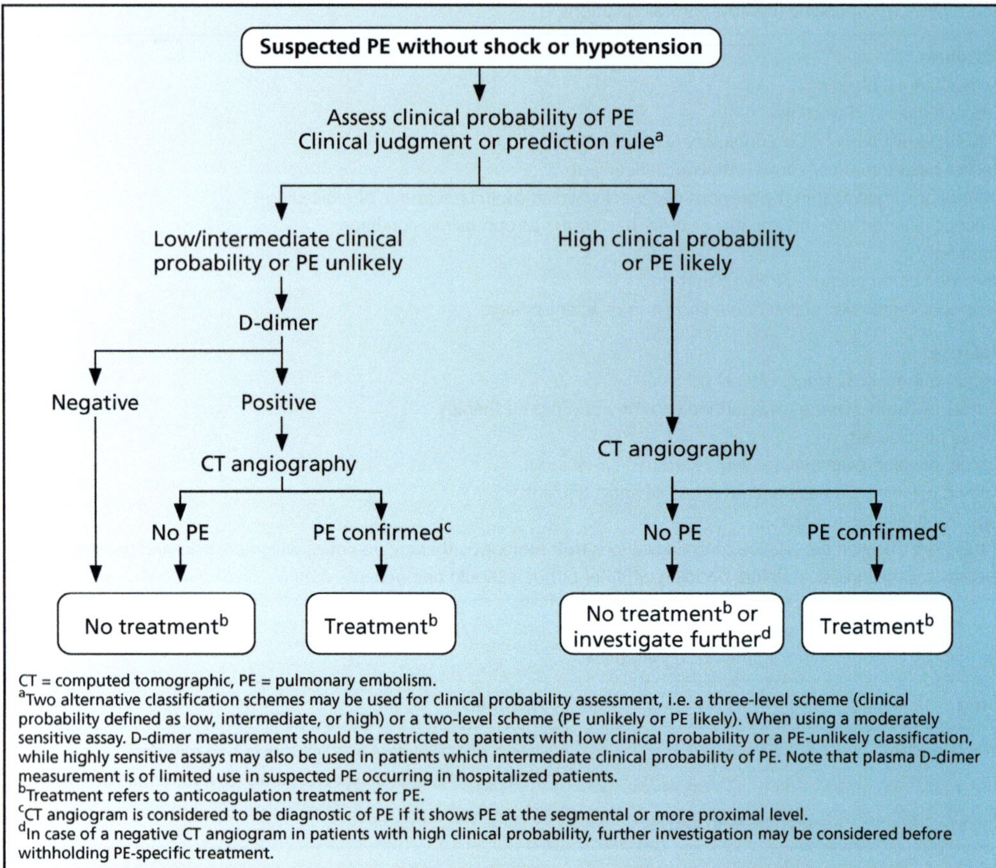

Figure 31.2 Suspected pulmonary embolism with shock or hypotension. Source: Konstantinides SV, Torbicki A, Agnelli G *et al.* (2014) 2014 ESC Guidelines on the diagnosis and management of acute pulmonary embolism. *Eur Heart J* 35, 3033–3080. Reproduced with permission of Oxford University Press.

- Once a thrombolytic drug is administered, cardiopulmonary resuscitation (CPR) must be continued for 60–90 minutes and the patient should be managed in ICU
- Consider VA (veno-arterial) ECMO, where available, in patients with persistent shock or refractory cardiac arrest despite initiation of thrombolysis

VTE in pregnancy

VTE is one of the leading direct causes of maternal death in the United Kingdom, and should be suspected in patients who are pregnant or <6 weeks postpartum.

If the history or clinical examination is suggestive of VTE, proceed as below.

If clinical concern for PE, a chest X-ray should be performed.

ESC guidelines continue to recommend D-dimer testing in low probability (Wells' score<4) cases. However, Royal College of Obstetricians and Gynaecologists (RCOG) guidelines have moved away from using D-dimer and pre-test probability scores in pregnant patients. Follow local guidance.

Compression proximal duplex ultrasound is the initial specific imaging of choice. A positive test for DVT will eliminate the need for any further thoracic imaging/radiation exposure if the patient is in the low-risk treatment category for PE, as treatment will be similar for both.

If ultrasound is negative for DVT, but PE still suspected, proceed to specific further diagnostic imaging (V/Q or CTPA). The modality of choice will depend on local availability and protocols.

Although extremely low baseline risk, VQ SPECT may carry a very slightly increased risk of childhood cancer (1/280,000 versus less than 1/1,000,000). CTPA is associated with a higher risk of maternal breast cancer (lifetime risk increased by up to 13.6%, background risk of 1/200 for the study population); in both situations, the absolute risk is very small. Where feasible, women should be involved in the decision to undergo CTPA or VQ SPECT.

The risk of undiagnosed maternal PE to a mother and her foetus far outweighs any risk from radiation exposure through diagnostic imaging.

Pregnant patients with a confirmed VTE should be treated with LMWH and referred to a multidisciplinary service for managing PE in pregnancy.

High-risk patients should have escalation of treatment considered as per the non-pregnant patient (see above), and also be assessed by a consultant obstetrician.

Long term sequelae

Chronic thromboembolic pulmonary hypertension (CTEPH)

CTEPH is the most serious long-term sequelae of PE and affects 2–4% of PE survivors.

Patients may present months or years after the initial acute presentation with PE.

Common presenting symptoms are:

- Dyspnoea (99%)
- Oedema (41%)
- Fatigue (32%)

Signs of right heart failure occur in advanced disease stages.

If CTEPH is suspected, refer for further investigations which may include echocardiogram, V/Q or CTPA and possibly right heart catheterisation.

Further reading

Konstantinides SV, Meyer G, Becattini C, *et al.* (2019) ESC Guidelines for the diagnosis and management of acute pulmonary embolism developed in collaboration with the European Respiratory Society (ERS). *Eur Heart J* 2020(41), 543–603.

Howard LSGE, Barden S, Condliffe R, *et al.* (2018) British Thoracic Society Guideline for the initial outpatient management of pulmonary embolism (PE). *Thorax* 73, ii1–ii29.

NICE guideline [NG158]. Venous thromboembolic diseases: diagnosis, management and thrombophilia testing. Published: 26 March 2020; Last updated: 2 August 2023.

Royal College of Obstetricians & Gynaecologists (2015). Thromboembolic disease in pregnancy and the puerperium: acute management. Green-top Guideline No. 37b.

Gastroenterology and Hepatology

CHAPTER 32
Abdominal pain

SIMON ANDERSON

Surgical causes of acute abdominal pain are typically due to gastro-intestinal obstruction, peritonitis or vascular emergencies (Table 32.1).

- Visceral pain arising from the gut, biliary tract or pancreas is poorly localized to the body surface. In contrast, the pain of peritoneal irritation (due to inflammation or infection) is well localized (unless there is generalized peritonitis) and constant, and associated with discrete abdominal tenderness.

Table 32.1 Causes of acute severe abdominal pain with shock.

Cause	Pathologies	Comments
Generalized peritonitis	Perforation of viscus mesenteric vascular occlusion leading to intestinal infarction and secondary peritonitis inflammatory conditions with localized, followed by generalized peritonitis (e.g. appendicitis, cholecystitis, diverticulitis, Crohn's disease abscess, pancreatitis) Late intestinal obstruction (most commonly due to large bowel tumour, adhesions, hernia or volvulus).	Perforated duodenal ulcers are now relatively uncommon; when caused by NSAIDs, use the signs may be misleadingly mild. Perforated colonic (or less commonly, small bowel) diverticula may be encountered. Most cases of perforation of the upper and lower GI tract are related to endoscopic procedures (e.g. polypectomy, endoscopic retrograde cholangiopancreatography [ERCP]). Elderly patients and those on long-term corticosteroids may not manifest typical symptoms of peritonitis and signs may be misleadingly mild.
Mesenteric infarction	Thrombosis: atherosclerotic disease of the mesenteric arteries, polycythaemia, sickle cell disease, cryoglobulinaemia and amyloidosis. Embolism: cardiac condition (e.g. atrial fibrillation, endocarditis). Aortic dissection (Chapter 18). Vasculitis.	Always consider a cardiac source of emboli in patients with atherosclerosis who present with features suggestive of acute mesenteric ischaemia. Polyarteritis nodosa is often overlooked as a cause of vasculitic mesenteric infarction as the autoantibody screen is typically negative.
Acute severe pancreatitis	Common causes are gallstones (50% cases) and alcohol (20%). Less common causes include ERCP and severe hyperlipidaemias.	See Chapter 43 for assessment and management of acute pancreatitis.
Ruptured abdominal aortic aneurysm	Atherosclerotic and inflammatory factors contribute to the pathogenesis of abdominal aortic aneurysm. Risk of rupture greatly increased in male smokers >65 years and in aneurysms >5.5 cm in diameter.	Typically causes acute severe abdominal, flank or back pain. Syncope without prominent pain can be a presentation. May also result in leg or spinal cord ischaemia.

Acute Medicine: A Practical Guide to the Management of Medical Emergencies, Sixth Edition.
Edited by Mridula Rajwani, Leila Vaziri, and Ivie Gbinigie.
© 2026 John Wiley & Sons Ltd. Published 2026 by John Wiley & Sons Ltd.

Acute abdominal pain – alerts.

> The most important initial decision is whether the cause is 'surgical' or 'medical'. Only after surgically treatable causes have been excluded should other conditions be considered.
>
> A careful history is paramount as symptoms may evolve with time, for example evolution of periumbilical 'visceral' pain to right iliac fossa pain in acute appendicitis, or partial/intermittent intestinal obstruction progressing to complete bowel obstruction. In addition, patients on immunosuppressants (including corticosteroids) and with comorbidities (particularly renal disease, diabetes and atherosclerosis) and the elderly, may present with atypical signs.

- Gastro-intestinal obstruction usually manifests with pain, bloating, nausea and vomiting with absent or high-pitched bowel sounds.
- Peritonitis manifests as severe pain, often unresponsive to analgesia, with abdominal tenderness to light touch or movement, 'guarding' and rebound tenderness (Blumberg's sign).

Priorities

1 If the patient has severe abdominal pain and cardiovascular compromised (systolic BP <90 mmHg, tachycardia and cool peripheries), the likely diagnosis is generalized peritonitis, perforated viscus (see below), mesenteric infarction, acute severe pancreatitis or ruptured abdominal aortic aneurysm (Table 32.1). The patient will need:
   - Vigorous fluid resuscitation, initially via a peripheral or central IV line, with monitoring of the urine output by bladder catheter.
   - Antibiotic therapy based on the local antibiotic guidelines; could consider starting cefotaxime 1–2 g 6-hourly IV + metronidazole 500 mg 8-hourly IV.
   - An urgent surgical opinion. If there are obvious signs of a ruptured abdominal aortic aneurysm (painful aortic pulsation and hypotension), emergency laparotomy is needed, before any radiological examination.
2 History needs to establish the characteristics of the abdominal pain, and the patient's other medical problems (Table 32.2):
   - When and how did the pain start – gradually or abruptly?
   - Where is the pain felt, and has it moved since its onset?
   - How severe is the pain?
   - Has there been vomiting, and when did vomiting begin in relation to the onset of the pain?
   - Women of childbearing age should be asked about their pregnancy and menstrual history (last menstrual period, last normal menstrual period, previous menstrual period, cycle length) and use of contraception. A pregnancy test should be done. Establish if there has been vaginal discharge or bleeding, dyspareunia or dysmenorrhea.
3 As well as a careful examination of the abdomen (Table 32.2), you should:
   - Check the temperature, pulse, jugular venous pressure (JVP) and blood pressure.
   - Listen to the heart and the lung bases.
   - Give oxygen if the patient has severe pain, is breathless or if oxygen saturation by pulse oximetry is <94%.
   - Insert an IV cannula and take blood for urgent investigations (Table 32.3).
   - Relieve severe pain with morphine 5–10 mg IV plus an antiemetic, for example prochlorperazine 12.5 mg IV.
   - Start an infusion of crystalloid, at a rate determined by the volume status of the patient.
   - Arrange appropriate imaging (Table 32.3).

See Figure 32.1 for an overview of management of acute abdominal pain.

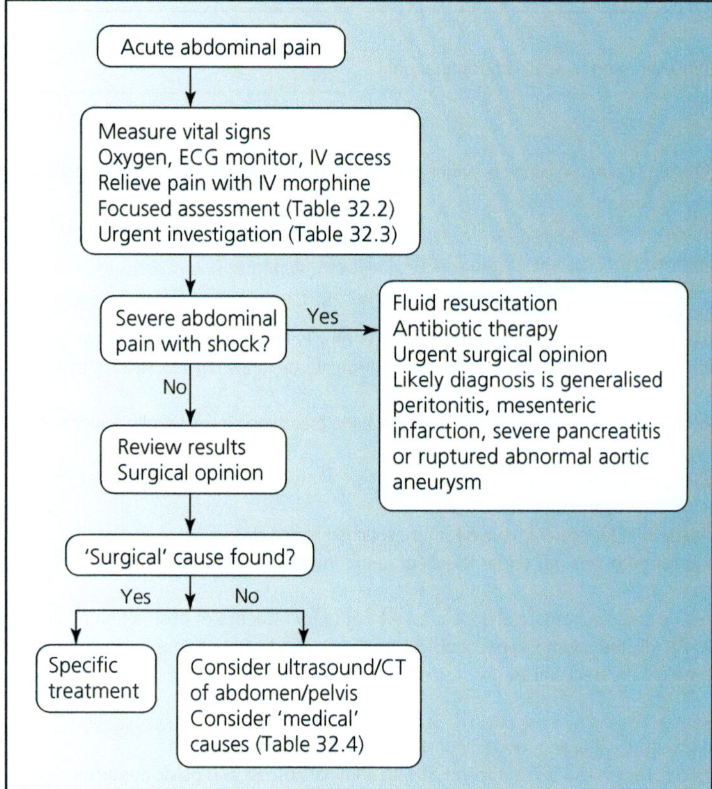

Figure 32.1 Management of acute abdominal pain.

Table 32.2 Focused assessment in acute abdominal pain.

History

When did the pain start and how did it start – gradually or abruptly?

Where is the pain, and has it moved since its onset? Visceral pain arising from the gut, biliary tract or pancreas is poorly localized. Peritoneal pain (due to inflammation or infection) is well localized (unless there is generalized peritonitis), constant and associated with abdominal tenderness.

How severe is the pain?

Has there been vomiting, and when did vomiting begin in relation to the onset of the pain?

What is the nature of the vomitus?

Haematemesis suggests a gastroduodenal lesion. Recent swallowed food could indicate a gastric outflow obstruction. Feculent vomiting suggests a distal small bowel obstruction of a fistula.

Previous abdominal surgery, and if so what for?

Other medical problems?

Examination

Key observations:

Abdominal distension?

Presence of abdominal scars? If present, check what operations have been done; adhesions from previous surgery may cause obstruction

Tenderness: localized or generalized?

Palpable organs, aorta or masses?

Hernial orifices (inguinal, femoral and umbilical) clear?

Femoral pulses present and symmetrical?

Bowel sounds

Rectal examination

Lungs and heart: signs of basal pneumonia? Signs of an inferior MI?

Table 32.3 Urgent investigation in acute abdominal pain.

All patients

Full blood count

Clotting screen if there is purpura or jaundice, prolonged oozing from puncture sites or a low platelet count

C-reactive protein

Group and screen

Blood glucose

Sodium, potassium, urea and creatinine

Liver function tests, albumin and calcium

Serum amylase (raised in pancreatitis, perforated ulcer, mesenteric ischaemia and severe sepsis)

Other tests to confirm or exclude pancreatitis if indicated (serum lipase; urine dipstick test for trypsinogen-2 [which has a high negative predictive value])

Arterial gases and pH if hypotensive or oxygen saturation <94% breathing air (metabolic acidosis seen in generalized peritonitis, mesenteric infarction and severe pancreatitis)

Blood culture if febrile or suspected peritonitis

Urine: stick test, MC&S and pregnancy test

12-lead ECG particularly if known cardiac disease or unexplained upper abdominal pain

Erect chest X-ray – looking for free gas under the diaphragm, indicating perforation, and evidence of basal pneumonia

Abdominal X-ray (supine and erect or lateral decubitus) – looking for evidence of obstruction of large and/or small bowel; ischaemic bowel (dilated and thickened loops of small bowel); cholangitis (gas in biliary tree); radio-dense gallstones; radio-dense urinary tract stones

Selected patients

A CT scan is the most sensitive imaging modality particular for intestinal obstruction.

Abdominal ultrasonography can assess for appendicitis, abdominal abscess and pelvic abnormalities without radiation exposure. Ultrasonography is also the first-line investigation for right upper quadrant pain, to exclude gallstones and other biliary pathology.

Further management

Further management will be determined by the results of investigations and surgical assessment. 'Medical' causes of abdominal pain are summarized in Table 32.4.

Table 32.4 'Medical' causes of acute abdominal pain.

Site of pain	Pathologies to consider	Comment
Right upper quadrant	Right basal pneumonia (Chapter 25) Pulmonary embolism (Chapter 31) Hepatic congestion due to congestive Heart failure Acute alcoholic hepatitis Acute viral hepatitis	Always listen for basal lung signs (pleural rub, crackles).
	Acute gonococcal perihepatitis (Fitz–Hugh–Curtis syndrome) Liver abscess Budd–Chiari syndrome Portal vein thrombosis	Fitz–Hugh–Curtis syndrome usually presents with right upper quadrant pain (which may radiate to the shoulder) and minimal pelvic signs. Think of Budd–Chiari syndrome in patients with acute or chronic upper abdominal pain, hepatomegaly and deranged liver enzymes.

Table 32.4 (*Continued*)

Site of pain	Pathologies to consider	Comment
Epigastric	Acute gastritis Gastroparesis Peptic ulcer disease Gastro-oesophageal reflux disease Acute inferior myocardial infarction (Chapter 12) Acute pericarditis (Chapter 16) Aortic dissection (Chapter 18) Acute pancreatitis (Chapter 43)	Pain in the distal oesophagus related to reflux oesophagitis can be difficult to distinguish from epigastric pain from gastric causes. An ECG should always be performed in patients with acute upper abdominal pain.
Left upper quadrant	Left basal pneumonia Pulmonary embolism Splenic infarction, Splenic abscess	Splenic causes are relatively uncommon but should be considered in patients with haemoglobinopathies such as sickle-cell disease and in procoagulant states.
Lower abdomen	Ileitis: • Infections, for example Yersinia • Crohn's disease • NSAID-enteropathy Diverticulitis (usually causes left iliac fossa pain but may present with right iliac fossa pain) Ureteric obstruction or stones Cystitis In women: • Pelvic inflammatory disease • Adnexal disease (e.g. ectopic pregnancy, cysts, torsion) • Uterine disease (endometritis, complications of leiomyomas)	Ovarian cysts are commonly encountered on ultrasound and may not be the cause of pain. Always consider other causes such as appendicitis or ileitis.
Central or diffuse	Viral or bacterial gastroenteritis (Chapter 34) Acute inflammatory bowel disease (Chapter 40) Spontaneous bacterial peritonitis Diabetic ketoacidosis (Chapter 44) Acute adrenal insufficiency (Chapter 47) Aortic dissection (Chapter 18) Acute intermittent porphyria Vaso-occlusive crisis of sickle cell disease Henoch–Schoenlein purpura (colicky pain with arthralgia, purpuric rash on buttocks and legs and sometimes bloody diarrhoea) Retroperitoneal haemorrhage (complicating anticoagulant therapy, bleeding disorder, leaking abdominal aortic aneurysm or vertebral fracture) Familial Mediterranean Fever	Crohn's disease can present with acute abdominal pain with minimal preceding symptoms. Spontaneous bacterial peritonitis can occur in patients with relatively mild ascites. Acute intermittent porphyria is rare but should be considered if recurrent unexplained generalized pain.

Further reading

Badger SA, Harkin DW, Blair PH, *et al*. (2016) Endovascular repair or open repair for ruptured abdominal aortic aneurysm: a Cochrane systematic review. *BMJ Open* 6, e008391. doi: 10.1136/bmjopen-2015-008391.

Bala M, Catena F, Kashuk J. (2022) *et al*, Acute mesenteric ischemia: updated guidelines of the World Society of Emergency Surgery. *World J Emerg Surg* 17(1), 54.

Bhangu A, Søreide K, Di Saverio S, *et al*. (2015) Acute appendicitis: modern understanding of pathogenesis, diagnosis, and management. *Lancet* 386, 1278–1287.

Clair DG, Beach JM. (2016) Mesenteric ischemia. *N Engl J Med* 374, 959–968.

Gans SL, Pols MA, Stoker J, *et al*. (2015) Guideline for the diagnostic pathway in patients with acute abdominal pain. *Dig Surg* 32, 23–31. http://www.karger.com/ Article/FullText/371583.

Lankisch PG, Apte M, Banks PA. (2015) Acute pancreatitis. *Lancet* 386, 85–96.

Murali N, El Hayek SM. (2021) Abdominal pain mimics. *Emerg Med Clin North Am* 39(4), 839–850.

Szatmary P, Grammatikopoulos T, Cai W, *et al*. (2022) Acute pancreatitis: diagnosis and treatment. *Drugs* 82(12), 1251–1276.

CHAPTER 33

Nausea and vomiting

SIMON ANDERSON

Acute vomiting in an adult is usually due to gastrointestinal infection, or an adverse effect of medication or pregnancy, although it may be a feature of a broad range of disorders (Table 33.1). Management is summarized in Figure 33.1. The cause is usually apparent in clinical assessment (Table 33.2). Choice of tests should be guided by the duration and severity of vomiting, and associated symptoms (Table 33.3).

Table 33.1 Causes of acute vomiting.

Infections
Gastroenteritis: viral (e.g. norovirus), bacterial (e.g. *Staphylococcus aureus and Bacillus cereus*)
Acute viral hepatitis
Systemic infections
Meningitis

Drugs and toxins
Chemotherapy:
severe – cisplatinum, dacarbazine, nitrogen mustard nitrogen mustard compounds; moderate – etoposide, methotrexate, cytarabine; mild – fluorouracil, vinblastine, tamoxifen
NSAIDs, colchicine, antibiotics (erythromycin, tetracycline), azathioprine, theophylline, opioids
Alcohol, illicit drug use or drug overdose, cannabis hyperemesis syndrome
Radiotherapy to upper abdomen or chest
Anaesthetic agents

Abdominal disorders
Mechanical obstruction: gastric outflow or small bowel
Functional disorders: idiopathic gastroparesis, chronic idiopathic pseudo-obstruction, functional dyspepsia, cyclical vomiting syndrome
Organic abdominal disorders: pancreatitis, peptic ulcer disease, cholelithiasis, mesenteric ischaemia, peritonitis

Neurological disorders
Migraine
Intracranial haemorrhage (subarachnoid haemorrhage, intracerebral haemorrhage, cerebellar haemorrhage)
Cerebellar infarction
Raised intracranial pressure (Chapter 64)
Labyrinthine disorders: vestibular neuritis, Ménière's disease

Psychiatric disorders
Psychogenic vomiting
Bulimia nervosa
Anxiety disorders

(Continued)

Acute Medicine: A Practical Guide to the Management of Medical Emergencies, Sixth Edition.
Edited by Mridula Rajwani, Leila Vaziri, and Ivie Gbinigie.
© 2026 John Wiley & Sons Ltd. Published 2026 by John Wiley & Sons Ltd.

Table 33.1 (*Continued*)

Metabolic and endocrine disorders
Pregnancy
Uraemia
Diabetic ketoacidosis (Chapter 44)
Hyper- or hypoparathyroidism
Adrenal insufficiency (Chapter 47)
Hyperthyroidism
Acute intermittent porphyria

Intrathoracic disorders
Inferior myocardial infarction

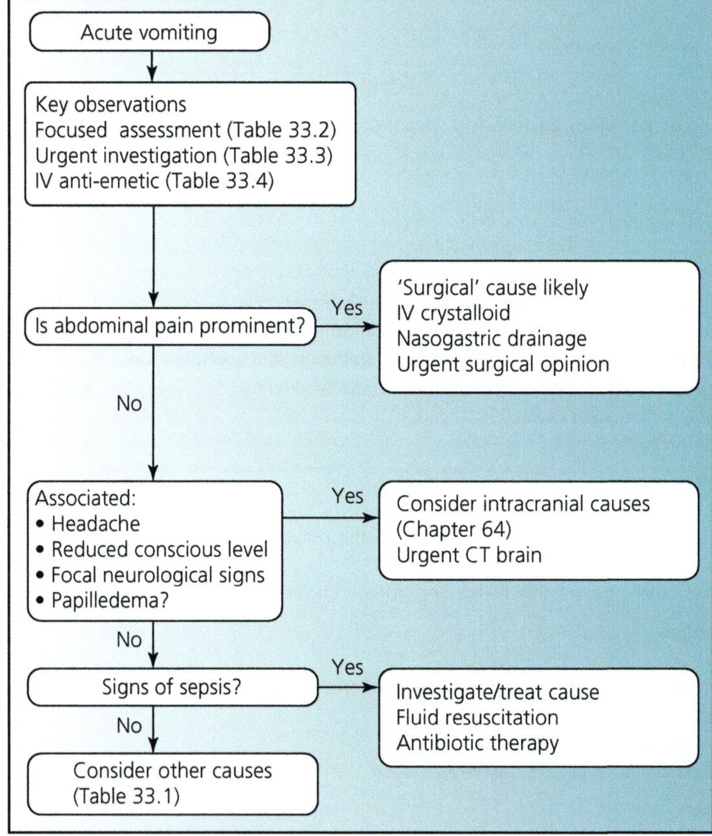

Figure 33.1 Management of the patient with acute vomiting.

Abdominal pain suggests a mechanical obstruction, particularly if the pain precedes vomiting. Other causes, such as acute pancreatitis or mesenteric ischaemia also need to be considered in such circumstances (see Chapter 32). Vomiting with diarrhoea suggests a viral or bacterial gastroenteritis (see Chapter 34).

Pregnancy and diabetic ketoacidosis are important causes often overlooked. Always consider the latter in an unwell diabetic patient with vomiting.

Table 33.2 Clinical assessment of the patient with vomiting.

History

Abdominal pain? Consider causes of an 'acute abdomen', specifically cholelithiasis, peptic ulcer disease, acute pancreatitis.

Early morning nausea and vomiting? Characteristic of pregnancy.

Abdominal pain with distension and tenderness? Suggests bowel obstruction, either mechanical (e.g. adhesions and strangulated hernia) or functional (pseudo-obstruction – Ogilvie's syndrome).

Headache? May indicate migraine. If worse with change in body position and associated with neurological signs (which may be subtle), suggests raised intracranial pressure due to, for example brain tumour or haemorrhage.

Nature of the vomitus? Vomiting food eaten several hours earlier indicates a gastric outflow obstruction or gastroparesis. Feculent vomiting, usually with pain, suggests a complete small bowel obstruction or gastro-colic fistula.

Heartburn and nausea? May indicate gastro-oesophageal disease.

Vertigo, nystagmus, gait disturbance? Typical of vestibular neuritis, and if unilateral hearing deficit, labyrinthitis. Other cranial nerve deficits are typically absent in these conditions.

History of repeated episodes of stereotypical symptoms lasting three to six days, asymptomatic between events? Characteristic of cyclical vomiting syndrome. This usually occurs in school-age children but can occur in adults.

Examination

Are there signs of volume depletion or sepsis?

Are there signs pointing to a specific disorder (Table 33.1)? Check carefully for features of neurological disease. Consider bulimia if signs of dental enamel erosion, lanugo-like hair, parotid enlargement.

Table 33.3 Investigation of the patient with acute severe vomiting.

All patients

Blood glucose

Sodium, potassium, urea and creatinine

Liver function tests, amylase, albumin, CRP and calcium

Full blood count

Urinalysis

Depending on clinical setting

Arterial blood gases and toxicology screen; pregnancy test, thyroid-stimulating hormone (TSH).

Chest X-ray

ECG

Abdominal X-ray if suspected intestinal obstruction/ileus (supine and erect or lateral decubitus); CT abdomen

CT brain

Blood culture

In patients with a history of recurrent episodes of vomiting, consider cyclic vomiting syndrome or cannabis hyperemesis syndrome as possible causes.

Priorities

Review the clinical observations and make a focused assessment (Table 33.2).

In the patient with acute severe vomiting, put in an IV cannula, arrange urgent investigations (Table 33.3), give IV anti-emetic (Table 33.4), and start IV crystalloid.

Further management is directed by the working diagnosis. If a 'surgical' cause is likely, insert a nasogastric tube, and seek urgent advice from the surgical team.

Table 33.4 Anti-emetic therapy.

Condition	Medication	Comments
Gastroenteritis	Metoclopramide 10 mg IV 8-hourly	Dopamine antagonist. May cause extrapyramidal side effects (ranging from mild restlessness, dystonia and rarely oculogyric crisis, particularly in children, women and elderly. Treat with procyclidine 5 mg IV.
	Domperidone 10 mg PO	Dopamine antagonist. Less likely to cause sedation and dystonic reaction. Small risk of cardiac adverse events (avoid in those >60 and/or on QT-prolonging medication)
	Ondansetron 4 mg IV 8-hourly as slow infusion over 15 min	5-HT3 antagonist. Second-line treatment. Use with caution in those with prolonged QT-interval.
Pregnancy-induced vomiting	Promethazine 25 mg IM or slow IV infusion; or cyclizine 50 mg PO/IM or IV	Antihistamine with anti-emetic and sedative properties.
	Metoclopramide 10 mg IV 8-hourly or Ondansetron 4 mg IV 8-hourly	Second-line treatment.
	Vitamin B6 and ginger	For nausea.
Migraine with vomiting	Metoclopramide (see above) or Prochlorperazine 12.5 mg IM	
	followed after 6 h if needed with 10 mg PO	Phenothiazine. Also available as a sublingual tablet.
Opioid-induced vomiting	Cyclizine 50 mg IV/IM or PO 8-hourly	Histamine H_1 – receptor antagonist.
	Prochlorperazine 12.5 mg IM	
Chemotherapy-induced vomiting	Ondansetron 8 mg IV (4 mg if >75 years old)	Can also be used prophylactically.
	Dexamethasone 8 mg IV OD.	Used as concomitant treatment with ondansetron.
	Prochlorperazine or metoclopramide	Second-line agents.
Post-operative nausea and vomiting	Metoclopramide 10 mg IV 8-hourly	See above.
	Ondansetron 4–8 mg IV 8-hourly	
Vestibular neuritis	Prochlorperazine 12.5 mg IM followed after 6 h with 10 mg PO if needed	
	Lorazepam 1 mg PO	Adjunctive treatment if needed.

Further reading

Heckroth M, Luckett RT, Moser C, *et al.* (2021) Nausea and vomiting in 2021: a comprehensive update. *J Clin Gastroenterol* 55(4), 279–299.

Perisetti A, Gajendran M, Dasari CS, *et al.* (2020) Cannabis hyperemesis syndrome: an update on the pathophysiology and management. *Ann Gastroenterol* 33(6), 571–578.

Venkatesan T, Levinthal DJ, Tarbell SE, *et al.* (2019) Guidelines on management of cyclic vomiting syndrome in adults by the American Neurogastroenterology and Motility Society and the Cyclic Vomiting Syndrome Association. *Neurogastroenterol Motil* 31(Suppl 2), e13604.

CHAPTER 34

Diarrhoea

SIMON ANDERSON

Definition

Diarrhoea is the passage of loose or liquid stools (types 5, 6 or 7 (entirely liquid) on the Bristol Stool Chart). Severe diarrhoea is the passage of four or more loose or liquid stools daily.

Acute diarrhoea is ≤14 days, persistent diarrhoea 15–30 days, and chronic diarrhoea >30 days in duration.

Acute diarrhoea is usually due to intestinal infection or an adverse effect of medication. **All unexplained cases of diarrhoea should be regarded as potentially infectious**, although both infective and non-infective agents can cause both diarrhoea and vomiting. *Clostridium difficile* followed by norovirus infection are the main causes of fatal illness and should always be considered in hospitalized patients. Norovirus is the commonest cause overall (around 20% of all cases). The commonest bacterial causes are due to *Salmonella* and *Campylobacter or E. coli*. Inflammatory bowel disease should be excluded if there is bloody diarrhoea (see Chapters 39 and 40). An overview of the management of acute diarrhoea is outlined in Figure 34.1.

Priorities

Establish the differential diagnosis from the history and examination (Table 34.1). Strict infection control protocols must be followed (including barrier nursing and hand-washing). Investigations needed urgently are given in Table 34.2.

- Features of community-acquired infective diarrhoea are given in Table 34.3 and hospital-acquired diarrhoea in Table 34.4.
- Particular causes to consider in the returning traveller are summarized in Table 34.5, and those in patients with HIV/ADS or immunosuppression in Table 34.6.

If the patient is severely ill (impaired consciousness level, severe volume depletion, marked abdominal distension or tenderness):
- Start vigorous fluid resuscitation with crystalloid, initially via a peripheral IV line, and correct electrolyte abnormalities.
- Start antibiotic therapy according to your local antimicrobial guidelines. On possible regimen is ciprofloxacin 400 mg 12-hourly IV and metronidazole 500 mg 8-hourly IV (immunocompetent patients) or gentamicin 5 mg/kg IV (immunosuppressed patients).

Acute Medicine: A Practical Guide to the Management of Medical Emergencies, Sixth Edition.
Edited by Mridula Rajwani, Leila Vaziri, and Ivie Gbinigie.
© 2026 John Wiley & Sons Ltd. Published 2026 by John Wiley & Sons Ltd.

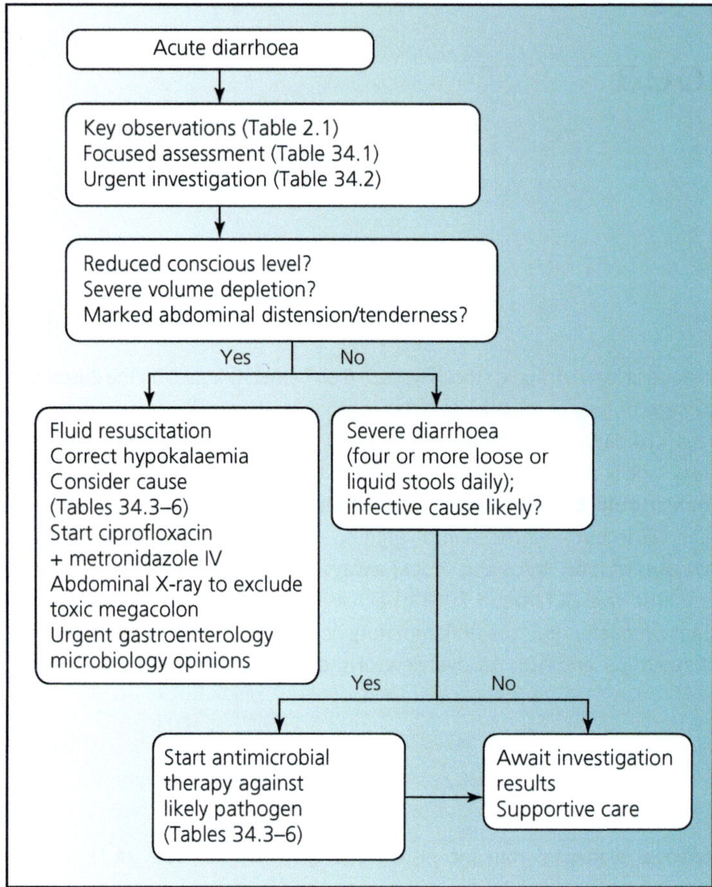

Figure 34.1 Management of acute diarrhoea.

Table 34.1 Focused assessment of the patient with acute diarrhoea.

History

Mode of onset (abrupt, sub-acute or gradual) and duration.

Frequency and nature of the stools (watery or containing blood and mucus). Bloody stools are a common feature of shigellosis, salmonellosis, severe *Campylobacter* enteritis and ulcerative colitis, and are rare (5%) in *C. difficile* infection.

Have others in the same household or who have shared the same food also developed diarrhoea?

Other symptoms (malaise, fever, vomiting and abdominal pain)?

Current or recent hospital inpatient (at risk of *C. difficile* infection)?

Travel abroad in the past six months?

Previous significant gastro-intestinal symptoms or known GI diagnosis?

Medications (in particular antibiotics) taken in the six weeks before the onset of diarrhoea?

Any other medical problems?

HIV/AIDS or other immunosuppression? (Table 34.6)

Examination

Severity of illness and degree of volume depletion (mental state, temperature, heart rate, blood pressure lying and sitting).

Signs of toxic megacolon (marked abdominal distension and tenderness)? (May complicate many forms of infective colitis (including *C. difficile*) as well as colitis due to inflammatory bowel disease.)

Extra-abdominal features (e.g. rash, arthropathy and uveitis)?

Table 34.2 Urgent investigation in acute severe diarrhoea.

Stool microscopy and culture
Test for *Clostridium difficile* toxin in stool
Full blood count
C-reactive protein
Blood glucose
Sodium, potassium, urea and creatinine
Liver function tests, albumin
Blood culture if febrile
Sigmoidoscopy if bloody diarrhoea
Abdominal X-ray if marked distension or tenderness (toxic megacolon)

Table 34.3 Causes of community-acquired diarrhoea.

Cause	Clinical features	Diagnosis/treatment (if indicated)
***Campylobacter* enteritis** (*C. jejuni*)	Incubation period two to six days. Associated fever and abdominal pain. Diarrhoea initially watery, later may contain blood and mucus. Usually, self-limiting, lasting two to five days. May be followed after one to three weeks by Guillain-Barré syndrome (Chapter 59)	Culture of *C. jejuni* from stool. Azithromycin 500 mg od PO for five days or Erythromycin 500 mg 12-hourly PO for five days.
Non-typhoid salmonellosis (Salmonella species)	Incubation period one to two days. Associated fever, vomiting and abdominal pain. Diarrhoea may become bloody if colon involved. Usually self-limiting. More severe in immunosuppressed.	Culture of *Salmonella* species from stool. Ciprofloxacin 500 mg 12-hourly PO for five days or trimethoprim 200 mg 12-hourly PO for five days.
Escherichia coli O157:H7 (enterohaemorrhagic *E. coli*)	Incubation period one to three days. Associated vomiting and abdominal pain. May have low-grade fever. Watery diarrhoea which may become bloody. May be complicated by haemolytic uraemic syndrome from 2 to 14 (mean 7) days after onset of illness.	Culture of *E. coli* O157 from stool (using sorbitol MacConkey agar; missed by standard culture). Supportive treatment. Antibiotic therapy unhelpful.
***Clostridium difficile* colitis**	Typically causes diarrhoea in hospital, often after antibiotic use but may also occur in the community. See Table 34.4.	Stool *C difficile* PCR and toxin EIA positive. Treat according to local guidelines.
Norovirus	Usually short incubation time (one to two days). Diarrhoea with vomiting is typical, with fever less common. Infections during outbreaks are more severe, with the elderly at particular risk of excess mortality.	The diagnosis is made by PCR analysis of stool and vomitus and the exclusion of other causes. Treatment is supportive.

- Obtain an abdominal X-ray to check for segmental or total colonic distension indicative of toxic megacolon.
- Seek urgent help from a microbiologist.
- Nurse the patient with standard isolation technique in a single room until the diagnosis is established.

All other patients:

- Further management will be determined by the results of microscopy and culture of the stool, and other investigations.

Table 34.4 Causes of hospital-acquired diarrhoea.

Cause	Clinical features	Diagnosis/treatment
Clostridium difficile colitis	Diarrhoea usually begins within 4–10 days of antibiotic treatment, but may not appear for four to six weeks. Presentations range from mild self-limiting watery diarrhoea to (rarely) acute fulminating toxic megacolon. Low-grade fever and abdominal tenderness are common. Although the rectum and sigmoid colon are usually involved, in 10% of cases colitis is confined to the more proximal colon.	Diagnosis is based on PCR testing and detection of *C. difficile* toxins A and B in the stool. In severe colitis, sigmoidoscopy may show adherent yellow plaques (2–10 mm in diameter). Supportive treatment and isolation of the patient to reduce the risk of spread. Stop antibiotic therapy and proton pump inhibitors if possible. If diarrhoea is mild (one to two stools daily), symptoms may resolve within one to two weeks without further treatment. Refer to local treatment guidelines. In general, if moderate diarrhoea (three or more stools daily), give Fidaxomicin 200 mg twice a day PO for 10 days. If severe infection (usually associated with hypoalbuminemia and/or ileus), give metronidazole 500 mg 3 times a day IV plus vancomycin 500 mg 4 times a day PO for 10–14 days (IV vancomycin should not be used as significant excretion into the gut does not occur). Around 20% of patients will have a relapse after initial treatment, due to germination of residual spores within the colon, re-infection with *C. difficile* or further antibiotic treatment. A second course of the same initial treatment is recommended.
Drugs	Many drugs may cause diarrhoea, including chemotherapeutic agents, proton pump inhibitors, metformin and laxatives in excess.	Diarrhoea resolves after treatment completed or with withdrawal of the causative drug.
Norovirus	See Table 34.3.	See Table 34.3.

Table 34.5 Causes of acute diarrhoea following recent travel abroad.

Cause	Clinical features	Diagnosis/treatment
Giardiasis (*Giardia lamblia*)	Widespread distribution. Explosive onset of watery diarrhoea one to three weeks after exposure.	Identification of cysts or trophozoites in stool or jejunal biopsy.
Amoebic dysentery (*Entamoeba histolytica*)	Mexico, South America, South Asia, West and South-East Africa. Diarrhoea may be severe with blood and mucus.	Metronidazole 400 mg 8-hourly PO for five days. Identification of cysts in stools. Metronidazole 750 mg 8-hourly PO for five days.
Schistosomiasis (*S. mansoni* and *japonicum*)	*S. mansoni*: South America and Middle East; *S. japonicum*: China and the Philippines. Diarrhoea onset two to six weeks or longer after exposure.	Identification of ova in stool. Praziquantel (seek expert advice).
Shigellosis (*Shigella* species)	Incubation period one to two days. Associated fever and abdominal pain. Diarrhoea may be watery or bloody.	Culture of *Shigella* species from stool. Ciprofloxacin 500 mg 12-hourly PO for five days or Trimethoprim 200 mg 12-hourly PO for five days.
Non-typhoid salmonellosis	See Community-acquired diarrhoea, Table 34.3.	

Table 34.6 Acute diarrhoea in the immunosuppressed/HIV-positive patient: specific pathogens to consider.

Cause	Clinical features	Diagnosis/treatment
Cryptosporidiosis (***Cryptosporidium* species**)	Subacute onset Associated abdominal pain Severe diarrhoea	Identification of oocysts in stool Seek expert advice on treatment
Isosporiasis (*Isospora belli*)	Incubation period: one week Associated fever, abdominal pain, diarrhoea with fatty stools	Identification of oocysts in stool, duodenal aspirate or jejunal biopsy Seek expert advice on treatment
Cytomegalovirus	Diarrhoea may be accompanied by fever, systemic illness and hepatitis	Serological tests for cytomegalovirus Seek expert advice on treatment

- If the patient has a fever, is dehydrated or is immunocompromised, start azithromycin 500 mg OD PO or ciprofloxacin PO or IV whilst awaiting the stool test results. The choice will depend upon your local antibiotic guidelines. (*Campylobacter* is currently the most common bacterial cause and most strains are resistant to ciprofloxacin. Moreover azithromycin-resistant *Shigella* infections are common in certain high-risk patients.)
- Anti-motility drugs such as loperamide are best avoided but can be given for short-term symptomatic relief. They are absolutely contraindicated in patients with shigellosis or dysentery (bloody stools and fever) due to the risk of a toxic megacolon.

Further management

This is directed by the working diagnosis.

Always consider the possibility of *C. difficile* infection and norovirus – involve the Infectious Diseases team early.

A flexible sigmoidoscopy and biopsies are not routinely needed, but if a new presentation of IBD is a possibility, a gastroenterology opinion should be sought (see below).

Could this be inflammatory bowel disease?

- This should be considered if there is blood or if the diarrhoea is chronic or recurrent or if there are systemic signs (e.g. rash, arthropathy and uveitis).
- Ulcerative colitis may present with acute diarrhoea, usually bloody. Vomiting does not occur, and abdominal pain is not a prominent feature. Diagnosis is by exclusion of infective causes (particularly *C. difficile*) and typical histological appearances on rectosigmoid biopsies.

- Crohn's disease is associated with less severe diarrhoea and blood is not prominent but there may be abdominal pain and tenderness particularly in the lower right quadrant.
- See Chapter 40 for further management of inflammatory bowel disease.

Could this be faecal impaction with overflow?

- This should be suspected in patients at risk of faecal impaction, for example the elderly, bed-bound, in those taking opioid analgesics.

- There is no vomiting or systemic illness. Rectal examination discloses hard-impacted faeces.
- Treatment is with laxatives/enemas.

Further reading

Guery B, Galperine T, Barbut F. (2019) Clostridioides difficile: diagnosis and treatments. *BMJ* 20(366), l4609.

Riddle MS, DuPont HL, Connor BA. (2016) ACG clinical guideline: diagnosis, treatment, and prevention of acute diarrheal infections in adults. *Am J Gastroenterol* 111(5), 602–622.

CHAPTER 35

Jaundice

BEN WARNER AND LYNN AFFARAH

Jaundice can be caused by a number of different pathologies, which can be sub-divided into pre-hepatic (excessive red cell breakdown), intra-hepatic (hepatocellular dysfunction) and post-hepatic (impaired hepatic excretion or obstruction of the biliary tree) (see Table 35.1).

Priorities

As with any clinical presentation, the aetiology is usually elicited by a detailed history (Table 35.2) and arranging appropriate investigations (Table 35.3).

- **Look for signs of sepsis**
- Give IV crystalloid, take blood (and ascitic fluid, if present) for culture, and start empirical IV antibiotic therapy to cover Gram-negative and anaerobic bacteria, in accordance with local guidelines (e.g. piperacillin-tazobactam or meropenem). Further management of sepsis is described in Chapter 5.
- **Assess for hepatic encephalopathy**
- The combination of jaundice and encephalopathy is characteristic of acute liver failure, but is also seen in other disorders (Table 35.3). If you suspect acute liver failure, seek urgent advice from a hepatologist. See Chapter 42 for further management of acute liver failure and decompensated chronic liver disease.

Table 35.1 Causes of jaundice.

Pre-hepatic	Intra-hepatic	Post-hepatic
Haemolysis	Viruses: hepatitis, EBV	Primary biliary cholangitis
Gilbert's syndrome	Alcoholic hepatitis	Primary sclerosing cholangitis
Crigger-Najjar syndrome	Autoimmune hepatitis	Intra-luminal causes such as gallstones
Drugs: Rifampicin, contrast	Sepsis/septicaemia	Mural causes such as strictures
agents and some anti-malarials	Alpha-1-antitrypsin deficiency	cholangiocarcinoma or biliary
	Vascular causes: Budd-Chiari syndrome	Extrinsic compression: pancreatic
	Wilson's disease	cancer, lymph nodes at porta hepatis
	Chronic liver disease/cirrhosis	Drug-induced cholestasis: flucloxacillin,
	Drugs: paracetamol overdose,	co-amoxiclav, nitrofurantoin
	isoniazid, statins, sodium valproate	

Acute Medicine: A Practical Guide to the Management of Medical Emergencies, Sixth Edition.
Edited by Mridula Rajwani, Leila Vaziri, and Ivie Gbinigie.
© 2026 John Wiley & Sons Ltd. Published 2026 by John Wiley & Sons Ltd.

Table 35.2 Focused assessment of the jaundiced patient.

History

Duration and time course of jaundice and other symptoms (e.g. fever and abdominal pain)

Known liver or biliary tract disease?

Itching/pruritus?

Constitutional symptoms: weight loss, low-grade fever, lymphadenopathy and fatigue?

Full drug history: including all non-prescription drugs, herbal remedies, dietary supplements, mushroom ingestion or khat, taken over the past year

Risk factors for viral hepatitis (foreign travel, IV drug use, men who have sex with men, multiple sexual partners, body piercing and tattoos, blood transfusion and blood products, needle-stick injury in health-care worker)?

Sexual history

Pregnancy?

Usual and recent alcohol intake?

Other medical problems (e.g. cardiovascular disease, transplant recipient, cancer, HIV/AIDS, haematological disease and inflammatory bowel disease)?

Family history of jaundice/liver disease, malignancy?

Examination

Physiological observations and systematic examination

Conscious level and mental state; grade of encephalopathy if present (see Chapter 42)

Signs of chronic liver disease?

Right upper quadrant tenderness (Table 35.4)?

Liver enlargement (seen in early viral hepatitis, alcoholic hepatitis, malignant infiltration, congestive heart failure and acute Budd–Chiari syndrome)?

Splenomegaly?

Signs associated with coagulopathy: bruising, petechiae, purpura

Ascites (Chapter 36)?

Lymphadenopathy?

Signs of upper gastrointestinal bleeding: melaena (digital rectal examination), haematemesis

Patients with suspected acute liver failure and grade 3 or 4 encephalopathy should be managed in an intensive care unit.

- **Assess for abdominal pain, distension or tenderness**
- These can be seen in a range of medical and surgical disorders (Chapter 36). Obtain an urgent surgical opinion.

Further management

Further management is directed by the working diagnosis.

- If there is evidence of haemolytic anaemia (anaemia with increased reticulocyte count, abnormal blood film, elevated plasma lactate dehydrogenase (LDH) and low plasma haptoglobin), seek urgent advice from a haematologist.
- Patients with presumed viral hepatitis can be discharged home with early clinic follow-up arranged, provided all the following criteria are met:
  - They are clinically stable and not encephalopathic.
  - Paracetamol poisoning, drug toxicity and other disorders that result in high AST/ALT levels have been considered and excluded (Table 35.4).
  - In women of child-bearing age, a pregnancy test is negative.
- If imaging demonstrates obstructive jaundice, early hepatobiliary intervention to achieve biliary decompression is needed: see Chapter 43.

Table 35.3 Urgent investigation in acute jaundice.

Full blood count and film
Coagulation screen
Blood glucose
Sodium, potassium, urea and creatinine
Liver function tests: bilirubin (total and unconjugated), aspartate aminotransferase, alanine aminotransferase, gamma
Glutamyl transpeptidase, alkaline phosphatase, albumin
Paracetamol level (Chapter 8)
Serum lactate dehydrogenase (LDH) and haptoglobin if suspected haemolysis
Blood culture if febrile
Urine stick test, microscopy and culture
Markers of viral hepatitis (anti-HAV IgM, HBsAg, anti-HBc IgM, anti-HCV, anti-HEV and EBV)
Test for HIV
Autoimmune screen (ANA, AMA, SMA, ANCA and immunoglobulins)
Microscopy and culture of ascites if present (aspirate 10 mL for cell count (use EDTA tube) and culture (inoculate blood
culture bottles) (see Chapter 24)
Ultrasound of liver, biliary tract and hepatic/portal vein and consider cross-sectional imaging (CT or MRI)
Pregnancy test in women of child-bearing age
Consider copper studies in young adults (Wilson disease, see Table 42.1)

AMA, anti-mitochondrial antibody; ANA, anti-nuclear antibody; ANCA, anti-neutrophil cytoplasmic antibody. EBV, Epstein-Barr Virus; EDTA, ethylene diaminetetra-acetic acid; HAV, hepatitis A virus; HBc, hepatitis B core; HBsAg, hepatitis B surface antigen; HCV, hepatitis C virus; HEV, hepatitis E virus; HIV, human immunodeficiency virus; IgM, immunoglobulin M; LDH, lactate dehydrogenase; SMA, smooth muscle antibody.

Table 35.4 Causes of plasma aspartate and alanine transaminase levels of more than 1000 units/L.

Common
Acute viral hepatitis, Ischaemic hepatitis
Acute drug or toxin-related liver injury (most commonly paracetamol)

Less common or rare
Acute exacerbation of autoimmune chronic active hepatitis
Reactivation of chronic hepatitis B
Acute Budd–Chiari syndrome
Veno-occlusive disease
HELLP syndrome of pregnancy (haemolysis, elevated liver enzymes and low platelet count)
Acute fatty liver of pregnancy
Hepatic infarction (may complicate HELLP syndrome)
Hepatitis delta in a chronic carrier of hepatitis B
Acute Wilson disease
Massive lymphomatous infiltration of the liver
Parasitic biliary obstruction

Further reading

National Institute for Care and Health Excellence (2014) Gallstone disease: diagnosis and management Clinical guideline: https://www.nice.org.uk/guidance/cg188?unlid=10194680392016226172055.
Roy-Chowdhury N, Roy-Chowdhury J. (2016) Diagnostic approach to the adult with jaundice or asymptomatic hyperbilirubinemia. UpToDate https://www.uptodate.com/contents/diagnostic-approach-to-the-adult-withjaundice-or-asymptomatic-hyperbilirubinemia?source=search_result&search=acute%20jaundice&selectedTitle=1~150.
Ryan DP, Hong TS, Bardeesy N. (2014) Pancreatic adenocarcinoma. *N Engl J Med* 371, 1039–1049. DOI: 10.1056/NEJMra1404198.

CHAPTER 36

Abdominal swelling, mass and hepato-splenomegaly

Ben Warner and Lynn Affarah

Abdominal examination may elicit a number of findings including abdominal masses or organomegaly or ascites (Figure 36.1).

Other considerations:

- Pelvic masses may be fibroids, bladder, ovarian cysts or gynaecological malignancies
- Masses in the right iliac fossa may be appendiceal, abscesses, features of Crohn's disease, tuberculosis, transplanted kidney or malignancy

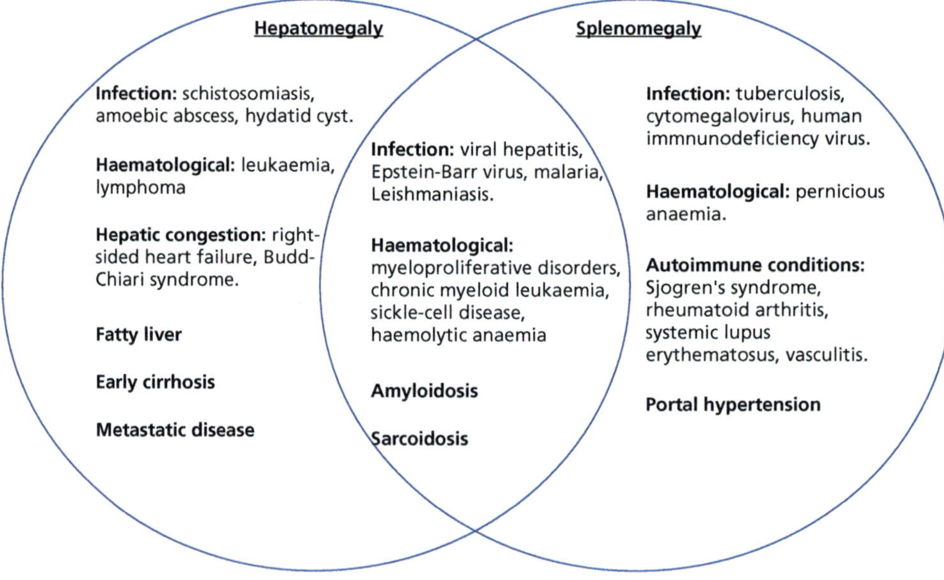

Figure 36.1 Causes of hepato- and splenomegaly.

Acute Medicine: A Practical Guide to the Management of Medical Emergencies, Sixth Edition.
Edited by Mridula Rajwani, Leila Vaziri, and Ivie Gbinigie.
© 2026 John Wiley & Sons Ltd. Published 2026 by John Wiley & Sons Ltd.

Ascites

Abdominal swelling may be caused by the accumulation of fluid within the peritoneal cavity, known as ascites. The clinical features, together with findings on diagnostic paracentesis (of which the serum-to-ascites albumin gradient (SAAG) is of particular importance), will narrow the differential diagnosis and direct further investigation. Assessment and management of the patient with ascites is summarised in Figure 36.2.

- The commonest causes for ascites seen in the emergency department are decompensated chronic liver disease, advanced heart failure and cancer.
- Patients who develop ascites as a complication of cirrhosis have a poor prognosis (two-year survival 50%), and should be referred to a hepatologist for consideration of liver transplantation.

Priorities

- Perform a diagnostic aspirate (30–50 mL) immediately on admission for new-onset ascites or if there is evidence of sepsis. The technique of diagnostic paracentesis is described in Chapter 112. Diagnostic tests on ascitic fluid are summarised in Table 36.1.
- If there is clinical or radiological evidence of cirrhosis, the cause of decompensation must be identified and treated: see Chapter 42.
- The management of spontaneous bacterial peritonitis is summarised in Section SBP below.

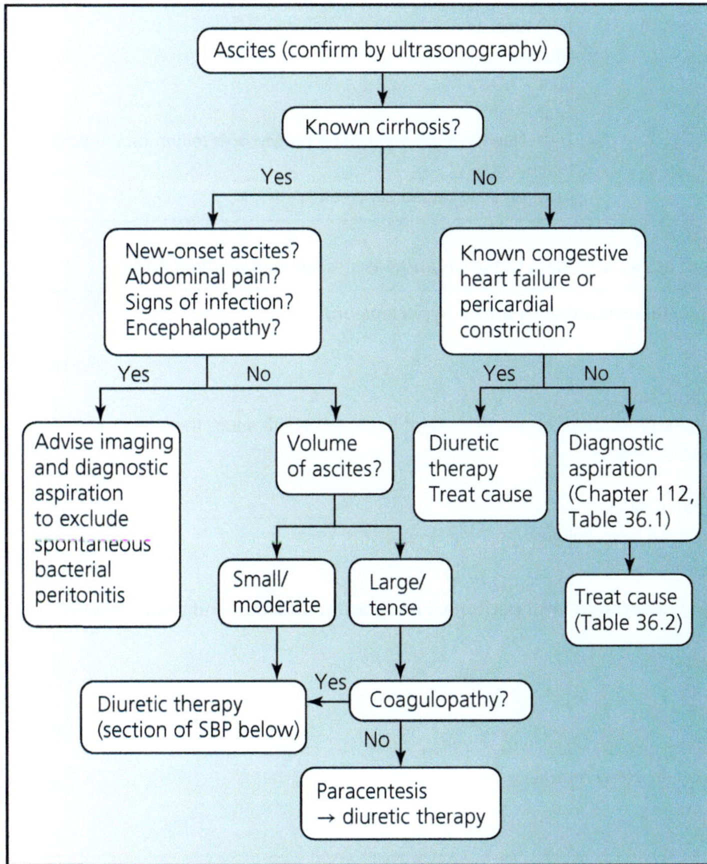

Figure 36.2 Assessment and management of the patient with ascites.

Table 36.1 Ascites: diagnostic tests.

Test	Comment
Visual inspection	Ascites due to cirrhosis are usually clear yellow, but may be cloudy when complicated by spontaneous bacterial peritonitis.
Albumin concentration	Measure the albumin concentration in ascites and serum and calculate the SAAG (serum minus ascitic albumin concentration). A SAAG of 11 g/L or greater indicates portal hypertension with 97% accuracy, while a SAAG of <11 g/L indicates the absence of portal hypertension. Causes of ascites according to the SAAG are given in Table 36.2.
Total and differential	Send a sample in an EDTA tube to the haematology laboratory for total and differential white cell count.
White cell count	In uncomplicated cirrhosis, the total white cell count is <500/mm³ and neutrophil count <250/mm³. Spontaneous bacterial peritonitis is associated with a neutrophil count of >250/mm³. In peritoneal tuberculosis, the white cell count is usually 150–4000/mm³, predominantly lymphocytes.
Bacterial culture	Send ascites for culture in patients with new-onset ascites or if you suspect infection (fever, abdominal pain, confusion, renal failure or acidosis). Inoculate aerobic and anaerobic blood culture bottles with 10 mL per bottle of ascites.
Cytology	Send a sample for cytology if you suspect malignancy or if the SAAG is <11 g/L. Cytology is usually positive in the presence of peritoneal metastases, but these are found in only about two-thirds of patients with ascites related to malignancy.
Other tests	Total protein Glucose LDH Gram stain Ziehl–Neelsen stain and testing for *Mycobacterium tuberculosis* DNA if suspected tuberculosis Amylase if suspected pancreatitis

Table 36.2 Causes of ascites according to the serum-to-ascites albumin gradient (SAAG).

High SAAG (≥11 g/L) (associated with portal hypertension)

Cirrhosis

Alcoholic hepatitis

Hepatic outflow obstruction:

- Budd-Chiari syndrome (thrombosis of one or more of the large hepatic veins, the inferior vena cava, or both)
- Hepatic veno-occlusive disease

Cardiac ascites:

- Severe tricuspid regurgitation
- All causes of right-sided heart failure
- Constrictive pericarditis

Low SAAG (<11 g/L) (associated with peritoneal neoplasms, infection and inflammation)

Peritoneal carcinomatosis

Peritoneal tuberculosis

Pancreatitis

Serositis

Nephrotic syndrome

Chylous ascites (lymphatic vessel rupture)

Myxoedema

Meig's syndrome

- Budd–Chiari syndrome is suspected in patients who present with sudden onset ascites in the absence of a known chronic liver disease. Presentation can range from asymptomatic to fulminant liver failure. Similarly, portal vein thrombosis can be asymptomatic, but typically presents with abdominal pain or features of portal hypertension such as varices or ascites. It is more common in patients with known chronic liver disease or who are in a hypercoagulable state. Duplex ultrasonography can be done if these are suspected, although computed tomography (CT) and magnetic resonance imaging (MRI) are more diagnostic.
- Ascites may complicate cardiac disease (severe tricuspid regurgitation, other causes of right-sided heart failure, and constrictive pericarditis). If the jugular venous pressure is raised, or there are other features of heart disease, check plasma brain natriuretic peptide (BNP)/N-terminal (NT)-proBNP and arrange echocardiography.
- Nephrotic syndrome as the cause of ascites can be confirmed or excluded by measurement of urinary protein excretion on a 24-h urine collection (>3.5 g/day is nephrotic-range proteinuria) or by calculating the albumin-to-creatinine ratio (ACR) in a spot urine sample (ACR is usually >220 mg/mmol in nephrotic syndrome).

Further management of ascites due to cirrhosis

In all patients with ascites, avoid nephrotoxic drugs, including NSAIDs, angiotensin-converting enzyme (ACE) inhibitors and α-adrenergic blockers.

Grade 1 or 2 (mild or moderate) ascites

Unless the ascites is new or complicated, both of these grades of ascites can be managed as an outpatient. Restrict dietary sodium intake to 80–120 mmol/day.

Start diuretic therapy with spironolactone 100 mg daily and increase by 100 mg weekly with monitoring of electrolytes and creatinine to a maximum of 400 mg daily. If spironolactone resistant, add furosemide 40 mg daily and increase weekly by 40 mg to a maximum of 160 mg with biochemical monitoring.

Monitor daily weight. Target weight loss is 0.5 kg daily in patients without peripheral oedema and 1 kg daily in those with peripheral oedema.

Aim for the minimum dose of diuretics once ascites have resolved.

Complications from diuretics include gynaecomastia (amiloride 10–40 mg daily can be substituted for spironolactone), renal failure, hyperkalaemia (either reduce the spironolactone or add in furosemide) and encephalopathy. Stop diuretics if plasma sodium levels fall below 120 mmol/L as this may be consistent with diuretic-induced hypovolaemic hyponatraemia (Chapter 52).

Grade 3 (large volume) ascites, or diuretic-resistant ascites

Severe ascites can cause breathlessness and this can be alleviated by paracentesis. If there are tense ascites, consider a single paracentesis, followed by dietary sodium restriction and diuretic therapy. Human albumin solution (100 mL of 20% HAS per 2 L of ascites removed) should be given IV during paracentesis. Seek advice from a hepatologist – see Chapter 42.

In the case of diuretic-resistant ascites and where the urinary sodium concentration remains below 30 mmol/L, the patient should be referred for a transjugular intrahepatic portosystemic shunt (TIPS) or consideration of liver transplantation.

Spontaneous bacterial peritonitis (SBP)

Definition
Spontaneous bacterial peritonitis (SBP) is defined as an infection of ascitic fluid without evidence of an intraabdominal surgically treatable source; depending on the clinical context, imaging by CT may be needed to exclude such a source.

Background
SBP is a common complication of ascites due to cirrhosis; the lower the ascitic fluid albumin concentration (prior to infection), the higher the risk. Aerobic Gram-negative bacteria, especially *Escherichia coli*, are the most common causative organisms. Features of SBP include fever (70%), abdominal pain (60%), abdominal tenderness (50%) and change in mental state (50%). It may be complicated by the hepatorenal syndrome (in up to 30%).

EDTA, ethylene diaminetetra-acetic acid; LDH, lactate dehydrogenase.

Diagnosis

The diagnosis of SBP is based on the finding of >250 neutrophils/mm³ in ascitic fluid. If the neutrophil count is less than this, but there are features of sepsis, treatment should be given for SBP, pending the result of culture; if the patient is well, hold off antibiotic therapy and remeasure the cell count in 48 h.

Management

- Treat with third-generation cephalosporin, for example cefotaxime 2 g 8-hourly IV for five days, followed by a quinolone PO for five days.
- If serum creatinine is >88 µmol/L, urea is >10.7 mmol/L, or bilirubin is >68 µmol/L, give human albumin solution 1.5 g/kg IV at diagnosis and 1 g/kg 48 h later to reduce the incidence of hepatorenal syndrome.
- Repeat diagnostic paracentesis at 48 h: if the neutrophil count has not reduced by 25% or the patient has ongoing signs of sepsis, discuss changing the antibiotic regimen with your microbiologist.

Antibiotic prophylaxis

This is indicated for:
- Patients with cirrhosis who present with gastrointestinal bleeding (Chapters 38 and 39).
- Patients with cirrhosis and ascites, with ascitic fluid protein <10 g/L, who require hospital admission for another reason.
- Patients with cirrhosis and ascites, with ascitic fluid protein <15 g/L and:
  - Impaired renal function (serum creatinine >106 µmol/L or urea >8.9 mmol/L)
  - Low plasma sodium ≤130 mmol/L or
  - Liver failure (Child–Pugh score ≤9 and serum bilirubin ≤51 µmol/L)
- Patients who have had one or more episodes of SBP, in whom the recurrence rate is up to 70% at one year.

Discuss the choice of prophylaxis with a hepatologist or microbiologist.

Further reading

Hernaez R, Hamilton JP. (2016) Unexplained ascites. *Clin Liver Dis* 7, 53–56. http://onlinelibrary.wiley.com/doi/10.1002/cld.537/full.

Pericleous M, Sarnowski A, Moore A, *et al.* (2016) The clinical management of abdominal ascites, spontaneous bacterial peritonitis and hepatorenal syndrome: a review of current guidelines and recommendations. *Eur J Gastroenterol Hepatol* 28, e10–e18.

Solà E, Solé C, Ginès P. (2016) Management of uninfected and infected ascites in cirrhosis. *Liver Int* 36(suppl 1), 109–115.

CHAPTER 37

Acute oesophageal disorders

GRACE BARNES AND ARIF HUSSENBUX

The differential for acute oesophageal disorders is wide. Initial presentation to the acute medical take can include dysphagia, pain (odynophagia, epigastric or retrosternal) or haematemesis.

Important oesophageal pathology to consider in these patients include:

- Gastro-oesophageal reflux disease
- Variceal bleeding, secondary to portal hypertension
- Malignancy
- Mallory–Weiss tear
- Oesophageal perforation
- Food bolus obstruction
- Oesophageal spasm

Other conditions to consider which may affect the oesophagus include motility disorders (e.g. achalasia), intrinsic oesophageal pathology (e.g. pharyngeal pouch), neuromuscular disorders (e.g. myasthenia gravis) and extrinsic pressure on the oesophagus (e.g. large retrosternal goitre).

Oesophageal perforation

Oesophageal perforation is a serious and potentially life-threatening emergency, caused by transmural disruption of the oesophageal wall. The thoracic oesophagus is most commonly affected, followed by cervical and then abdominal oesophageal sections.

Perforation can occur spontaneously, as a result of trauma, or following instrumentation (see Table 37.1). Recognition is key, to ensure timely investigation and urgent management.

Differential diagnoses to consider include:

- Cardiac causes – Myocardial infarction, pericarditis
- Respiratory causes – Pneumothorax, pulmonary embolism, pneumonia
- Vascular causes – Aortic dissection
- Abdominal causes – Perforated peptic ulcer disease, acute pancreatitis

If oesophageal perforation is suspected, perform a focused history and examination, looking for the following presenting features:

- Severe retrosternal chest pain following vomiting, straining, coughing or hiccupping
- Dysphagia and/or odynophagia

Acute Medicine: A Practical Guide to the Management of Medical Emergencies, Sixth Edition.
Edited by Mridula Rajwani, Leila Vaziri, and Ivie Gbinigie.

Table 37.1 Summary of potential causes of oesophageal perforation, and the clinical features to consider for each cause.

Causes of oesophageal perforation	Features
Spontaneous oesophageal rupture (Boerhaave syndrome)	Often perforation is on the left side of the lower thoracic oesophagus, with a leak into the left pleural cavity Often following vomiting or straining
Blunt chest trauma	Look for additional injuries/consider if high impact mechanism of injury
Foreign body obstruction	Includes obstructing foreign body from ingestion or invading/obstructing tumour
Ingestion of corrosive substance	Clarify any history of ingestion of toxic substance, metal object or battery
Recent oesophageal surgery	Including laparoscopic procedures
Recent oesophageal instrumentation	Very low risk with diagnostic endoscopy Risk increases with endoscopic procedure such as dilatation, endoscopic mucosal resection, oesophageal stent insertion and radiofrequency ablation.
Recent cardiac radiofrequency ablation of left atria (for atrial fibrillation)	Associated with the risk of developing atrio-oesophageal fistula

- Dyspnoea
- Haemodynamic instability
- Subcutaneous emphysema over chest wall
  - If pneumomediastinum present
- Reduced/absent air entry on auscultation of chest
  - If pleural effusion or pneumothorax present
- Rigid/tender abdomen

Urgent investigations to arrange:
- Observations
  - Is there evidence of haemodynamic instability?
  - Include blood pressure on both arms *(differential: aortic dissection)*
- Bloods
  - Full blood count (FBC), C-reactive protein (CRP), clotting profile, group and save and an arterial blood gas
  - Include troponin and D dimer *(differential: pulmonary embolism(PE), myocardial infarction (MI), aortic dissection)*
- Electrocardiogram (ECG)
  - Is there evidence of cardiac ischaemia? *(differential: myocardial infarction (MI), pericarditis)*
- Chest X-ray
  - Look for evidence of pneumomediastinum/pneumoperitoneum, widened mediastinum, subcutaneous emphysema, pleural effusion or pneumothorax
  - Give water-soluble oral contrast (gastrograffin) to localise perforation (always seek surgical opinion prior to requesting this)
- Computed tomography (CT) chest
  - Cross-sectional imaging can highlight area of perforation/oesophageal damage, with water-soluble oral contrast (gastrograffin) to confirm site and extent of extravasation as a definitive test.

Initial management of oesophageal perforation includes resuscitation, analgesia and broad-spectrum antibiotic cover (including anaerobic cover). Patients should be kept 'nil by mouth' with IV fluids, pending urgent surgical review, and often need to be nursed in a high-dependency setting, such as high-dependency unit (HDU) or intensive care unit (ICU).

Although small perforations can be managed conservatively, definitive management of oesophageal perforation often relies on surgical intervention. There is increasing evidence for the role of endoscopic intervention in management of oesophageal perforation, including endoscopic application of clips, endovac procedures and covered stents.

Mallory–Weiss syndrome

Mallory-Weiss syndrome arises following mucosal disruption in the gastrointestinal (GI) tract leading to formation of mucosal tears. Commonly this arises at the gastro-oesophageal junction (often right lateral wall, following lesser curvature of the stomach) due to rapid changes in pressure and discoordination of muscle contraction. This disruption leads to exposure of submucosal vessels and formation of one or more longitudinal mucosal tears.

Mucosal damage can result in bleeding and often presents as a non-variceal upper GI haemorrhage – see Chapter 38 for management of an acute upper GI haemorrhage.

Risk factors for Mallory–Weiss syndrome:
- Repetitive retching and/or vomiting following excessive alcohol intake or a large meal.

Investigations:
- Blood tests
  - Including haemoglobin, clotting profile and group and save
- Endoscopic evaluation
  - Mallory–Weiss tear confirmed with direct visualisation of the mucosal tear

Initial management of bleeding from a Mallory–Weiss tear is the same as for any acute GI haemorrhage, including haemodynamic stabilisation and resuscitation, and management of any coagulopathy.

In most cases, bleeding from a Mallory-Weiss tear will stop spontaneously, and re-bleeding is uncommon. Rarely, endoscopic therapy may be required to stop bleeding if high-risk stigmata are present, such as a visible bleeding vessel.

Food bolus obstruction

Food bolus obstruction is not uncommon on the acute medical take. Patients often present with sudden onset dysphagia, chest pain and sensation of a blockage, which has occurred whilst eating. The food bolus gets stuck in the oesophagus, blocking any further oral intake into the stomach and subsequent oral intake is regurgitated. Pain is due to oesophageal spasm.

Common causes of a food bolus include large pieces of meat, or small bones (chicken or fish). Most food boluses pass spontaneously (with subsequent immediate resolution of symptoms); however, 10–20% of cases will require endoscopic intervention.

Oesophageal pathology that can predispose to obstructing food bolus:
- Eosinophilic oesophagitis
  - Strong association with food bolus obstruction in adults
  - Typically affects young males
  - There may be a history of atopy
  - Diagnosed on tissue biopsy taken at time of endoscopy (showing eosinophilic infiltration in oesophageal tissue)
  - Management with proton pump inhibitor (PPI) therapy or topical steroid therapy

- Oesophageal strictures
  - Often visualised during endoscopic procedure
  - May require subsequent procedure for endoscopic dilatation if proven to be benign
- Dysmotility
  - Macroscopically and microscopically normal mucosa
  - Requires further investigation (e.g. Barium swallow for diagnosis of achalasia)
  - Consider non-GI tract pathology (e.g. neuromuscular disorder)
  Management of a food bolus:

- History
  - Confirm with patient what they were eating and time of symptom onset
  - Is there dysphagia to solids, fluids or saliva?
- Arrange key investigations
  - Blood tests
    - Including full blood count (FBC), renal profile and clotting profile
  - X ray imaging
    - Are there small radio-opaque bones?
    - Is there evidence of free air in the mediastinum?
- Nil by mouth
- IV maintenance fluid
- Analgesia (not via oral route)
- Endoscopy ideally within 12 h
  - To reduce risk of localised ischaemia in the oesophagus.
  - Food bolus is manually broken down and removed using endoscopic tools such as grasping forceps, roth nets and snares.
  - Endoscopy can also aid in diagnosis of underlying oesophageal pathology (see Table 37.1).
  Once the food bolus has been removed and the patient is safely tolerating oral intake, they are usually able to be safely discharged home on the same day.

Barrett's oesophagus

Barrett's oesophagus is a pre-malignant condition, where the normal squamous epithelium of the oesophagus is replaced by columnar mucosa, often secondary to longterm gastro-oesophageal reflux. If left untreated, there is a high risk of dysplasia progressing to malignancy (adenocarcinoma).

The mainstay of treatment involves PPI therapy to treat underlying gastro-oesophageal reflux. Radiofrequency ablation and endoscopic resection can also be considered to treat affected areas.

If Barrett's oesophagus is identified during endoscopy, then patients should undergo ongoing regular surveillance endoscopy (with biopsy), to look for malignant change. Frequency of surveillance is dependent on the extent of mucosal involvement; if <3 cm this is performed every five years, and if >3 cm and <10 cm, this increases to every three years. If histology confirms dysplasia, ongoing management and surveillance should be discussed in a multi-disciplinary setting.

Oesophageal malignancy

It is important to remember that presentation of acute oesophageal disorders can also highlight underlying oesophageal malignancy, with approximately 9000 new cases diagnosed every year in the United Kingdom.

There are two forms of oesophageal carcinoma; adenocarcinoma and squamous cell carcinoma (SCC). SCC typically affects the upper third of the oesophagus, with risk factors including tobacco smoking. Adenocarcinoma affects the lower third of the oesophagus, with risk factors including reflux and Barrett's oesophagus.

Symptomatic oesophageal malignancy often presents with progressive painless dysphagia, initially to solids which progresses to liquids. If suspected, urgent endoscopy should be requested on a two-week wait pathway, with tissue biopsy to confirm the diagnosis, and subsequent staging CT chest, abdomen and pelvis.

Management is determined via a multidisciplinary approach; this can range from radical oesophagectomy and neoadjuvant chemotherapy, to localised radiotherapy and oesophageal stenting.

Further reading

BSG: Guidelines on the diagnosis and management of eosinophilic oesophagitis.https://gut.bmj.com/content/71/8/1459.

Endotherapy of leaks and fistula.https://www.ncbi.nlm.nih.gov/pmc/articles/PMC4482829/.

Nature Disease Primers – Non-variceal upper gastrointestinal bleeding.https://www.nature.com/articles/nrdp201820.

NICE Guideline: Barrett's oesophagus and stage 1 oesophageal adenocarcinoma.https://www.bsg.org.uk/getmedia/04aee08d-e3d0-4139-aec5-f37ef5eb39b8/barretts-oesophagus-and-stage-1-oesophageal-adenocarcinoma-monitoring-and-management-pdf-66143891094469.pdf?ext=.pdf.

The etiology, diagnosis and management of oesophageal perforation.https://www.sciencedirect.com/science/article/abs/pii/S1091255X23015123?via%3Dihub.

CHAPTER 38

Haematemesis and melaena

Udi Shmueli

About 90% of non-variceal bleeds and 50% of variceal bleeds stop spontaneously. Mortality is around 7–10% in patients with non-variceal bleeds, and 30% in those with variceal bleeds. Almost all deaths occur in patients >65 years and those with major comorbidities, most often from multi-organ failure secondary to hypovolaemia/hypotension.

Priorities

1 **Make a rapid clinical assessment**, to include an estimate of the volume of blood lost (Table 38.2). Put in a large-bore IV cannula (e.g. green or grey Venflon), and take 20 mL of blood for urgent investigations (Table 38.3). Initial fluid resuscitation should be with IV crystalloid. Give blood when available if the patient is shocked, or actively bleeding with a haemoglobin of <90 g/L.

Table 38.1 Causes of upper gastrointestinal haemorrhage.

Common
Gastric or duodenal peptic ulcer
Oesophageal or gastric varices
Erosive oesophagitis, gastritis or duodenitis
No lesion identified (10–15% cases; usually because the lesion is obscured by blood, difficult to identify, such as Dieulafoy's lesion, or healed by the time of the gastroscopy)

Less common or rare
Portal hypertensive gastropathy
Angiodysplasia
Gastric antral vascular ectasia (GAVE), (long red stripes arising from the pylorus, also known as 'watermelon' stomach)
Mass lesions (polyp or cancer)

Mallory-Weiss syndrome (Chapter 37)
Dieulafoy's lesion (an abnormally large submucosal vessel that erodes the gastric epithelium bleeding intermittently; there is no primary ulcer and so in the absence of bleeding it is difficult to see)
Haemobilia (bleeding from the bile duct)
Haemosuccus pancreaticus (bleeding from the pancreatic duct)
Aorto-enteric fistula (fistula between aneurysmal aorta or aortic graft and the gut, most often duodenum; endoscopy is primarily to exclude bleeding from other causes; the fistula may not be visualised)
Cameron lesions (linear ulcers within the sac of a hiatus hernia at the diaphragmatic impression)

Acute Medicine: A Practical Guide to the Management of Medical Emergencies, Sixth Edition.
Edited by Mridula Rajwani, Leila Vaziri, and Ivie Gbinigie.
© 2026 John Wiley & Sons Ltd. Published 2026 by John Wiley & Sons Ltd.

Table 38.2 Focused assessment in acute upper GI bleeding.

History

Has there been haematemesis, melaena or both? Did vomiting precede the first haematemesis (suggesting Mallory–Weiss tear, although this history is absent in 50% of cases)? Was bleeding associated with syncope?

Has there been previous upper gastrointestinal bleeding? What was the cause?

Current and recent drug therapy: ask specifically about non-steroidal anti-inflammatory drugs (NSAIDs), aspirin, clopidogrel, warfarin and direct-acting oral anticoagulants

Usual and recent alcohol intake

Known chronic liver disease

Other medical problems, for example heart disease, chronic kidney disease, haematological conditions.

Examination

Estimate the volume of blood loss from the physiological observations:

Major bleed (>1500 mL; >30% of blood volume)	**Minor bleed (≤750 mL; <15% of blood volume)**
Pulse ≤120/min	Pulse <100/min
Systolic BP <120 mmHg (note this is influenced by age and usual blood pressure)	Systolic BP ≤120 mmHg, with postural fall <20 from lying to sitting
Cool or cold extremities	Normal perfusion of extremities
Tachypnoea (respiratory rate >20/min)	Normal respiratory rate
Abnormal mental state: agitation, confusion, reduced conscious level	Normal mental state
Signs of chronic liver disease?	
Abdominal tenderness or masses?	
Hepatomegaly, splenomegaly or ascites?	

Table 38.3 Urgent investigation in acute upper GI bleeding.

Full blood count

Group and screen serum: crossmatch at least 4 units of whole blood if there is shock, significant blood loss or initial haemoglobin <100 g/L

Coagulation screen

Sodium, potassium, urea and creatinine

Liver function tests

ECG

Chest X-ray

Box 38.1 Manifestations of acute upper GI bleeding

Haematemesis is the vomiting of red blood and indicates moderate or severe acute upper gastrointestinal (GI) bleeding.

Coffee-ground vomiting is the vomiting of dark brown vomitus that resembles coffee grounds. It results from the oxidation of haem to haematin by gastric acid and indicates minor upper GI bleeding that has slowed or stopped.

Melaena is black, tarry stool and typically indicates upper GI bleeding. Small intestinal or right colon bleeding can also cause melaena (Chapter 39). Upper GI bleeding of >50–100 mL is required to cause melaena, which may persist for several days after bleeding has ceased. Black stool that is not melaena may result from ingestion of iron or some foods.

Haematochezia is the passage of liquid blood or clots per rectum, and usually indicates lower GI bleeding (Chapter 39), but sometimes can result from severe upper GI bleeding with rapid transit of blood through the gut.

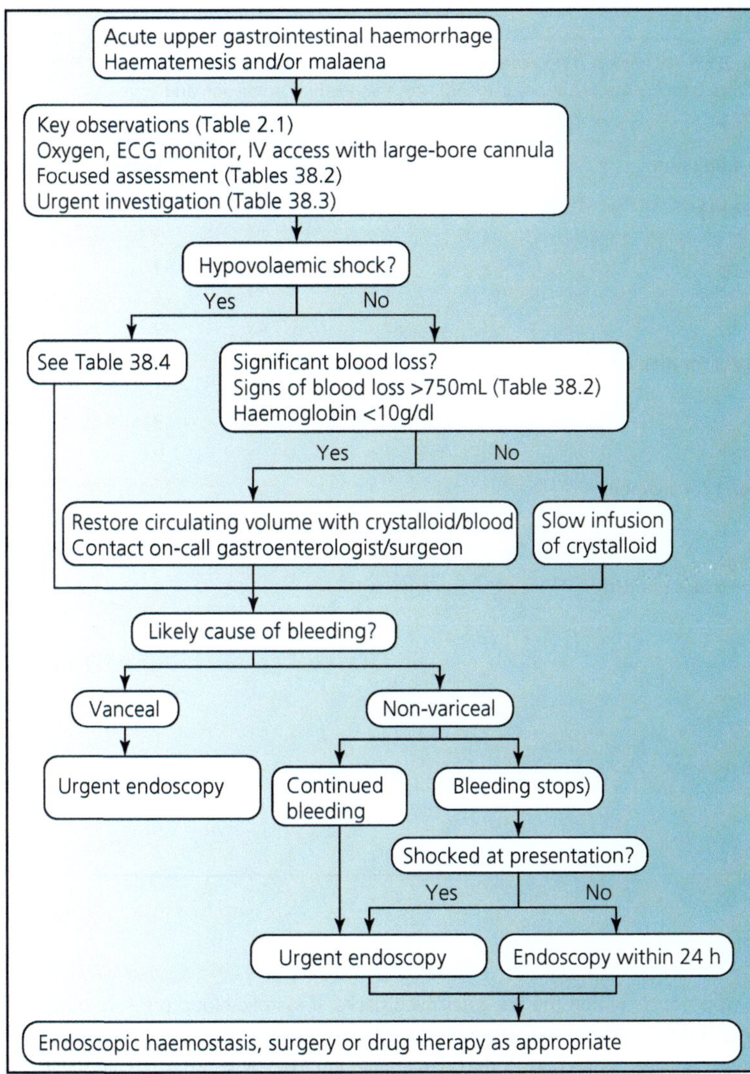

Figure 38.1 Management of acute upper GI bleeding.

The Blatchford score (Table 38.4) is a screening tool to assess the probability that endoscopic intervention or blood transfusion will be needed, and is helpful when discussing the patient's management with colleagues.

2 **If there is hypovolaemic shock** (systolic blood pressure ≤90 mmHg, pulse ≤100/min, cold extremities):

- Give oxygen 60–100% and attach an electrocardiogram (ECG) monitor.
- Obtain help:
  - Inform gastroenterology/surgical and critical care colleagues, and contact the on-call endoscopy service, to arrange an urgent endoscopy.
  - Put out a major haemorrhage call.

Table 38.4 Blatchford score.

Add the scores for each risk marker. If no value applies to a particular marker, score 0. A total score can range from 0 to 23. A score above zero indicates the need for admission and inpatient endoscopy.

Risk marker on admission	Score
Blood urea (mmol/L)	
≤6.5 <8.0	2
≤8.0 <10.0	3
≤10.0 <25	4
≤25	6
Haemoglobin (g/L) for men	
≤120 <130	1
≤100 <120	3
<100	6
Haemoglobin (g/L) for women	
≤100 <120	1
<100	6
Systolic blood pressure (mmHg)	
100–109	1
90–99	2
<90	3
Other markers	
Pulse ≤100/min	1
Presentation with melaena	1
Presentation with syncope	2
Hepatic disease	2
Heart failure	2

- Transfuse blood products within the pre-assembled packs. If systolic blood pressure remains <100 mmHg, use uncrossmatched O Rhesus negative blood (Rhesus positive blood is acceptable for males and post-menopausal females). Start transfusing crossmatched blood as soon as it is available, via a second IV cannula. Use a blood warmer if infusing at >50 mL/kg/h.
- Correct clotting abnormalities (see below).
- Consider inserting a urinary catheter to monitor the urine output (aim for urine output of 0.5 mL/kg/h).

3 Managing anticoagulants, antiplatelet agents and coagulopathies (Chapter 85) and Platelets

Holding and reversal of these agents should be individualised, bearing in mind the risks of thromboembolic events.

Emergency Endoscopy should not be delayed for reversal of anticoagulation.

- Warfarin
  - Hold warfarin if there is minor bleeding, or the bleeding has stopped.
  - With serious or life-threatening bleeding reverse warfarin with Prothrombin complex concentrate (PCC) and vitamin K 5-10 mg by intravenous injection: discuss with haematologist.
- Directly acting oral anticoagulants (DOACs)
  - Ask when the last dose was taken as the half-life of these drugs is usually only 8–12 h. It is usually sufficient to just hold the DOAC.

- If necessary due to instability prothrombin complex concentrate can help reverse DOACs: discuss with haematologist
- In life-threatening emergencies dabigatran can be reversed with idarucizumab. Rivaroxaban, edoxaban and apixaban can be reversed with the even more expensive Andexanet alfa. They work in minutes but there is a significant risk of thromboembolic events: discuss with haematologist.
- Low dose aspirin
  - Taken for secondary prevention low dose aspirin (75 mg) can be continued.
  - Taken for primary prevention it could be stopped.
- Dual antiplatelet therapy
  Continue the aspirin, stop the second antiplatelet agent, but discuss with cardiology and restart as soon as possible preferably within five days.
- If the platelet count is <50 × 10^9/L, and the patient is actively bleeding, give platelet concentrate: discuss with a haematologist.
4 **If you suspect bleeding oesophageal or gastric varices** (because of a past history of variceal bleeding or chronic liver disease):
- Give terlipressin 2 mg IV followed by 1–2 mg 4–6 hourly until bleeding is controlled, for up to five days.
- Give IV antibiotic as per your local guidelines (e.g. co-amoxiclav 1.2 g 8-hourly IV or tazocin 4.5 g 8-hourly IV), to prevent bacterial infection (including spontaneous bacterial peritonitis, Chapter 36), which is a common complication.
- Contact the endoscopy service for urgent endoscopy, anaesthetic/critical care support may be required if there is continued bleeding or any impairment in conscious level.
- If there is continued variceal bleeding (and the airway is protected by endotracheal intubation), a Sengstaken–Blakemore tube can be inserted by an experienced operator.
- Other supportive measures for patients with decompensated chronic liver disease are discussed in Chapter 42.
5 **In patients without shock but with evidence of significant blood loss (e.g. syncope in association with bleeding; clinical signs of blood loss >750 mL) or haemoglobin <100 g/L:**
- Start an infusion of crystalloid to maintain systolic blood pressure >100 mmHg.
- Transfuse blood if the initial haemoglobin is <70 g/L. Correct clotting abnormalities (see above).
- Contact the on-call endoscopy service to arrange endoscopy within 24 h.

Further management

Blood transfusion
Once the volume deficit has been corrected, recheck the haemoglobin and transfuse blood if this is 70 g/L or below. The target haemoglobin is 70–100 g/L.

Endoscopy
- Urgent endoscopy is needed for patients with shock on admission (but not before adequate resuscitation), with known varices or signs of chronic liver disease, or evidence of continued bleeding.
- Other patients should have endoscopy within 24 hours of admission (with the exception of those with a Blatchford score of zero, who can be considered for discharge with outpatient endoscopy). They can be allowed to eat, but must be nil by mouth for >4 h prior to endoscopy.

Drug therapy
- Stop nonsteroidal anti-inflammatory drugs (NSAIDs).
- Anticoagulant and antiplatelet therapy see above.

- There is no evidence that starting a proton pump inhibitor (PPI) before endoscopy alters outcome. Treatment with a PPI makes testing for *Helicobacter pylori* unreliable. But pre-endoscopy high-dose intravenous PPI therapy can be considered, to downstage endoscopic stigmata and thereby reduce the need for endoscopic therapy.
- Tranexamic acid is not helpful.

Management after endoscopy

- Calculate the Rockall score (Table 38.5). Those with a score ≤2 can be discharged (predicted mortality <1%). Those with a score ≥3 should remain in hospital for close observation.
- Further management is determined by the endoscopic diagnosis and should be discussed with a gastroenterologist.

Peptic ulcer

- Patients with low-risk peptic ulcer bleeding based on clinical and endoscopic criteria (e.g. clean ulcer base) can be discharged on the same day as endoscopy.
- Most patients with high-risk peptic ulcer bleeding based on clinical and endoscopic criteria (e.g. stigmata of recent haemorrhage) should remain hospitalised for at least 72 h.
- Start a PPI. If the patient is stable and able to tolerate oral medication, this can be administered by mouth (e.g. omeprazole 40 mg PO 12-hourly). If the patient is at high risk of further bleeding (high Rockall score) or unable to tolerate oral medication, give a bolus of omeprazole (or pantoprazole) 80 mg IV followed by an infusion of 8 mg/h for 72 h.
- Rebleeding after an initial endoscopy requires either a repeat endoscopy or referral to interventional radiology, depending on the initial findings at endoscopy. If interventional radiology is not promptly available, refer for surgery.
- Full-dose PPIs should be given for at least four weeks.

Table 38.5 Rockall score post-endoscopy.

Add the scores at the top of each column for each of the variables to derive a total risk score. The total score can range from 0 to 11.

	Score			
	0	1	2	3
Age shock on admission?	<60 no shock (systolic blood pressure ≤100, pulse <100)	60–79 Tachycardia (systolic BP ≤100, pulse ≤100)	≤80 Hypotension (systolic BP <100)	
Comorbidity	None		Heart failure, ischaemic heart disease, any other comorbidity	Renal failure, liver failure, disseminated malignancy
Diagnosis at endoscopy	Mallory–Weiss tear, no lesion seen, no signs of recent bleeding	All other diagnosis	Malignancy of upper GI tract	
Major stigmata of recent bleeding at endoscopy	None or dark spot only		Blood in upper GI tract, adherent clot, visible or spurting vessel	

- Most patients with gastric ulcers should have a repeat endoscopy at six to eight weeks to confirm healing and exclude malignancy.
- If *Helicobacter pylori* positive, start eradication treatment according to local protocols. Most ulcers not due to NSAIDs or aspirin are associated with *H. pylori* infection. As the Clotest taken at endoscopy may be falsely negative when taken at the time of an acute bleed, a high index of suspicion should be kept and a urease breath test or faecal antigen test (off PPIs for two weeks) should be ordered after the acute event when appropriate. Gastric biopsies taken for histology at the time of the initial endoscopy can also improve the detection rate.
- Anticoagulant and antiplatelet therapy: NSAIDs should be stopped; low-dose aspirin, if needed for secondary prevention of vascular events or coronary stent thrombosis, can be continued with concomitant PPI therapy. Other antiplatelet agents (e.g. clopidogrel) should be stopped temporarily and timing of restarting discussed with the appropriate specialist (cardiologist or stroke physician).

Erosive gastritis

There are two groups of patients:

- Previously well patients in whom erosive gastritis is related to aspirin, NSAIDs or alcohol. Bleeding usually stops when these agents are withdrawn and no specific treatment is needed. A short course of a PPI can be given to limit concomitant damage from acid exposure. *H. pylori* should be treated if present.
- In critically ill patients with stress ulceration, in whom the mortality is high, correct clotting abnormalities and give a PPI. Sucralfate is also an option.

Oesophagitis and oesophageal ulcer

Give a PPI for at least four weeks. Oesophagitis may require indefinite treatment with PPI.

Oesophageal and gastric varices

- Variceal bleeding stops spontaneously in 50% of patients. The risk of further bleeding can be substantially reduced by follow-up endoscopic therapy to obliterate residual varices and administration of a non-selective beta blocker (e.g. propranolol or carvedilol).
- Discuss management of the varices and the underlying cause of portal hypertension with a gastroenterologist or hepatologist.

Mallory-Weiss tear

- Bleeding usually stops spontaneously and rebleeding is rare.
- If bleeding continues, the options are repeated endoscopy with a view to endotherapy (argon-plasma coagulation, application of haemostasis clip), tamponade using a Sengstaken–Blakemore tube, or interventional radiology for embolization.

Negative endoscopy

- In 15–20% of patients, the first endoscopy does not reveal a source of bleeding. Discuss repeating the endoscopy, especially if blood or food obscured the views obtained, or the patient has chronic liver disease (as varices which have recently bled may not be visible).
- Patients who presented with melaena alone, should be investigated for a small bowel or proximal colonic source of bleeding (Chapter 39). A normal blood urea suggests a colonic cause of melaena, except in patients with chronic liver disease (in whom urea levels are often low).
- Computed tomography (CT) angiography can be useful after two negative endoscopies, but only if performed when the patient is actively bleeding.

Further reading

Gralnek IM, Stanley AJ, Morris AJ, *et al.* (2021) Endoscopic diagnosis and management of nonvariceal upper gastrointestinal hemorrhage (NVUGIH): European Society of Gastrointestinal Endoscopy (ESGE) Guideline – Update 2021. *Endoscopy* 53(3), 300–332.

Stanley AJ, Laine L. (2019) Management of acute upper gastrointestinal bleeding. *BMJ* 364, l536.

Siau K, Hearnshaw S, Stanley AJ, *et al.* (2020) British Society of Gastroenterology (BSG)-led multisociety consensus care bundle for the early clinical management of acute upper gastrointestinal bleeding. *Frontline Gastroenterol* 11, 311–323.

Gerson LB, Fidler JL, Cave DR, Leighton JA. (2015) American College of Gastroenterology Clinical Guideline: diagnosis and management of small bowel bleeding. *Am J Gastroenterol* 110, 1265–1287.

National Institute for Health and Care Excellence (2015) *Blood transfusion*. NICE guideline (NG24). https:// www.nice.org.uk/guidance/ng24.

National Institute for Health and Care Excellence (2016) *Acute upper gastrointestinal bleeding in over 16s: management*. Clinical guideline (CG141). https://www.nice.org.uk/guidance/cg141? unlid=122385053201610212730.

Tripathi DJ, Stanley AJ, Hayes PC. (2015) UK guidelines on the management of variceal haemorrhage in cirrhotic patients. *Gut* 64, 1680–1704. doi: 10.1136/gutjnl-2015-309262.

CHAPTER 39

Lower gastrointestinal bleeding

Nathan Spence

This refers to any bleeding into the gastrointestinal (GI) tract that occurs distal to the ligament of Treitz. Lower GI bleeding is variable in its presentation, ranging from minor clinical concern to life-threatening emergency. This chapter will provide a comprehensive overview of the key aspects of lower GI bleeding, including its epidemiology, common causes, assessment protocols and management strategies for both unstable and stable cases, along with considerations for patient discharge.

Lower GI bleeding affects a considerable portion of the population, with an incidence of approximately 50 per 100,000 individuals annually and is a common cause of hospital admissions. It accounts for approximately 3% of all emergency surgical referrals in the United Kingdom, and carries a 3% mortality rate. The incidence of lower GI bleeding increases with age, and it is often associated with significant comorbidities, particularly in elderly patients. It is extremely uncommon for such patients to require emergency laparotomy.

The causes of lower GI bleeding are varied, but the most common include:

Diverticulosis: Diverticular disease is the leading cause of significant lower GI bleeding in the United Kingdom, especially in older adults. Diverticula are small pouches that form in the walls of the colon, most typically in the sigmoid colon. Bleeding occurs when a vessel within the diverticulum erodes into the diverticular sac, leading to abrupt, painless, and often massive bleeding. Although bleeding from diverticula usually resolves spontaneously, it can recur and may require intervention in some cases.

Anorectal conditions: Benign anorectal conditions such as haemorrhoids, anal fissures and rectal ulcers are also common causes of lower GI bleeding. Haemorrhoids are swollen veins in the lowest part of the rectum and anus, and their rupture can lead to bright red blood in the stool. While this type of bleeding is usually mild and self-limiting, it can be distressing for patients and may occasionally require treatment.

Angioectasia: Angioectasias are vascular malformations that are often found in the caecum and ascending colon, but can be found throughout the lower GI tract. These abnormal blood vessels are fragile and prone to bleeding, particularly in older patients or those with chronic kidney disease. Angioectasias can cause recurrent, intermittent bleeding that may be difficult to diagnose without specialised imaging or endoscopy.

Colitis: Colitis refers to inflammation of the colon, which can result from various causes, including infectious agents, inflammatory bowel disease (IBD) and ischaemic injury.

Colorectal cancer and polyps: Neoplastic lesions, including colorectal cancer and polyps, are important causes of lower GI bleeding, especially in older adults, but increasingly seen in all age groups. Polyps are benign growths on the inner lining of the colon that can become ulcerated and bleed. Colorectal cancer is a critical diagnosis to consider in patients with unexplained lower GI bleeding.

Acute Medicine: A Practical Guide to the Management of Medical Emergencies, Sixth Edition.
Edited by Mridula Rajwani, Leila Vaziri, and Ivie Gbinigie.
© 2026 John Wiley & Sons Ltd. Published 2026 by John Wiley & Sons Ltd.

Assessment

The initial assessment of a patient presenting with lower GI bleeding is essential in determining severity and, in turn, initial management. The history should focus on the onset, duration and characteristics of the bleeding. Key questions include the colour of the blood (bright red, maroon or dark), the presence of clots, and whether the bleeding is associated with pain or changes in bowel habits.

A past medical history of conditions such as diverticular disease, colorectal cancer or IBD should be elicited. Physical examination should include a thorough abdominal examination and an assessment of the patient's vital signs to identify any signs of hemodynamic instability. The digital rectal examination (DRE) is a simple but crucial part of the initial assessment. It can provide immediate information about the presence and type of blood in the rectum, which can help localise the source of bleeding. All patients should have standard laboratory investigations including an full blood count (FBC), urea and electrolytes (U&Es), liver function tests (LFTs) and clotting studies. A group and save should be urgently sent for crossmatch.

The first determination in patients presenting with lower GI bleeding is establishing any evidence of haemodynamic instability. This can be achieved by calculating the shock index. This is a quick and effective tool for identifying patients who require urgent intervention and more aggressive resuscitation. It is calculated by dividing the heart rate by the systolic blood pressure. A shock index greater than 1 is indicative of hemodynamic instability and suggests that the patient may be at risk for significant blood loss. Such patients are described as unstable and require urgent intervention.

Management

The primary focus of management in unstable patients is resuscitation, monitoring and rapid diagnosis to facilitate timely therapeutic intervention. The initial step is aggressive resuscitation. This involves the administration of intravenous fluids, such as crystalloids, to restore circulating volume and improve tissue perfusion. In cases of significant blood loss, transfusion of packed red blood cells (PRBCs) may be necessary. Clinicians should have a low threshold to activate the major haemorrhage protocol to access an adequate volume of blood products.

Once initial resuscitation is underway, it is critical to identify the source of bleeding as quickly as possible. Computed tomography angiography (CTA) is the preferred diagnostic tool in unstable patients with lower GI bleeding. CTA is a non-invasive imaging modality that can rapidly localise the site of active bleeding, allowing for targeted interventions. In cases where CTA identifies a bleeding source, therapeutic options such as endoscopic therapy or interventional radiology procedures can be immediately considered.

It should be noted that patients who take anticoagulation will need to have it paused or reversed in the context of acute bleeding. This is covered elsewhere in the book.

If the patient is deemed stable enough, therapeutic endoscopy can be performed to control bleeding. Techniques such as clipping, thermal coagulation and injection therapy can be used to achieve haemostasis. Endoscopy also allows for direct visualisation of the bleeding site, which can inform ongoing management decisions. Alternatively, interventional radiology procedures such as embolisation may be employed. Embolisation involves the targeted delivery of materials to occlude the bleeding vessel to stop bleeding. This is particularly useful in cases where the bleeding site is inaccessible or where surgical intervention is not an option due to anaesthetic risk.

As stated earlier, patients should only be considered for emergency surgery if all endoscopic and radiological management options have been exhausted.

Finally, in unstable patients, it is essential to consider the possibility of an upper GI source. Up to 11–15% of patients initially suspected to have lower GI bleeding are eventually found to have an upper GI source. This is especially true in cases where the patient presents with hemodynamic instability, as brisk upper GI bleeding can manifest with significant fresh PR bleeding. A patient with a known history of peptic ulcer disease, cirrhosis or oesophageal varices are at higher risk for upper GI bleeding. Clinicians should also pay close attention to serum urea. This laboratory finding is often associated with upper GI bleeding, where the digestion and absorption of blood lead to an increase in urea production. All patients with unstable GI bleeding should be considered for oesophago-gastroduodenoscopy (OGD) after initial resuscitation.

Stable lower GI bleeding is characterised by hemodynamic stability. In these cases, the bleeding is often less severe and allows for a more measured approach to diagnosis and management. The focus in stable bleeding is on accurately diagnosing the source of the bleeding and selecting the appropriate therapeutic interventions, while also considering the potential for outpatient management.

Patients who are assessed as stable still may have experienced significant blood loss and need red cell transfusion. Restrictive transfusions targets should be used to reduce the risk of transfusion-related complications, such as transfusion-associated circulatory overload (TACO) and transfusion-related acute lung injury (TRALI). Red cell transfusion should be offered to patients with a Hb of <70 g/L with a target of 70–90 g/L. Special consideration should be given to patients with a history of cardiovascular disease. These patients warrant a more relaxed transfusion target of 80 g/L and a target of 100 g/L.

Inpatient versus outpatient management

A key consideration in patients with stable bleeding is whether they can be managed as an outpatient or whether they warrant hospital admission. The Oakland score (Table 39.1) is a validated risk stratification tool specifically designed to risk-stratify patients with lower GI bleeding. It is calculated based on seven variables: age, gender, previous admission for lower GI bleeding, findings on DRE, heart rate, systolic blood pressure and haemoglobin levels.

Using the Oakland score, patients can be split into two groups – those having 'minor' bleeds and those having 'major' bleeds (Table 39.2).

Minor bleeding can be considered as suitable for outpatient management and investigation. Although the timing of this can be decided based on local availability, it should be noted that of patients presenting with lower GI bleed, 6% will eventually be found to have colorectal cancer. For this reason, patients should strongly be considered for "urgent outpatient colonoscopy".

Major bleeding should be managed with inpatient admission to allow for close observation and expedited management. These patients should have urgent inpatient endoscopy. The choice of colonoscopy versus sigmoidoscopy will be based on suspected underlying diagnosis and local hospital availability. There is no good evidence to recommend the timing of endoscopy – good bowel preparation significantly improves diagnostic yield so this should be a priority. There is limited evidence to suggest the benefit of 'immediate' colonoscopy – it is generally considered that the 'next available list' is appropriate. If a bleeding lesion is detected on endoscopy, then it can be readily treated.

Patients who undergo endoscopy during which no bleeding point or lesion is seen warrant a trial of observation. If there is no further bleeding observed then patients can be discharged with outpatient follow-up. Clinical teams may wish to repeat endoscopy after discharge to ensure no lesions were missed on the initial attempt. Those patients that do not stop bleeding will need specialist discussion with gastroenterology with regards to second-line investigations such as capsule endoscopy or labelled red cell scanning.

An important caveat to the above approach is patients presenting with post-polypectomy bleeding. Given that the likely diagnosis is already known, colonoscopy should be the first step in diagnosis and treatment rather than CT angiography.

Table 39.1 The Oakland score.

Criteria	Score
Age	
<40	0
40–69	1
≥70	2
Gender	
Female	0
Male	1
Previous lower gastrointestinal bleeding (LGIB) admission	
No	0
Yes	1
DRE findings	
Blood	0
No blood	1
Heart rate (bpm)	
<70	0
70–89	1
90–109	2
≥110	3
Systolic BP (mmHg)	
≥160	0
130–159	2
120–129	3
90–119	4
<90	5
Hb (g/L)	
≥160	0
130–159	4
110–129	8
90–109	13
70–89	17
<70	22

Table 39.2 Factors to help differentiate minor and major bleeding.

Minor bleeding	Major bleeding
Oakland score ≤ 8	Oakland score > 8
Self-limiting bleeding	Ongoing bleeding
No co-morbidities	Significant cardiovascular co-morbidities

Further reading

Gerson LB, Fidler JL, Cave DR, Leighton JA. (2015) ACG clinical guideline: diagnosis and management of small bowel bleeding. *Am J Gastroenterol* 110(9), 1265–1287. doi: 10.1038/ajg.2015.246.

Oakland K, Chadwick G, East JE, *et al.* (2019) Diagnosis and management of acute lower gastrointestinal bleeding: guidelines from the British Society of Gastroenterology. *Gut* 68(5), 776–789. doi: 10.1136/gutjnl-2018-317807.

Oakland K, Desborough MJ, Murphy MF, *et al.* (2019) Rebleeding and mortality after lower gastrointestinal bleeding in patients taking antiplatelets or anticoagulants. *Clin Gastroenterol Hepatol* 17(7), 1276–1284. e3. doi: 10.1016/j.cgh.2017.12.032.

Olaussen A, Blackburn T, Mitra B, Fitzgerald M. (2014) Review article: shock index for prediction of critical bleeding post-trauma: a systematic review. *Emerg Med Australas* 26(3), 223–228. doi: 10.1111/1742-6723.12232.

CHAPTER 40

Inflammatory bowel disease

GRACE BARNES AND ARIF HUSSENBUX

Introduction to IBD

Inflammatory bowel disease (IBD) is a chronic, inflammatory condition affecting the gastrointestinal (GI) tract. The prevalence of IBD has increased over time, with 1 in 200 individuals diagnosed in Western countries. IBD is classified into two principal forms; Crohn's disease (CD) and ulcerative colitis (UC). At a minimum, the diagnosis of UC or CD is based on a combination of clinical, biochemical, endoscopic and histological investigations. Key features are summarised in Table 40.1.

IBD can present as an indolent disease, or more acutely with a flare. Its symptom burden and degree of inflammation can vary between patients, and over the lifetime of an affected individual.

Consider investigating for IBD in any patient presenting with at least a six-week history of the following symptoms:

- Abdominal pain, especially if localised to the right lower quadrant
- Change in bowel habit (typically diarrhoea with or without bleeding)

Table 40.1 Key features of IBD.

	Crohn's disease	**Ulcerative colitis**
Area of GI tract affected	Mouth to anus, but most commonly affects the terminal ileum and proximal colon. Upper GI tract more commonly affected in paediatric population.	Rectum, colon and terminal ileum (rarely).
Clinical features	Abdominal pain, weight loss, non-bloody diarrhoea, fever. Extra-intestinal manifestations of IBD.	Bloody diarrhoea (greater than 6 weeks). Extra-intestinal manifestations of IBD.
Radiological appearances	Abscess, fistula or stricture formation. Skip lesions/wall thickening affecting the GI tract.	Colitis. In severe disease, toxic megacolon.
Endoscopic appearances	Skip lesions. Cobblestone appearances. Serpiginous ulceration.	Continuous inflammation starting at the rectum, extending proximally. Loss of vascular pattern. Superficial erosions and ulceration.
Mucosal involvement	Transmural inflammation.	Mucosal inflammation only.
Histopathological features	Granuloma formation. Crypt abscess formation. Fissuring ulceration.	Active chronic colitis limited to the mucosa. Crypt atrophy. Lack of granuloma or fissuring ulcers.

Initial investigations for IBD include:

- Blood tests including full blood count, C-reactive protein and albumin
- Faecal calprotectin
- Stool culture and *Clostridium difficile* toxin assay
- Direct visualisation via ileocolonoscopy with biopsy

Patients with IBD should be referred to a gastroenterologist for specialist input within 4 weeks of a suspected IBD diagnosis.

Recognition of IBD flare

Patients with IBD (either known or new diagnosis) can also present acutely with a flare in their underlying disease.

Consider an IBD flare as a differential in a patient presenting with:

- Diarrhoea (in particular, bloody diarrhoea) – see also Chapter 34
- Abdominal pain – see also Chapter 32
- Systemic upset (fever and tachycardia)

To diagnose an acute flare in IBD, a focused history, examination and appropriate investigations should be performed.

Important differentials to consider

- Infective diarrhoea
  - More likely if acute presentation, recent travel or unwell contacts
  - Infection *must* be excluded prior to consideration of immunosuppression
- Ischaemic colitis
  - More likely in patients with atrial fibrillation and/or peripheral vascular disease
- Diverticular disease
  - Acute diverticulitis classically presents with left lower quadrant abdominal pain, fever and raised white cell count
- Malignancy
  - Should be considered for any adult presenting with a change in bowel habit
- Pancreatitis

Focused history – key questions to include

- Onset and duration of symptoms
- Any precipitating factors (including dietary triggers) or unwell contacts
  - Helping to exclude an infective cause
- Frequency, volume and consistency of stool, including presence of blood or mucus
- Nocturnal symptoms
- Evidence of urgency or tenesmus
- Associated pain (and relation to defecation)
- Extra-intestinal manifestations
  - New rash, joint pain, visual symptoms and/or oral ulceration
- Family history
- Smoking history

Focused examination – key signs to elicit

- Physiological observations – in particular, check temperature and heart rate
- Nutritional status
  - Is there evidence to suggest malabsorption?
- Extra-intestinal manifestations
  - Arthritis, uveitis/iritis, pyoderma gangrenosum or erythema nodosum
- Abdomen
  - Scars, masses, bowel sounds or guarding/peritonism
- Perianal/rectal examination
  - Is there perianal disease?
  - Is there any alternate cause for blood in stool (i.e. haemorrhoid or anal fissure)?

Key investigations

- Full blood count (FBC)
  - Haemoglobin – is there evidence of anaemia?
  - White cell count – could be elevated with infection, IBD flare or steroids.
  Consider neutropaenia if already on immunomodulator therapy and unwell.
- Urea and electrolytes (U&Es)
  - Creatinine – is there evidence of renal impairment secondary to fluid loss?
  - Electrolytes – is there derangement with high GI tract losses?
- C-reactive protein (CRP)
  - Is there evidence of an underlying inflammatory process?
- Albumin
  - A reduced albumin may be associated with increased disease activity.
- Amylase
  - Rule out pancreatitis – even if known IBD, as treatment may have led to secondary pancreatitis (e.g. recent steroid course).
- ECG
  - Is there atrial fibrillation? (If so, consider ischaemic colitis.)
- Stool culture (including *Clostridium difficile* toxin)
  - Need to exclude infection before considering immunosuppression – even if known IBD, superadded infection can precipitate a flare.
- Abdominal x-ray (AXR)
  - Is there evidence of dilated bowel loops/toxic megacolon (defined as total or segmental non-obstructive dilatation of the colon ≥5.5 cm)?
- Erect chest x-ray (CXR)
  - Is there an intercurrent chest infection?
  - Is there free air under the diaphragm, raising concern of perforation?
- Consider computed tomography (CT) imaging
  - May need to proceed to CT if differential includes surgical pathology, or concern about obstruction.
  - Be mindful that IBD diagnosis can mean high lifetime exposure to radiation with serial scans/imaging, and therefore consider radiation risk.

If an IBD flare is suspected, please refer to the gastroenterology team/IBD team for review.

Immediate management of IBD flare in inpatient

1 Establish a stool chart
  - Patients can often keep a record themselves – give paper at the bedside
  - Summarise as number of bowel motions in 24 h period +/- presence of blood, consistency and volume.

2 Prescribe venous thromboembolism (VTE) prophylaxis
  - Even in the presence of bloody diarrhoea if the patient remains haemodynamically stable – IBD is associated with an increased VTE risk.

3 Prescribe steroid
  - IV hydrocortisone 100 mg every 6 h (IV preferred over PO, as there will be poor enteral absorption in acute flare). Early gastroenterology involvement is required if systemic corticosteroids are being considered.
  - This can be started with clinical suspicion of an acute flare, even whilst stool samples are pending.

4 Prescribe IV fluid
  - Likely significant GI losses leading to dehydration if opening bowels >6 times per day.
  - Replace electrolytes intravenously, especially potassium.

5 Discontinue opioids, non-steroidal anti-inflammatory drugs (NSAIDs) and anti-diarrhoeal agents
  - Likely to worsen symptoms.

6 Endoscopic evaluation of severity if no features of obstruction
  - Tissue biopsies taken during endoscopy, to confirm underlying pathology and presences of inflammation.

7 Refer to dietetics team for nutritional support
  - May require supplementation with nasogastric feeding, or dietary modification.

8 Assess response to therapy at 72 h

If there is an appropriate response to therapy:
- Consider stepping down to oral steroid therapy (e.g. Prednisolone 40 mg OD)
  - Will need a weaning course for steroid treatment on discharge.
  - Remember to always cover with proton pump inhibitor (PPI) and bone protection.
  - Ensure the patient has appropriate gastroenterology follow-up.
- Consider long-term agent for disease control
  - See below for specific therapies for Crohn's and UC.

If there is no response/limited response to steroid therapy:
- Consider repeat investigation (e.g. repeat AXR and CT scan).
- Consider rescue therapy (biologic agent such as infliximab or ciclosporin).
  - Choice of agent guided by gastroenterology team.
- Early referral to surgical team

Ulcerative colitis – further management (Figure 40.1)

Severe colitis fulfils the Truelove and Witts criteria, including bloody stool frequency of ≥ 6 per day and any of:
- Tachycardia (>90 beats/min)
- Temperature (>37.8)
- Anaemia (haemoglobin < 10.5 g/dL)
- C-reactive protein (CRP) or erythrocyte sedimentation rate (ESR) > 30

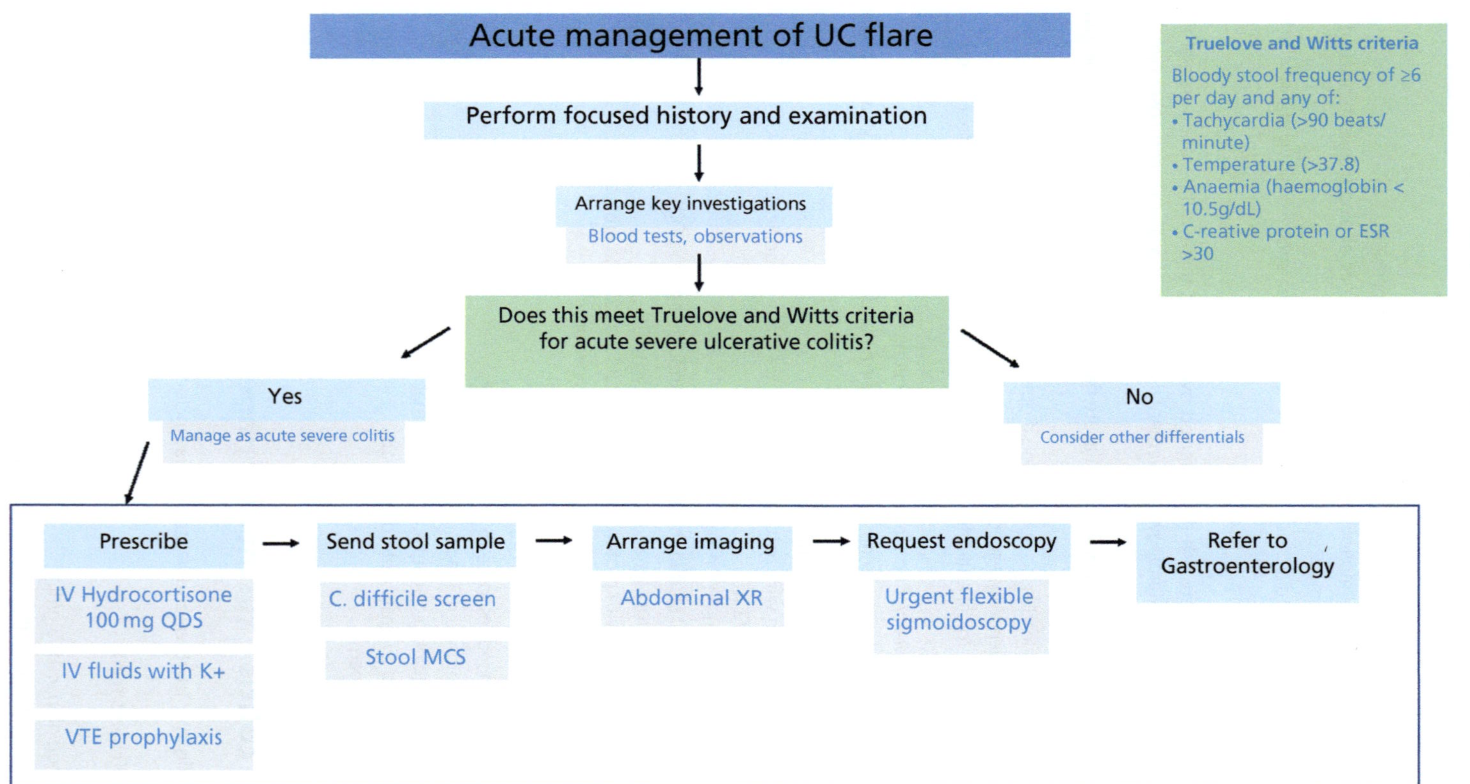

Figure 40.1 Acute management of UC flare.

An urgent flexible sigmoidoscopy should be requested to grade the severity of disease. Response to therapy should be assessed at 72 h following initiation of intravenous steroids.

For UC, this can be done using the Travis criteria:

- Frequency of stools
  - <6 stools per day indicates appropriate response.
- C-reactive protein (CRP) level
  - <45 indicates appropriate response.
- Systemic features
  - Resolution of pyrexia and tachycardia indicates appropriate response.

There is no evidence that prolonged intravenous steroids are helpful. For patients who meet the Travis criteria, second-line therapy should be considered. This includes infliximab, ciclosporin or a referral for a sub-total colectomy with ileostomy formation.

Following treatment of an acute flare, patients with UC should be considered for long-term therapy.

Drug therapy in ulcerative colitis

Initial management of mild to moderate active UC should be managed with oral and/or topical 5-aminosalicylic acid (5-ASA), depending on the extent of disease. Renal function should be monitored. If there is limited response, consider a course of oral corticosteroid (prednisolone, or budesonide if systemic effects of steroids need to be minimised). If 5-ASA therapy fails, or multiple steroid courses have been prescribed within a year, then escalation of a steroid sparing agent is indicated. Options that can be considered by the gastroenterology team include:

- Thiopurines – e.g. azathioprine and 6-mercaptopurine
- Anti-tumour necrosis factor (anti-TNF) therapy – e.g. infliximab and adalimumab
- Anti-integrin therapy – e.g. vedolizumab
- Janus kinase (JAK) inhibitor – e.g. tofacitinib

Surgery in ulcerative colitis

As UC is restricted to the colon, a sub-total colectomy is a curative procedure for these patients. This results in stoma formation (end ileostomy); an ileo-rectal anastomosis can be considered at a later date. Surgical resection is often reserved for patients who have failed to achieve disease control with pharmacological therapies. It is also vitally important that the diagnosis of UC is correct, as surgical resection is not curative if there is CD or an alternative diagnosis.

Crohn's disease – further management (Figure 40.2)

As CD is a lifelong disease, therapy aims to induce remission in the short term and maintain remission in the long term. In patients with active, moderate to severe CD, systemic corticosteroids should be prescribed. Early gastroenterology involvement is required for consideration of biological therapy and appropriate multi-disciplinary team (MDT) discussion.

Investigations for CD also include dedicated imaging of the small bowel, as this is not amenable to direct endoscopic evaluation. This includes considering capsule endoscopy, or magnetic resonance imaging (MRI) enterography – both typically performed as an outpatient study.

Drug therapy in Crohn's disease

Initial management of mild to moderate CD can be non-pharmacological, via an exclusive enteral nutrition (EEN) diet. Early dietitian involvement is crucial as compliance can be challenging due to EEN being an exclusive liquid diet. For mild to moderate disease limited to the ileum and ascending colon, budesonide can be

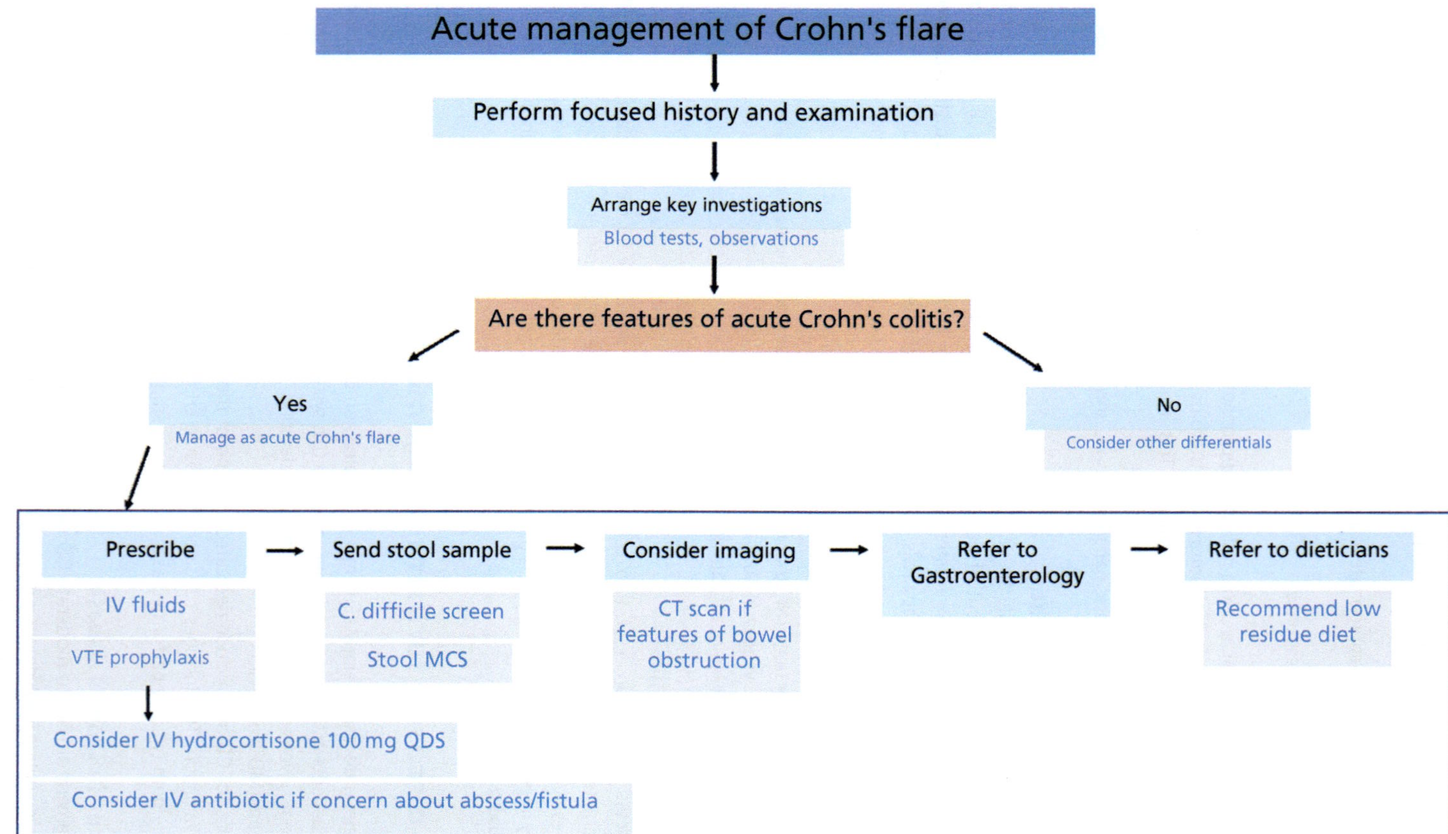

Figure 40.2 Acute management of Crohn's disease flare.

considered. 5-ASA therapy is not effective in CD. Patient should be established on a steroid-sparing agent early in their management. Options that can be considered by the gastroenterology team include:

- Immunomodulator therapy – e.g. azathioprine and 6-mercaptopurine
- Anti-TNF therapy – e.g. infliximab and adalimumab
- Anti-integrin therapy – e.g. vedolizumab
- JAK inhibitor – e.g. tofacitinib

Surgery in Crohn's disease

As CD can affect the entire length of the GI tract, there are no curative surgical options. A specialist MDT approach is mandatory for these patients. Fistulating disease, stricturing, abscess formation and peri-anal disease require early surgical involvement. Multiple small bowel resections can lead to short bowel syndrome and subsequent intestinal failure.

Further reading

BSG consensus guidelines on management of IBD. https://gut.bmj.com/content/68/Suppl_3/s1.

Nature Reviews Disease Primers – Crohn's disease. https://www.nature.com/articles/s41572-020-0156-2#citeas.

Nature Reviews Disease Primers – Ulcerative colitis. https://www.nature.com/articles/s41572-020-0205-x.

Ng SC, Shi HY, Hamidi N, *et al.* (2017) Worldwide incidence and prevalence of inflammatory bowel disease in the 21st century: a systematic review of population-based studies. *Lancet* 390, 2769–2778. https://www.sciencedirect.com/science/article/pii/S0140673617324480?via%3Dihub.

NICE guidelines on the management of IBD. https://www.nice.org.uk/guidance/qs81/chapter/ Quality-statement-1-Specialist-assessment.

CHAPTER 41

Alcohol-related liver disease and acute medical complications

BEN WARNER AND LYNN AFFARAH

Alcohol-related liver disease (ARLD) refers to a spectrum of liver pathology caused by alcohol excess, which ranges from steatosis (alcoholic fatty liver), steatohepatitis (alcohol hepatitis), progressive fibrosis and cirrhosis, and eventually the development of hepatocellular cancer (HCC).

Common presentations of ARLD in the emergency department include decompensated ARLD cirrhosis (see Chapter 42) and alcohol hepatitis, which when severe, is the most florid form of ARLD and can be life-threatening.

Alcoholic hepatitis is characterized by

- A recent history of heavy alcohol use (within three months of presentation) (see Table 41.4).
- Progressive jaundice, with or without other signs of liver decompensation (ascites and/or encephalopathy)
- An AST: ALT ratio of ≥2, which is rarely seen in other forms of liver disease
- In its severe forms, it can cause prolonged prothrombin time, hypoalbuminaemia and thrombocytopaenia
- See Table 41.1

Seek urgent advice from a hepatologist or gastroenterologist if you suspect alcoholic hepatitis.

The mainstay of treatment is supportive (see Table 41.2): treating infection (which is the leading cause of mortality in this patient group), managing alcohol withdrawal and optimising nutrition.

Steroid therapy may be indicated in patients with severe alcoholic hepatitis (DF > 32, see Table 41.1), but its role remains controversial due to the increased risk of infection and gastrointestinal bleeding. This should only be commenced by or following discussion with a consultant hepatologist.

Table 41.1 Alcoholic hepatitis: diagnosis.

Clinical features and blood results

- Jaundice
- Prolonged history of alcohol excess (within three months)
- Stigmata of chronic liver disease may be present
- Fever
- Tender hepatomegaly and a hepatic bruit
- Ascites
- Raised white cell count (may be >20×10^9/L) and C-reactive protein
- Prothrombin time prolonged >5 s over control
- Mildly raised AST and ALT (typically 2–3 times level of normal, AST: ALT ratio of ≥2; increases of >10 times suggests viral hepatitis or drug toxicity)
- Raised gamma-glutamyl transpeptidase and serum IgA
- Raised bilirubin

Acute Medicine: A Practical Guide to the Management of Medical Emergencies, Sixth Edition.
Edited by Mridula Rajwani, Leila Vaziri, and Ivie Gbinigie.
© 2026 John Wiley & Sons Ltd. Published 2026 by John Wiley & Sons Ltd.

Table 41.1 (*Continued*)

- Raised ferritin (often > 1000 micrograms/L)
- Low sodium, low potassium, low urea, variable creatinine, low haemoglobin, high MCV, low platelet count

Identification of clinically severe alcoholic hepatitis
- An index of severity ('discriminant function', DF) can be calculated: DF = ([patient's prothrombin time − control] × 4.6) + (bilirubin (μmol/L) ÷ 17.1)
- A DF of > 32 identifies patients with severe alcoholic hepatitis (mortality ~50%) who may need intensive care and who may benefit from corticosteroids in the absence of sepsis or other contraindications to steroids.

ALT, alanine aminotransferase; AST, aspartate aminotransferase; IgA, immunoglobulin A; MCV, mean corpuscular volume.

Table 41.2 Alcoholic hepatitis: management.

- Seek advice from a gastroenterologist/hepatologist
- Avoid diuretics and ensure adequate volume replacement (use 4.5% human albumin solution and/or salt-poor albumin; avoid normal saline)
- Supportive management of alcohol withdrawal
- Optimise nutrition with a low threshold for starting nasogastric feeding, aiming for 35–40 kcal/kg of body weight per day
- Give oral/IV thiamine
- Start broad-spectrum antibiotics after taking cultures of blood, urine and ascites
- Check renal function and prothrombin time daily until there is a consistent improvement
- A full liver screen must be done to exclude other causes of hepatitis
- Give thromboprophylaxis if there are no signs of bleeding and platelet count is >50 × 10^9/L
- Consider early transjugular liver biopsy
- Corticosteroid therapy in patients with DF >32 (prednisolone 40 mg daily for 28 days, with gastroprotection and bone protection) should be considered by a Gastroenterologist or Hepatologist

DF, discriminant function (see Table 41.1).

Other alcohol-related problems presenting acutely

Common acute medical issues in patients who consume alcohol heavily (Table 41.3) include the importance of taking a thorough alcohol history (Table 41.4) as well as the management of alcohol withdrawal syndrome and Wernicke's encephalopathy (Table 41.5) outlined below:

Table 41.3 Common acute medical problems in the patient who drinks heavily.

System	Problems
Neuropsychiatric	Alcohol withdrawal syndrome
	Major seizures related to alcohol withdrawal Wernicke encephalopathy (thiamine deficiency)
	Polyneuropathy
	Depression/anxiety Self-poisoning
Respiratory	Pneumonia (including aspiration pneumonia)
	Smoking-related disorders (~80% of patients with alcohol dependence smoke)
Cardiovascular	Acute atrial fibrillation
	Alcoholic cardiomyopathy
Liver and pancreas	Alcoholic hepatitis
	Acute pancreatitis
	Cirrhosis
	Decompensated chronic liver disease

(*continued*)

Table 41.3 (*Continued*)

System	Problems
Alimentary tract	Variceal bleeding
	Alcoholic gastritis
	Poor diet with consequent vitamin deficiencies
Musculoskeletal	Myopathy
	Fractures
Haematological	Macrocytosis
	Anaemia
	Thrombocytopenia
	Leucopenia

Table 41.4 Taking an alcohol history.

Information needed	Questions to ask
Average weekly alcohol consumption and pattern of drinking • One unit of alcohol equals 10 mL by volume (8 g by weight) of pure alcohol. • The percentage alcohol by volume (abv) of any drink equals the number of units in 1 L of that drink (e.g. a bottle (750 mL) of wine (12% abv) contains 9 units). • Higher-risk drinking is defined as regularly consuming >50 units/week for men and >35 units/week for women.	Do you ever drink alcohol? What do you usually drink? How many times each week do you drink? How much do you have on these occasions? Are there times when you drink more heavily than this?
Is there alcohol dependence?	Do you drink every day? What time of day is your first drink? If you do not drink for a day or miss your first drink of the day, how do you feel? How would you rate alcohol as one of your priorities? Is it sometimes hard to think of anything else? Have you ever needed medication to stop drinking?
Has alcohol caused medical, psychiatric or social problems?	Has alcohol ever caused you any problems in the past? What were these? Has anyone close to you expressed worries about your drinking? Did this cause difficulties between you? Are you concerned about your alcohol use? Has alcohol ever affected your work or ability to sort things out at home? Has alcohol ever got you into trouble with the police (e.g. drinkdriving offence)? Is your alcohol use leaving you short of money?

Source: McIntosh C, Chick J (2004) Alcohol and the nervous system. *J Neurol Neurosurg Psych* 75 (III), 16–21. Reproduced with permission of BMJ Publishing Group Ltd.

Table 41.5 Management of alcohol withdrawal syndrome and Wernicke encephalopathy.

Problem	Features	Management
Alcohol withdrawal syndrome	Signs of autonomic hyperactivity (appear within hours of the last drink, usually peaking within 24–48 h): tremor, sweating, nausea, vomiting, anxiety, agitation Alcohol withdrawal delirium (delirium tremens): acute confusional state, auditory and visual hallucinations, marked autonomic hyperactivity Delirium tremens may be complicated by hyperthermia, hypovolaemia, electrolyte derangement and respiratory infection	Manage severe alcohol withdrawal syndrome on the high-dependency unit General supportive measures: fluid replacement if needed; exclusion of hypoglycaemia; treatment of intercurrent illness (e.g. pneumonia, alcoholic hepatitis); vitamin supplements (vitamin B compound, strong, two tablets daily, thiamine 100 mg 12 hourly PO, and vitamin C 50 mg 12-hourly PO) Mild or moderate withdrawal symptoms: treat with reducing doses of oral chlordiazepoxide Severe withdrawal symptoms: treat initially with IV lorazepam (monitor respiratory rate and oxygen saturation)

Table 41.5 (*Continued*)

Problem	Features	Management
Seizures related to alcohol withdrawal	One to six tonic-clonic seizures without focal features which begin within 48 h of stopping drinking May occur up to seven days after stopping drinking if the patient has been taking benzodiazepines	Usually brief and self-limiting and do not require specific treatment. Consider lorazepam to reduce the risk of further seizures. If frequent or prolonged, manage as status epilepticus (Chapter 57). Avoid phenytoin. Exclude/treat hypoglycaemia
Wernicke encephalopathy	Confusional state Nystagmus VI nerve palsy (unable to abduct the eye) Ataxia with wide-based gait; may be unable to stand or walk	Treat with IV thiamine (Pabrinex IV highpotency injection, containing thiamine 250 mg per 10 mL (two ampoules): two pairs of ampoules 8-hourly for two days, then one pair daily for five days, followed by oral thiamine. IV Pabrinex should be given by infusion over 30 min; may cause anaphylaxis.

Further reading

Connon JP, Haber PS, Hall WD. (2016) Alcohol use disorders. *Lancet* 387, 988–998.

Simpson SA, Wilson MP, Nordstrom K (2016) Psychiatric emergencies for clinicians: emergency Department management of alcohol withdrawal.

Thursz M, Morgan TR. (2016) Treatment of severe alcoholic hepatitis. *Gastroenterology* 150, 1823–1834.

CHAPTER 42

Acute liver failure and decompensated chronic liver disease

BEN WARNER AND LYNN AFFARAH

Liver failure

The term liver failure is applied to two distinct syndromes: acute liver failure (ALF) and decompensated chronic liver disease. Management of suspected liver failure is summarised in Figure 42.1.

ALF is defined as severe acute liver injury (ALI) with encephalopathy and impaired liver synthetic function (international normalised ratio $\geq$1.5) in the absence of pre-existing liver disease; an illness duration of <26 weeks distinguishes acute from chronic liver failure. ALF has an annual incidence of around 5 per million in the United Kingdom. Causes are given in Table 42.1.

Decompensated chronic liver disease (acute on chronic liver failure) is defined as a syndrome in patients with chronic liver disease, with or without previously diagnosed cirrhosis, characterised by acute hepatic decompensation resulting in liver failure (jaundice and prolongation of the prothrombin time/international normalised ratio), and one or more extrahepatic organ failures. Management is focused on identification and treatment of the precipitant(s) (Table 42.6) while providing supportive care.

Acute liver failure

Consider ALI in any patient with liver damage (serum aminotransferases 2–3× upper limit of normal) and impaired liver function with jaundice and/or coagulopathy. The development of hepatic encephalopathy with/after ALI is suggestive of ALF. Particular aetiologies favour ALF (e.g. paracetamol toxicity). Common causes for ALF are shown in Table 42.1.

The prognosis of ALF is related to the time taken for encephalopathy to develop and the aetiology. Hyperacute liver failure (the development of encephalopathy <7 days after jaundice) is associated with a better prognosis than ALF (jaundice to encephalopathy between 8 and 28 days) and sub-ALF (jaundice to encephalopathy in 4–12 weeks). Aetiologies with the worst prognosis include non-A, non-B causes for ALF, while paracetamol toxicity and pregnancy-related syndromes have the most favourable outcomes.

Priorities

If you suspect ALF:

1 Check the blood glucose, as hypoglycaemia is a common complication.
   - If <4.0 mmol/L, give 100 mL of 20% glucose or 200 mL of 10% glucose over 15–30 min IV. Recheck blood glucose after 10 min, if still <4.0 mmol/L, repeat the above IV glucose treatment.

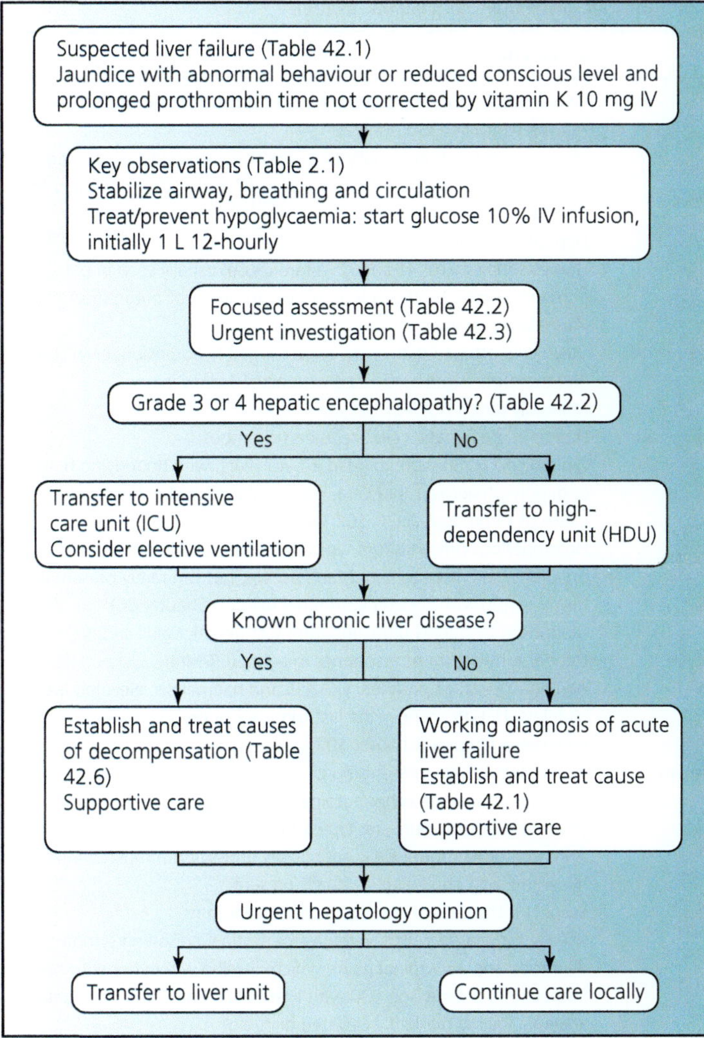

Figure 42.1 Management of suspected acute liver failure.

- Start an IV infusion of 10% glucose, initially 1 L/12 h, to prevent hypoglycaemia; use a large peripheral vein as it can cause thrombophlebitis.

2 Make a focused clinical assessment (Table 42.2), including a detailed drug history (including any herbal and over-the-counter medications) from the patient or family members, and arrange urgent investigations (Table 42.3).

3 Start N-acetylcysteine (NAC) without delay using the standard regimen (Chapter 8) even in non-paracetamol poisoning, as it can be hepato-protective.

4 If there is grade 3 or 4 encephalopathy, transfer the patient to an ICU for elective intubation and ventilation. Other patients with ALF should be nursed in a high-dependency unit.

5 Obtain advice on management from a hepatologist or your regional liver unit, with the investigation results to hand when you make the phone call.

Table 42.1 Causes of acute liver failure (fulminant hepatic failure).

Cause	Comment
Drug-related	Paracetamol poisoning is the commonest cause of ALF in the United Kingdom; AST/ALT are typically >3500 units/L
	Idiosyncratic reaction (usually occurs within six months of starting drug); many drugs implicated, including Co-Amoxiclav, Flucloxacillin, chemotherapy agents, statins, phenytoin, carbamazepine
Viral hepatitis	Hepatitis A, B or E virus
	Herpes simplex virus -1 and -2 (a rare cause; usually seen in patients taking immunosuppressive therapy or in third trimester of pregnancy)
	Varicella zoster virus
Ischaemic hepatitis ('shock liver')	May occur after cardiac arrest or prolonged hypotension, or in severe heart failure, and therefore often associated with acute kidney injury
	Markedly raised AST/ALT
Acute Budd-Chiari syndrome	Due to acute hepatic vein occlusion (thrombosis)
	Typically occurs in women aged 20–40 years, with underlying haematological disorder (e.g. polycythaemia rubra vera, paroxysmal nocturnal haemoglobinuria) or other cause of thrombophilia (P. 567 Table 100.6)
	Heterogenous presentation: typically presents in a more chronic form with right upper quadrant pain, hepatomegaly and ascites, but can rarely present with fulminant liver failure (often with concomitant renal failure) (Chapter 86)
	Diagnosed by duplex ultrasonography of hepatic veins and IVC or computed tomography/magnetic resonance imaging (CT/MRI)
Pregnancy-related	Acute fatty liver of pregnancy (AFLP) and haemolysis, elevated liver enzymes, low platelets (HELLP) occur in the last trimester of pregnancy and are often associated with pre-eclampsia (Chapter 103)
Autoimmune hepatitis (AIH)	About 25% of AIH presentations occur acutely/sub-acutely
	Consider if there are other autoimmune disorders (e.g. haemolytic anaemia, idiopathic thrombocytopenic purpura, type 1 diabetes, thyroiditis, coeliac disease)
	Autoantibodies (antinuclear antibodies, anti-smooth muscle antibodies) and hypergammaglobulinaemia usually present
***Amanita phalloides* poisoning**	Suspect if the patient has eaten wild mushrooms
	Usually associated with severe gastrointestinal poisoning symptoms (nausea, vomiting, diarrhoea and abdominal pain), which develop within hours to one day of ingestion
Wilson disease	Suspect in a patient age <30 with liver failure and Coombs-negative haemolytic anaemia (giving markedly elevated bilirubin)
	Kayser-Fleischer rings are present in ~50%
	Serum ceruloplasmin is typically low (but may be normal in ~15% and is often reduced in other forms of ALF) and serum/urinary copper levels high
	Alkaline phosphatase and urate are low
Malignant infiltration	May occur in breast cancer, small cell lung cancer, lymphoma and melanoma
	Associated with hepatomegaly
	Diagnosis made by imaging and biopsy
	Consider haemophagocytic lymphohistiocytosis (HLH) in lymphoma
Cause unclear	Retake the drug history
	Consider transjugular liver biopsy

ALF, acute liver failure; ALT, alanine aminotransferase; AST, aspartate aminotransferase; IVC, inferior vena cava.

Determining the cause of ALF (Table 42.1)

- In the United Kingdom, paracetamol poisoning causes around 50% of ALF, and viral hepatitis around 40%. The mortality of patients with paracetamol poisoning who reach medical attention is 0.4%. Where ALF occurs due to viral hepatitis, mortality is around 40% and 60% due to non-A, non-B viral hepatitis.

Table 42.2 Focused assessment of the patient with possible acute liver failure.

History

Duration and time course of jaundice and other symptoms (e.g. fever and abdominal pain)

Known liver or biliary tract disease?

Full drug history: including all non-prescription drugs, herbal remedies, dietary supplements, mushroom ingestion or khat, taken over the past year

Risk factors for viral hepatitis (foreign travel, IV drug use, men who have sex with men, multiple sexual partners, body piercing and tattoos, blood transfusion and blood products and needle-stick injury in health-care worker)?

History of depression, previous drug overdoses or previous attempts of suicide

Pregnancy?

Usual and recent alcohol intake?

History of substance misuse or recreational drugs

Other medical problems (e.g. cardiovascular disease, transplant recipient, cancer, human immunodeficiency virus/ acquired immunodeficiency syndrome (HIV/AIDS) and haematological disease)?

Family history of jaundice/liver disease?

Examination

Physiological observations and systematic examination

Conscious level and mental state; grade of encephalopathy if present:

Grading of hepatic encephalopathy	
Grade	**Clinical features**
Subclinical	Impaired work, personality change, sleep disturbance
	Abnormal findings on psychomotor testing
Grade 1	Mild confusion, agitation, apathy, oriented in time and place
	Fine tremor, asterixis
Grade 2 Grade 3	Drowsiness, lethargy, disoriented in time Asterixis, dysarthria
	Sleepy but rousable, disoriented in time and place
	Hyperreflexia, hyperventilation
Grade 4	Responsive only to painful stimuli or unresponsive

Asterixis? Ask the patient to hold the arms outstretched with the wrists extended and fingers spread apart, and eyes closed, for 30 s or longer. The sign is positive if after a brief latent period, there is a sudden lapse of maintenance of the posture.

Hepatic foetor?

Signs of chronic liver disease?

Right upper quadrant tenderness?

Liver enlargement (seen in early viral hepatitis, alcoholic hepatitis, malignant infiltration, congestive heart failure and acute Budd–Chiari syndrome)?

Splenomegaly?

Ascites (Chapter 36)?

- Consider mushroom (*Amanita phalloides*) poisoning in patients with a compatible history; severe nausea, vomiting, diarrhoea and abdominal pain develop within hours to one day of ingestion. Penicillin G 300,000 units/kg/day and milk thistle (silibinin) 30–40 mg/kg/day PO or IV are recognised treatments.

- Wilson's disease and autoimmune hepatitis, although both forms of chronic liver disease, can be treated as if they are ALF. Wilson's classically presents with Coombs-negative haemolytic anaemia and a high bilirubin to ALP ratio. The diagnosis is confirmed by high urinary copper levels. Treatment aims to lower serum copper levels via haemofiltration. Penicillamine is not recommended acutely. Autoimmune hepatitis should be treated with 40–60 mg prednisolone PO per day.

- The presence of a nodular liver on imaging in a patient suspected of having ALF does not necessarily indicate that the patient has pre-existing cirrhosis. Nodularity can occur with benign conditions. As the severity of

Table 42.3 Urgent investigation in suspected acute liver failure.

Needed urgently

Arterial blood gases, pH, lactate

Blood glucose

Prothrombin time (PT)/international normalised ratio (INR) and activated partial thromboplastin time (APTT)

Full blood count and reticulocyte count

Sodium, potassium, urea and creatinine (urea may be low because of reduced hepatic synthesis; if markedly elevated with a normal creatinine, suspect upper gastrointestinal bleeding)

Liver function tests: bilirubin (including split bilirubin), aspartate transaminase, alanine transaminase, gamma-glutamyl transpeptidase, alkaline phosphatase and albumin

Amylase and lipase

Paracetamol level (even if history is not suggestive, should always be performed)

Septic screen including:

- Blood culture
- Urine stick test, microscopy and culture
- Microscopy and culture of ascites if present (aspirate 10 mL for cell count (use EDTA tube) and culture (inoculate blood culture bottles) (see Chapter 36)
- Chest X-ray
- Fungal screen (beta D glucan and galactomannan)

CT head (to rule out other causes of altered consciousness besides hepatic encephalopathy)

Abdominal imaging: ultrasound of liver, biliary tract and hepatic/portal veins or CT abdomen/liver with triple phase to assess vasculature

ECG

Pregnancy test in women of childbearing age

For later analysis

Markers of viral hepatitis (anti-HAV IgM, HBsAg, anti-HBc IgM, anti-HCV, anti-HDV, anti-HEV, anti-HSV and anti-VZV)

HIV test

Autoimmune profile (antinuclear antibodies, antismooth muscle antibodies and immunoglobulins)

Plasma ceruloplasmin in patients aged <50 (to exclude Wilson's disease)

Serum (10 mL) and urine (50 mL) for toxicological analysis if needed

Blood group and screen

EDTA, ethylene diaminetetra-acetic acid; HAV, hepatitis A virus; HBc, hepatitis B core; HBsAG, hepatitis B surface antigen; HCV, hepatitis C virus; HDV, hepatitis D virus; HEV, hepatitis E virus; HSV, herpes simplex virus; VZV, varicella zoster virus; IgM, immunoglobulin M.

fibrosis increases, so, too, does the diagnostic accuracy of ultrasound in detecting cirrhosis. The gold standard for diagnosing cirrhosis is liver biopsy, or non-invasively by a Fibroscan.

- ALF in women in the third trimester of pregnancy is most commonly due to haemolysis, elevated liver enzymes, low platelets (HELLP) syndrome (coexistent hypertension and proteinuria) or acute fatty liver of pregnancy (AFLP) (see Chapter 32). AFLP can be confirmed by hepatic steatosis on imaging. Other causes of ALF, however, also occur in pregnancy. Treatment is alongside maternity staff and commonly involves prompt delivery of the foetus.

Further management of acute liver failure before transfer to a Liver Unit

General care and monitoring

- Nurse the patient with 30 head-up tilt in a quiet area of an ICU or high-dependency unit, avoiding unnecessary disturbance.
- Monitor the conscious level, pulse, blood pressure, temperature and plasma glucose 1–4-hourly. Monitor oxygen saturation by pulse oximeter and give oxygen by mask to maintain SaO_2 >90%.

- Give platelet concentrate before placing central venous and arterial lines if the platelet count is <50 × 10^9/L. Avoid giving fresh frozen plasma (FFP) unless there is active bleeding, as this affects coagulation tests – the best prognostic marker – for several days, and can precipitate fluid overload. If correction of coagulopathy is needed, discuss with your local haematologist: typically, FFP is given in combination with recombinant activated factor VIIa.
- If encephalopathy is grade 2 or more, or if systolic BP is <90 mmHg, central venous pressure monitoring and a urinary catheter will be required. Fluid resuscitation should be with 4.5% human albumin solution (HAS) or normal saline unless the blood glucose levels are low.
- If encephalopathy progresses to grade 3 or 4, arrange elective intubation and ventilation.
- If there is any evidence of sepsis, then commence antibiotics and antifungals after a full septic screen.
- Give lactulose to assist in ammonia excretion and prevent worsening encephalopathy. Avoid any potentially nephrotoxic agents.
- Put in a nasogastric tube for gastric drainage if the patient is vomiting or is ventilated. Start enteral feeding early or parenteral feeding if required. Replace potassium, magnesium and phosphate as needed (Chapter 52).

Management of complications

Complications of ALF and management of complications are summarised in Table 42.4.

- Give mannitol 20% 100–200 mL (0.5–1.0 g/kg) IV over 10 min alongside maintenance of mean arterial pressure (MAP) at >75 mmHg using vasopressors, with a cerebral perfusion pressure of 60–80 mmHg.
- Increase plasma sodium to 145–155 mmol/L with hypertonic normal saline (Chapter 52).
- Avoid seizures by using phenytoin alongside short-acting benzodiazepines.
- Consider therapeutic hypothermia 32–34 °C as a bridge to transplantation.

Table 42.4 Major complications of acute liver failure and their management.

Complication	Management
Cerebral oedema	See text
Hypotension	Correct hypovolaemia with blood or 4.5% human albumin solution
	Use epinephrine, norepinephrine or dopamine infusion (Chapter 2) to maintain mean arterial pressure >60 mmHg
Acute kidney injury	Correct hypovolemia
	Stop nephrotoxic medication
	Avoid high-dose furosemide
	See Hepatorenal syndrome below
	Start renal replacement therapy if anuric or oliguric with plasma creatinine >400 μmol/L
Hypoglycaemia	Give glucose 10% IV 1 L 12-hourly to prevent hypoglycaemia
	Check blood glucose 1–4 hourly
	If blood glucose is <4.0 mmol/L, give 100 mL of 20% glucose or 200 mL of 10% glucose over 15–30 min IV; recheck blood glucose after 10 min, if still <4.0 mmol/L, repeat
Coagulopathy	Give vitamin K 10 mg IV daily
	Prophylactic correction of coagulopathy with fresh frozen plasma and platelet transfusion is not recommended (may increase risk of thrombosis or transfusion-related lung injury). Consider in special circumstances such as invasive procedures or active bleeding.
	Review venous thrombosis prophylaxis daily
Anaemia	Transfuse if haemoglobin <70 g/dL

(continued)

Table 42.4 (*Continued*)

Complication	Management
Gastric stress ulceration	Prophylaxis with proton pump inhibitor, ranitidine or sucralfate
Hypoxaemia	Many possible causes: inhalation/aspiration, infection, pulmonary oedema, atelectasis and intrapulmonary haemorrhage.
	Increase inspired oxygen
	Ventilate with positive end-expiratory pressure if SaO_2 remains <92%
Sepsis	Daily culture of blood, sputum and urine
	Early treatment of presumed infection with broad-spectrum antibiotic therapy: discuss with microbiologist
	Consider antifungal therapy if fever with negative blood cultures
Nutrition	Oral nutrition should be encouraged
	Low threshold to commence enteral nutrition or parenteral nutrition

Cerebral oedema occurs in 75–80% of patients with grade 4 encephalopathy and is often fatal. It may result in paroxysmal hypertension, dilated pupils, sustained ankle clonus and sometimes decerebrate posturing (papilloedema is usually absent). Intracranial pressure (ICP) should be maintained below 25 mmHg. To avoid raised ICP.

Criteria for liver transplantation

These are summarised in Table 42.5.

Management of decompensated chronic liver disease

Priorities

Search for and treat precipitants (Tables 42.6).

- Spontaneous bacterial peritonitis (SBP) is common and may not be accompanied by abdominal tenderness. If there are ascites, aspirate 10 mL for cell count and microscopy and culture (inoculate blood culture bottles).

SBP is defined as **ascitic fluid with >250 white blood cells/mm³** of which **>75% are polymorphs**

Table 42.5 Criteria for transplantation in acute liver failure (ALF) (King's College Hospital)*.

ALF due to paracetamol poisoning	ALF due to non-paracetamol poisoning
- Arterial pH <7.3 after volume resuscitation	- INR >6.5 Or any three of the following features:
- International normalized ratio (INR) >6.5	- Non-A, non-B viral hepatitis, drug-induced, Wilson or indeterminate aetiology of ALF
- Creatinine >300 µmol/L	- Time from jaundice to encephalopathy >7 days
- Grade 3 or 4 encephalopathy	- Age <10 or >40
	- INR >3.5
	- Serum bilirubin >200 micromol/L
Absolute contraindication to transplantation	**Relative contraindications to transplantation**
- Extrahepatic malignancy	- Age >70
- Irreversible brain injury	- Active alcohol/substance misuse
- Advanced cardiopulmonary disease	- Severe psychiatric disorder
- Cholangiocarcinoma	- Portal vein thrombosis
	- Pulmonary hypertension

*Contraindications (absolute or relative) should not preclude transfer to a Liver Unit.

Table 42.6 Precipitants of decompensated chronic liver disease.

Intercurrent infection, especially spontaneous bacterial peritonitis (Chapter 36)
Acute gastrointestinal bleeding (variceal and non-variceal) (Chapter 38)
Drugs: diuretics, hypnotics, sedatives and opioid analgesics
Alcoholic hepatitis
Viral hepatitis
Major surgery and anaesthesia
Liver ischaemia secondary to hypotension
Acute portal vein thrombosis or Budd–Chiari syndrome (hepatic vein obstruction)
Hypokalaemia and hypoglycaemia
Constipation
Development of hepatocellular carcinoma
No cause apparent (in up to 40% of patients)

- If there is suspicion of SBP, commence antibiotic treatment with a third-generation cephalosporin, for example Cefuroxime 1 g 8-hourly IV while your ascitic tap results are pending.
- Once confirmed, continue IV antibiotics for five days, followed by a quinolone PO for five days.
- SBP should also be treated with HAS (20%), giving 1.5 g/kg of HAS on day 1 and 1 g/kg of HAS on day 3 (100 mL of 20% HAS = 20 g).
- Consider secondary prophylaxis for SBP in these patients on discharge.
- A rectal examination must be performed to exclude melaena. Evaluation and management of acute upper and lower gastrointestinal bleeding is described in Chapters 38 and 39.

Other considerations

1 Reduce the intestinal nitrogenous load
- Lactulose 10–30 mL, 2–3× per day, aiming for at least two soft stool motions per day

2 Optimise nutrition
- Early inpatient dietetic review.
- Advise to eat little and often, every 2–3 h with a bedtime snack, to prevent a hypercatabolic state, and to adhere to a low-salt diet, particularly if there are ascites.
- Low threshold to consider enteral feeding via nasogastric tube if there are any barriers to eating and drinking (e.g. hepatic encephalopathy).
- Monitor re-feeding electrolytes and replace as needed. Consider starting intravenous Pabrinex (vitamin B complex), two pairs twice a day.

3 Maintain blood glucose >4.0 mmol/L

4 Fluid balance
In the absence of renal impairment and/or infection, treat ascites with spironolactone combined with a loop diuretic if necessary, aiming for weight loss of 0.5 kg/day. If ascites is refractory to diuretic therapy, use paracentesis with IV infusion of 100 mL of 20% HAS. See Chapter 36 for further management of ascites.

5 Thromboprophylaxis
Patients remain at high risk of venous thromboembolism even when prothrombin time is prolonged, prescribe low-molecular-weight heparin prophylaxis unless there is active bleeding or the platelet count is $<50 \times 10^9$/L.

6 Medications
Avoid sedatives and opioids. Other drugs that are contraindicated are listed in the *British National Formulary*.

7 Seek advice on further management from a hepatologist or gastroenterologist.

Hepatorenal syndrome

Definition

Hepatorenal syndrome (HRS) is a type of renal failure in patients with acute or chronic liver disease with portal hypertension, usually in the setting of marked abnormalities in arterial circulation which lead to renal hypoperfusion. It is usually made after other causes of acute kidney injury (AKI) have been excluded (see Chapter 86).

Background

HRS occurs in around 20–25% of patients with ALF and decompensated chronic liver disease. SBP (Chapter 36) is complicated by AKI in 30–40% of cases and is a common precipitant of HRS.

Diagnosis

AKI (see Chapter 86 for definition and staging)

Exclusion of other causes of AKI

No or minimal proteinuria

Normal or near-normal urine microscopy

Urine sodium concentration <10 mmol/L (if not taking diuretic); urine osmolality greater than plasma osmolality

Failure of renal function to improve after withdrawal of diuretics and with volume expansion with HAS 1 g/kg (up to 100 g) IV daily for two days.

Management

Seek advice from a hepatologist

Treat the underlying liver disease

Exclude/treat SBP (Chapter 36)

General management of AKI (Chapter 86)

Consider treatment with terlipressin (0.5–2.0 mg IV every 4–12 h) for 5–15 days plus human albumin solution, 1 g/kg (up to 100 g) IV on days 1 and 2, followed by 20–40 g daily, for 5–15 days.

Further reading

Baekdal M, Ytting H, Larsen FS. (2016) Acute liver failure. *J Hepatol Gastroint Dis* 2(3). (open access).

Bernal W, Wendon J. (2013) Acute liver failure. *N Engl J Med* 369, 2525–2534.

Bernal W, Jalan R, Quaglia A, *et al.* (2015) Acute on chronic liver failure. *Lancet* 386, 1576–1587.

National Institute for Health and Care Excellence (2016) Cirrhosis in over 16s: assessment and management NICE guideline (NG50). https://www.nice.org.uk/guidance/ng50.

Wijdicks EFM. (2016) Hepatic encephalopathy. *N Engl J Med* 375, 1660–1670.

CHAPTER 43

Biliary tract disorders and acute pancreatitis

BEN WARNER AND LYNN AFFARAH

Gall stones occur in around 10% of the population and is mostly asymptomatic. However, they can cause pain (biliary colic), acute cholecystitis, choledocholithiasis, cholangitis and pancreatitis (see Tables 43.1 and 43.2).

Table 43.1 Biliary tract disorders: clinical features and management.

Clinical features	Investigations	Management
Biliary colic		
Severe pain, typically in RUQ or epigastrium (may be retrosternal) Can last between 20 min and 6 h Associated nausea and vomiting Usually precipitated by fatty foods	Blood results: Normal Imaging: Abdominal ultrasound to look for gallstones	• Analgesia • Low-fat diet • Elective referral to surgical team for consideration of cholecystectomy
Acute calculous cholecystitis		
Severe pain, typically RUQ, lasts more than12 h Febrile at presentation (usually low-grade fever) History of biliary colic	Blood results: Elevated WCC and CRP Liver function tests and amylase normal or mildly raised ALT rises before alkaline phosphatase Imaging: Abdominal ultrasound to look for features of cholecystitis	• Analgesia • Antibiotic therapy (usually to cover Gram-negative bacteraemia) • Keep nil by mouth pending urgent surgical review
Acute cholangitis		
Charcot triad: abdominal pain (RUQ), jaundice and fevers/rigors Reynold's pentad: above with septic shock and altered mental status May present post-ERCP	Blood results: Elevated WCC and CRP Abnormal liver function tests and raised bilirubin Amylase often raised **Imaging**: Abdominal ultrasound may show a dilated common bile duct but cross-sectional imaging is preferable (CT/MRCP)	• Analgesia • Antibiotic therapy (as above) • Fluid replacement/resuscitation • Keep nil by mouth pending urgent surgical/gastroenterology opinion • Biliary drainage (usually by ERCP)

ALT, alanine aminotransferase; CRP, C-reactive protein; ERCP, endoscopic retrograde cholangiopancreatography; RUQ, right upper quadrant; WCC, white-cell count.
Hepatology at a Glance by Dr Deepak Joshi (page 94 Biliary Disorders).

Table 43.2 Acute pancreatitis: clinical features and management.

Element	Comment
Common causes	Gallstones
	Alcohol
Less common causes	Complication of ERCP
	Hyperlipidaemia
	Drugs (e.g. thiopurines and sodium valproate) Hypercalcaemia
	Pancreas divisum
	Abdominal trauma
	HIV infection
	Genetic predisposition: Mutations in SPINK1, CFTR and PRSS1
Clinical features and blood results	Epigastric pain, typically sudden in onset when due to gallstones, may increase in severity over a few hours in other causes, may last for several days
	Nausea and vomiting
	Abdominal tenderness/guarding
	Fever at presentation may reflect cytokine-mediated systemic inflammation or acute cholangitis
	Shock, respiratory failure, renal failure and multiorgan failure may occur
	Raised amylase and lipase
	Raised white cell count and C-reactive protein Abnormal liver function tests (elevated ALT more than three times the upper limit of normal is highly predictive of gallstone pancreatitis if alcohol is excluded)
	Hypoglycaemia, hypocalcaemia, hypomagnesaemia and disseminated intravascular coagulation may occur
Identification of severe (10–15%) Acute pancreatitis	APACHE II score of 8 or more
	Persistent organ failure (shock, respiratory failure and renal failure) and of SIRS

ALT, alanine aminotransferase; APACHE II, severity of illness scoring system based on acute physiology and chronic health evaluation; ERCP, endoscopic retrograde cholangiopancreatography; SIRS, systemic inflammatory response. Hepatology at a Glance by Dr Deepak Joshi (page 96 Pancreatic Disorders).

Management of acute pancreatitis

Early fluid resuscitation with 250–500 mL/h (with careful monitoring of fluid status) of Ringer's lactate or Hartmann's solution aiming to maintain low urea and haematocrit levels.

ICU referral for patients with organ failure, and those with conditions that will make fluid management difficult (e.g. chronic kidney disease and heart failure).

Urgent abdominal ultrasound to confirm the diagnosis. CT/MRCP for those who fail to improve or deteriorate at 48–72 h.

In the absence of gallstones and alcohol excess, measure triglyceride levels (>1000 mg/dL suggests primary or secondary hypertriglyceridaemia as the cause). Urgent discussion with Endocrinology, as these patients often require insulin therapy to bring down their triglyceride levels.

Consider pancreatic tumours in patients over the age of 40.

Analgesia with opioid and anti-emetics.

Antibiotic therapy is indicated only for patients with evidence of infected necrosis or extrapancreatic sepsis, for example chest or urinary sepsis.

ERCP within 24 h for patients with gallstone pancreatitis in whom biliary obstruction is suspected on the basis of raised bilirubin and clinical cholangitis.

Nutritional support: in mild AP, oral feeding with low-fat solid food is sufficient. In severe AP a nasogastric/nasojejunal tube may be required in the context of vomiting and/or gastric-outlet obstruction. Parenteral feeding should be avoided if possible.

Infected necrosis is considered in cases where SIRS persists beyond 7–10 days of hospitalization and is confirmed by CT.

Antibiotics are recommended as the first line in the stable patient, followed by endoscopic/surgical/radiographical intervention if required but not before four weeks.

The unstable patient requires earlier intervention.

Further reading

Deepak Joshi. Hepatology at a Glance.
Lankisch PG, Apte M, Banks PA. (2015) Acute pancreatitis. *Lancet* 386, 85–96.
National Institute for Health and Care Excellence (2014) Gallstone disease: diagnosis and management. Clinical guideline (CG188). https://www.nice.org.uk/guidance/cg188?unlid=78410445201622195914.
Updated Tokyo Guidelines for acute cholangitis and acute cholecystitis (2013) (open access). http://link. springer.com/journal/534/20/1/page/1.

Endocrinology and Metabolic Disorders

CHAPTER 44

Diabetic emergencies: DKA and HHS

Vimal Venugopal

Diabetic ketoacidosis (DKA)

Consider DKA in any ill patient with diabetes, especially if nausea, vomiting or abdominal pain are prominent. DKA most often occurs in patients with type 1 diabetes but is also increasingly seen in those with type 2 diabetes.

Priorities

1 Is this DKA?

- Clinical assessment and investigation of the patient with suspected DKA are summarized in Tables 44.1 and 44.2.
- Examination typically shows signs of volume depletion (average deficit 10% of body weight) and tachypnoea due to metabolic acidosis. There may also be features of an associated disorder that has precipitated DKA.
- DKA is confirmed by a blood glucose >11 mmol/L or a history of known diabetes mellitus, serum ketones >3 mmol/L and venous blood pH <7.3 and/or bicarbonate <15 mmol/L.
- Venous blood gases are preferred to arterial blood gases as venous sampling is easier and less painful for the patient. The differences in venous and arterial pH and bicarbonate levels are not significant enough to affect management. Capillary blood glucose and capillary blood ketones are sufficiently accurate for monitoring.

2 If DKA is confirmed, start treatment immediately

- The treatment of DKA (Tables 44.3–44.5) involves fluid replacement to restore the circulating volume, replacement of lost potassium and the use of fixed-rate intravenous insulin infusion to clear the ketonaemia.
- If the patient is taking a long-acting insulin, this should be continued, as this allows earlier weaning from the infusion.
- If the patient has a continuous subcutaneous insulin infusion pump, this should be disconnected unless you are instructed not to do so by a specialist diabetes team.

3 Identify and treat the precipitant of DKA

- Infection is a common precipitant (~40% cases) and complication of DKA and may not cause fever. Check carefully for a focus of infection, including examination of the feet and perineum.
- Seek a surgical opinion if abdominal pain or abnormal signs do not resolve with correction of acidosis.

Table 44.1 Focused assessment in suspected diabetic ketoacidosis.

History
Diabetes history (duration, treatment and complications)
Polydipsia, polyuria, weight loss?
Nausea, vomiting, abdominal pain?
Possible precipitant of DKA? Consider:
* Inappropriate reduction in, or poor compliance with, insulin therapy
* Error in insulin prescription or administration
* Alcohol or substance use
* Emotional stress
* Infection
* Acute coronary syndrome
Comorbidities
Pregnancy?

Examination
Physiological observations
Focus of infection? Check feet and perineum
Abdominal signs?

* Other causes of DKA are an inappropriate reduction in, or poor compliance with, insulin therapy (~25% cases), errors in insulin prescription or administration, surgery, acute coronary syndrome, alcohol or substance use and emotional stress.
* DKA may also be the first presentation of type 1 (and, less commonly, type 2) diabetes.

4 **Consider admission to ICU/HDU if the patient**
* Is aged 18–25 years (as higher risk of cerebral oedema) or >70 years (as higher risk of fluid overload)
* Has a reduced conscious level or hypotension which is not corrected by fluid replacement
* Has cardiac or renal failure
* Is pregnant
* At presentation has one or more of the following features:
  * Plasma ketones >6.0 mmol/L
  * Venous bicarbonate <5 mmol/L
  * Venous pH <7.0
  * Plasma potassium <3.5 mmol/L
  * Anion gap >16 mOsmol/kg (calculated as [(plasma sodium+potassium)-(plasma chloride+bicarbonate)])
  * Depressed level of consciousness or GCS<12
  * New hypoxia with SpO2 <92%
  * Hypotension (systolic BP<90)
  * Heart rate >100 bpm or <60 bpm

Table 44.2 Urgent investigation in suspected diabetic ketoacidosis.

Glucose – checked in capillary blood and venous plasma
Capillary blood ketones
Sodium, potassium, urea and creatinine
Venous blood gases
Full blood count
C-reactive protein
Two blood cultures
Urine dipstick, microscopy and culture
Chest X-ray
ECG

Table 44.3 Fluid replacement in diabetic ketoacidosis.

This must take account of:
- The likely fluid deficit (typically 100 mL/kg body weight)
- The blood pressure, central venous pressure and urine output
- Coexisting cardiac or renal disease

1. If systolic BP <90 mmHg, give normal saline 500 mLs IV over 15 min, if no improvement of BP, can repeat another infusion of 500 mLs of normal saline. Consider placement of a central line to monitor central venous pressure (CVP) in patients with cardiac or renal failure.
2. If/once systolic BP more than 90 mmHg, infuse 1 L of normal saline without added potassium followed by further normal saline infusion with added potassium (calculated based on potassium monitoring results), a typical regime is outlined below
    - 1 L normal saline over 1 h
    - 1 L normal saline (with added potassium) over the following 2 h
    - 1 L normal saline (with added potassium) over the following 2 h
    - 1 L normal saline (with added potassium) over the following 4 h
    - 1 L normal saline (with added potassium) over the following 4 h
    - 1 L normal saline (with added potassium) over the following 6 h
3. Once blood glucose level falls <14 mmol/L, glucose 10% should be given at a rate of 125 mL/h alongside the saline infusion, at the rate required to correct fully the fluid deficit.

Table 44.4 Potassium replacement in diabetic ketoacidosis*.

Plasma potassium (mmol/L)	Potassium added (mmol/L)
<3.5	Regimen needs review**
3.5–5.5	40
>5.5	None

*Check plasma potassium on admission, 60 min, 120 min, and then 2-hourly from then on.
**Can increase the rate of the overall fluid infusion if fluid balance permits, infusion rates of up to 20 mmol/h of potassium can be given peripherally. If there is persistent hypokalaemia, rates of up to 40 mmol/h can be given via a central venous catheter, with monitoring in a high-dependency unit.

Table 44.5 Fixed rate insulin infusion in diabetic ketoacidosis.

Continue basal insulin in patients on basal bolus insulin regimen.
Switch off continuous subcutaneous insulin pump if the patient has one.

1. Make 50 units of soluble insulin up to 50 mL with normal saline (i.e. insulin 1 unit/mL). Flush 10 mL of the solution through the line before connecting to the patient (as some insulin will be adsorbed onto the plastic).
2. Start the infusion at 0.1 units/kg/h. Check hourly capillary blood glucose and ketones, and send venous glucose if capillary blood glucose meter reads 'high'.
3. Aim for blood ketones to fall by 0.5 mmol/L/h. If blood ketones do not fall, increase insulin infusion in 1 unit/h increments until blood ketones fall by at least 0.5 mmol/L/h. If there is no fall in blood ketones or glucose, confirm that the pump is working and the IV line is connected properly. Consult diabetes specialist team if blood ketone levels are still not falling.
4. If blood glucose drops below 14 mmol/L, consider reducing rate of fixed-dose insulin infusion to 0/05 units/kg/h

Further management
Supportive care

- Place a nasogastric tube if the patient is too drowsy to answer questions or there is a gastric succussion splash. Aspirate the stomach and leave on continuous drainage. Inhalation of vomit is a potentially fatal complication of DKA.
- Use graduated compression stockings and prophylactic low-molecular-weight heparin to reduce the risk of deep vein thrombosis.

Monitoring

- Continuous display of ECG and oxygen saturation
- Check hourly:
  - Conscious level (e.g. by AVPU or Glasgow Coma Scale score) until fully conscious
  - Respiratory rate and blood pressure until stable and then 4-hourly
  - Fluid balance
  - Capillary blood glucose and plasma ketones
  - Venous blood glucose by laboratory measurement until capillary blood glucose is <20 mmol/L
- Check venous pH, bicarbonate and potassium on admission, at 60 min, 120 min and then 2-hourly on a blood gas analyser
- Put in a bladder catheter if no urine has been passed after 1 h, or if the patient is incontinent, but not otherwise

Insulin infusion

- The blood glucose should fall with the administration of IV insulin. However, as long as ketoacidosis persists, the fixed rate insulin infusion must be continued even if the blood glucose enters the normal range. When blood glucose is <14 mmol/L, start an infusion of 10% glucose to prevent hypoglycaemia (the commonest complication of treatment of DKA)
- If blood glucose falls below 14 mmol/L, consider reducing fixed rate insulin infusion to 0.05 units/kg/h
- Once the exit criteria for DKA are met, and the patient is eating and drinking, the IV insulin infusion can be weaned off (Table 44.6).
- Prophylactic-dose low-molecular-weight heparin (LMWH) (chapter 85).
- Resolution of HHS is characterized by serum osmolality <300 mOsm/kg, blood glucose <15 mmol/L, resolution of hypovolaemia and a return to the baseline cognitive status.

Table 44.6 Switching from IV to SC insulin after resolution of diabetic ketoacidosis.

1. Resolution of DKA requires a venous pH >7.3 and blood ketones <0.6 mmol/L.
2. In patients already on basal bolus regime, the basal dose should have been continued throughout the DKA treatment.
3. In patients newly diagnosed with diabetes, start a long-acting insulin 0.25 units/kg and request diabetes specialist team input.
4. When starting a basal bolus insulin regime for type 1 diabetes, half of the total daily dose should be as long-acting insulin SC at evening. Divide the remaining half into three to calculate the dose of rapid-acting analogue insulin SC before meals.
5. Once DKA has resolved and patient is able to eat, give the fast-acting insulin with a meal and stop the intravenous fixed rate insulin one hour later.
6. Check blood glucose before meals and at 2200 h, and adjust doses of insulin as needed, aiming for levels 4–7 mmol/L.
7. Refer to diabetes team for advice on further management.

Most patients will require subcutaneous insulin post resolution of HHS. If the total daily requirement falls below 20 units an oral hypoglycaemic can be considered. Consult the inpatient diabetes team on an appropriate regimen before discharge.

Hyperosmolar hyperglycaemic state (HHS)

Consider HHS in any ill patient with diabetes, especially if volume depletion and drowsiness are prominent.

- HHS typically occurs in older patients with type 2 diabetes, but can also occur in teenagers and young adults. Any illness that leads to a reduced fluid intake can precipitate HHS, which may be the first presentation of diabetes.
- The onset of HHS is usually over a number of days, and slower compared to DKA. However, an overlap syndrome with features of both HHS and DKA may be seen.
- Fluid losses (100–220 mLs/kg) are greater than in DKA
- Mortality of patients with HHS is high (up to 20%), with the major causes of death being the precipitating illness, thromboembolism and aspiration pneumonia.

Hyperosmolar hyperglycaemic state does not have a precise definition but is characterized by

- Blood glucose $\geq$30 mmol/L, but no ketoacidosis (plasma ketones $\leq$3 mmol/L, venous bicarbonate $\geq$15 mmol/L) and
- Plasma osmolality $\geq$320 mOsmol/kg (normal range 285–295 mOsmol/kg); this can be measured directly or calculated from the formula: plasma osmolality = [2 (plasma Na) + glucose + urea].

Management

Clinical assessment, investigation and management are as for DKA, with the differences noted below. Identify and treat any precipitating illness.

- The goals of treatment are to normalize osmolality, glucose as well as replace fluid and electrolyte deficits
- Use normal saline to correct the fluid deficit. Switch to 0.45% sodium chloride solution if plasma osmolality is not falling despite adequate fluid replacement. Plasma sodium may rise initially but this is not an indication to use 0.45% sodium chloride solution.
- The change in serum sodium should be below 10 mmol/24 h
- The rate of fall of osmolality should not exceed 8 mOsm/kg/h.
- The fall in blood glucose should be no more than 5 mmol/L/h.
- Subcutaneous long-acting insulin should be continued if already part of patient's insulin regimen. Intravenous insulin (0.05 units/kg/h) should only be administered if there is significant ketonaemia/ketonuria (plasma ketones >1 mmol/L or urine ketones greater than 2+), or if blood glucose is not falling despite correction of the fluid deficit. If ketones >3 mmol/L and ph<7.3, treat using DKA protocol
- Starting intravenous insulin too early risks greater changes in osmolality than desired leading to potential severe neurological complications
- Aim for a positive fluid balance of 3–6 L by 12 h and the remaining replacement of estimated fluid losses within next 12 h (average deficit in HHS is 10 L). Encourage the patient to drink when conscious level allows safe swallowing.
- The risk of foot ulceration is high, particularly if the patient has a reduced conscious level. The heels should be protected and the feet checked daily.
- The risk of thromboembolism is high. Unless contraindicated (e.g. recent stroke), give Prophylactic-dose LMWH (Chapter 85) until mobile.

- Resolution of HHS is characterized by serum osmolality<300 mOsm/kg, blood glucose <15 mmol/L, resolution of hypovolaemia and a return to the baseline cognitive status

Most patients will require subcutaneous insulin post resolution of HHS, if the total daily requirement falls below 20 units, when an oral hypoglycaemic can be considered. Consult the inpatient diabetes team on an appropriate regimen before discharge.

Further reading

JBDS 02 The Management of Diabetic Ketoacidosis in Adults.
Joint British Diabetes Societies Inpatient Care Group (2022) The management of the hyperosmolar hyperglycaemic state (HHS) in adults with diabetes.

CHAPTER 45
Hyperglycaemic states

VIMAL VENUGOPAL

Blood glucose should ideally be tested in all inpatients as part of initial observations on admission. Further glucose monitoring should continue in patients

- with diabetes mellitus.
- if initial blood glucose monitoring was abnormal or any patient with a clinical state in which derangements of blood glucose are common or must be excluded (Table 45.1).
- Hyperglycaemia is defined as plasma glucose concentration >11 mmol/L.
- Patients with significant frailty may have blood glucose target range allowing glucose up to 15 mmol/L.

Plasma blood glucose >11 mmol/L or above individual target range

- Assess the conscious level and state of hydration and establish if the patient is taking treatment for diabetes.
- If the patient is unwell or blood glucose above 18 mmol/L, check urine or capillary blood for ketones. If there is ketonuria 2+ or greater, or capillary ketones ≥1.5 mmol/L, and the patient is unwell, check venous plasma bicarbonate concentration.
- The patient can now be placed in one of three groups (Table 45.2):
- Diabetic ketoacidosis or hyperosmolar hyperglycaemic state: see Chapter 44
- Newly diagnosed or poorly controlled insulin-treated diabetes: see below

Further management of newly diagnosed or poorly controlled diabetes

- If the patient is already on treatment for diabetes, consider increasing the doses of current medication: seek specialist advice.
- If blood glucose is persistently >18 mmol/L, give 4–6 units of rapid-acting insulin SC, repeated every 4 h, until blood glucose is <18 mmol/L. Check capillary blood glucose (CBG) 1–2 hourly.
- Use a variable-rate insulin infusion (VRII; 'sliding scale') (Table 45.3) if the patient:
  - Is critically unwell
  - Is vomiting

Acute Medicine: A Practical Guide to the Management of Medical Emergencies, Sixth Edition.
Edited by Mridula Rajwani, Leila Vaziri, and Ivie Gbinigie.
© 2026 John Wiley & Sons Ltd. Published 2026 by John Wiley & Sons Ltd.

Table 45.1 Clinical states in which derangements of blood glucose must be excluded.

Coma or reduced conscious level
Transient loss of consciousness
Seizures
Delirium/acute behavioural disturbance
Suspected stroke/TIA
Poisoning
Metabolic acidosis
Severe hyponatraemia
Liver failure
Hypothermia
Parenteral nutrition
Corticosteroid therapy
Acute coronary syndrome

Table 45.2 Categorization of the patient with blood glucose >11 mmol/L.

	Blood glucose (mmol/L)	Ketonaemia/ Ketonuria	Venous bicarbonate (mmol/L)	Dehydration	Drowsiness
DKA	>11	3+	<15	++	+/++
HHS	>30	1+	>15	++++	+++
Diabetes*	>11	to 2+	>15	/+	

DKA, diabetic ketoacidosis; HHS, hyperosmolar hyperglycaemic state.
*Either newly diagnosed or poorly controlled.

- Is unable to eat and drink (e.g. in perioperative period)
- Has a complication of pregnancy
- Acute coronary syndrome if CBG above 11 mmol/L
- If the patient is normally on long-acting insulin, this should be continued while the VRII is being administered. Aim to switch back from VRII to patient's usual diabetes regimen as soon as the patient is eating and critical illness resolving.
- If the patient is usually on continuous subcutaneous insulin infusion (CSII) and the decision is made to start VRII, leave CSII running for 30 min after VRII started, then disconnect CSII.

Stepping down from variable-rate insulin infusion

- If the patient is already on insulin or to be newly started on insulin, VRII must be continued 30 min after the administration of basal insulin before being taken down.
- Ask advice from a diabetologist on long-term management. In general:
  - Insulin-treated DM, with good control (HbA1c <7.5%): return to usual regime.
  - Insulin-treated DM, with poor control (HbA1c >7.5%): review regimen.
  - Oral therapy with good control (HbA1c <7.5%): return to usual therapy.
  - Oral therapy with poor control (HbA1c >7.5%): transfer to insulin.
  - Newly diagnosed DM: individualized treatment.

Table 45.3 Variable-rate insulin infusion ('sliding scale').

Regimens must be individualized.

If the patient is already receiving a long-acting insulin analogue, this should be continued. Obese patients require more insulin per hour because of insulin resistance. CBG measurement should be used to determine the initial insulin infusion rate and checked hourly to ensure that the infusion rate is appropriate.

1. Make 50 units of soluble insulin up to 50 mL with normal saline (i.e. 1 unit/mL). Flush 10 mL of the solution through the line before connecting to the patient (as some insulin will be adsorbed onto the plastic).
2. Check blood glucose and start the insulin infusion at the appropriate rate (see below).
3. Administer 1 L of 0.45% saline with 5% glucose at 125 mL/h IV (83 mL/h if heart or renal failure).
4. Co-administer potassium chloride IV at an appropriate rate if plasma potassium is <5.5 mmol/L.
5. Check CBG hourly. Adjust the insulin infusion rate as needed, aiming to keep blood glucose between 6 and 10 mmol/L.
   - If CBG is within the target range or falling towards it, continue same rate of insulin infusion.
   - If CBG remains over >12 mmol/L for 3 consecutive readings and is not dropping by 3 mmol/L/h or more the rate of insulin infusion should be increased.
   - If CBG drops to below 4.0 mmol/L, the insulin infusion should be stopped and hypoglycaemia should be treated irrespective of whether the patient has symptoms. Insulin infusion should be restarted at a stepped-down rate once CBG is >4.0 mmol/L.

Capillary blood glucose (mmol/L)	Insulin infusion rate (1 unit/mL)		
	Insulin sensitive	**Standard**	**Insulin resistant**
<4.0	Stop infusion and treat for hypoglycaemia if indicated (Chapter 46). When CBG is >4.0 mmol/L, restart infusion at a lower rate.		
4.1–8.0	0.5	1	2
8.1–12.0	1	2	4
12.1–16.0	2	4	6
16.1–20.0	3	5	7
20.1–24.0	4	6	8
>24.0	6	8	10

- If starting insulin in an insulin naïve patient
  - Estimate the daily insulin requirement from the total dose given by infusion over the previous 6h (provided blood glucose stable). Divide the total amount given in the last 6 h by 6 and multiply by 20 to give a total daily dose (TDD). Give half the TDD as long-acting background insulin subcutaneously (SC) once daily. Divide the remaining half into three and give as rapid-acting insulin SC before meals.
  - Monitor plasma glucose pre-prandially and at 2200 h and adjust doses of insulin as needed.

Further reading

American Diabetes Association. (2016) Classification and diagnosis of diabetes. *Diabetes Care* 39(Suppl. 1), S13–S22. DOI: 10.2337/dc16-S005.

Palmer BF, Clegg DJ. (2015) Electrolyte and acid-base disturbances in patients with diabetes mellitus. *N Engl J Med* 373, 548–559.

The use of variable rate intravenous insulin infusion (VRIII) in medical inpatients JBDS-IP October 2014.

CHAPTER 46

Hypoglycaemia

VIMAL VENUGOPAL

In hospital inpatients with diabetes, hypoglycaemia is defined as a blood glucose <4.0 mmol/L and it should be corrected.

In a person without diabetes, the diagnosis of hypoglycaemia is based on Whipple's triad:

- Symptoms of hypoglycaemia (Table 46.1)
- Simultaneous demonstration of low blood glucose (<3.5 mmol/L)
- Resolution of symptoms with correction of low blood glucose

Hypoglycaemia must be excluded in any patient with seizures, abnormal behaviour, delirium, reduced conscious level or abnormal neurological signs. Hypoglycaemia is most often due to the treatment of diabetes mellitus, but other causes should be considered (Table 46.2).

Priorities

- If hypoglycaemia is suspected in inpatients with diabetes, check a bedside capillary blood glucose and if this is <4 mmol/L, treat as hypoglycaemia without delay.
- Some pregnant patients with diabetes mellitus may have individualized glucose target ranges that allow blood glucose as low as 3.5 mmol/L.
- Consider sending a venous sample for laboratory testing. Capillary blood glucose (CBG) may be falsely low in patients with reduced perfusion of the extremities.
- Consider sending serum insulin and C-peptide levels along with plasma glucose to help investigate unexplained hypoglycaemia.

Asymptomatic (incidental) or mildly symptomatic hypoglycaemia

Give 15–20 g of oral glucose (as a sugary drink, snack (e.g. five soft sweets) or glucose gel). Repeat capillary blood glucose measurement in 10 min and if still below 4 mmol/L, repeat the oral glucose administration (up to three times). If CBG does not improve above 4 mmol/L proceed with intravenous replacement as below.

If the patient is drowsy or fitting (this may sometimes occur with mild hypoglycaemia, especially in young patients with diabetes):

- Give 100 mL of 20% glucose or 200 mL of 10% glucose over 15 min IV and consider glucagon 1 mg IV/IM/SC.
- Recheck blood glucose after 10 min, if still below 4.0 mmol/L, repeat the above IV glucose treatment.

Table 46.1 Manifestations of hypoglycaemia.

Autonomic	Neuroglycopaenic
Dizziness	Irritability
Sweating	Confusion
Palpitations	Transient loss of consciousness
Tremor	Seizures
Blurred vision	Coma
Anxiety	Focal neurological abnormalities
Hunger	
Paraesthesia	

Table 46.2 Causes of hypoglycaemia.

In patients with diabetes mellitus

Excess insulin
Incorrect insulin injection technique
Increased exercise (relative to usual)
Gastroparesis and malabsorption
Excess insulin secretagogues (e.g. sulphonylureas)
Development of renal failure (with reduced clearance of insulin and sulphonylurea)
Development of other endocrine disorders (adrenal insufficiency, hypothyroidism and hypopituitarism)
Early pregnancy and breast-feeding

In patients with or without diabetes mellitus

Alcohol binge (inhibits hepatic gluconeogenesis)
Starvation
Severe liver disease (Chapter 42)
Sepsis (Chapter 5)
Salicylate poisoning
Adrenal insufficiency (Chapter 47)
Hypopituitarism (Chapter 48)
Other drugs known to cause hypoglycaemia (e.g. propranolol, salicylates and disopyramide)
Falciparum malaria (Chapter 75)
Insulinoma
Nesidioblastosis (acquired hyperinsulinism due to beta cell hyperplasia)
Insulin autoimmune hypoglycaemia
Accidental or non-prescribed use of insulin or insulin secretagogues
Factitious hypoglycaemia

- In patients with malnourishment or alcohol-use disorder, there is a remote risk of precipitating Wernicke encephalopathy by a glucose load: prevent this by giving thiamine 100 mg IV before or shortly after glucose administration.

  When the patient is alert and able to swallow, and blood glucose is >4 mmol/L, give a long-acting carbohydrate (usually 20 g, increase to 40 g in those given glucagon) of the patient's choice, for example two biscuits, one slice of bread/toast or a 200–300 mL glass of milk.

- If unable to eat or to remain nil by mouth, start an IV infusion of glucose 10% at 100 mL/h via a central or large peripheral vein. Adjust the rate to keep the blood glucose level at 5–10 mmol/L.

- After excess sulphonylurea therapy, maintain the glucose infusion for 24–36 h as the risk of hypoglycaemia may persist for up to 24–36 h following the last dose, especially if there is concurrent renal impairment.

If hypoglycaemia is only partially responsive to glucose 10% infusion
- Give glucose 20% 100 mL/h IV via a central vein.
- If the cause is intentional insulin overdose, consider local excision of the injection site.

Prevent further or recurrent hypoglycaemia

- This is a fundamental step in all patients with DM and a crucial one in those with hypoglycaemia unawareness.
- Implicated drugs should be discontinued or amended. Consider referral to the diabetes team for prescription of continuous glucose monitoring systems.
- Specific conditions (e.g. insulinoma and cortisol deficiency) should be directly addressed wherever possible, but this will require specialist input.

Further management

- Identify and treat the cause (Table 46.2).
- In patients without diabetes presenting with blood glucose levels below 3.5 mmol/L with symptoms and no obvious cause, check simultaneous insulin and C-peptide levels. Elevated insulin and C-peptide levels indicate endogenous hyperinsulinaemia, whereas low C-peptide levels in the presence of elevated insulin levels suggest exogenous insulin as the cause of hypoglycaemia.
- Full blood count, renal and liver function tests should be checked in all patients. Additional testing will be directed by the clinical picture and differential diagnosis.
- Give advice to the patient about driving (consult Driver and Vehicle Licensing Authority guidance). Patients with diabetes treated with insulin or oral therapy can continue to drive a car, provided they have adequate awareness of hypoglycaemia, and have had no more than one episode of severe hypoglycaemia (requiring assistance from another person) in the preceding 12 months.

Further reading

Joint British Diabetes Societies Inpatient Care Group (2023) The hospital management of hypoglycaemia in adults with diabetes mellitus.

CHAPTER 47

Adrenal disorders

Zaw Ye Htet

Acute adrenal insufficiency/adrenal crisis

Consider this diagnosis in any patient with unexplained hypotension and suggestive clinical features (Table 47.1), particularly if not responsive to initial fluid resuscitation. Prompt recognition and glucocorticoid replacement may be a life-saving treatment in a critically unwell patient, and should not be delayed while awaiting test results.

Acute adrenal insufficiency most commonly occurs as an acute exacerbation of an underlying chronic or subacute insufficiency, triggered by concomitant illness such as infection.

Underlying conditions

Primary adrenal insufficiency is caused by loss of function of the adrenal gland itself, for example due to autoimmune-mediated destruction of adrenocortical tissue or surgical removal of the adrenal glands or due to inborn disruption of adrenal cortisol production in congenital adrenal hyperplasia. Also due to infection (Tuberculosis, infiltration (sarcoidosis, lymphoma, metastasis, etc) and adrenolytic drugs (metyropone, keto-conazole, mitotane, etc)

Table 47.1 Clinical features of adrenal insufficiency.

Primary (Addison's disease) and secondary adrenal insufficiency
Tiredness, weakness, anorexia, weight loss
Hypotension/postural hypotension or dizziness
Nausea, vomiting
Hyponatraemia, hypoglycaemia, mild normocytic anaemia, lymphocytosis, eosinophilia

Primary adrenal insufficiency and associated disorders only
Hyperpigmentation, especially in areas exposed to mechanical shear stress: palmar crease, knuckles, scar, oral mucosa
Hyperkalaemia
Vitiligo
Autoimmune thyroid disease

Secondary adrenal insufficiency and associated disorders only
Pale skin without marked anaemia
Amenorrhea, decreased libido and potency
Scanty axillary and pubic hair
Small testicles
Secondary hypothyroidism
Headache, visual symptoms
Features of AVP deficiency (diabetes insipidus): Polyuria, loss of ability to concentrate urine

Acute Medicine: A Practical Guide to the Management of Medical Emergencies, Sixth Edition.
Edited by Mridula Rajwani, Leila Vaziri, and Ivie Gbinigie.
© 2026 John Wiley & Sons Ltd. Published 2026 by John Wiley & Sons Ltd.

Secondary adrenal insufficiency is caused if the regulation of adrenal cortisol production by the pituitary is compromised, for example due to pituitary tumour, infection (Tuberculosis), infiltration (neurosarcoidosis, haemochromatosis etc), hypophysitis (IgG4, checkpoint inhibitor immunotherapy etc), pituitary apoplexy, Sheehan's Syndrome, previous pituitary surgery or radiotherapy, abrupt withdrawal of long-term exogenous corticosteroid treatment (prednisolone >5 mg daily or equivalent for ≥four weeks).

In secondary adrenal insufficiency, haemodynamic compromise may not be accompanied by typical electrolyte disturbance as aldosterone is unaffected.

Priorities

In the patient presenting with acute circulatory collapse and suspected adrenal insufficiency (Tables 47.1 and 47.2), the following goals should be achieved in the first hour of treatment:

- Rapid assessment of airway, breathing, circulation and conscious level in a high dependency or critical care environment, with continuous monitoring of heart rate, blood pressure and oxygen saturation.
- Airway management if the airway is compromised or the Glasgow Coma Scale score is less than 8.
- Supplemental oxygen if needed to maintain oxygen saturation >94%.
- Intravenous access, with blood sent for urgent investigations (Table 47.3).
- Fluid resuscitation with normal saline to correct the volume deficit.
- Place a bladder catheter for monitoring of urine output.
- Look for a MedicAlert® or similar bracelet/necklace as this may reveal the diagnosis.
- Give hydrocortisone (immediate bolus injection of 100 mg hydrocortisone IV or IM followed by continuous intravenous infusion of 200 mg hydrocortisone per 24 h (alternatively 50 mg hydrocortisone per IV or IM injection every 6 h). Fludrocortisone is not required in addition, as this dose of hydrocortisone has sufficient mineralocorticoid action.
- Give a broad-spectrum antibiotic after taking blood and urine for culture, in case the trigger is infection.
- If the patient is well enough, take a detailed history of the symptoms of adrenal insufficiency and commonly associated disorders (Table 47.1). Look for clinical signs, especially hyperpigmentation suggestive of elevated adrenocorticotropic hormone (ACTH), to differentiate primary from secondary adrenal insufficiency. Hyperpigmentation is best seen over the palmar creases, knuckles, old scars and the oral mucosa.

Once stabilized, transfer the patient to an appropriate care area.

Table 47.2 Urgent investigation in suspected acute adrenal insufficiency.

Urea, creatinine, sodium, potassium and glucose*
Venous blood gas and lactate
Plasma cortisol (in patients not already known to have adrenal failure)
Plasma corticotrophin (ACTH) in patients not already known to have adrenal failure (taken in EDTA tube, for later analysis; transport immediately to the laboratory for freezing)
Thyroid function tests
Full blood count
Coagulation screen
C-reactive protein
Blood culture
Urine microscopy and culture
Chest X-ray
ECG

* Typical biochemical findings in acute adrenal insufficiency are raised creatinine, low sodium (120–130 mmol/L), raised potassium in primary adrenal insufficiency (5–7 mmol/L), low glucose.

Table 47.3 Short tetracosactrin (Synacthen) test.

- The test should be done when the patient has recovered from acute illness, as glucocorticoid (but not fludrocortisone) must be hold before the test. Final dose of hydrocortisone should be at midday, on the day prior to the test. If on, prednisolone, the dose in the morning of the test should be delayed till after the test, so no dose needs to be omitted before the test.
- The patient should be resting quietly but need not fast prior to the test. Tetracosactide may exacerbate bronchospasm in those with asthma. Oestrogens, for example in oral contraceptives, should be stopped six weeks before the test.
- Give 250 μgm of tetracosactide IV or IM before 10 am. Measure plasma cortisol immediately before, and 30 and 60 min after the injection. Baseline plasma ACTH should also be measured.
- With normal adrenal function, the baseline plasma cortisol is over 140 nmol/L, and the 30 or 60-min level is over 500 nmol/L and at least 200 nmol/L above the baseline level. (note: cut-off values are dependent on the assay used check local values with your laboratory)
- In patients with primary hypoadrenalism, tetracosactrin does not stimulate cortisol secretion, because the adrenal cortex is already maximally stimulated by endogenous corticotropin. In severe secondary hypoadrenalism, plasma cortisol does not increase because of adrenocortical atrophy. **However, in secondary hypoadrenalism which is mild or of recent onset, the test may be normal.**

Box 47.1 Acute adrenal insufficiency – alerts.

- Adrenal insufficiency can be a difficult diagnosis to make in an acutely unwell patient as the diagnostic tests are not valid in this population and apparently normal plasma cortisol level may not be appropriately elevated for the degree of metabolic stress present.
- Delay in administration of high-dose glucocorticoid leads to excess morbidity and mortality in critically unwell patients with adrenal insufficiency.
- Newly diagnosed patients with adrenal insufficiency require careful education regarding sick-day rules and may need an emergency injection pack and training before discharge.

Further management
Steroid replacement

- If in doubt, hydrocortisone replacement should continue until adrenal sufficiency can be conclusively confirmed or excluded. In the acutely unwell patient, give hydrocortisone 50 mg 6-hourly IV or IM.
- After treatment of any underlying concomitant illness and when the patient is feeling well, parenteral hydrocortisone can be stepped down to a double-physiological dose of oral hydrocortisone, approximately 40 mg daily in divided doses. When completely recovered, physiological replacement can commence.
- Mineralocorticoid replacement **for primary adrenal insufficiency** is normally achieved with a dose of fludrocortisone 50–200 μgm PO once daily and is started at 100 μgm. Adequacy of dose can be assessed by an absence of clinical signs of hypovolaemia (e.g. postural hypotension) and normal electrolytes.

Making the patient safe for discharge

- Educating the patient on what to do in the presence of acute illness is of paramount importance and may be a life-saving intervention. Patient information resources can be found and reproduced free of charge at the website of the Addison's Disease Self-help Group, www.addisonsdisease.org.uk, and are based on the advice of an expert panel.
- Patients should be advised:
- Sick day rule 1: the need to double daily oral glucocorticoid dose during illness with fever that requires bed rest and/or antibiotics

- Sick day rule 2: the need to administer glucocorticoids per IV or IM injection during prolonged vomiting or diarrhoea, during preparation for colonoscopy or in case of acute trauma or surgery
- Teach the patient and partner/parents how to self-administer and inject hydrocortisone and provide them with a **Hydrocortisone Emergency Injection kit** (100 mg hydrocortisone sodium succinate for injection; hyperlink to ADSHG and Pit foundation where there are picture tutorials on using this); check regularly that their kit is up to date.
- If a cause of permanent adrenal insufficiency is confirmed, the patient should be strongly advised to wear an identity bracelet to alert health-care professionals to their condition and potential need for immediate hydrocortisone in the event of an emergency.

Confirming the diagnosis

When well, definitive determination of adrenal status can be sought. If primary adrenal insufficiency is suspected (ACTH elevated at presentation), a short Synacthen test is done (Table 47.3). Alternative investigations (e.g. an insulin stress test) may be necessary for secondary adrenal insufficiency; seek advice from an endocrinologist.

Determining the cause

- If primary adrenal insufficiency is confirmed, further investigations such as adrenal autoantibodies and imaging of adrenal glands are required to elucidate the aetiology. Seek advice from an endocrinologist.
- If secondary adrenal insufficiency is identified, a thorough search for a history of exogenous steroid is the first step. Inhaled and topical steroids can be absorbed systemically in sufficient quantities to result in adrenal insufficiency if stopped abruptly. Glucocorticoids are also found in commercially available skin-lightening creams and are a common cause of Cushing's syndrome (followed by adrenal insufficiency after cessation) in certain demographic groups.
- In the absence of exogenous steroid, first-line investigations are directed at the pituitary gland. Seek advice from an endocrinologist.

Phaeochromocytoma/paraganglioma crisis

- Phaeochromocytomas/paragangliomas are tumours of chromatin cells, derived from neural crest tissues. They most commonly occur in the adrenal medulla in which instance they are called phaeochromocytomas.
- They often secrete catecholamines (adrenaline, noradrenaline and dopamine) but may secrete other hormones as well.
- Usually present between the ages of 20 and 50 years, with earlier presentation increasing the likelihood that they are due to a genetic syndrome.
- They can present with life-threatening catecholamine-induced crises (Table 47.4).

Table 47.4 When to consider a catecholamine-induced crisis.

Severe hypertension
Headache, palpitation and sweating
Acute pulmonary oedema
Acute regional ischaemia (limb/mesenteric)
Encephalopathy with hypertension
Acute chest pain with hypertension
Heart failure with hypertension
Acute kidney injury with hypertension
Any acute presentation in a patient with known genetic associate: neurofibromatosis, von Hippel-Lindau, MEN 2, previous paraganglioma (SDH mutation)

- Crises may be triggered by administration of drugs, such as dopamine antagonists, tricyclic antidepressants, radiocontrast media or anaesthetic agents.
- Manipulation of the tumour is likely to trigger a crisis in a patient without sufficient alpha-adrenergic blockade and exclusion of catecholamine excess is necessary prior to surgery on any tumour located at a site typical for paraganglioma and phaeochromocytoma.
- Usually, sporadic but are also associated with several genetic syndromes including multiple endocrine neoplasia (type 2A or 2B), von Hippel-Lindau disease, succinate dehydrogenase (SDH) mutations and neurofibromatosis type 1.

Priorities

In the patient presenting with a suspected catecholamine-induced crisis (Table 47.4), the following goals should be achieved in the first hour of treatment:

- Rapid assessment of airway, breathing, circulation and conscious level in a high dependency or critical care environment, with continuous monitoring of heart rate, blood pressure and arterial oxygen saturation. Consider an arterial line for invasive monitoring.
- Airway management if the airway is compromised or the Glasgow Coma Scale score is less than 8.
- Supplemental oxygen if needed to maintain SaO_2 >94%.
- Intravenous access with blood sent for urgent investigations (Table 47.5).
- Assess for organ failure:
  - Cardiovascular: arrhythmias, heart failure, ischaemic stroke, intracranial bleed, vasospastic peripheral ischaemia, myocardial infarction, aortic dissection or aneurysmal rupture
  - Respiratory: pulmonary oedema
  - Neurological: encephalopathy
  - Renal: acute kidney injury
  - Haematological: disseminated intravascular coagulation
- In the absence of organ failure, see further management for advice on commencing alpha blockade with oral phenoxybenzamine. If organ failure is present, intravenous alpha blockade may be necessary. Phentolamine is the preferred agent, delivered as a slow IV bolus 5–15 mg every 5–15 min as necessary (after the initial test dose of 1 mg) or continuous infusion (100 mg in 500 mL of 5% dextrose water and rate titrated with blood pressure monitoring via an arterial line. Caution is required; the circulating volume may be substantially reduced as a physiological response to increased vascular resistance. When reversed rapidly,

Table 47.5 Investigation of suspected catecholamine-induced crisis.

Urgent
ECG
Echocardiography
Chest X-ray
Arterial blood gases, pH and lactate (high lactate not necessarily indicative of ischaemic tissue, may be raised by direct effect of catecholamines on cellular metabolism)
Blood metadrenaline, normetadrenaline and dopamine concentration
Full blood count
Coagulation screen
Biochemical profile
Triple-phase adrenal CT scan (or in and out of phase adrenal MRI)

Later
Base of skull to pelvis imaging if adrenal imaging negative
Nuclear medicine imaging ([123] I-mIBG)
Further investigation to be directed by neuroendocrine tumour multidisciplinary team

a dramatic fall in blood pressure may ensue. Intravenous alpha blockade must be accompanied by aggressive intravenous filling to replace this missing volume as the arterial resistance falls.

- Identify the precipitant and commence appropriate management.
- Common ITU interventions to be avoided: Labetalol for BP control (at least not as initial therapy) and noradrenergic inotropic support.
- Involve a specialist endocrinology team at the earliest opportunity.

Further management
Biochemical confirmation

If organ failure is not present, confirmation of pathological elevation of catecholamines should be sought by measuring catecholamines or their metabolites (metanephrines) in the urine or blood. Plasma metanephrine levels are the most specific of these tests and less susceptible to the effects of intercurrent illness than levels of adrenaline or noradrenaline themselves. The vast majority of paragangliomas will secrete one or both of these hormones, pure dopamine-secreting paragangliomas are very rare.

Imaging

Dedicated cross-sectional imaging (CT or MRI) of the adrenal glands should be undertaken to localize the tumour. If negative, imaging from neck to pelvis is required.

Functional imaging is also useful as it may identify metastases and/or confirm uptake of a tracer by malignant paragangliomas, which may then be utilized in targeted radiotherapy should this be necessary post-surgery (peptide-receptor radionuclide therapy). ^{131}I-meta-IodoBenzylGuanidine (mIBG) is most commonly used.

Adrenergic blockade

Alpha blockade using phenoxybenzamine at an initial dose of 10 mg 12-hourly PO should be initiated once the diagnosis is confirmed. This carries a risk of inducing profound hypotension and is best undertaken as an inpatient. This allows for more rapid up-titration of the dose and more accurate fluid replacement as the degree of alpha blockade increases. The dose is sequentially increased until normotension is achieved or adverse effects (chiefly nasal congestion and postural hypotension) become intolerable.

Beta blockade to control tachycardia or tachyarrhythmia only to be commenced once adequate alpha blockade is in place.

There is no specific consensus on blood pressure and heart rate targets; however, it is recommended to reach a seated blood pressure target <130/80 mmHg. Targets for heart rate should be 60–70 bpm in a seated and 70–80 bpm in an upright position, respectively.

Multidisciplinary management

Early involvement of the surgical team to plan surgery is important, and management of paragangliomas/phaeochromocytomas is best under a multidisciplinary team of endocrinologists, endocrine surgeons, radiologists and nuclear medicine physicians.

Consider a genetic syndrome

In those with a family history or who are aged <60, the possibility of a genetic syndrome should be considered. Evidence of neurofibromatosis type 1 (café-au-lait spots, cutaneous neurofibromata), multiple endocrine neoplasia type 2A (medullary thyroid cancer, hyperparathyroidism) or type 2B (as for type 2A plus Marfanoid habitus, and mucosal ganglioneuromas) and von Hippel Lindau (haemangioblastoma, renal cell cancer, pancreatic islet cell tumours) should be sought.

If genetic testing confirms a diagnosis of these conditions or of SDH mutation, appropriate cascade screening of family members is necessary and referral to a clinical geneticist is required.

Genetic testing criteria for inherited phaeochromocytoma and paraganglioma excluding NF1

Testing of individual (proband) affected with disease where the individual +/− family history meets one of the following criteria. The proband has:

1 Phaeochromocytoma <60 years, OR

2 Any paraganglioma OR metastatic phaeochromocytoma at any age, OR

3 3.Phaeochromocytoma/paraganglioma with loss of staining for SDH proteins on IHC, OR

4 Bilateral phaeochromocytoma (any age), OR

5 Phaeochromocytoma and renal cell carcinoma (any age), OR

6 Phaeochromocytoma/paraganglioma (any age) AND ≥1 relative (first/second/third degree relative) with phaeochromocytoma/paraganglioma/renal cell cancer (any age)/gastrointestinal stromal tumour

Further reading

Charmandari E, Nicolaides NC, Chrousos GP. (2014) Adrenal insufficiency. *Lancet* 383, 2152–2167.

Lenders JWM, Duh Q-Y, Graeme Eisenhofer G, *et al*. (2014) Phaeochromocytoma and paraganglioma: an Endocrine Society clinical practice guideline. *J Clin Endocrinol Metab* 99, 1915–1942.

Society for Endocrinology (2016). Endocrine Emergency Guidance. Emergency management of acute adrenal insufficiency (adrenal crisis) in adult patients. http://www.endocrineconnections.com/content/5/5/G1.

CHAPTER 48

Disorders of anterior and posterior pituitary

ZAW YE HTET

Pituitary apoplexy

Pituitary apoplexy is a rare clinical syndrome comprising sudden-onset severe headache accompanied by visual deficit, extraocular muscle nerve palsy or reduced conscious level. It may be misdiagnosed as meningitis or subarachnoid haemorrhage.

Pituitary apoplexy results from haemorrhage into or infarction of a pre-existing pituitary tumour, and is almost invariably associated with hypopituitarism. A prior diagnosis of pituitary tumour is usually absent, with the apoplexy representing the first presentation of a previously unrecognized tumour in 80% of cases.

Patients with pituitary apoplexy should, once stabilized, be transferred to a neurosurgical centre for the multidisciplinary management of an experienced pituitary surgeon, neuro-ophthalmologist and endocrinologist.

Priorities
Consider the diagnosis

- Headache is usually frontal, although may take any form. It is primarily caused by pressure effects in the pituitary fossa and often induces nausea and vomiting.
- If blood escapes into the subarachnoid space, this may be accompanied by meningism. Cranial nerve III, IV and VI palsies result from compression of the adjacent cavernous sinuses, and visual field/acuity deficits from compression of the optic chasm lying superior to the fossa. Haemorrhage and the resultant pressure effects may not be maximal at presentation and repeated examination is essential to detect progressive neurological deficit, the presence of which may trigger escalation to emergency neurosurgical intervention.
- Some degree of pituitary hormone insufficiency is a feature of most cases of apoplexy, with adrenocorticotropic hormone (ACTH) and consequently cortisol insufficiency being both common, and the most important of these. If severe enough this may manifest as haemodynamic instability, since the lack of glucocorticoid obtunds the pressor effect of catecholamine signals. Delay in glucocorticoid replacement in these patients may be fatal.
- Apoplexy may be precipitated by many factors; hypertension, major surgery, especially coronary artery bypass grafting, dynamic testing of the pituitary gland, anticoagulation therapy, coagulopathies, pregnancy and head trauma.

Resuscitate the patient

In the first hour of treatment the following goals should be achieved:

- Rapid assessment of airway, breathing, circulation and conscious level.
- Airway management if the airway is compromised or the Glasgow Coma Scale score is less than 8.
- Supplemental oxygen, if needed to achieve arterial saturation 94–96%.
- Fluid resuscitation in the shocked or otherwise haemodynamically compromised patient, with the addition of immediate administration of a sufficient dose of glucocorticoid on the presumption of ACTH insufficiency, for example 100–200 mg intravenous hydrocortisone to be followed by 50–100 mg every 6 h (preferably by intramuscular injection as this provides a predictable pharmacokinetic profile and therefore more consistent glucocorticoid activity when compared to intravenous boluses) or 200 mg per 24 h infusion after bolus dose.
- Also, consider empirical steroid replacement in patients with altered conscious level, reduced visual acuity and severe visual field defect.
- Visual field examination by confrontation (with a red pin if available), Snellen chart visual acuity and cranial nerve III, IV, Va and VI examination. Document these clearly in the notes for later comparison.
- Request urgent dedicated pituitary imaging, preferably magnetic resonance imaging (MRI) as this is the most sensitive modality. General cerebral imaging not dedicated to the pituitary fossa cannot be relied upon to reveal the diagnosis, with CT demonstrating a pituitary mass in less than 80% of cases and pituitary haemorrhage in only 20%.
- Other investigations needed urgently are given in Table 48.1.

Further management

- Once stabilised, take a history, seeking symptoms of pituitary hormone insufficiency, including menstrual changes, sexual dysfunction, any constitutional changes in weight, skin, hair, bowel habit, energy levels and symptoms of specific hormone excess, including those of acromegaly, Cushing's syndrome, hyperprolactinaemia (galactorrhoea, oligomenorrhoea and hypogonadism) and thyrotoxicosis.
- Once recovered from acute episode, hydrocortisone should be tapered to standard maintenance oral dose, that is 20 mg/day in divided doses.
- You should liaise with the local centre of expertise to arrange a safe and early transfer.
- Surgical intervention should be considered in
  - Severely reduced visual acuity
  - Severe and persistent visual field defects
  - Deteriorating level of consciousness

Table 48.1 Urgent investigations in suspected pituitary apoplexy.

Urea, creatinine and electrolytes

Blood glucose

Venous blood gas and lactate

Baseline pituitary profile: cortisol and ACTH (before hydrocortisone), thyroid stimulating hormone (TSH) and free T4, prolactin, growth hormone, insulin-like growth factor-1

luteinizing hormone, follicular-stimulating hormone and testosterone (male) or oestradiol (female)

Full blood count

Coagulation screen

C-reactive protein

Blood culture

Urine microscopy and culture

Chest X-ray

ECG

MRI brain

Studies have shown significantly greater improvement in visual acuity and visual field defects in patients who had early surgery (within eight days).

- Urine output should be carefully monitored and if averaging more than 200 mL/h for two consecutive hours may indicate posterior pituitary impairment and the onset of arginine vasopressin (AVP) deficiency (cranial diabetes insipidus). Co-existing ACTH and cortisol deficiency can mask AVP deficiency, which can become more prominent after staring steroid replacement. Paired serum and urine osmolalities should be sent (and processed) urgently. If plasma osmolality is >285 mOsmol/L and urine osmolality is <300 mOsmol/L (inappropriately diluted urine), desmopressin can be given, for example as a 1 µgm subcutaneous injection. A urinary catheter must be inserted for fluid balance monitoring. In all but those with no adverse signs, hourly neurological assessment should be carried out (to include Glasgow Coma Scale and cranial nerve examination with visual fields) until stability has been established.
- Formal neuro-ophthalmological assessment in the form of visual fields (Humphrey or Goldmann perimetry) and gaze palsy assessment (e.g. Hess chart) should be completed as soon as is practicable and daily thereafter.
- If serial neurological examination reveals rapidly deteriorating signs or reducing conscious level, repeat contact with the neurosurgical team is required to arrange transfer for emergency surgery.
- If the patient is clinically stable or improving, continue conservative management.
- In case of secondary hypothyroidism, it is important to rule out cortisol deficiency or ensure adequate steroid replacement first before starting levothyroxine.
- Prior to discharge, provide Steroid Emergency Card, education on sick days rules (see Box 48.1) and hydrocortisone emergency injection kit.
- Long-term follow-up by endocrine and neurosurgical teams.

Box 48.1 Pituitary apoplexy – alerts.

- Consider pituitary apoplexy in any patient with sudden onset severe headache.
- Once stabilized, the patient with pituitary apoplexy should be managed by a specialist multidisciplinary team of neurosurgeons, ophthalmologists and endocrinologists.
- Glucocorticoid replacement is a life-saving intervention and should be administered without delay in patients with cardiovascular compromise.

Hypophysitis

Hypophysitis is a rare inflammatory condition of the pituitary.

Causes include infection: (TB, syphilis), infiltration (sarcoidosis), autoimmune (lymphocytic hypophysitis) and immunotherapy/checkpoint inhibitor induced.

With increased usage of checkpoint inhibitor immunotherapy such as ipilimumab (CTLA-4 inhibitor), nivolumab and pembrolizumab (PD-1 inhibitors) as they significantly improve prognosis in a number of cancers, immune-mediated hypophysitis has become a more common presentation to acute medicine, and can be life threatening if not recognised and treated appropriately.

Clinical features

Hypophysitis can present with hormonal defects, mass effect or both.

Hypopituitarism (ACTH and TSH deficiency, less commonly gonadotrophin and GH deficiency).

Posterior pituitary can also be involved resulting in AVP deficiency (Cranial Diabetes Insipidus).

Mass effect: headache, visual field defect, cranial nerves palsy.

Investigations

Random cortisol and ACTH (before any steroid treatment)

FBC, CRP, U&E, LFT, glucose

TSH, T4, LH, FSH, oestradiol/testosterone, prolactin

MRI Pituitary as soon as possible, but urgently if there is mass effect

Management

- Features of acute cortisol deficiency may be non-specific, and patients receiving checkpoint inhibitors and acutely unwell should be assumed to have acute cortisol deficiency (can also be from checkpoint inhibitor-induced adrenalitis, but management is the same in the acute setting) until proven otherwise, and treated with empirical steroid replacement until serum cortisol result is available.
- Fluid resuscitation.
- Hydrocortisone 100 mg IV or IM stat followed by infusion of 200 mg per 24 h. Alternatively, 50 mg of hydrocortisone IM or IV 6 hourly.
- Random cortisol level >450 nmol/L excludes cortisol deficiency, and steroids can be stopped and reassessment of the causes of signs and symptoms is required. (The cortisol cut-off value may vary depending on the assay, and consultation with local laboratory/biochemistry is recommended.)
- If cortisol <450 nmol/L, continue IV/IM/infusion hydrocortisone until clinically stabilised (usually 24–48 h) and then tapered to oral maintenance dose, that is 20 mg/day in divided doses.
- It is important to obtain a good drug history with regards to recent glucocorticoid use to enable correct interpretation of cortisol result.
- Methylprednisolone is usually not required for acute cortisol deficiency but may be beneficial if there is mass effect: visual field defect, cranial nerves palsy and intractable headache. Additional hydrocortisone is not required if methylprednisolone is used for these indications.
- Immunotherapy can be continued once the patient is clinically stable on steroid replacement.
- If there is significant polyuria (>200 mL per hour for 2 consecutive hours), polydipsia and hypernatraemia after steroid replacement, AVP deficiency (cranial diabetes insidious) from posterior pituitary involvement should be considered. Urgently send paired serum osmolality and urine osmolality. If serum osmolality >285 mOsmol/L and urine osmolality <300 mOsmol/L, AVP deficiency is likely. Consider SC desmopressin 1 mcg stat with close monitoring of intake output, and seek endocrine input.
- Short Synacthen Test can be falsely reassuring if it is done within 6–12 weeks of acute hypophysitis.
- Before discharge, patients should be provided with a Steroid Emergency Card, education with regards to 'sick day rules' (see Box 48.2), and a hydrocortisone emergency injection kit.
- Follow up with endocrinology on discharge.

Box 48.2 Sick day rules.

Sick day rule 1: the need to double daily oral glucocorticoid dose during illness with fever that requires bed rest and/or antibiotics

Sick day rule 2: the need to administer glucocorticoids per IV or IM injection during prolonged vomiting or diarrhoea, during preparation for colonoscopy or in case of acute trauma or surgery

Further reading

Society for Endocrinology (2016). Endocrine Emergency Guidance. Emergency management of pituitary apoplexy in adult patients. http://www.endocrineconnections.com/content/5/5/G12.
Society for Endocrinology (2018). Endocrine Emergency Guidance: Endocrine Emergency Guidance for the acute management of the endocrine complications of checkpoint inhibitor therapy.

CHAPTER 49

Thyroid emergencies

GEETHA BHAT AND MICHELLE STEFANELLI

Thyroid storm

The diagnosis of thyroid storm should be considered in any patient with fever, abnormal mental state, sinus tachycardia or atrial fibrillation, who may have signs of thyrotoxicosis.

- Thyroid storm is an acute life-threatening metabolic emergency caused by extremely high levels of thyroid hormone activity and is characterized by exaggerated manifestations of thyrotoxicosis.
- It usually occurs in inadequately treated thyrotoxic patients often triggered by severe stress and manifested by decompensation of multiple organs.
- It is associated with a high mortality rate (20%) if not treated promptly.
- If the diagnosis is suspected, antithyroid treatment must be started before biochemical confirmation. Adequate beta blockade to neutralize the associated autonomic overdrive is also essential.
- It is important to note that Thyroid Stimulating Hormone (TSH) levels do not distinguish thyroid storm from thyrotoxicosis.

Thyrotoxicosis is the syndrome resulting from supranormal thyroid hormone activity, and is usually the result of hyperthyroidism, defined as increased thyroid hormone production by the native thyroid gland. Causes are summarized in Table 49.1.

Priorities

Is this thyroid storm?

- The diagnosis of thyroid storm is clinical, and rests on the identification of actual or impending decompensation of organ function due to thyrotoxicosis (Table 49.2).
- The most common system used to help diagnose thyroid storm early is the Burch–Wartofsky score. Using this system, the following criteria must be met:
  - Elevated Free T3 (FT3) and/or Free T4 (FT4)
  - At least one CNS manifestation- restlessness, delirium, psychosis, lethargy or coma
  - One or more other symptoms
    - Fever 38 °C or higher
    - Tachycardia (130 bpm or more/ Afib)
    - Heart failure – pulmonary edema (NYHA class III or IV)
    - Gastrointestinal dysfunction

Table 49.1 Causes of hyperthyroidism.*

Autoimmune	Graves' disease**
	Hashitoxicosis
	Postpartum thyroiditis
Immune check point inhibitor	Use of immune check point inhibitor
Infectious	Subacute thyroiditis
	Pyogenic thyroiditis
Nodular	Solitary adenoma
	Toxic multinodular goiter
Neoplastic	Differentiated thyroid carcinoma (rare, mostly follicular)
Secondary	TSHoma
	Thyroid hormone resistance
	Hyperemesis gravidarum
	Hydatidiform mole/choriocarcinoma
Destructive	Amiodarone-induced thyrotoxicosis type 2 (AIT-2)
	Trauma
	Irradiation
	Lithium
Iodine excess	Amiodarone-induced thyrotoxicosis type 1 (AIT-1)
(Jod-Basedow phenomenon)	Iodine contrast
	Dietary (moving from iodine deficient to iodine rich area)

*Other causes are oversupply of exogenous thyroid hormone in patients taking levothyroxine or other thyroid supplements, and very rarely, ectopic thyroid hormone production by an ovarian teratoma (struma ovarii).
**Pathognomonic features of Graves' disease include the presence of thyroid eye disease, pretibial myxedema, thyroid acropachy, or a bruit over the enlarged thyroid gland.

- Can also meet diagnostic criteria with labs indicative of thyrotoxicosis plus 3 or more other non-CNS manifestations
- Elderly patients may not show typical symptoms of thyrotoxicosis and hepatic manifestations (nausea, vomiting, diarrhoea)

What has triggered the thyroid storm?

- Thyroid storm may occur in the course of the natural history of an underlying thyrotoxic process but is more often related to decompensation caused by an intercurrent precipitating illness. This is most frequently an infection but may also be surgery (particularly thyroid surgery or occasionally non-thyroid surgery), other critical illness or childbirth.
- Other iatrogenic causes include radioactive iodine therapy in patients with insufficiently controlled hyperthyroidism, abrupt cessation of antithyroid medications (usually due to non-adherence), administration of iodine-containing pharmaceuticals (e.g. amiodarone or contrast agents), or induction of anesthesia.

Immediate management and stabilization

Thyroid storm is an acutely life-threatening condition and must be managed in a higher dependency setting (resuscitation area/ HDU/ICU). The immediate management priorities in the first hour are:

- Rapid assessment of airway, breathing, circulation and level of consciousness. Continuous monitoring of blood pressure, heart rate and ECG.
- Airway management by experienced staff if the airway is compromised or the Glasgow Coma Scale score is less than 8.
- Supplemental oxygen as needed, to maintain arterial oxygen saturation 94–96%.
- Hemodynamic stabilization. Hypotension may be due to high output cardiac failure or a compromising tachyarrhythmia (usually supraventricular). DC cardioversion may well be unsuccessful for A.Fib in a severely

Table 49.2 Burch and Wartofsky score for diagnosis of thyrotoxic storm in a patient with elevated thyroid levels

Criteria	Points
Thermoregulatory dysfunction	
Temperature	
Less than 37.2 °C (99.0 °F)	0
37.2–37.7 °C (99.0–99.9 °F)	5
37.8–38.2 °C (100.0–100.9 °F)	10
38.3–38.8 °C (101.0–101.9 °F)	15
38.9–39.3 °C (102.0–102.9 °F)	20
39.4–39.9 °C (103.0–103.9 °F)	25
40.0 °C or higher (104 °F or higher)	30
Cardiovascular	
Heart rate	
Less than 100	0
100–109	5
110–119	10
120–129	15
130–139	20
140 or higher	25
Atrial fibrillation	
Absent	0
Present	10
Congestive heart failure	
Absent	0
Mild	5
Moderate	10
Severe	20
Gastrointestinal/hepatic dysfunction	
Manifestation	
Absent	0
Moderate (diarrhoea, abdominal pain, nausea/vomiting)	10
Severe (jaundice)	20
Central nervous system disturbance	
Manifestation	
Absent	0
Mild (agitation)	10
Moderate (delirium, psychosis, extreme lethargy)	20
Severe (seizure/coma)	30
Precipitant history	
Status	
Present	0
Absent	10
Interpretation	
Total score	**Interpretation**
<25	Thyrotoxic storm unlikely
25–45	Impending thyrotoxic storm
>45	Thyrotoxic storm confirmed

Source: Burch HB, Wartofsky L (1993) Life-threatening hyperthyroidism: thyroid storm. *Endocrinol Metab Clin North Am* 22, 263–277. Reproduced with permission of Elsevier.

hyperthyroid patient. Unless there is clinical suspicion of underlying cardiomyopathy, rate-related failure may be managed with a short-acting beta blocker (e.g. IV esmolol) with prompt withdrawal if clinical state worsens. Patient with thyroid storm and heart failure to be managed in an intensive care environment, with continuous BP and CVP monitoring.

- Assessment for common precipitants of thyroid storm: sepsis, diabetic ketoacidosis, or myocardial infarction (see above). If identified, appropriate management should be initiated. When no precipitating factor is apparent, broad-spectrum antibiotics are warranted until intercurrent infection has been excluded. Other precipitating causes can be managed in the usual manner.
- Cooling measures should be employed to correct fever, initially with paracetamol (acetaminophen) 1000 mg PO/IV.
- Transfer to the Intensive Care Unit (ICU) for further management.

Further management

The treatment of thyroid storm can be broken down into categories based on the effect on thyroid hormone. The management is directed towards blocking further production of thyroid hormone, blocking its release, blocking conversion of the inactive T4 to active T3 and limiting the adrenergic effects of high thyroid hormone activity. Eventually all patients will need definitive therapy which is either radioactive iodine ablation or thyroidectomy.

Refer to Table 49.3 for additional information on route and dosing of medications.

- Thionamides are initiated to prevent production of new thyroid hormone. Propylthiouracil is the preferred agent due to its additional benefit in reducing peripheral conversion of T4 to T3. Due to Propylthiouracil's association with fulminant hepatitis, a rare but potentially fatal complication, methimazole should be considered in those with known liver disease. These medications are given orally or via a feeding tube. Rectal and IV formulations may be considered when the oral route is contraindicated.
- Beta blockers should be used to negate the catecholaminergic effects of thyrotoxicosis. In the setting of acute thyrotoxic storm for rapid onset of action and inability to take oral medications, intravenous esmolol should be used. Consider an arterial line for continuous blood pressure monitoring if IV beta blockers are initiated. The dose is titrated according to cardiovascular parameters. Once the patient is stable and able to tolerate oral medications, propranolol is the preferred agent given its additional capacity to block peripheral T4 to T3 conversion.
- Glucocorticoids in the form of IV hydrocortisone are critical in supporting circulation and reducing the peripheral effects of thyroid hormone by decreasing peripheral conversion of T4 to T3.
- Therapy against thyroid hormone release such as 'Cold' iodine (i.e. non-radioactive iodine) can be administered in the form of Lugol's solution (5% elemental iodine, 10% potassium iodide in distilled water) or a saturated solution of potassium iodide (SSKI) diluted in water. These make use of the Wolff-Chaikoff effect in which high doses of iodine result in a blockade of the incorporation of iodine into thyroglobulin. This should be administered at least 1 hour after administration of thionamides to prevent the iodine from being used as substrate. Effectiveness of iodine solutions is time-limited to around ten days, after which the thyroid escapes this effect by down-regulating iodine transporters.
- Finally, thyroid hormone clearance can be enhanced through using medications such as cholestyramine.
- In extreme treatment refractory thyrotoxicosis, plasmapheresis has been used to clear circulating thyroid hormones to allow a window for emergency thyroidectomy to be performed safely.

Myxoedema coma

At the opposite end of the spectrum to thyroid storm lies the rare endocrine emergency of myxoedema coma, which has a prevalence of less than 1 per million per year, and is largely a disease of the elderly. The physical signs of hypothermia from whatever cause closely resemble those of myxoedema coma; however, if there is

Table 49.3 Therapy for thyroid storm.

Therapy against new thyroid hormone production – Thionamides	Dose/route/frequency for loading and maintenance
Propylthiouracil	PO loading dose of 500–1000 mg followed by 250 mg every 4 h OR Rectal dose of 400–600 mg every 6 h
Methimazole	IV 10–30 mg every 8–6 h OR PO 60–120 mg/day in 4–6 doses OR Rectal 20–40 mg every 8–6 h
Carbimazole	PO 20–30 mg every 4–6 h
Therapy blocking the catecholaminergic affects	
Esmolol	IV loading dose of 250–500 mcg/kg followed by 50–100 mcg/kg/min
Propranolol	IV 0.5–1.0 mg over 10 min followed by 10–2.0 mg over 10 min every few hours OR PO 60–120 mg every 4–6 h
Glucocorticoids blocking peripheral conversion	
Hydrocortisone	IV loading dose of 300 mg followed by 100 mg every 8 h
Therapy against thyroid hormone release (administer at least 1 h after thionamide)	
SSKI	PO 5 drops every 6 h OR Rectal 250–500 mg every 6 h
Lugol's solution	PO 8 drops every 6 h OR Rectal 5–10 drops every 8–6 h (max 80 drops/day)
Sodium iodide	IV 0.5 g every 12 h
Lithium	PO 300 mg every 4–6 h
Therapy enhancing thyroid hormone clearance	
Cholestyramine	1–4 g twice/day

other evidence of hypothyroidism, then thyroid hormone and hydrocortisone prior (in case there is coexisting autoimmune adrenal insufficiency) should be given. Even with treatment, mortality is high as 25%.

Priorities

Is this myxoedema coma?

- Hypothermia and altered mental status are the cardinal features (although most patients are not actually comatose, i.e. Glasgow Coma Scale score <8).
- A history of hypothyroidism, previous radioactive iodine treatment, thyroidectomy (look for scar on neck), and proceeding symptoms of hypothyroidism (weight gain with reduced appetite, dry skin and hair loss) are indications that myxedema coma should be considered.
- Bradycardia, bradypnea, hypoxemia and hypotension are common.
- Hyponatremia, hypercapnia, hypercalcemia, hypoglycemia and elevated creatinine kinase are often present.

Table 49.4 A score >60 highly suggestive/diagnostic of myxedema coma. A score 25–59 supportive of diagnosis of myxedema coma. A score <25 myxedema coma unlikely.

Thermoregulatory dysfunction (temperature °F/°C)	Points	Cardiovascular dysfunction	Points
>95/35	0	**Bradycardia/Heart rate (beats/min)**	
89.6–95/32–35	10	Absent	0
<89.6/32 20	20	50–59	10
		40–49	20
Central nervous system effects		<40	30
Absent	0		
Somnolent/Lethargy	10	ECG changes (QT prolongation, BBB, low voltage, heart block, ST changes)	10
Obtunded	15	Pericardial/pleural effusion	19
Stupor	20	Pulmonary edema	15
Coma/seizures	30	Cardiomegaly	15
		Hypotension	20
Gastrointestinal findings			
Anorexia/abdominal pain/constipation	5	**Metabolic disturbances**	
Decreased intestinal motility	15	Hyponatremia	10
Paralytic ileus	20	Hypoglycemia	10
		Hypoxemia	10
Precipitating event		Hypercarbia	10
Absent	0	Decrease in GFR	10
Present	10		

- It is important to note that the degree of TSH elevation may not indicate the severity of hypothyroidism, as there may be variable suppression of the hypothalamic-pituitary axis.
- A diagnostic scoring system for myxedema coma can be useful in establishing a diagnosis (Table 49.4).

What has caused myxoedema coma?

- Myxedema coma is usually precipitated by an event causing an increased metabolic demand which outstrips the adaptive mechanisms compensating for chronic hypothyroidism, such as infection or trauma.
- Other triggers include cold weather, sedative agents, general anesthesia, acute coronary syndrome, and stroke.

Immediate management

- ABCDE assessment
- **Airway**: may be compromised by oedema of the upper respiratory tract structures. Airway adjuncts or intubation may be required.
- **Breathing**: ventilatory failure is common and should be confirmed with arterial blood gas analysis. Assisted ventilation is often necessary for the first 24–48 h.
- **Circulation**: cautious fluid resuscitation, bearing in mind the likely impairment of cardiac contractility, can be employed. Glucocorticoids should be administered at least 1 h prior to thyroid hormone replacement (50–100 mg every 6-h IV) as severe hypothyroidism may impair ACTH response to stress. The possibility of undiagnosed autoimmune adrenal insufficiency as a comorbidity must be recognized and treated promptly to prevent precipitating acute adrenal crisis. Correct hypoglycemia using intravenous glucose
- Identify the precipitant and initiate treatment. Investigation needed urgently is given in Table 49.5.
- Infection may be occult and sepsis is unlikely to be accompanied by an elevated temperature. If in doubt, administer broad spectrum antibiotics.

Table 49.5 Urgent investigation in suspected myxedema coma.

Blood glucose
Creatinine and electrolytes
Plasma calcium and phosphate
Liver function tests
Creatine kinase
Full blood count
C-reactive protein
Arterial pH, gases and lactate
Blood and urine culture
Thyroid function tests (TSH, free T4, free T3)
Plasma cortisol
ECG
Chest X-ray
CT head

- The ECG will be abnormal and usually shows bradycardia, small voltage QRS complexes and flattened or inverted T-waves. Varying degrees of heart block may be present. Measure the QTc interval, which may be prolonged, bringing a risk of polymorphic ventricular tachycardia (torsades de pointes; see Chapter 13). Assess for evidence of myocardial ischemia or infarction.
- Cerebellar signs may be the result of severe hypothyroidism, but assess for evidence of an acute stroke.
- Assess for evidence of an upper gastrointestinal bleed.
- **Obtain a collateral history**: there will usually be a history of hypothyroidism, thyroid ablation, and/or medication non-compliance.
- Review the drug history for new medications, which may have precipitated the acute presentation. Alert the critical care team and transfer to an appropriate ICU.

Further management/thyroid hormone replacement

- Restoration of thyroid hormone activity is essential. There is no high-grade evidence to suggest how this is best achieved, but initial replacement via the intravenous route is strongly recommended following the administration of intravenous glucocorticoids if the concern for concurrent adrenal insufficiency has not been ruled out.
- Restoring normal target tissue thyroid hormone activity as soon as possible to reverse life-threatening disturbance of body systems must be weighed against the possibility of inducing fatal tachyarrhythmias with rapid correction.
- Initial treatment should be with intravenous levothyroxine, with a loading dose of 200–400 mcg. For patients who are older, smaller, or have a history of cardiovascular disease smaller doses should be considered, as the associated rapid increase in thyroid hormone receptor signaling may induce adverse cardiac events.
- Following the initial loading dose, patients can be treated with oral levothyroxine at weight-based dosing of 1.6 mcg/kg per body weight. The dose should be reduced to 75% of the calculated dose with intravenous administration.
- Administration of concurrent intravenous liothyronine at a loading dose of 5–20 mcg (followed by a dose of 2.5–10 mcg every 8 h) can be considered to combat the concern of decreased conversion to triiodothyronine in patients with myxedema coma. This is a weak recommendation with low-quality evidence. This should be dosed with caution as there is an association of high serum triiodothyronine with mortality.
- Once the patient improves clinically, treatment may be switched to oral therapy or another enteral route if oral administration is not possible. Treatment with liothyronine could be discontinued.

- Improvements in mental status, improved cardiac function, and pulmonary function can be expected within a week. Measurements of thyroid hormone levels every 1–2 days showing improvement can be reassuring. Failure of TSH to downtrend and thyroid hormone levels to improve may indicate a need for dosage adjustments. High serum T3 levels may indicate a need to decrease dose, but the TSH may take weeks to months to normalize completely. Over-replacement should be avoided as there is risk of tachyarrhythmias.

Supportive care

- Hypothermia should not be treated with active rewarming since this will induce peripheral vasodilatation, negating the compensatory diversion of blood flow to the vital organs. Passive rewarming with a blanket is preferred.
- Glucocorticoids should be continued until coexisting adrenal insufficiency (Chapter 47) has been excluded. Once patient is clinically improved, a Cosyntropin stimulation test can be performed, obtaining cortisol levels before and after administration of synthetic ACTH.
- Ongoing supportive management of organ failure (e.g. mechanical ventilation or vasopressors) while awaiting response to thyroid hormone replacement is a key determinant of outcome. The time to recovery may be variable depending on the duration of severe hypothyroidism. A multidisciplinary team approach is essential in successful management of these thyroid emergencies.

Further reading

Chiong YV, Bammerlin E, Mariash CN. (2015) Development of an objective tool for the diagnosis of myxedema coma. *Transl Res* 166, 233–243. DOI: 10.1016/j.trsl.2015.01.003.

De Leo S, Lee SY, Braverman LE. (2016) Hyperthyroidism. *Lancet* 388, 906–918.

Dixit S. (2014) A rare case of myxedema coma with neuroleptic malignant syndrome (NMS). *J Clin Diagn Res*. DOI: 10.7860/jcdr/2015/13008.5868.

Jonklaas J, Bianco AC, Bauer AJ, *et al*. (2014) Guidelines for the treatment of hypothyroidism: prepared by the American thyroid association task force on thyroid hormone replacement. *Thyroid* 24(12), 1670–1751. DOI: 10.1089/thy.2014.0028.

Matfin G, MSc (Oxon), MD ChB, FASCE, FACP (2014) A Clinician's guide Endocrine and metabolic Medical Emergencies 2014 by Endocrine society.

Sharp CS, Wilson MP, Nordstrom K. (2016) Psychiatric emergencies for clinicians: the Emergency Department management of thyroid storm. *J Emerg Med* 51, 155–158.

CHAPTER 50

Parathyroid disorders

AYE CHAN MAUNG AND CHRISTINE J.H. MAY

Hyperparathyroidism

Primary hyperparathyroidism (PHPT) is one of the most common causes of hypercalcemia particularly in ambulatory care settings. It is characterized by hypercalcemia due to autonomous overproduction of parathyroid hormone (PTH) (Table 50.1).

The overwhelming majority of PHPT patients are asymptomatic and often diagnosed incidentally on routine blood tests done for other medical indications. However, patients may present with symptoms of hypercalcaemia particularly when adjusted calcium is more than 3 mmol/L (Table 50.2, Figure 50.1).

Parathyroid crisis is a rare and potentially fatal complication of PHPT in which patients develop severe symptoms and signs of hypercalcemia. It is characterized by a serum calcium level usually greater than 3.5 mmol/L resulting from marked elevation of PTH with multiple organ dysfunction. It is associated with profound dehydration and impaired renal function, gastrointestinal and psychological disturbances. Cardiac arrhythmias, pancreatitis and neuromuscular disturbance can also occur. It is an endocrine emergency that requires aggressive medical therapy and early surgical treatment.

PHPT is most commonly due to solitary adenoma (80%), less commonly due to four-gland hyperplasia or multiple adenomas and very rarely due to parathyroid carcinoma (<1%). Although it is relatively rare, it can be associated with germline mutation especially when diagnosed at a younger age or with multiple gland involvement.

Table 50.1 Causes of hypercalcaemia.

PTH mediated
- Primary hyperparathyroidism (Sporadic or Familial)
- Familial hypocalciuric hypercalcaemia (Positive family history and calcium/creatinine clearance ratio <0.01)
- Tertiary hyperparathyroidism (in advanced chronic kidney disease patients)
- Lithium induced

Non-PTH mediated
- Malignancy (bony metastases, humoral hypercalcaemia and multiple myeloma)
- Medications (thiazides, PTH analogues, vitamin A or D overdose)
- Endocrine diseases (hyperthyroidism, Addison's disease, acromegaly and pheochromocytoma)
- Granulomatous diseases (sarcoidosis and tuberculosis)
- Miscellaneous (immobilisation and Milk alkali syndrome)

Acute Medicine: A Practical Guide to the Management of Medical Emergencies, Sixth Edition.
Edited by Mridula Rajwani, Leila Vaziri, and Ivie Gbinigie.

Table 50.2 Focused assessment in primary hyperparathyroidism patient.

History taking	Examination
Symptoms of hypercalcaemia (Ca > 3 mmol/L)	Signs of dehydration
Fatigue, lethargy, muscle weakness	Altered mental status
Polyuria, polydipsia	Band keratopathy
Depression, confusion	Neck lump, cervical lymphadenopathy
Constipation, abdominal pain, nausea, vomiting, anorexia	Blood pressure – can be elevated
Complications of PHPT	**Underlying aetiology**
Renal: Renal stones, nephrocalcinosis, renal impairment	Cutaneous lichen amyloidosis (MEN2)
Skeletal: Fragility fractures, osteoporosis, osteitis fibrosa cystica	Fibromas in the mandible/maxilla
Gastrointestinal: Peptic ulcer, pancreatitis	(PHPT-jaw tumour syndrome)
Underlying aetiology	
Personal/family history of hypercalcaemia or multiple endocrine neoplasia	
Drugs (lithium and thiazides)	

Familial hypocalciuric hypercalcemia (FHH) can show a similar biochemical picture, but usually, the degree of hypercalcemia and elevation in PTH are mild. Fractional excretion of urinary calcium is typically low (<1%) in FHH.

Tertiary hyperparathyroidism can manifest with raised PTH levels together with raised creatinine and phosphate levels in patients with end-stage kidney disease.

Lithium alters the set point of calcium-sensing receptor at the parathyroid glands for PTH secretion and induces parathyroid hyperplasia. The onset of hypercalcemia after initiation of lithium treatment could vary from months to years.

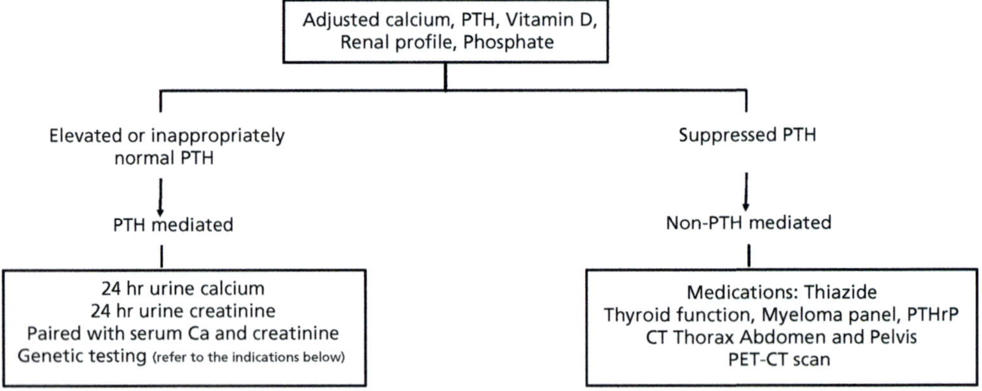

Figure 50.1 Initial biochemical work-up of a hypercalcaemic patient.

Treatment considerations

- The initial management of severe hypercalcaemia includes intravascular volume expansion with intravenous fluids, and parathyroidectomy if meeting surgical criteria (see below).
- Other treatment options depending on local protocols include subcutaneous calcitonin (if available) to promote calciuresis, intravenous bisphosphonate to exert strong anti-osteoclastic action and cinacalcet. Management of hypercalcaemia was discussed more detail in Chapter 52.
- The treatment of choice in symptomatic PHPT is parathyroid surgery (Table 50.3). Surgery remains the only definitive treatment. Localization studies (Figure 50.2) can provide useful information to the endocrine

surgeon in pre-operative planning and achieve successful focused parathyroidectomy. The success rate is greater than 95% in high-volume centres with experienced surgeons.

- Vitamin D deficiency is common in patients with PHPT. Pre-operative replacement with vitamin D (1000–2000 units of cholecalciferol daily) is safe and unlikely to exacerbate hypercalcaemia. Vitamin D optimisation reduces post-op hypocalcaemia.

Table 50.3 Indications for referral for surgery in asymptomatic primary hyperparathyroidism.

1. Age <50 years
2. Serum calcium >0.25 mmol/L above upper limit of normal range
3. Reduction in eGFR or creatinine clearance <60 mL/min
4. Nephrolithiasis or renal stone – symptomatic or identified on imaging
5. Bone mineral density (BMD) T-score ≤−2.5 at any site or previous fragility fracture or both

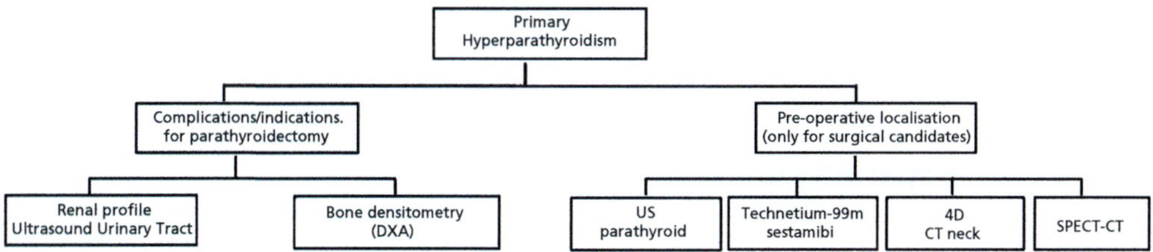

Figure 50.2 Investigations in a patient with confirmed PHPT.

Genetic testing in primary hyperparathyroidism

NHS England has developed eligibility criteria and available genetic panels for rare/inherited diseases. The current genetic testing criteria for PHPT based on version 6 (published 8 January 2024) includes:

i. age of diagnosis <50 years
   OR
ii. any age with:
   - a confirmed or relevant family history, OR
   - multiglandular disease or hyperplasia in the presence of relevant family history, OR
   - parathyroid carcinoma or atypical or cystic adenoma, OR
   - ossifying fibroma(s) of the maxilla and/or mandible.

Medical management of primary hyperparathyroidism

- Medical therapy can be considered in patients with PHPT who meet surgical criteria but are either unfit or unwilling to undergo surgery (Table 50.4).
- The choice of pharmacological agents depends on the primary indication and its intended effect on bone metabolism.
- Combination therapies could be considered if there is more than one clinical indication.

Table 50.4 Medical management of primary hyperparathyroidism.

Drug	Dose	Indication	Side effects
Cinacalcet	30 mg once – twice daily (maximum 960 mg/day)	Ca > 2.85 mmol/L with symptoms or Ca > 3 mmol/L	Headache, nausea, vomiting, dizziness
Bisphosphonates	E.g. Alendronate 70 mg weekly	Osteoporosis	Reflux and dyspepsia, rarely osteonecrosis of jaw, atypical femoral fractures
Denosumab	Subcutaneous 60 mg every six months	Osteoporosis	Cellulitis, eczema, hypocalcaemia

Monitoring in asymptomatic primary hyperparathyroidism

1 Serum calcium and renal profile – annually
2 Dual-energy X-ray absorptiometry (DXA) (ideally including distal 1/3 radius) and vertebral fracture assessment (VFA) – every two to three years
3 Ultrasound scan (US) of urinary tract – if renal stone suspected

Hypoparathyroidism

Hypoparathyroidism is due to either absent or deficient production of PTH in response to hypocalcaemia. It can present with acute hypocalcaemia to the acute medical take.

Severe hypocalcaemia is a life-threatening medical emergency and hence timely intervention is essential.

Causes of Hypoparathyroidism

- The most common cause of hypoparathyroidism is post-surgical (75%), with nonsurgical causes accounting for the remaining 25% of cases (Figure 50.3). Postoperative hypocalcaemia after anterior neck surgery is usually transient and resolves within six weeks after surgery in approximately 2/3 of cases.
- If hypoparathyroidism persists six months after neck surgery, it can be considered chronic or permanent.
- Serum magnesium level should always be checked as hypomagnesemia (particularly below 0.4 mmol/L) causes suppression as well as resistance to PTH action.

The clinical manifestations of hypoparathyroidism can vary from mild (perioral numbness, muscle cramps) to severe symptoms (seizure, laryngospasm and arrhythmias) depending on the severity and the rapidity of hypocalcaemia. Patients with long-standing hypocalcaemia due to chronic hypoparathyroidism can be asymptomatic despite significant biochemical derangements (Table 50.5).

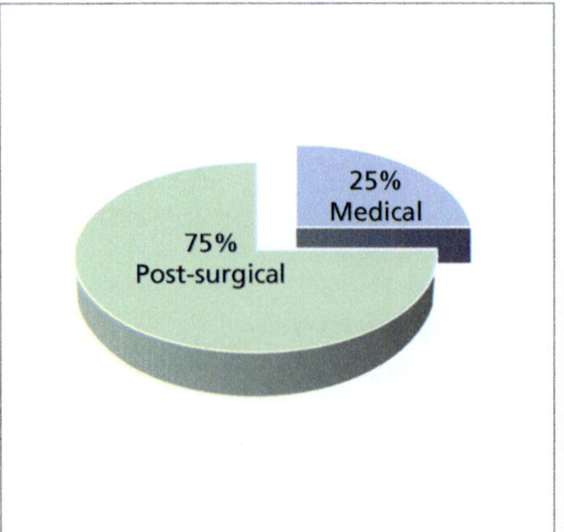

Figure 50.3 Causes of hypoparathyroidism.

Table 50.5 Focused assessment in hypoparathyroidism patient.

History taking	Examination
Symptoms of hypocalcaemia	**Signs of neuromuscular excitability**
Perioral or distal extremities paraesthesia	Trousseau's sign
Muscle cramps/weakness	Chvostek's sign
Tetany (carpopedal spasm)	Myoclonic jerks
Laryngospasm/Bronchospasm	Prolonged QTc on ECG
Confusion, Seizure	
Underlying aetiology	**Underlying aetiology**
History of neck surgery or radiation	Surgical neck scar
Personal/family history of autoimmune disease	Vitiligo, oral mucosa or nail bed candidiasis
Head and neck cancer	(Autoimmune polyendocrine syndrome)
Family history of hypoparathyroidism	Dysmorphic features, deafness (genetic causes)
Drugs (proton pump inhibitors [PPI], cinacalcet, immunotherapy)	Signs of chronic liver disease (Haemochromatosis, Wilson's disease)

Biochemical parameters suggesting hypoparathyroidism

- Hypocalcaemia: either adjusted total calcium or ionized calcium
- PTH: undetectable or inappropriately low/normal in the context of hypocalcaemia
- Hyperphosphatemia

Acute management

Mild hypocalcaemia (adjusted calcium >1.9 mmol/L) and asymptomatic

Oral calcium (e.g. AdCal, Calcichew, SandoCal etc) providing elemental calcium 2000–3000 mg in divided doses can be used with/without vitamin D supplements.

Severe hypocalcaemia (adjusted calcium <1.9 mmol/L) or symptomatic

1 Cardiac monitoring: risk of QTc prolongation and cardiac arrhythmias
2 10 mL of 10% calcium gluconate in 100 mL of 0.9% sodium chloride or 5% dextrose intravenously over 15 min with ECG monitoring.
3 This can be repeated until patient is asymptomatic.
4 Correct hypomagnesemia (if any) as per local trust guidelines
5 If persistently hypocalcaemic, consider intravenous infusion of calcium gluconate via central or large peripheral vein (prepare 100 mL of 10% calcium gluconate in 1 L of 0.9% sodium chloride and start at 50–100 mL/h and titrate to aim for adjusted calcium around 2.1–2.3 mmol/L)
6 Monitor serum calcium every 4–6 hours
7 Switch to oral calcium therapy once serum calcium stabilised, consider starting activated Vitamin D

Chronic management

- Patients with hypoparathyroidism have a deficiency of both PTH as well as 1,25 hydroxyvitamin D due to a lack of stimulation of 1α-hydroxylase enzyme in renal tubular cells in the absence of PTH (Table 50.6).
- Hence, 1-alpha hydroxylated vitamin D metabolites are necessary to correct the hypocalcaemia and facilitate the intestinal absorption of calcium. Calcitriol is approximately two times more potent than alfacalcidol in maintaining serum calcium within the target range.
- It is recommended to maintain serum calcium close to the lower limit of normal to reduce the risk of kidney stones and nephrocalcinosis.

Table 50.6 Medical management in hypoparathyroidism.

Medication	Dose
Calcium	1000–2000 mg of elemental calcium in divided doses
Calcium carbonate (40% elemental Ca): should be taken with food	
Calcium citrate (21% elemental Ca): preferred in achlorhydria, patients on PPI or post-bariatric surgery	
Active vitamin D	
Alfacalcidol	0.5–4 mcg daily
Calcitriol	0.25–2 mcg daily
Parental vitamin D	800–2000 IU daily
Cholecalciferol (vitamin D3)	
Ergocalciferol (vitamin D2)	

Treatment goals in chronic hypoparathyroidism

- Aim for a low normal adjusted calcium (2.0–2.25 mmol/L) and free of symptoms of hypocalcaemia
- Avoid hypercalciuria (can consider low calcium diets, limit sodium intake and Thiazide if hypercalciuric)
- Maintain normal serum phosphate
- Maintain vitamin D level >50 nmol/L
- Maintain normal magnesium level

Monitoring in chronic hypoparathyroidism

- Assessment of symptoms of hypocalcaemia and hypercalcaemia
- Bone profile (calcium, magnesium phosphate) and renal profile – every 6–12 monthly, (sooner, i.e. within one to two weeks after medication changes or acute admission related to hypocalcaemia or hypercalcaemia)
- 24-hour urine calcium – annually
- Ultrasound urinary tract – if renal stone suspected

Patient support groups

These are a great resource for both patients and clinicians.

Parathyroid UK – https://parathyroid uk.org gives information on both hypoparathyroidism and hyperparathyroidism.

Further reading

Hyperparathyroidism

Bilezikian JP, Silverberg SJ, Bandeira F, *et al.* (2022) Management of primary hyperparathyroidism. *J Bone Miner Res* 37(11), 2391–2403. DOI: 10.1002/jbmr.4682. Epub 2022 Oct 17. PMID: 36054638.

Bollerslev J, Rejnmark L, Zahn A, *et al.* (2022) European expert consensus on practical management of specific aspects of parathyroid disorders in adults and in pregnancy. *Eur J Endocrinol* 186(2), R33–R63. DOI: 10.1530/EJE-21-1044. PMID: 34863037; PMCID: PMC8789028.

NHS England – National Genomic Test Directory https://www.england.nhs.uk/wp-content/uploads/2018/08/Rare-and-inherited-disease-eligibility-criteria-version-6-January-2024.pdf.

Hypoparathyroidism

Bollerslev J, Rejnmark L, Marcocci C, *et al.* (2015) European society of endocrinology clinical guideline: treatment of chronic hypoparathyroidism in adults. *Eur J Endocrinol* 173(2), G1–G20. DOI: 10.1530/EJE-15-0628. PMID: 26160136.

Khan AA, Bilezikian JP, Brandi ML, *et al.* (2022) Evaluation and management of hypoparathyroidism summary statement and guidelines from the second international workshop. *J Bone Miner Res* 37(12), 2568–2585. DOI: 10.1002/jbmr.4691. Epub 2022 Nov 14. PMID: 36054621.

CHAPTER 51

Pancreatic endocrine disorders (non-diabetic)

SHANI A.D. MATHARA DIDHENIPOTHAGE AND BAHRAM JAFAR-MOHAMMADI

The endocrine pancreas constitutes discrete islets of Langerhans, that are composed of different cell types (alpha, beta, delta, epsilon, and F cells) secreting hormones that are essential for life; glucagon, insulin, somatostatin, and pancreatic polypeptide. Disorders of the endocrine pancreas are rare yet need to be suspected in common clinical presentations in the acute general medicine (AGM) department for early diagnosis and specialised management.

Functional pancreatic neuroendocrine neoplasms (P-NENs) that could present with common clinical syndromes to AGM are described in this chapter. Insulinomas and gastrinomas are the most common functional P-NENs, whilst glucagonomas and VIPomas, including other very rare functional P-NENs (somatostatinomas, GRHomas, ACTHomas) represent less than 10% of all P-NENs.

A patient presenting with recurrent severe hypoglycaemia (non-diabetic): Could this be an insulinoma?

Hypoglycaemia (Plasma glucose (PG) <3 mmol/L) is a common presentation to AGM. Recurrent hypoglycaemia fulfilling Whipple's triad (a) Symptoms/signs consistent with hypoglycaemia, b) Low PG measured at the time of the symptoms/signs, c) Relief to symptoms/signs when PG is raised to a normal level) in a patient with no diagnosis of diabetes mellitus, needs further evaluation to exclude insulinoma.

Symptoms of hypoglycaemia are classified as follows: a) autonomic symptoms; sweating, hunger, paraesthesia, tremor, anxiety, palpitations, and nausea; b) neuroglycopenic symptoms (PG < 2.2 mmol/L): dizziness, confusion, fatigue, difficulty in speaking or concentrating, headache, changes in vision, seizures, and loss of consciousness.

To confirm true hypoglycaemia, a plasma sample is recommended as capillary or continuous glucose monitoring devices may not be accurate at low levels. The patient's clinical history will help to establish the first investigations to be undertaken. If the episodes are after a fast, it is more likely to be related to an insulinoma (provided there are adequate glycogen stores). Post prandial hypoglycaemia, may necessitate a mixed meal test. If the patient has presented with hypoglycaemia, it may be an opportune time to check PG, insulin and c-peptide as per the figure below. However, in most cases a prolonged fast (up to 72 h), may be needed to establish the diagnosis.

Insulinomas are the commonest hormone secreting P-NENs, yet are still rare (Incidence 0.7- 4 cases per million per year), hence it is recommended to exclude more common causes of hypoglycaemia during evaluation (Figure 51.1 and Table 51.1). Most insulinomas are small, benign, and solitary pancreatic tumours. They commonly present in the 5th decade of life, however, can present earlier (2nd -3rd decade) when associated with multiple endocrine neoplasia type 1(MEN 1). Insulinomas associated with MEN 1 (16%) are usually bigger, multiple, and have high malignant risk (25%) and recurrence rate (Table 51.2).

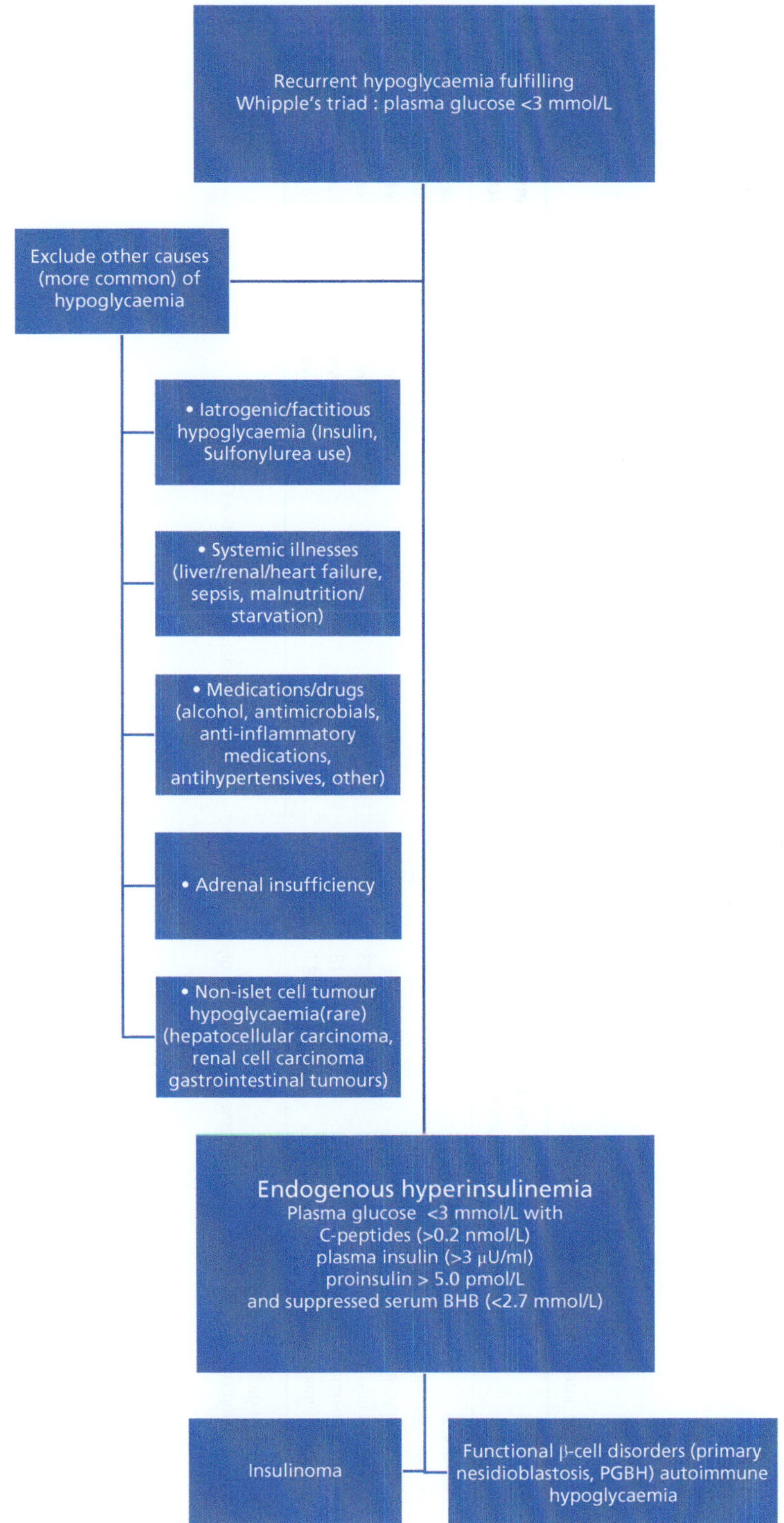

Figure 51.1 Hypoglycaemia. BHB, β-hydroxybutyrate; PGBH, post gastric bypass hypoglycaemia.

Table 51.1 Interpretation of biochemical tests in hypoglycaemia evaluation.

Diagnosis	Plasma glucose (mmol/L)	Insulin (pmol/L)	C-peptide (pmol/L)	Pro-insulin (pmol/L)	β-Hydroxybutyrate (mmol/L)	Blood hypoglycaemic agent screen	Insulin autoantibodies screen
Insulinoma	<3	≥18	≥200	≥5	≤2.7	Negative	Negative
Primary nesidioblastosis, PGBH	<3	≥18	≥200	≥5	≤2.7	Negative	Negative
Oral hypoglycaemic agent	<3	≥18	≥200	≥5	≤2.7	Positive	Negative
Exogenous insulin	<3	>>18	<200	<5	≤2.7	Negative	Negative
Insulin autoimmune syndrome	<3	>>18	>>200	>>5	≤2.7	Negative	Positive
Non-insulin mediated hypoglycaemia	<3	<18	<200	<5	>2.7	Negative	Negative

PGBH, post gastric bypass hypoglycaemia.

Source: Adopted from Evaluation and management of adult hypoglycaemic disorders: an Endocrine Society Clinical Practice Guideline

Table 51.2 Characteristics of insulinoma.

Clinical presentation	Diagnosis	Tumour localisation	Treatments		Prognosis
			Symptom control	**Specific treatment**	

• Recurrent hypoglycaemia (Fasting: 73%, post-prandial: 6%, both fasting and post-prandial: 21%)
• Weight gain
	• Biochemical interpretation as in Table 51.1
	• Provocative tests recommended if no spontaneous onset hypoglycaemia
	
	  i. over-night unsupervised fast
	  ii. 72 h prolonged supervised fast*
	  iii. mixed meal test: more post prandial symptoms
		• CECT/MRI pancreas
		• Endoscopic ultrasonography
		• ^{68}Gallium-DOTATATE-PET/CT
		• selective intraarterial calcium stimulation test (rarely performed If no visible disease)
			• Treat acute hypoglycaemia as per local guidelines
			• Frequent small meals with complex carbohydrates and food with low glycaemic index
			• Oral Diazoxide
			• SSA (Octreotide, Lanreotide)
			• PRRT
			• Everolimus
				• Surgery (±resection of metastases) is the only curative option
				• Liver directed therapy for metastases
				• PRRT
				• Chemotherapy
					• Good prognosis with benign tumours: 10-year survival ~88%
					• High recurrence rate with MEN 1 syndrome (21% in MEN 1 versus 7% in sporadic at 20 years)

CECT, Contrast enhanced computer tomography; MEN1, Multiple endocrine neoplasia 1, MRI, Magnetic resonance imaging; PG, plasma glucose; PRRT, Peptide Receptor Radionuclide Therapy; SSA, Somatostatin analogue.

A patient presenting with severe/recurrent peptic ulcer disease (PUD) or acute upper gastrointestinal (UGI) bleeding: Could this be a gastrinoma?

Acute PUD and UGI bleeding are common presentations to AGM. Gastrinomas are the most common functional, and malignant P-NENs (Incidence 0.5–2 cases per million per year), that are characterised by autonomous release of gastrin from tumour cells leading to a clinical syndrome of gastric acid hypersecretion: a) peptic ulcers that are multiple, located in uncommon anatomical sites, treatment resistant, less associated with H. pylori infections, and not associated with non-steroidal anti-inflammatory drugs (NSAIDs), b) complications of PUD; bleeding, perforation, pyloric stenosis, c) heart burn, d) dysphagia due to erosive gastritis, and e) chronic watery diarrhoea. Zollinger-Ellison syndrome (ZES) is the characteristic clinical syndrome of gastrinoma a) ulceration in unusual locations in UGI tract or recurrent ulcerations, b) gastric acid hypersecretion, c) non-beta islet tumours of the pancreas.

Gastrinoma evaluation pathway summarised in Figure 51.2. They (Table 51.3) usually present in the 4th -5th decade of life and commonly (85%) occur as solitary tumours in the 'gastrinoma triangle' (an anatomical area that is defined, superiorly by the confluence of the cystic and common bile duct, inferiorly by the junction of the second and third portions of the duodenum, and medially, by the junction of the neck and body of the pancreas). Up to 25% associated with MEN 1 syndrome and present earlier in life. At presentation, 36% can have localised or locally advanced disease with lymph node metastases. Liver is the commonest site of distant metastases (~35%).

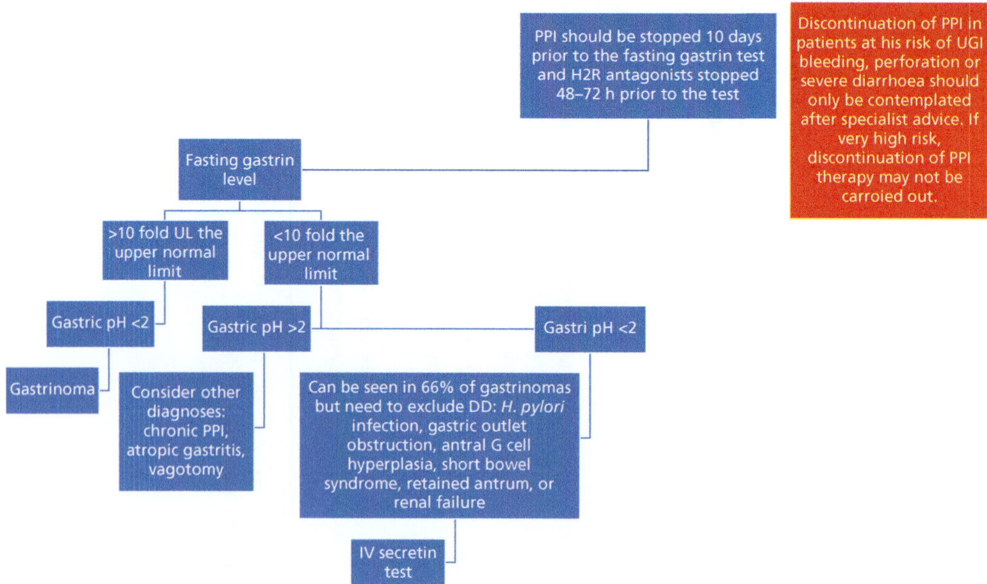

Figure 51.2 Suspected gastrinoma. DD, differential diagnoses; H2R, Histamine H2-receptor; PPI, proton pump inhibitors; UGI, upper gastrointestinal tract.

Table 51.3 Characteristics of gastrinoma.

Clinical presentation	Diagnosis	Tumour localisation	Treatment		Prognosis
			Symptom control	Specific treatment	
• 80%: recurrent, severe and treatment resistant PUD • 50–60%: heart burn and dysphagia • 40–70% PPI responsive chronic watery diarrhoea • Ectopic Cushing syndrome (very rare)	• A fasting serum gastrin level of >10-fold the upper ncrmal limit in the presence of gastric p H<2 or basal acid output >15 mmol/h	• CECT/MRI abdomen • [68]Gallium-DOTATATE-PET/CT • Endoscopic ultrasonography • Esophagogastroduodenoscopy (OGD) • Selective intraarterial calcium/ secretin stimulation test (rarely performed If no visible disease)	• PPI are first line treatment • H2R blockers if not tolerating PPI • SSA (Octreotide, Lanreotide)	• Surgical resection/ debulking • Liver directed therapy • PRRT • Chemotherapy	• The 15-year survival rate in patients either sporadic or MEN-1 gastrinomas and localized disease: >90% • Five-year survival with liver metastases: 50–70%

CECT, Contrast enhanced computer tomography; MEN1, Multiple endocrine neoplasia 1; MRI, Magnetic resonance imaging; PPI, Proton pump inhibitors; PRRT, Peptide Receptor Radionuclide Therapy; PUD, Peptic ulcer disease; SSA, Somatostatin analogue.

A patient presenting with severe watery diarrhoea and hypokalaemia: Could this be a VIPoma?

Profuse chronic watery diarrhoea is a rare presentation to AGM. Verner Morrison syndrome (VMS) or WDHA (watery diarrhoea hypokalaemia achlorhydria) is a rare differential diagnosis of this presentation (Table 51.4). VMS is characterised by profuse, refractory watery diarrhoea, severe hypokalaemia and dehydration that is associated with Vaso intestinal polypeptide (VIP) secreting (VIPomas) P-NENs (Incidence 0.05–0.2 cases per million per year).

A patient presenting with new onset diabetes/worsening glycaemic control in a previously controlled diabetes with erythematous skin rash: Could this be a glucagonoma?

Severe hyperglycaemia and weight loss associated with new onset diabetes in an adult should raise the suspicion of pancreatic neoplasm. Glucagonomas (Incidence 0.01–0.1 cases per million per year) are rare P-NENs that are associated with excessive secretion of glucagon, hence leading to hyperglycaemia (Table 51.5).

Multiple Endocrine Neoplasia type 1

Multiple endocrine neoplasia type 1 (MEN1) syndrome is characterised by combined occurrence of tumours involving parathyroid glands, pancreatic islet cells and the anterior pituitary gland, that is inherited as autosomal dominant syndrome due to germline MEN1 mutation.

MEN1 syndrome should be suspected in patients who are diagnosed with functional P-NENs, and serum calcium level is a useful screening tests as primary hyperparathyroidism is one of the commonest and earliest endocrine manifestation of MEN 1.

Table 51.4 Characteristics of VIPoma.

Important clinical points	Clinical presentation	Diagnosis	Tumour localisation	Treatment		Prognosis
				Symptom control	Specific treatment	
• Usually present in the 3rd-5th decade of life • 90% located in the pancreas • 5% associated with MEN 1 • 40–70% are malignant	• Profuse watery diarrhoea, not resolve with fasting, associated with hypokalaemia and dehydration (90–100%) • Hypercalcaemia, hyperglycaemia, Hypomagnesaemia • Facial flushing (8%)	Raised fasting VIP with characteristic clinical syndrome	• CECT abdomen • MRI abdomen • Endoscopic ultrasonography • ^{68}Gallium-DOTATATE-PET/CT • FDG PET	• Correction of electrolyte abnormalities and re-hydration with IV fluids • SSA -short acting IV or SC octreotide • Glucocorticoids	• Surgical resection/debulking • Long acting SSA (Octreotide, Lanreotide) • Liver directed therapy • PRRT • Chemotherapy	Five-year survival up to 68%

CECT, Contrast enhanced computer tomography; IV, intravenous; MEN1, Multiple endocrine neoplasia 1; MRI, Magnetic resonance imaging; PRRT, Peptide Receptor Radionuclide Therapy; SC, subcutaneous; SSA, Somatostatin analogue; VIP, Vaso intestinal polypeptide.

Table 51.5 Characteristics of glucagonoma.

Important clinical points	Clinical presentation	Diagnosis	Tumour localisation	Treatment		Prognosis
				Symptom control	Specific treatment	
• Usually present in the 5th decade of life • 3% associated with MEN1 • ~80% have metastases at presentation • 100% located in the pancreas	• 55–75% hyperglycaemia • 82% Necrolytic migratory erythema (erythematous, well-demarcated, pruritic, and painful plaques, that often involve the intertriginous areas, perineum, and buttocks) • 71% weight loss or cachexia	Raised fasting plasma glucagon with clinical symptoms and pancreatic tumour	• CECT abdomen • MRI abdomen • ^{68}Gallium-DOTATATE-PET/CT • FDG PET	• Short acting SSA (octreotide) • Insulin to control blood glucose	• Surgical resection/ debulking • Long acting SSA (Octreotide, Lanreotide) • Liver directed therapy • PRRT • Chemotherapy	• Five-year survival: ~85% in benign disease, and ~60% in malignant disease

CECT, Contrast enhanced computer tomography; MEN1, Multiple endocrine neoplasia 1; MRI, Magnetic resonance imaging; PRRT, Peptide Receptor Radionuclide Therapy; SSA, Somatostatin analogue.

Further reading

Cryer, P.E., Axelrod, L., Grossman, A.B. et al. (2009). Evaluation and management of adult hypoglycemic disorders: an endocrine society clinical practice guideline. *J Clin Endocrinol Metab* 94 (3): 709–728. DOI: 10.1210/jc.2008-1410. Epub 2008 Dec 16. PMID: 19088155.

Falconi, M., Eriksson, B., Kaltsas, G. et al. (2016). ENETS consensus guidelines update for the management of patients with functional pancreatic neuroendocrine tumors and non-functional pancreatic neuroendocrine tumors. *Neuroendocrinology* 103 (2): 153–171. DOI: 10.1159/000443171.

Wass, J., Arlt, W., and Semple, R. (ed.) (2022; online edn). *Oxford Textbook of Endocrinology and Diabetes 3e*, 3e. Oxford: Oxford Academic 1 Jan. 2022), https://doi.org/10.1093/med/9780198870197.001.0001.

CHAPTER 52
Electrolyte disorders

Martin Crook, Praveen Weeratunga, and Pramith Ruwanpathirana

Human cells are immersed in a solution of water, electrolytes and organic molecules. Maintaining tight control of the electrolyte concentration is vital for the optimal functioning of cells. Electrolyte abnormalities can lead to multi-organ dysfunction and, if left untreated, can culminate in death.

Disorders of plasma sodium (reference range 135–145 mmol/L)

Disorders of plasma sodium concentration are amongst the most common electrolyte disturbances encountered in clinical practice. Increased sodium concentrations lead to 'hypernatraemia', while decreased sodium concentrations leads to 'hyponatraemia'. True changes in plasma sodium concentrations are always associated with changes in plasma osmolality. For example, hypernatraemia with hypertonicity and hyponatraemia with hypotonicity. Plasma osmolality determines the movement of water between the intracellular and extracellular compartments; hence, plasma sodium disorders are closely linked to changes in cell volume. The degree of cell volume change parallels the rapidity of the change in plasma sodium concentration.

Hyponatraemia

Hyponatraemia is due to excess plasma water relative to the plasma sodium. It occurs due to loss of Na^+ in excess of water through the kidneys, intestine or sweat glands; retention of free water in the body through increased water resorption by the kidneys; and excessive consumption of electrolyte-free water. Therefore, hyponatraemia can occur with hypovolaemia, euvolaemia and hypervolaemia. Except for long-term consumption of electrolyte-free fluids (such as beer), all other causes of hyponatraemia are associated with increased antidiuretic hormone (ADH) activity.

True hyponatraemia is always associated with a low plasma osmolality (measured serum osmolality <275 mOsm/kg). If the plasma osmolality is normal or high, it indicates pseudo-hyponatraemia, where another osmotically active particle has attracted water into the plasma, diluting Na^+. Examples are hyperglycaemia, hyper protein anaemia eg paraprotein, and hyperlipidaemia. The following discussion will apply only to true hyponatraemia.

Clinical manifestations

Clinical manifestations of hyponatraemia depend on the rapidity of plasma $[Na^+]$ change. Acute hyponatraemia is associated with cerebral oedema, whereas patients can tolerate lower levels of $[Na^+]$ if this develops gradually over many days or weeks. In acute hyponatraemia, the cells have not adapted to the low sodium milieu and, therefore, can be reversed rapidly. Still, cell lysis occurs if the $[Na^+]$ is normalised rapidly in chronic hyponatraemia. Hyponatraemia is considered acute if it develops within 48 h.

Acute Medicine: A Practical Guide to the Management of Medical Emergencies, Sixth Edition.
Edited by Mridula Rajwani, Leila Vaziri, and Ivie Gbinigie.
© 2026 John Wiley & Sons Ltd. Published 2026 by John Wiley & Sons Ltd.

Table 52.1 Severity categories of hyponatraemia.

Hyponatraemia severity	Serum [Na$^+$]*/mmol/L	Symptoms**
Mild hyponatraemia	135–130	Mild non-specific symptoms
Moderate hyponatraemia	130–125	Nausea without vomiting
		Confusion
		Headache
Profound hyponatraemia	<125	Vomiting
		Cardio-respiratory distress
		Deep somnolence
		Seizures
		Coma

*Measured by ion-specific electrode.

**The symptoms do not always parallel the [Na$^+$]. The rapidity of the lowering of plasma [Na$^+$] contributes to the symptom severity. Some patients with chronic severe hyponatraemia developed over a long period can have only mild symptoms. Although the symptoms are non-specific, chronic hyponatraemia is associated with osteoporosis, falls, cognitive decline and death.

Clinical features of hyponatraemia range from non-specific symptoms to coma and death. A serum [Na$^+$]< 135 mmol/L is defined as hyponatraemia, and the clinical features worsen with the reduction in [Na$^+$] (Table 52.1).

Causes of hyponatraemia

The causes of hyponatraemia can be divided according to the patient's volume status, with management strategies varying according to the specific type (refer to Table 52.2).

SIADH warrants special consideration. It is a diagnosis of exclusion. Hypo cortisolism and hypothyroidism should be excluded in euvolaemic hyponatraemia before diagnosing SIADH. Once SIADH is confirmed, the underlying cause should be evaluated. The causes of SIADH are listed in Table 52.3.

Management of hyponatraemia

Differentiating true hyponatraemia from pseudohyponatraemia is the first step of management. This can be established by measuring the serum osmolality.

The treatment of hyponatraemia requires balancing the risk of cerebral oedema (which can lead to death and permanent brain damage) with severe hyponatraemia and osmotic demyelination syndrome (ODS) with rapid correction of [Na$^+$] (results in locked-in syndrome). The severity of hyponatraemia should be a composite assessment of the serum [Na$^+$] and the symptoms. If the symptoms and the Na$^+$ concentration are not congruent, attributing the causality of symptoms to hyponatraemia should be done cautiously.

Managing severe hyponatraemia

The overarching principle is that the risk of cerebral oedema outweighs the risk of ODS in this group of patients. Therefore, prompt correction of [Na$^+$] is necessary. However, [Na$^+$] correction should remove the patient from the risk of cerebral oedema and not completely normalise [Na$^+$]. This can be achieved by increasing the [Na$^+$] by 4–5 mmol/L (Table 52.4).

Management of mild to moderate hyponatraemia

When treating the underlying cause of hyponatraemia (in mild to moderate hyponatraemia or after achieving a 5 mmol/L increment in severe hyponatraemia), the serum [Na$^+$] should not be increased by more than 10 mmol/L in the first 24 h and 8 mmol/L in subsequent days. Therapy should continue until the serum [Na$^+$] exceeds 130 mmol/L.

Table 52.2 Hyponatraemia according to the extracellular fluid status.

Hyponatraemia type	Causes	Laboratory parameters**		Management
		Spot urine osmolality/mOsm/kg	Spot urine [Na$^+$]/mmol/L	
Hypovolaemic hyponatraemia	Renal losses: diuretic use, salt wasting syndromes	>100*	>30	Reducing the dose, stopping diuretics, fluid resuscitation with isotonic crystalloids
	Non-renal losses: vomiting, diarrhoea, excessive sweating	>100*	<30	Fluid resuscitation with isotonic crystalloids
Euvolaemic hyponatraemia	Excessive water intake (beer potomania, primary polydipsia)	<100	<30	Treat the underlying condition.
	SIADH Hypocortisolism Hypothyroidism Acute intermittent porphyria	>100*	>30	Water restriction for the management of SIADH
Hypervolaemic hyponatraemia	Heart failure d-ACLD Nephrotic syndrome	>100*	<30	Manage and optimise the underlying condition Water restriction considered
	Chronic kidney disease	Varies over a wide range		

d-ACLD, decompensated advanced chronic liver disease; SIADH, Syndrome of inappropriate cortisol secretion.

*Urine osmolality should be more than the plasma osmolality, indicating ADH secretion.

**Other laboratory investigations that can be used are serum urea concentration, serum uric acid concentration, fractional sodium excretion, fractional uric acid excretion, fractional urea excretion and plasma copeptin concentration.

Table 52.3 Diagnostic criteria and causes of SIADH.

Criteria for diagnosis of SIADH
- Hyponatraemia and reduced plasma osmolality
- Urine sodium concentration >30 mmol /L and urine osmolality greater than plasma osmolality or not maximally dilute
- No oedema or signs of hypovolaemia
- Normal renal, thyroid and adrenal function
- The patient is not taking diuretics or purgatives

Causes of SIADH

Malignant disease

Small cell carcinoma of bronchus, thymoma, lymphoma, sarcoma, mesothelioma, carcinoma of the pancreas and duodenum

Pulmonary disorders

Pneumonia, tuberculosis, empyema, asthma, pneumothorax, positive-pressure ventilation

Neurological disorders

Meningitis, encephalitis, head injury, brain tumour, cerebral abscess, subarachnoid haemorrhage, Guillain–Barré syndrome

Drugs

Antidepressants, carbamazepine, cytotoxics, MDMA ('ecstasy'), NSAIDs, opioids, oxytocin, phenothiazines, thiazides Vincristine

Others

Post-operative state
HIV infection
Idiopathic
Reset osmostat
Acute intermittent porphyria

Table 52.4 Steps of managing severe hyponatraemia.

Step	Action
Step 1	IV 3% saline 150 mL** over 20 min
Step 2	Check serum [Na+].
Step 3	If serum [Na+] has increased by 5 mmol/L or the symptoms have improved, stop further saline infusions. Initiate workup for the cause of hyponatraemia.*
Step 4	If the serum [Na+] has not increased by 5 mmol/L, repeat steps 1 and 2. Three consecutive 150 mL† of 3% saline infusions can be given over 24 h. †There is no consensus on whether to give 3% saline as a continuous infusion over 4–6 h or a slow IV injection over 20 min.
Step 5	If the symptoms persist despite an increase of 5 mmol/L in [Na+], a 3% saline infusion should be started, targeting a rise of 1 mmol/L/h in the serum [Na+]. The infusion should be stopped when the [Na+] concentration increases by 10 mmol/L or the serum sodium concentration reaches 130 mmol/L, whichever occurs first. Titration of the 3% saline infusion can be calculated using the following formula, although it is prone to error. Four hourly serum [Na+] evaluations should be done to prevent over-correction.

$$\text{Change in serum Na}^+ = \frac{\left(\text{Infusate Na}^+ + \text{Infusate K}^+\right) - \text{serum Na}^+}{\text{Total body water}\,(l) + 1}$$

Figure 1. Adrogue Madias formula
Adapted from Adrogue and Madias[6]   *((308 mmol – 115 mmol) / ((60 kg × 0.6) + 1) = 5.2 mmol/L)*

*The symptoms might take time to recover. Hence, do not aim at complete reversal of symptoms immediately.
**Reduce the dose if the patient is thin-built and <50 kg.

It should be noted that the risk of ODS is higher in patients with a history of alcohol abuse, liver disease, use of thiazides or antidepressants, and concomitant hypokalaemia. If these risk factors are present, a lower increment of [Na+] should be targeted.

If the serum [Na+] increases beyond the target, it can be reversed by infusing 5% dextrose or administering intravenous or nasal desmopressin.

Hypernatraemia

Hypernatraemia is a serum [Na+] > 145 mmol/L. The serum osmolality should be raised (>300 mOsm/kg) in all cases of true hypernatraemia. It occurs either with excessive loading of Na+ or loss of body water more than the loss of body Na+.

Excessive Na+ loading is usually iatrogenic and caused by overtreatment with Na+-containing solutions such as 3% NaCl, 8.4% $NaHCO_3$, or IV Albumin solution etc.

Causes of hypernatraemia

Loss of body water more than Na+ can occur through renal or extra-renal routes. Diabetes insipidus (cranial, nephrogenic or gestational) is a common cause. Osmotically active particles (glucose and mannitol) will drag water into the tubules and lead to water loss exceeding Na+ loss. In contrast to secretory diarrhoea, where Na+ is lost through the gut (leading to hyponatraemia), osmotic diarrhoea drags body water into the gut lumen, resulting in hypernatraemia.

The natural response to hypernatraemia is the thirst response and increased ADH secretion, to reabsorb free water from the renal collecting ducts. Therefore, elderly or critically ill patients with impaired thirst response are prone to develop hypernatraemia. Except in cases of cranial diabetes insipidus, plasma ADH should be elevated in all causes of hypernatraemia.

Clinical features

Similar to hyponatraemia, the clinical features of hypernatremia are primarily neurological (confusion, altered mental status and coma). Hypernatraemia leads to a shift of water from the brain cells to the extracellular compartment, leading to brain shrinkage. In children, this can result in intracranial haemorrhages, while in adults, this leads to osmotic demyelination. Similar to hyponatraemia, rapid correction of Na$^+$ in chronic hypernatraemia is harmful and results in brain oedema. (the opposite consequences of hyponatraemia). Rhabdomyolysis has been described with severe hypernatraemia.

Management

The target drop of serum [Na$^+$] is 10 mmol/L per day in chronic hypernatraemia. Acute hypernatraemia (<48 h from onset) can be usually rapidly corrected without the risk of developing brain oedema.

The principle of correcting hypernatraemia is to provide the body with salt-free water, either enterally or parenterally. The free water deficit and the amount of fluid required for correction can be calculated using the following formula:

$$\text{Free Water Deficit} = \left[(\text{serum Na} - 140) / 140\right] \times 0.6 \text{ Body Weight (kilograms)}$$

$$\text{TBW : Total body water or body weight in kilograms} \times 0.6$$

$$[\text{Calculating the Effect of 1 liter of an Intravenous Solution on Serum Sodium}$$

$$\text{Change in serum Na} = \{[\text{Na] infused} - [\text{Na] serum}\} / (\text{total body water} + 1)]$$

Management strategies for specific causes of hypernatraemia are summarised in Table 52.5.

Table 52.5 Causes for and management of hypernatraemia.

Cause	Diagnostic features	Management
Hypovolaemic causes		
Cranial diabetes insipidus*	Inappropriately dilute urine** Polyuria (>3 L/day) Urine osmolality increases >50% with DDAVP	Treat the underlying cause. Regular DDAVP supplementation
Nephrogenic diabetes insipidus*	Inappropriately dilute urine** Polyuria (>3 L/day) Urine osmolality does not increase >50% with DDVP	Remove secondary cause (Li$^+$, hypercalcaemia, hypokalaemia and obstructive uropathy) Cautious use of thiazides and NSAIDS Excessive water intake
Diuresis due to osmotically active particles (glucose and mannitol)	Concentrated urine (>800 mOsm/kg) Increased urine volume Low urine [Na$^+$]	Treat the underlying cause Hypotonic crystalloids (5% dextrose, ½ normal saline) infusions and increased oral/enteral free water (In hyperglycaemic hyperosmolar state, the serum osmolality is higher than 0.9% saline. Therefore, 0.9% saline is the preferred crystalloid)
Osmotic diarrhoea	Concentrated urine. (>800 mOsm/kg) Oliguric (<500 mL/day)	Treat the underlying cause Hypotonic crystalloids (5% dextrose and ½ normal saline) infusions
Reduced thirst	Concentrated urine. (>800 mOsm/kg) Oliguric (<500 mL/day)	Increase oral free water intake
Hypervolaemic causes		
Excessive Na$^+$ loading	Concentrated urine Increased urine volume Increased urinary [Na$^+$]	Increase enteral-free water intake If severe, consider hypotonic crystalloids (5% dextrose and ½ normal saline).

DDAVP, Desmopressin.
*In the presence of hypernatraemia, a water-deprivation test is contraindicated.
**Urine osmolality is lower than the serum osmolality.

Disorders of plasma potassium (reference range 3.5–5.5 mmol/L)

Disorders of potassium can occur due to three reasons:

1 Excess or reduced intake into the body.
2 Excess or reduced excretion from the body.
3 Movement between intracellular and extracellular compartments.

While sodium disorders primarily lead to neurological manifestations, potassium disorders often result in cardiac manifestation; and sudden death is possible. Therefore, managing potassium disorders is a vital skill for clinicians.

Hyperkalaemia

A serum potassium (K^+) level greater than 5.5 mmol/L is defined as hyperkalaemia.

The most common cause of hyperkalaemia is reduced potassium excretion from the body, making it a significant complication of kidney disease. Drug-induced hyperkalaemia due to mineralocorticoid receptor antagonists, ACE inhibitors and angiotensin receptor blockers is also commonly seen in clinical practice.

The causes of hyperkalaemia are detailed in Table 52.6.

Clinical manifestations

Cardiac arrhythmia are an important clinical consequence of hyperkalaemia. The severity of hyperkalaemia and associated electrocardiograph (ECG) changes are shown in Figure 52.1.

Management

The management of hyperkalaemia depends in-part upon the severity and the presence of ECG changes.

If there is an imminent risk of cardiac arrhythmia (in cases of severe hyperkalaemia or the presence of ECG changes), it is crucial to stabilise the cardiac myocyte membrane promptly. Cardiac membrane stabilisation is

Table 52.6 Causes of hyperkalaemia.

Pseudohyperkalaemia[*]

Reduced excretion from the body
Acute kidney injury or chronic kidney disease
Mineralocorticoid deficiency:
• Adrenal insufficiency, hyporeninaemic hypoaldosteronism, renal tubular acidosis type 4
Drugs:
angiotensin-converting-enzyme inhibitors, angiotensin receptor blockers, potassium-sparing diuretics (spironolactone and amiloride), cyclosporine, tacrolimus, oral contraceptive pill, NAIDS and trimethoprim

The transition from the intracellular compartment to the extracellular compartment
Severe tissue damage:
• Rhabdomyolysis
• Tumour-lysis syndrome
Acidosis (non-anion gap) or hypoxia
Digoxin toxicity
Familial hyperkalaemic periodic paralysis (rare)

Excessive intake
Oral or intravenous potassium excess (drugs, supplements and food)
Red cell transfusions

[*]When intracellular K^+ leaks out of cells within the blood tubes, leading to a spuriously high K^+ level. (In haemolysis, leukaemia, cooling of blood, red cell membrane-transporter defects, muscle activity during venepuncture etc).

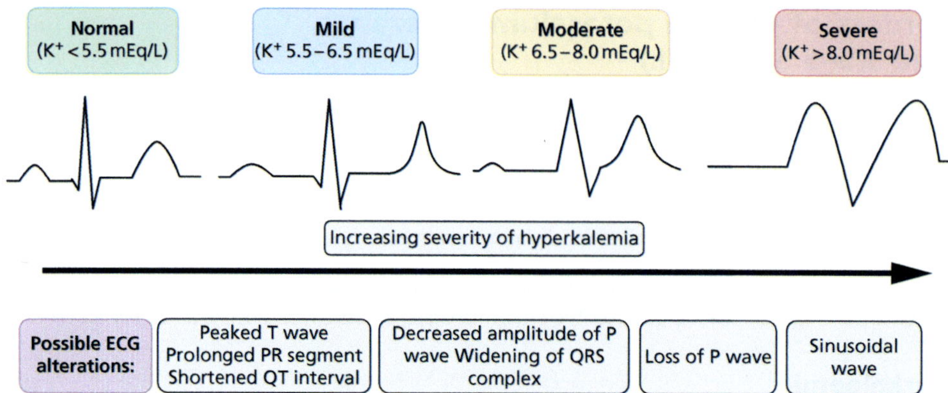

Figure 52.1 ECG changes of hyperkalaemia. The ECG changes, and the serum K^+ does not always parallel. In patients with chronic hyperkalaemia, the ECG changes might be absent.

achieved by administering IV calcium gluconate (30 mL) or IV calcium chloride (10 mL) over 2–3 min through a large cannula. This intervention does not reduce the plasma K^+ levels but prevents the development of cardiac arrhythmias. The patient should be transferred to a monitored bed equipped with continuous cardiac monitoring and defibrillation facilities. The ECG should be repeated after 5 min, and if the ECG changes have not been reversed, another dose of IV calcium should be administered.

Subsequently, measures should be taken to reduce the plasma K^+ levels.

1 Drive plasma K^+ into the cells (used to buy time as it has a quick action)
   a IV insulin and glucose infusion: add 10 units of human insulin to 50 mL of 50% glucose and infuse over 30 min. Avoid hypoglycaemia by monitoring blood glucose. The effect begins at 10 min, peaks at 30–60 min, and lasts 4–6 h.
   b Nebulised salbutamol: 10–20 mg (contraindicated in unstable angina or acute myocardial infarction). This effect starts at about 30 min, peaks at around 90 min, and lasts 2–6 h.
   c Intravenous sodium bicarbonate (isotonic or hypotonic) can be used in severe hyperkalaemia with severe acidosis. However, the effect is delayed and thus not very useful in the acute setting.
2 Remove K^+ from the body.
   a Gut potassium-binding resins: Options include calcium resonium (15 g three times daily orally or 30 g daily by retention enema), Patiromer (8.4 g daily orally) and sodium zirconium cyclosilicate (10 g three times daily for 72 h)
   b Haemodialysis
3 Reduce K^+ intake
   a Reduce K^+ rich meals (includes fresh fruits, green leaves and salt substitutes)
   b Omit K^+ supplementation
4 Treat the precipitating cause
   a Discontinue drugs that cause hyperkalaemia
   b Treat the underlying disease (kidney disease, rhabdomyolysis and tumour lysis syndrome)

Hypokalaemia

Hypokalaemia is a serum potassium level of less than 3.5 mmol/L. Hypokalaemia can result from either increased K^+ loss from the body or the movement of K^+ into the cells from the extracellular compartment. Hypokalaemia due to reduced intake is exceedingly rare (see Table 52.7). The body loses K^+ either through the kidneys or the gut.

Table 52.7 Causes of hypokalaemia.

Pseudo hypokalaemia – increased uptake of K+ into the cells in-vitro (in acute leukaemia)

Increased loss of body K+
Losses through kidney
Mineralocorticoid excess/apparent mineralocorticoid excess
- Conn's syndrome
- Cushing's syndrome
- Bartter/Gitelman's syndrome
- Liquorice excess
- Glucocorticoid therapy

Fanconi syndrome
Hypomagnesaemia
Drugs: loop diuretics, thiazides, carbonate dehydratase inhibitors, penicillin group antibiotics
Renal tubular acidosis type 1 and 2

Losses through the gut
Gastrointestinal loss:
Prolonged diarrhoea or vomiting
Intestinal fistula
Purgative abuse

Redistribution from the extracellular compartment to the intra-cellular compartment
Alkalosis
Catecholamines
Vitamin B12 therapy
Insulin
Beta-adrenergic drugs
Thyrotoxicosis
Rapidly growing tumours
Familial hypokalaemic periodic paralysis (rare)

Clinical manifestations

Hypokalaemia predisposes individuals to ECG QT prolongation, ventricular arrhythmias and death. Severe hypokalaemia, or hypokalaemia with ECG changes (see Figure 52.2), should be treated promptly with intravenous K+. In addition to its effects on the cardiac muscle, hypokalaemia affects the skeletal muscle, leading to proximal myopathy, areflexia and rhabdomyolysis. When the smooth muscles are affected, it results in paralytic ileus. Mild-to-moderate hypokalaemia can be treated with oral potassium chloride (KCl) supplementation.

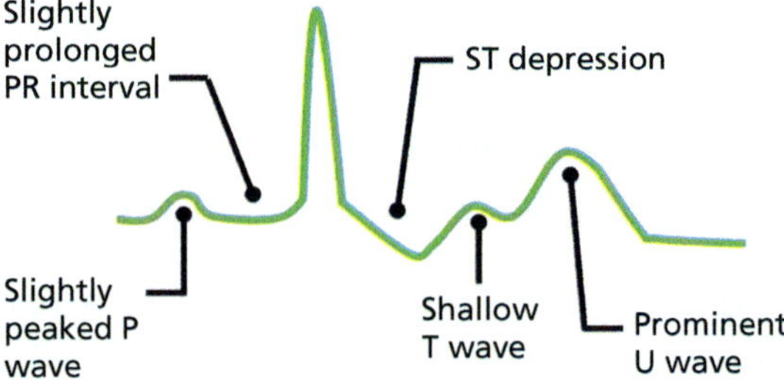

Figure 52.2 ECG changes of hypokalaemia.

Table 52.8 Aetiological evaluation of hypokalaemia.

Exclude obvious causes: diarrhoea, vomiting, diuretics, insulin and beta-agonists.

Look for urinary K^+ loss: the ideal test is a 24-h urinary collection to quantify K^+ (>15 mmol/L despite hypokalaemia suggesting renal loss). An alternative is the urinary K^+/creatinine ratio (>13 mmol/L/g → suggestive of renal loss). The patient should not be on diuretics.

If there is urinary K^+ loss, proceed to step 3.

Localise the pathology into the nephron segment: Disorders of all nephron segments can lead to hypokalaemia.

Segment of the nephron	Function	Condition	Blood pressure	Acid–base imbalance	Additional features
Proximal tubule	↓	Proximal RTA	↔	Acidosis	Glycosuria, aminoaciduria
Ascending limb of LOH	↓	Bartter's syndrome	↓	Alkalosis	Hypocalcaemia
Distal convoluted tubule	↓	Gitelman syndrome	↓	Alkalosis	Hypercalcaemia
Collecting ducts: principal cells	↑	Hyperaldosteronism	↑	Alkalosis	
		Syndrome of apparent mineralocorticoid excess			
		Liddle syndrome			
		Liquorice ingestion			
		Congenital adrenal hyperplasia types (17 alpha and 11 β hydroxylase deficiency)			
Collecting duct: intercalated cells	↓	Distal RTA	↔	Acidosis	Nephrocalcinosis, renal stones and alkaline urine

LOH, loop of Henle; RTA, renal tubular acidosis.

Evaluation

A complete discussion on evaluating the causes of hypokalaemia is beyond the scope of this book. However, a brief outline is provided in Table 52.8. The definitive treatment of hyperkalaemia is addressing the underlying cause.

Management

K^+ infusions can be painful and cause thrombophlebitis. If administered too rapidly, they can induce brady arrhythmias and cardiac arrest. Therefore, KCl should be given as a slow infusion at 20 mmol/h. KCl is constituted of 0.9% sodium chloride (NaCl) with a maximum concentration of 20 mmol/L. It should be infused through a central line. The body K^+ deficit can be calculated using the following formula:

$$K^+ \text{ deficit in } (mmol/L) = (desired)K^+ (mmol/L) - patient's \ K^+ (mmol/L) \times 0.4 \times body \ weight \ kg$$

It should be remembered that total body K^+ is usually normal in conditions where hypokalaemia is due to the shift of K^+ from the extracellular compartment to the intracellular compartment. Therefore, such patients risk developing rebound hyperkalaemia; hence, K^+ should be replaced only to prevent imminent cardiac arrhythmias.

Disorders of plasma calcium (reference range 2.20–2.60 mmol/L albumin corrected or adjusted)

Disorders of Ca^{2+} are mainly due to abnormalities of PTH secretion, vitamin D and bone metabolism. Calcium is bound to albumin (and other anions) in circulation. Therefore, the total serum Ca^{2+} level is a function of serum albumin. It's the free fraction of calcium that's physiologically important. Hence, for the management and evaluation of disorders of Ca^{2+}, the serum albumin corrected calcium or the serum ionised Ca^{2+} should be measured.

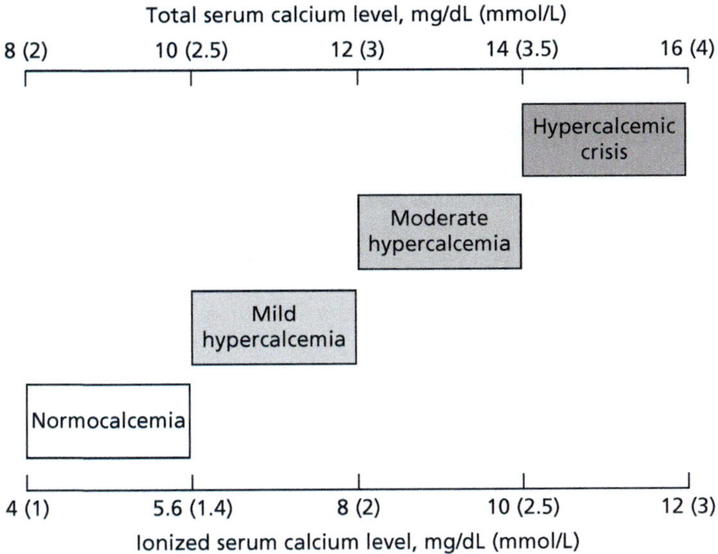

Figure 52.3 Definitions of hypercalcaemia severity categories.

The serum calcium correction formula (albumin corrected total calcium (mmol/L) = Total calcium (mmol/L) + 0.02 [40 (g/L) – albumin (g/L)])

Hypercalcaemia

The definitions of hypercalcaemia severity categories are illustrated in Figure 52.3.

Causes

Hypercalcaemia is a result of one of four mechanisms:

1 Increased PTH: Due to primary or tertiary hyperparathyroidism, familial hypocalciuric hypercalcaemia or PTH-related peptide secreted from malignancies.
2 Increased vitamin D: Caused vitamin D overdose or increased synthesis in granulomatous diseases (such as sarcoidosis or lymphoma)
3 Increased bone lysis: Seen in disseminated malignancy, multiple myeloma or thyrotoxicosis
4 Miscellaneous causes: Drug-induced (e.g. thiazides), milk-alkali syndrome, Addison's disease, VIPoma or pheochromocytoma

Clinical features

The clinical features of hypercalcaemia can be remembered by the phrase 'bones, groans, moans and stones.'

- **Bones:** Increased bone lysis can cause hypercalcaemia, predisposing to increased fracture risk (hyperparathyroidism, myeloma and bone metastasis)
- Abdominal **groans**: Due to gut dysmotility and renal colic
- Psychotic **moans**: Personality changes or depression due to the effect on the brain and
- Renal **stones**: Due to increased urinary filtration of Ca^{2+} (sometimes resulting in nephrocalcinosis and renal failure).

The ECG changes of hypercalcaemia include bradycardia, atrioventricular (AV) nodal block and short QT interval.

Hypercalcaemia can also cause nephrogenic diabetes insipidus and lead to polyuria and dehydration. Patients with severe hypercalcaemia are often profoundly dehydrated. Additionally, acute pancreatitis is a serious complication of severe hypercalcaemia.

Management of severe hypercalcaemia

Severe hypercalcaemia is a serum corrected/adjusted calcium greater than 3.40 mmol /L.

Aggressive hydration (4–6 L of 0.9% NaCl over 24 h) is the first and the most important step in managing severe hypercalcaemia.

After volume repletion, if the serum Ca^{2+} is still high,

- IV bisphosphonates (IV zoledronic acid 4 mg or IV pamidronate 60 mg),
- subcutaneous denosumab,
- IV steroids (hydrocortisone 100–300 mg daily),
- calcitonin
- haemodialysis can be used sequentially.

The definitive management is the aetiological evaluation and treatment of the underlying cause. Managing mild asymptomatic hypercalcaemia involves identifying and treating the underlying cause of hypercalcaemia.

Hypocalcaemia

Hypocalcaemia can be defined as an albumin adjusted or corrected serum calcium of less than 2.20 mmol/L.

Clinical features

Hypocalcaemia increases the excitability of neurons and muscles. It predisposes to seizures, prolongs the ECG QT interval of the heart (resulting in ventricular tachyarrhythmias), and causes smooth muscle contraction, which can lead to bronchospasms, laryngospasms, and death. Early symptoms include peri-oral numbness and paraesthesia of the hands and feet. Clinical signs that demonstrate neuronal hyper-excitability include the Chvostek's sign and the Trousseau's sign (Figure 52.4).

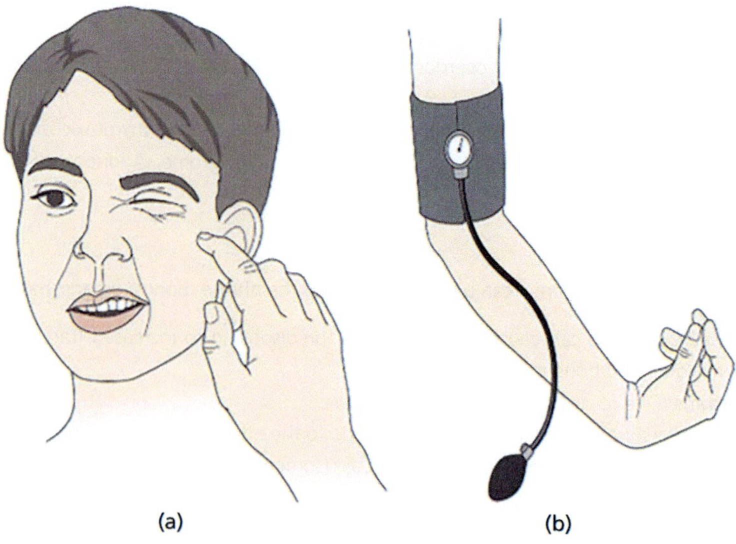

(a)   (b)

Figure 52.4 Clinical signs of hypocalcaemia. (a) Positive Chvostek's sign and (b) positive Trousseau's sign.

Chvostek's sign-tapping of facial nerve branches results in twitching of facial muscles. Trousseau's sign – Elicited by inflating the BP cuff on the upper arm to 20 mmHg above systolic pressure within 2–5 min. The carpal spasm occurs due to ulnar nerve ischaemia.

Causes

1 Reduced PTH levels – Hypoparathyroidism (post-thyroidectomy, autoimmune or due to Mg^{2+} deficiency) or pseudohypoparathyroidism (PTH).
2 Vitamin D deficiency includes rickets, osteomalacia or vitamin D resistance.
3 Mineral bone disease of chronic kidney disease
4 Miscellaneous causes – drug-induced (e.g., loop diuretics), burns, rhabdomyolysis, tumour lysis syndrome or acute pancreatitis.

Management

Hypocalcaemia should be treated promptly to prevent life-threatening complications. Severe hypocalcaemia is treated with 10% IV calcium gluconate (10 mL administered over 2–3 min). Mild to moderate hypocalcaemia is treated with oral calcium (such as calcium lactate, calcium carbonate and calcium acetate) and vitamin D supplementation.

Disorders of plasma magnesium (reference range 0.70-1.20 mmol /L)

Magnesium is essential for neuro-muscular activity, intracellular enzymatic reactions, energy metabolism, cell replication and nucleic acid metabolism. Similar to Ca^{2+} metabolism, Mg^{2+} is stored in the bone in large quantities. While Ca^{2+} is primarily an extracellular cation, Mg^{2+} is mainly intracellular.

Hypomagnesaemia

Causes

1 Reduced gastrointestinal absorption: due to malabsorption syndromes, proton pump inhibitors, and vitamin D deficiency.
2 Increased gastrointestinal loss: often due to diarrhoea
3 Increased renal loss: due to renal tubular dysfunction or drug-induced effects – such as the use of diuretics
4 Intracellular shift: seen in conditions like refeeding syndrome or diabetes ketoacidosis (similar to K^+, another intracellular cation)

Clinical manifestations

The neuromuscular features of hypomagnesaemia are tetany, tremor, seizures, muscle weakness, ataxia, nystagmus, vertigo, apathy, depression, irritability, delirium and psychosis. Cardiac features are sinus tachycardia, other tachyarrhythmias, QT prolongation, and ST and T wave changes.

Management

Treatment of hypomagnesaemia is to replace Mg^{2+}, identify the aetiology and address it.

Magnesium is replaced intravenously in severe hypomagnesaemia. IV $MgCl_2$ (50 mmol/day as a continuous infusion) or IV $MgSO_4$ can be used. The Mg^{2+} dose should be corrected for renal functions. Mild hypomagnesaemia is treated with oral Mg salts ($MgCl_2$, $Mg(OH)_2$, $MgSO_4$).

Certain causes of hypomagnesaemia are associated with simultaneous hypokalaemia or hypocalcaemia. As discussed earlier, Mg^{2+} replacement will aid in correcting K^+ and Ca^{2+}. However, in hypophosphatemia, Mg^{2+} replacement can further reduce the plasma PO_4^{3-}. This can be prevented by replacing Ca^{2+} simultaneously.

Hypermagnesaemia

Causes

The causes of hypermagnesaemia are sometimes the opposite of those for hypomagnesaemia.

- Increased gastrointestinal absorption: due to cathartics or antacids
- Reduced urinary excretion: in conditions such as familial hypocalciuric hypocalcaemia or renal failure
- Increased transition from the intracellular space to extracellular space: seen in tumour lysis syndrome, burns, or trauma
- Other causes: including adrenal insufficiency or hypothyroidism

Of the aforementioned causes, the commonest is iatrogenic – due to cathartics/antacids and treatment of asthma, eclampsia etc.

Clinical manifestations

Hypermagnesaemia is rare due to the kidney's ability to excrete large amounts of magnesium ions. However, when it occurs, it reduces the excitability of the neurons and muscles, relaxes the vascular smooth muscles and leads to refractory shock. The heart is also affected by severe hypermagnesaemia. It manifests as bradycardia (despite hypotension), prolongation of ECG PR, QRS, and QT intervals, and heart block. Gut mobility decreases. Muscle weakness and paralysis in hypomagnesaemia might escalate to respiratory failure in severe cases.

Management

Management of hypermagnesaemia is to treat the underlying cause. Hydration with normal saline is commonly practised to dilute the serum Mg^{2+}. In severe hypermagnesaemia, dialysis can be initiated for rapid correction.

Disorders of plasma phosphate (reference range 0.80–1.50 mmol/L)

Phosphate is an intracellular anion. It is absorbed from the gut along with Ca^{2+}, which is regulated by activated vitamin D. The bone is a large store of inorganic phosphate; many proteins and nucleic acids have phosphate incorporated into their organic structures. Phosphate is excreted via the kidneys, which PTH enhances, whereas phosphate reabsorption is promoted by activated vitamin D.

Causes

The causes of hyper and hypophosphatemia are summarised in Table 52.9.

Management

The management of phosphate disorders equates to the management of the underlying aetiology. For hypophosphataemia, oral or intravenous phosphate supplements are used to replace phosphate. Intravenous phosphate (9–18 mmol) should be constituted in 5% dextrose and be given over 6–12 h. The patient should be monitored for hypocalcaemia.

For hyperphosphataemia, gut phosphate binders (such as $CaCO_3$, sevelamer or lanthanum carbonate) are used to increase the elimination of phosphate from the body. Gut phosphate binders are the mainstay of treatment for hyperphosphataemia associated with renal bone disease.

Table 52.9 Causes for disorders of phosphate.

Disorder of plasma phosphate	Cause	Consequence
Hypophosphataemia	**Reduced absorption** Vitamin D deficiency (Rickets and osteomalacia) Malabsorption syndromes Anorexia nervosa **Increased urinary loss** Hyperparathyroidism Proximal tubular dysfunction (Fanconi's syndrome) X-linked hypophosphatemic rickets Oncogenic hypophosphataemia **Intracellular shifts** Insulin therapy in diabetes Refeeding syndrome	• Osteomalacia. • Myopathy • Rhabdomyolysis • Impaired diaphragmatic contractility • Cardiomyopathy • Seizures • Paraesthesia • Renal tubular impairment
Hyperphosphataemia	**Increased absorption** Vitamin D toxicity Phosphate containing laxatives **Reduced urinary loss** Hypoparathyroidism/ pseudohypoparathyroidism Renal failure **Extracellular shift** Tumour lysis syndrome Rhabdomyolysis Trauma	Phosphates bind with ionised Ca^{2+} and precipitate in the tissues. This leads to tissue calcification (calciphylaxis) and hypocalcaemia. Persistently elevated phosphate levels are a risk factor for atherosclerosis.

Acknowledgements

Sharmila Kugaperumal and Thamalee Palliyaguru for proofreading.

Further reading

Sterns RH. (2015) Disorders of plasma sodium – causes, consequences, and correction. *N Engl J Med* 372, 55–65.

Spasovski G, Vanholder R, Allolio B, *et al.* (2014) Clinical practice guideline on diagnosis and treatment of hyponatraemia The guidelines were peer-reviewed by the owner societies and by external referees before publication. *Eur J Endocrinol* 170(3), G1–G47. DOI: 10.1530/EJE-13-1020.

The Renal Association, Guideline for Management of Hyperkalaemia. 2020. https://www.ukkidney.org/ health-professionals/guidelines/treatment-acute-hyperkalaemia-adults.

Neurology

Headache syndromes: including subarachnoid haemorrhage and cerebral venous sinus thrombosis

SIMON RINALDI AND ROBERTO BELLANTI

The most common cause of acute headache in patients presenting to the emergency department is migraine. A minority have potentially life-threatening disorders such as subarachnoid haemorrhage, bacterial meningitis or cerebral venous sinus thrombosis. The clinical assessment (Table 53.1) enables you to place the patient in one of three groups, guiding differential diagnosis, investigation and further management.

1 Acute headache with 'red flag' features
- Red flag features include fever, reduced level of consciousness, optic disc swelling, neck stiffness, and focal neurological signs. Causes of headache with red flag features are given in Table 53.2.
- If the patient is febrile, or central nervous system (CNS) infection is highly suspected, take blood cultures and start antimicrobial therapy to cover bacterial meningitis and herpes simplex encephalitis. Next, obtain cerebrospinal fluid (CSF) to confirm the diagnosis, identify the pathogen, and direct further therapy. Computed tomography (CT) must be performed before lumbar puncture (LP) if any of the following are present:
  - Focal neurological signs
  - Altered consciousness
  - Optic disc swelling, which may be due to raised intracranial pressure (papilloedema)
  - Immunosuppression
  - Recent seizure(s), within two weeks
- Tuberculous and cryptococcal meningitis should be considered in high-risk groups. Meningism may be absent or mild in these diseases.
- Infectious diseases acquired abroad (e.g. malaria and typhoid) should be considered in patients with the relevant travel history.
- When subarachnoid haemorrhage is suspected (see below), CT is the initial investigation of choice and lumbar puncture is likely to be more useful if delayed until 12 h after the onset of headache.

2 Headache with local signs
- Causes and management are summarized in Table 53.3.

3 Acute headache without abnormal signs
- Causes are given in Table 53.4.
- Always consider subarachnoid haemorrhage and giant-cell arteritis (see below).
- Formal criteria state that a headache cannot be diagnosed as migraine or tension-type headache until multiple episodes have occurred. While such criteria highlight the increased difficulty in diagnosing a single episode, it may still be appropriate to treat migraine-like headache as such if other more serious causes have been satisfactorily excluded.

Acute Medicine: A Practical Guide to the Management of Medical Emergencies, Sixth Edition.
Edited by Mridula Rajwani, Leila Vaziri, and Ivie Gbinigie.
© 2026 John Wiley & Sons Ltd. Published 2026 by John Wiley & Sons Ltd.

Table 53.1 Focused assessment of the patient with acute headache.

History

Speed of onset: Was it sudden? How long did it take to reach maximum intensity?

Context of onset: Was it exertion-related, orgasmic, upon changing posture or waking up?

Duration: Is the headache still present? How long has it lasted?

Severity: How severe? Worst headache ever? Syncope at onset?

Distribution: Unilateral or bilateral? Frontotemporal or occipital?

Associated features: Was there associated nausea, vomiting, photo/phonophobia or pulsating quality? All are associated but not pathognomonic of migraine.

Associated systemic, neurological or visual symptoms (e.g. syncope/presyncope, limb weakness, speech disturbance, blurring of vision, transient blindness, diplopia, scalp tenderness, jaw claudication, malaise, myalgia/stiffness, scotomata and fortification spectra). Did these precede or follow the headache?

Background

Medication history and possible exposure to toxins

Recent travel abroad

Immunosuppressed or known malignancy

Disorders associated with increased risk of aneurysmal subarachnoid haemorrhage: polycystic kidney disease, Ehlers–Danlos syndrome type IV, pseudoxanthoma elasticum, fibromuscular dysplasia, sickle cell disease, alfa-1 antitrypsin deficiency

Family history of migraine or subarachnoid haemorrhage

Examination

Key observations: airway, respiratory rate, arterial oxygen saturation, heart rate, blood pressure, perfusion, consciousness level, temperature, blood glucose

Neck stiffness (in both flexion and extension)

Focal neurological signs

Horner syndrome – if complete or partial ptosis and constricted pupil are present, consider carotid artery dissection.

Visual acuity and fields defects

Fundi (disc swelling or retinal haemorrhage)

Signs of dental, ENT or ophthalmic disease

Temporal artery tenderness or loss of pulsation

Table 53.2 Causes of acute headache with 'red flag' features.

Cause

Vascular

- Subarachnoid haemorrhage
- Cerebral venous sinus thrombosis
- Intracranial haemorrhage
- Subdural haematoma
- Hypertensive encephalopathy
- Pituitary apoplexy
- Cerebral vasculitis

Infective

- Bacterial meningitis
- Viral encephalitis
- Brain abscess
- Subdural empyema
- Tuberculous meningitis
- Cryptococcal meningitis
- Toxoplasma encephalitis
- Systemic infection with headache/meningism

Others

- Poisoning with amphetamine/cocaine
- Other causes of raised intracranial pressure
- Hyperviscosity syndrome
- Severe hyponatraemia
- Malignant meningitis (carcinoma, melanoma, lymphoma and leukaemia)

Table 53.3 Causes of acute headache with local signs.

Cause	Comment/management
Acute sinusitis	Suspect if associated fever, facial pain especially on bending over, mucopurulent nasal discharge, and tenderness on pressure over the affected sinus. Obtain X-rays of the sinuses, looking for mucosal thickening, a fluid level or opacification. Treatment is with phenoxymethylpenicillin and steam inhalations if there are no life-threatening complications, or co-amoxiclav if the patient is systemically unwell (or if symptoms worsen after two to three days of first-line antibiotic). Doxycycline or clarithromycin should be prescribed in case of allergy to penicillin (refer to local guidelines). Discuss management with an ENT surgeon.
Acute angle-closure glaucoma	Usually unilateral; eye red and injected, visual acuity reduced due to corneal clouding, pupil fixed. Refer urgently to Ophthalmology.
Giant cell arteritis	See text
Temporomandibular joint disorder	A group of disorders affecting the temporomandibular joint (TMJ) and the masticatory muscles. Signs include limitation of jaw opening, tenderness to palpation of the TMJ and palpable spasm of masseter and internal pterygoid muscles. Seek advice from an oral surgeon.
Cervicogenic headache	Headache referred from disorders of the cervical spine.
Mucormycosis	Fungal infection may occur in severely immunocompromised patients. Periorbital and orbital cellulitis cause orbital and facial pain, proptosis, purulent nasal discharge and mucosal necrosis.

Table 53.4 Acute headache with no abnormal signs.

Cause	Comment
Tension-type headache	Usually described as pressure or tightness around the head. Does not have the associated symptoms or aura of migraine, although some patients may have both types of headaches.
Migraine	See Table 53.5 for diagnostic criteria.
Medication-overuse headache	Suspect in patients who have frequent or daily headaches and regularly use analgesics for headache.
Drug-related	Seen with nitrates, nicorandil, dihydropyridine calcium antagonists, and sildenafil.
Toxin exposure	Seen with carbon monoxide poisoning.
Subarachnoid haemorrhage	See text.
Giant cell arteritis	See text
Cerebral venous sinus thrombosis	Headache frequently precedes other symptoms, and can be the only symptom. Onset may be 'thunderclap', acute or progressive.
Pituitary apoplexy	Usually associated with ophthalmoplegia and reduced visual acuity.
Carotid or vertebral arterial dissection	Unilateral headache, which may be accompanied by neck pain. May follow neck manipulation or minor trauma. Usually accompanied by other signs (ischaemic stroke, Horner syndrome or pulsatile tinnitus).
Spontaneous intracranial hypotension	Due to CSF leak from spinal meningeal defects or dural tears. Headache worse on standing and relieved by lying down (like post-LP headache). May be accompanied by nausea and vomiting, dizziness, auditory changes, diplopia, visual blurring, interscapular pain and/or radicular pain in the arms or legs.
Benign (idiopathic) 'thunderclap' headache	Assumes subarachnoid haemorrhage and cerebral venous thrombosis have been excluded.

Table 53.5 Diagnostic criteria for migraine.

Migraine without aura
- At least five attacks lasting 4–72 h (in some cases may be longer than 72 h – 'status migrainosus')
- At least two of the following:
  - Unilateral
  - Pulsating
  - Moderate to severe
  - Aggravated by movement

  NB: migraine headache may be bilateral or vary unilateral/bilateral during a single episode, and may be continuous rather than pulsatile.
- At least one associated symptom:
  - Nausea or vomiting
  - Photophobia or phonophobia

Migraine with aura
- One or more transient focal neurological aura symptoms
- Gradual development of aura symptoms over >4 min, or several symptoms in succession
- Aura symptoms last 4–60 min
- Headache follows or accompanies aura within 60 min

Table 53.6 Suspected diagnoses and investigation required.

Suspected diagnosis	Investigation
CNS infection	Full blood count, CRP, blood cultures (if fever), CT head, LP
Intracranial haemorrhage	CT head, coagulation screen
Giant cell arteritis (GCA)	ESR, C-reactive protein
Sinus infection	Skull X-ray
Subarachnoid haemorrhage	CT head (high sensitivity within the first 6 h), LP (if no contraindication), CT angiogram (if LP positive for xanthochromia)
Cerebral venous sinus thrombosis	MR venogram (MRV), coagulation screen (subsequently targeted to investigate specific coagulation disorders if suspected)

CRP, C-reactive protein; CVST, cerebral venous sinus thrombosis; ESR, erythrocyte sedimentation rate; LP, lumbar puncture.

In the patient with headache, diagnostic tests should be chosen to answer targeted clinical questions. Table 53.6 lists the relevant tests to request when specific diagnoses are suspected.

Subarachnoid haemorrhage

Clinical features
- Subarachnoid haemorrhage (SAH) manifests with sudden-onset, thunderclap headache, typically described as the 'worst ever', reaching maximum intensity within minutes at most.
- Around 20% of patients with subarachnoid haemorrhage have acute headache with no other signs, but most have associated photophobia with nausea and/or vomiting. There may be neck stiffness and, on examination, patients with SAH may have positive Kernig's sign, suggestive of meningism.

Diagnosis
- SAH is diagnosed on the basis of clinical history, CT head, and CSF analysis if imaging does not show an acute bleed. CT is most sensitive for detection of subarachnoid haemorrhage if done within 6 h of onset of the headache. Examination of the CSF by spectrophotometry to detect bilirubin (a breakdown product of

haemoglobin) is the most reliable method of confirming or excluding subarachnoid haemorrhage. Bilirubin is reliably present in the CSF from 12 h to two weeks after haemorrhage (occasionally longer). Lumbar puncture should therefore be delayed to over 12 h after the onset of headache unless meningitis is also suspected.

- Once SAH is confirmed, the next step is to determine whether it is traumatic or non-traumatic, and imaging (CT angiogram or MR angiogram) is necessary.
- Non-traumatic SAH is secondary to aneurysms (berry or infectious), coagulation disorders, uncontrolled anticoagulation therapy, or dural arteriovenous fistulae (AVF).

Treatment

- Patients with confirmed SAH should be closely monitored in a high-dependency unit or ICU. The aims must be strict blood pressure control, prevention of SAH complications, and treatment of the underlying cause. Nimodipine should be commenced as soon as possible (PO/NG), usually 60 mg every 4 h if systolic BP is >100 mmHg or 30 mg every 2 h if SBP <100 mg. If SAH is aneurysmal, urgent referral to neurosurgery is needed for consideration of surgery (clipping or endovascular coiling, depending on site of the aneurysm, clinical picture, comorbidities and local practice) and further management.
- Complications of SAH include acute hydrocephalus, rebleeding and vasospasm. Acute hydrocephalus occurs from intraventricular extension of blood and subsequent obstruction of the cerebral aqueduct. Clinical manifestations include worsening headache, altered mental status, and coma. Hydrocephalus is treated with the placement of an intraventricular shunt. Rebleeding tends to occur early on, if the aneurysm has not been secured, and may cause mass effect if evacuation is not prompt and a haematoma forms, leading to uncal herniation. Vasospasm can occur between 3 and 15 days from the bleeding (the risk is highest between days 5 and 10), can cause ischaemia and delayed infarcts, and is the leading cause of morbidity and mortality in patients who survive initial SAH. Symptoms of vasospasm include headache, nausea, vomiting, changes in mental status, and focal neurological deficits. Transcranial Doppler ultrasound, CTA and digital subtraction angiography may be helpful in the diagnosis of vasospasm.

Cerebral venous sinus thrombosis

Clinical features

- Headache is the most common symptom of cerebral venous sinus thrombosis (CVST), occurs in up to 90% of cases, is the only manifestation in 25% of patients, and is due to raised intracranial pressure (ICP). CVST, however, has a wide range of potential manifestations, including focal neurological deficits, isolated cranial nerve palsies (most commonly VI palsy), seizures, altered mental status, and coma. CVST-related headache is usually progressive over hours to days (occasionally thunderclap, presumably related to SAH then leading to CVST), and worse lying flat. It can be localised or holocranial, and may have migrainous features. Patients may also describe transient visual obscurations upon lying down or bending over.
- On examination, patients may have focal neurological deficits and/or papilloedema. If thrombosis occurs in a cortical vein (not in a venous sinus), symptoms will typically be focal deficits (anatomically related) and/or seizures, and raised ICP is less common.

Diagnosis

- Patients with suspected CVST require urgent CT + CT venogram or MR + MR venogram, to confirm the diagnosis. Imaging should be done in patients with new-onset, persistent, progressive headache that has positional features and does not improve with regular analgesia, with or without focal deficits or optic disc swelling.
- Risk factors for CVST include pregnancy and puerperium, oral contraceptive pill, cancer and any prothrombotic states, ENT infections and known dural AVF.

- Lumbar puncture to measure opening pressure (which would be pathologically raised in CVST, >20 cmH$_2$0) is not required if the diagnosis can be made on the basis of imaging.

Treatment

- CVST is treated with anticoagulation, usually in the form of low molecular weight heparin (LMWH) followed by warfarin, and discussion with Haematology is advised. Still, there is not much evidence in using DOACs in CVST. Anticoagulation should be lifelong for patients with underlying prothrombotic states.
- If the patient does not improve or worsen despite LMWH, local thrombolysis should be considered, and referral to ICU and Neurosurgery made. Meanwhile, treat seizures and other associated symptoms.

Giant cell arteritis

- GCA should be considered in any patient aged 50 or over with headache, which will usually be of days or a few weeks in duration.
- Associated symptoms include malaise, weight loss, jaw claudication, scalp tenderness and visual changes (amaurosis fugax, diplopia and partial or complete loss of vision).
- If the ESR is >50 mm/h and/or CRP raised, or the temporal artery is thickened or tender (feel 2 cm above and 2 cm forward from the external auditory meatus), start prednisolone immediately. For patients with visual symptoms give 60 mg as a one-off dose; these patients should be seen by an ophthalmologist the same day. For those without visual symptoms, give 40–60 mg daily (minimum 0.75 mg/kg). Also give aspirin 75 mg daily, if not contraindicated, and a proton pump inhibitor for gastroprotection.
- Arrange an urgent review by a rheumatologist.

Migraine

- Recurrent attacks, lasting minutes, of (usually unilateral) fully reversible visual, sensory or other CNS symptoms. These tend to develop gradually, followed by headache and associated migraine symptoms. The first migraine headache usually occurs between the ages of 10 and 30.
- Aura symptoms may be visual, sensory, speech/language-related, motor, brainstem-related or retinal.
- Treatment of an acute attack is with an non-steroidal anti-inflammatory drug (NSAID), triptan, dispersible aspirin or paracetamol and an antiemetic, for example metoclopramide 10 mg IM or domperidone (available in suppository form). Combination therapy with a triptan and NSAID/paracetamol may be more effective.

Further reading

Headache Classification Committee of the International Headache Society (IHS). (2013) The international classification of headache disorders, 3rd edition (beta version). *Cephalalgia* 33, 629–808. https://www. ichd-3.org/.

Thilak S, Brown P, Whitehouse T, *et al.* (2024) Diagnosis and management of subarachnoid haemorrhage. *Nat Commun.* 15(1), 1850. Published 2024 Feb 29. DOI: 10.1038/s41467-024-46015-2.

Ulivi L, Squitieri M, Cohen H, *et al.* (2020) Cerebral venous thrombosis: a practical guide. *Pract Neurol.* 20(5), 356–367. DOI: 10.1136/practneurol-2019-002415.

CHAPTER 54

Weakness and paralysis

SIMON RINALDI AND ROBERTO BELLANTI

Paralysis is a complete loss of voluntary movement. Weakness is a reduction in the force of voluntary movement and is a result of pathology affecting the motor pathway at any point from the cerebral cortex to the muscle fibre (Box 54.1). Weakness can be life-threatening if respiratory muscles are involved.

- Stroke (Chapter 56), multiple sclerosis and spinal cord injury are the major central nervous system pathologies causing weakness.
- Guillain–Barré syndrome (GBS) (Chapter 59) is the most common cause of acute neuromuscular paralysis.

Pathologies at different localizations produce distinctive features (Table 54.1), broadly divided into upper motor neuron (UMN) or lower motor neuron (LMN) syndromes (Table 54.2).

Priorities

Prompt identification of patients

- with acute stroke, who may be candidates for thrombolysis or thrombectomy (Chapter 56)
- at risk of neuromuscular respiratory failure
- who require urgent imaging and/or neurosurgical opinion (Figure 54.1)

The clinical assessment is summarized in Table 54.3.

Diagnostic tests are directed by the clinical picture, although some tests should be considered for all patients (Table 54.4). Acute stroke and spinal cord/cauda equina syndromes require urgent neuroimaging.

Box 54.1 Medical Research Council (MRC) scale for assessment of muscle power.

Grade	Description
0	No contraction
1	Flicker or trace of contraction
2	Active movement with gravity eliminated
3	Active movement against gravity
4	Active movement against gravity and resistance
	Grades 4−, 4 and 4+ may be used to indicate movement against slight, moderate and strong resistance respectively
5	Normal power

Table 54.1 Localization of the cause of weakness by clinical syndrome.

Localization	Syndrome(s)	Additional features	Possible pathology
Brain	Hemiplegia	Homonymous hemianopia, ipsilateral sensory loss, dysphasia, dysphagia	Stroke, MS, tumour, migraine, post-ictal, hypoglycaemia
Brainstem	Crossed	Ipsilateral cranial nerve, contralateral arm/leg	Stroke, central pontine myelinolysis. MS
Spinal cord	Anterior cord	Para/quadriplegia, sensory level, sphincter disturbance, proprioception/vibration (relatively) spared	Anterior spinal artery thrombosis, cord compression, tumour, radiation
	Posterior cord	Sensory ataxia, vibration sensation loss	B12/copper deficiency, HIV, syphilis, tumour, dural metastasis, MS
	Brown Séquard (hemi-cord)	Ipsilateral weakness and loss of proprioception/vibration, contralateral loss of pain and temperature	MS, penetrating injury, tumour
	Conus medullaris	Prominent sphincter involvement, saddle anaesthesia, mixed UMN/LMN signs	Disc prolapse, tumour
Spinal roots	Cauda equina	Back/radicular pain, sphincter disturbance, dermatomal sensory loss	Disc prolapse, tumour, arachnoiditis, lumbar canal stenosis, infection
	Polyradiculopathy	Proximal and distal weakness, areflexia in affected limbs, back/radicular pain, sensory symptoms > sensory signs	GBS/CIDP, leptomeningeal infiltration (e.g. lymphoma), Lyme, VZV/viral
Plexus	Brachial or lumbosacral plexopathy	Pain (often in groin or shoulder) before weakness, patchy/minimal sensory loss	Diabetes, idiopathic, infiltrative (cancer/lymphoma), radiation, infective
Peripheral nerve	Demyelinating	Proximal and distal weakness without wasting, global areflexia, early vibration loss	GBS/CIDP, paraproteinaemic
	Axonal	Distal weakness and sensory loss, wasting, reflex loss in weak limbs/at ankles only	Alcohol, nutritional, diabetes, critical illness, paraneoplastic
	Multiple mono-neuropathies	Pain, systemic features of vasculitis	Vasculitis, lymphoma, sarcoid, amyloid, HIV, multiple pressure palsies
Neuro-muscular junction	Myasthenia	Fatigable facial/proximal weakness, diplopia, dysphagia, dysarthria, neuromuscular respiratory failure, no sensory loss	Autoimmune (myasthenia gravis), paraneoplastic, non-paraneoplastic (Lambert-Eaton), botulism
Muscle	Proximal myopathy	Myalgia, rash	Inflammatory (dermatomyositis), steroids, statins
	Rhabdomyolysis	Myalgia, dark urine/myoglobinuria	Crush injury, malignant hyperthermia, neuroleptics

AVM, arterio-venous malformation; CIDP, chronic inflammatory demyelinating polyradiculoneuropathy; MS, multiple sclerosis.

Table 54.2 Features of lower motor neuron (LMN) and upper motor neuron (UMN) weakness.

	LMN	UMN
Tone	Normal/decreased	Increased (spasticity)
Deep tendon reflexes	Suppressed/lost	Exaggerated
Plantar response	Flexor/mute	Extensor
Fasciculations	May be present	Absent
Atrophy	Pronounced (if axonal process)	Slight (reflecting disuse)
Distribution of weakness	Individual muscles may be affected, bilaterally innervated muscles can be involved	Groups of muscles affected, 'pyramidal' pattern;* bilaterally innervated muscles spared

* Extensors weaker than flexors in arms, flexors weaker than extensors in legs.

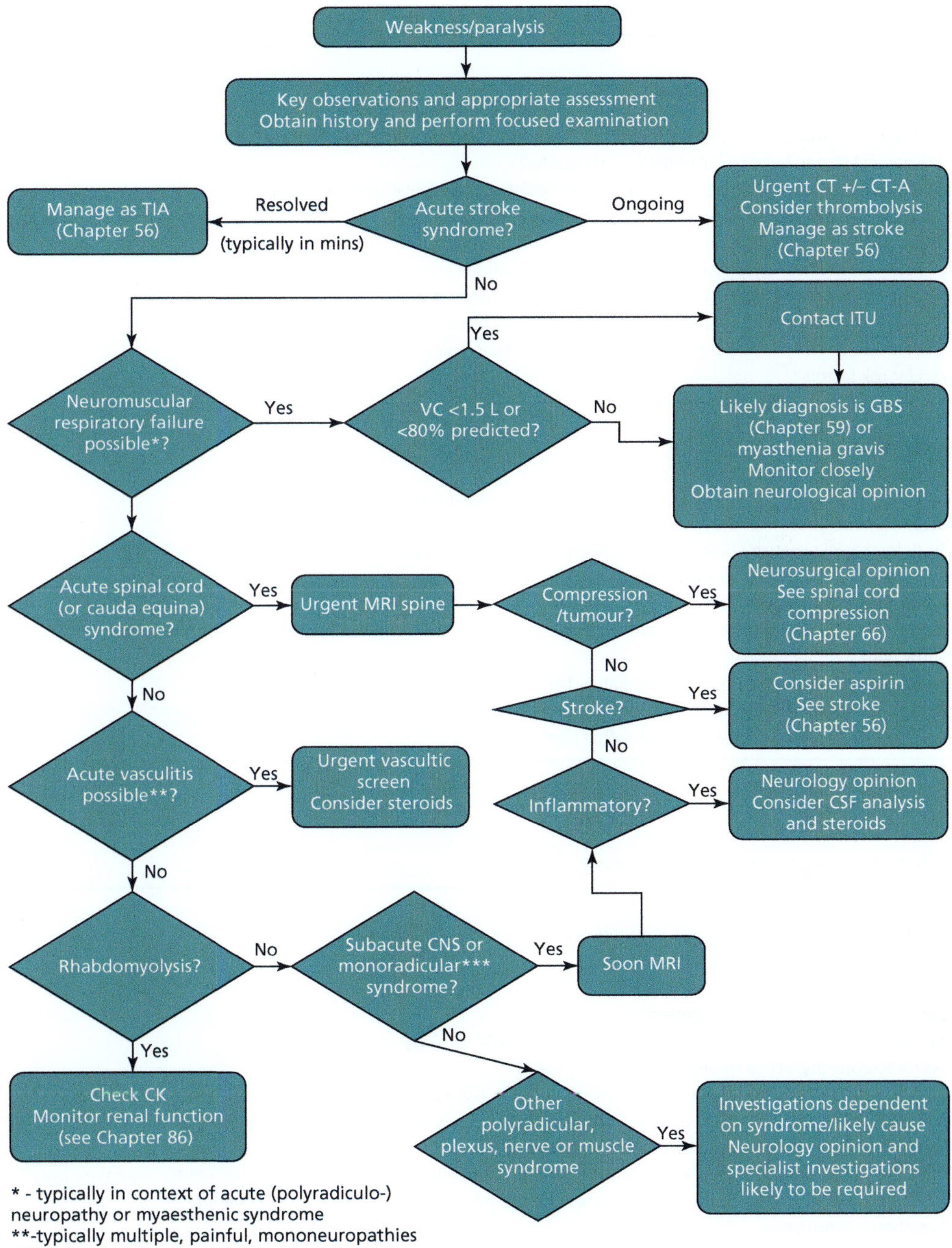

Figure 54.1 Assessment of the patient with weakness or paralysis.

Table 54.3 Focused assessment of the patient with weakness.

History

Time and speed of onset and progression (instant, seconds, hours, days, weeks; resolving, stable, fluctuating/fatigable, worsening)?

Distribution? (hemi-, quadri-, para-, monoplegia, localized, proximal, distal, axial) Cranial nerve distribution involvement? (facial, bulbar, ocular/diplopia) Headache?

Other associated pain? Character? Myelopathic (constricting)? Radicular (shooting/deep ache)? Localized to entrapment sites or plexus? Neuropathic (paraesthesia)? Myalgic?

Sensory loss? Distribution? Saddle?

Sphincter disturbance? Dysphasia/hemianopia/other cortical symptoms?

Functional impairment? Walking? Stairs/chairs? Fine motor tasks? Breathing?

Prodromal illness/infection? Trauma? Compression? Arising from sleep?

Systemic upset? Weight loss? Diet/malnutrition? Alcohol/drug/toxin exposure?

Vascular risk factors?

Past neurological or systemic disease?

Examination

Rapid assessment of ABC/vital signs/glucose

If acute stroke, possible CT scanning +/ thrombolysis now takes priority

Assess distribution of weakness, tone and reflex pattern per Table 54.2. Also see Box 54.2

Check for cranial nerve and higher mental dysfunction. Is there dysphasia?

Perform sensory testing with a hypothesis in mind

Test for fatigability if appropriate

Ptosis +/ diplopia developing or worsening with prolonged upgaze? Reduction in power after repetitive muscle contraction?

Check vital capacity if neuromuscular respiratory failure possible

General examination to look for cause

Bruit? AF? Rash? Cachexia? Lymphadenopathy? Organomegaly?

Table 54.4 Urgent investigation of the patient with weakness.

To consider in all patients

Glucose, FBC, U+Es, LFTs, Ca^{2+}/Mg^{2+}, ESR/CRP, clotting, TFTs, ABGs, cultures, ECG, CXR

If acute stroke possible

Urgent CT head and CT-A (refer to Chapter 56)

Spinal cord/cauda equina syndromes

MRI spine +/LP, B_{12}/folate, copper, syphilis, HIV, CMV and VZV serology

Polyradiculopathy/acute neuropathy

NCS, LP, blood film, B_{12}/folate/thiamine, Borrelia/*C. jejuni*/CMV/EBV/HIV/*Mycoplasma* serology, anti-ganglioside and paraneoplastic antibodies, serum and urine protein electrophoresis with immunofixation, urinary porphyrins

Multiple mononeuropathies/mononeuritis multiplex

ANA/ENA, ANCA, Cryoglobulins, ACE, HIV serology, paraneoplastic antibodies, blood film, NCS/EMG, Schirmer's test, LP, nerve biopsy, PMP22 genetics (of multiple pressure palsies), anti-GM1 antibodies (if pure motor)

Myasthenic syndromes

NCS/EMG (with repetitive stimulation/single fibre EMG), anti-acetylcholine receptor and anti-MuSK antibodies (myasthenia gravis), anti-voltage gated calcium channel antibodies (LEMS), CT thorax (both)

Box 54.2 Weakness and paralysis – alerts.

A common pitfall is to fail to distinguish true neurological weakness from its mimics. Patients with systemic illness, infections, cachexia and depression may report weakness when objective tests of strength are normal. Conversely, patients with systemic illness, pain, or functional disorders may have apparent weakness on examination without localised neurological dysfunction. In the latter group, the observation of give-way weakness, a positive Hoover sign, or inconsistency between the examination findings and functional performance may provide the diagnosis.

Further management

Further management is directed by the working diagnosis.
- Patients with acute stroke should be admitted to a specialist stroke unit, have an assessment of their swallow performed, and be regularly monitored for deterioration and the development of complications (Chapter 56).
- Patients with GBS (Chapter 59) and myasthenia (Chapter 61) need regular vital capacity checks and involvement of ICU in the event of deterioration, but may be suitable for the general ward in the absence of respiratory compromise.
- In all immobile patients, pressure sores, deep vein thrombosis, respiratory infection/aspiration and contractures need to be prevented and addressed.

Further reading

Asimos AW (2015) Evaluation of the adult with acute weakness in the emergency department. UpToDate, last updated Oct 2021. https://www.uptodate.com/contents/
evaluation-of-the-adult-with-acute-weakness-in-the-emergency-department

CHAPTER 55

Visual disturbance

TRISTAN MCMULLAN AND NIMRATH KAINTH

The visual pathway extends from the cornea to the occipital cortex (Figure 55.1). Visual disturbance may occur due to ocular, intracranial or systemic disease that requires prompt intervention to preserve sight. Clinical assessment (Table 55.1; Figure 55.2) will narrow the differential diagnosis and determine further management.

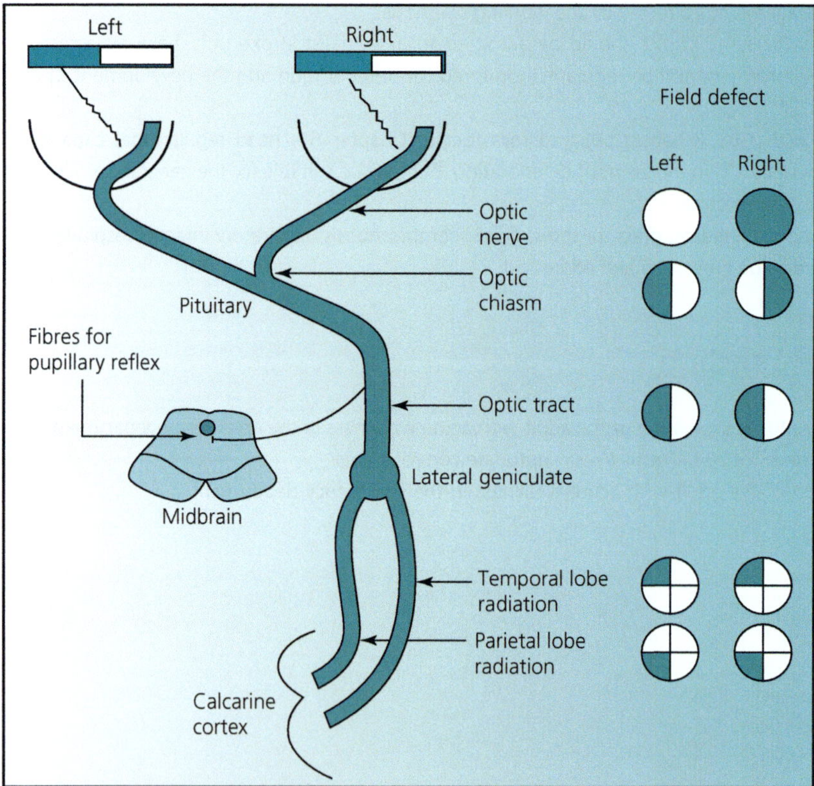

Figure 55.1 Visual pathway. The visual pathway. Characteristic field defects seen with lesions at various sites along the pathway are illustrated. The calcarine cortex in the occipital lobe is the location of the primary visual cortex. The occipital lobes are supplied by the posterior cerebral arteries, terminal branches of the basilar artery. The pupillary reflex is affected only if fibres proximal to the lateral geniculate body are damaged, or there is a lesion in the midbrain or of the III nerve. Source: Weiner HL, Levitt LP (1978). *Neurology for the house officer* 2e. William and Wilkins. Reproduced with permission of Wolters Kluwer Health.

Table 55.1 Focused assessment of the patient with visual loss.

History

See text: establish if the visual loss was:

- Sudden or gradual
- In one or both eyes
- Persistent or transient
- In the central or peripheral field
- Painful or painless; if painful, ache or gritty

Associated headache, nausea or vomiting?

Has the patient noticed new 'floaters' or photopsia?

Other neuro-ophthalmic symptoms?

Symptoms suggestive of polymyalgia rheumatica/giant cell arteritis (malaise, lethargy, anorexia, weight loss, night sweats, headache, occipital pain, jaw claudication, scalp tenderness)?

Other systemic symptoms?

Cardiovascular risk factors?

Past eye history, for example cataract surgery or previous uveitis; refractive state, myopic or hypermetropic?

Past medical history: diabetes? Thyroid disease? Immunosuppression? Connective tissue disease?

Drug history

Family history

Social history, to include occupation and driving and smoking status

Examination

Perform a general examination, with particular attention to heart, blood pressure, carotid and temporal arteries.

Eyes

- Red eye, discharge, photophobia, watering?
- Pupillary abnormalities?
- Ptosis, eyelid swelling, eyelid erythema, proptosis = exophthalmos?
- Nystagmus?
- Eye movements and assessment for diplopia
- Fundoscopy

Visual acuity

Check the visual acuity using a Snellen chart, in each eye, with the patient wearing their glasses or contact lenses, or looking through a pinhole. If visual acuity is lower than can be measured by the Snellen chart, determine if the patient can count fingers (CF), detect hand movement (HM) or perceive light (PL).

Visual fields

Visual field respecting the horizontal midline (i.e. superior or inferior defects) are seen with retinal vascular or optic nerve disorders, including glaucoma. Defects respecting the vertical midline represent a neurological lesion such as a stroke or compressive lesions.

Central defects are caused primarily by macular disease, such as age-related macular degeneration. In macular disease, the patient experiences a positive scotoma, that is, a 'spot' in the vision is seen and reported. Conversely, in optic nerve disease a negative scotoma is present, but not reported, that is, the defect is not 'seen' by the patient, but can be detected on examination.

Amsler grid

This is used to assess macular function. The patient should wear their glasses or contact lenses with any reading correction, if worn. Hold the grid at eye level around 33 cm away in good lighting. Cover one eye and ask the patient to focus on the central dot with the uncovered eye, then repeat with the other eye. Distortion will be reported if there is macular pathology (age-related macular degeneration or macular oedema). A central scotoma may be detected in optic nerve disease.

Colour vision

Ask the patient to assess the colour quality of a bright red object (e.g. top of red pen). A relative difference between the eyes indicates pathology affecting the optic nerve (e.g. optic neuritis); the red is desaturated or 'washed out' in the affected eye.

(continued)

Table 55.1 (*Continued*)

'Swinging flash light' test to detect a relative afferent pupillary defect (RAPD)
Normally, both pupils constrict symmetrically when a bright light is shone into one eye. When the torch is swung to the
other eye, the pupils remain the same size. A RAPD is present if the pupil dilates, when the torch is swung to the
affected eye. Both pupils constrict when the torch is swung back to the unaffected eye. A positive RAPD indicates severe
retinal and/or optic nerve injury in the affected eye.

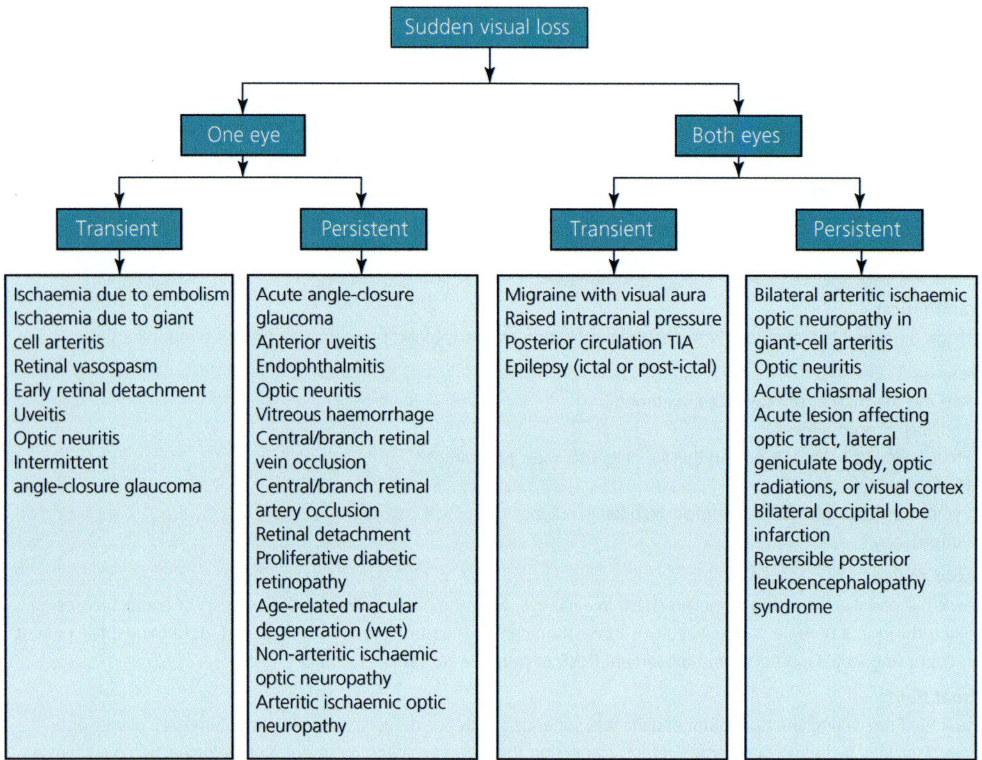

TIA, transient ischaemic attack

Figure 55.2 Analysis of sudden visual loss.

   Giant cell arteritis (GCA) should be considered in any patient over 50 with new-onset visual symptoms. It has
a varied presentation including transient visual loss (amaurosis fugax), persistent visual loss due to retinal or
optic nerve ischaemia (may rarely affect both eyes) or diplopia.

The history

Sudden versus gradual?
Sudden loss of vision typically (but not exclusively) reflects vascular disease, and gradual loss of vision, a
non-vascular disorder (Table 55.2).

Table 55.2 Differential diagnosis of gradual visual loss.

Cause	Key features
(a) Painful	
Optic neuritis	Subacute but rapid profound visual loss, with gradual recovery over six weeks.
	May be pain on eye movements, particularly convergence.
	Positive RAPD, if unilateral.
	Reduced colour vision or red desaturation.
	Central/centrocecal visual field defect.
	May be history of multiple sclerosis.
Corneal epitheliopathy:	Pain, watering, photophobia.
	Stains with fluorescein dye and visualised with blue light.
	Corneal sensation will be reduced.
Herpes keratitis	May display characteristic dendritic ulcer.
Scleritis	Deep ache with 'beefy' redness of the eye (best seen in daylight)
	Does not blanch with topical application of 10% phenylephrine drops.
	May be a history of connective tissue disease e.g. rheumatoid arthritis.
(b) Painless	
Keratoconus, corneal dystrophies	Blurring of vision and loss of acuity.
	May be family history.
Cataract	Gradual blurring/fogging of vision, glare and dazzle.
	No distortion.
Post-cataract surgery: cystoid macular oedema	Central blurring of vision, usually four to six weeks post-cataract surgery.
Posterior capsule opacification	Gradual fogging of vision post-cataract surgery.
Age-related macular degeneration (dry)	Decreased vision with loss of clarity – may be some distortion.
Diabetic maculopathy (exudative, ischaemic)	Decreased visual acuity and blurry vision.
Macular problems: epiretinal membrane, macular hole	Decreased vision with loss of clarity – some distortion likely.
Compressive optic neuropathy	Typically unilateral.
	Insidious visual field loss that may become apparent when the good eye is covered.
	Positive RAPD and variable loss of colour vision.
	Differential diagnosis: Thyroid orbitopathy
Drug-related: maculopathy, optic neuropathy	Decreased visual acuity and blurry vision.
	(See Table 55.5)

AION, anterior ischaemic optic neuropathy; CF, counting fingers; CWS, cotton wool spot; HM, hand movements; NPL, no perception of light; PL, perception of light; RAPD, relative afferent pupillary defect.

Unilateral versus bilateral?

Unilateral loss of vision indicates disease of that eye or optic nerve.

Bilateral visual loss occurs with systemic disease or focal disorders involving the visual pathway from the optic chiasm back to the occipital cortex.

Patients may report loss of vision in only one eye, even though both eyes are affected; with a homonymous hemianopia, the patient may only be aware of the visual loss in the eye with the temporal field defect, despite having a nasal visual field defect in the fellow eye.

Persistent versus transient?

Sudden, painless and persistent loss of vision is usually due to ischaemia/infarction or haemorrhage at some point along the visual pathway, but is also a feature of retinal detachment (Table 55.3). Sudden transient loss of vision has a range of ocular, vascular and neurological causes (Table 55.4).

Table 55.3 Differential diagnosis of sudden persistent visual loss.

Cause	Features
(a) Painful	
Acute angle-closure glaucoma	Sight-threatening, clinical emergency.
	Unwell patient – nausea/vomiting, periocular pain and headache.
	Congested eye with mid-dilated pupil.
	Iris details hazy due to corneal oedema.
	May be preceded by subacute attacks.
	High intraocular pressure, for example >35 mmHg.
	Likely hypermetropic = long sighted (patient's glasses make their eyes look bigger, to an observer, when worn)
Anterior uveitis	Brow ache, red eye – particularly perilimbal (around corneal limbus) injection. Pupil will likely be constricted.
	Hypopyon in severe cases.
Endophthalmitis	Sight-threatening, clinical emergency.
	Post-operative endophthalmitis: within 2–14 days of surgery.
	Pain, lid swelling, loss of vision, hypopyon.
	Endogenous endophthalmitis: seek infective source, for example infected central venous cannula, septic focus.
	May be immunosuppressed.
	Less of a hot eye.
	Clinical emergency.
Optic neuritis	May affect one eye or both eyes.
	Pain is less of a feature than visual loss. Maybe pain on eye movements.
	RAPD, if unilateral.
	Subacute dramatic vision loss over one to two days.
	Swollen hyperaemic optic nerve when acute; optic disc pallor when established. Visual field loss – typically central/centrocaecal.
	Uhthoff's sign – visual loss exacerbated by increased body temperature, for example hot bath. Frequently associated with multiple sclerosis (MS): 25–72% will develop MS at 15 years, depending on MRI findings.
	Subacute visual loss with pain on ocular movement and RAPD with field loss.
	Colour vision profoundly affected.
	May have MS or develop MS.
	Neurology input required.
(b) Painless affecting one eye	
Vitreous haemorrhage	Sudden onset of floaters and blurred vision.
	Red reflex may be absent if haemorrhage is significant.
	No RAPD.
	Caused by proliferative diabetic retinopathy, or retinal tear until proven otherwise in non-diabetics.
Central/branch retinal vein occlusion	Often presents in the morning with variable visual loss from mild to profound, depending on degree of ischaemia.
	RAPD if ischaemic.
	Dark blot haemorrhages in quadrants according to venous drainage involved e.g. supero-temporal if BRVO, whole fundus if CRVO; hemi-vein occlusion will cause haemorrhage in either superior or inferior retina.
	Respects horizontal meridian if not CRVO (in which case whole retinal involved).

Table 55.3 (*Continued*)

Cause	Features
Central/branch retinal artery occlusion	Retinal pallor and oedema with profound visual loss. May have cherry red spot if acute. Cattle-tracking of blood cells in retinal arterioles (segmentation of blood column denoting impaired, sluggish circulation). RAPD. Must exclude giant cell arteritis. Cardiovascular work up and referral to stroke team.
Retinal detachment	Sight-threatening, clinical emergency. May be preceded by flashes and floaters, symptomatic of posterior vitreous separation/ detachment (PVD). Field loss commensurate with retinal elevation – supero-temporal detachment causing infero-nasal field loss. White billowing retina seen on ophthalmoscopy.
Proliferative diabetic retinopathy	May be asymptomatic until tractional retinal detachment or vitreous haemorrhage supervene. Venous new vessel proliferation at optic nerve or along arcades or in watershed (ischaemic) area nasal to the optic nerve. Other diabetic changes will be present. If markedly asymmetric, consider coexisting carotid disease.
Age-related macular degeneration (wet)	Central visual loss with haemorrhage +/− exudate in central macula. May be bilateral. Variable visual loss from 6/6 to hand movement vision.
Non-arteritic ischaemic optic neuropathy (NAION)	Acute visual loss, typically in morning. Swollen disc with haemorrhagic component. RAPD, loss of colour vision and has associated field defect. Younger age group, 45–65. Small optic nerves, may be hypermetropic 'disc at risk'
Arteritic ischaemic optic neuropathy (AION)	As above but chalky white optic disc. Vision usually worse than NAION. Older age group >50, typically >75. May have associated symptoms and signs of giant-cell arteritis (but may be 'silent' GCA). If GCA suspected, treat with corticosteroid (see text).

AION, anterior ischaemic optic neuropathy; CF, counting fingers; CWS, cotton wool spot; HM, hand movements; NPL, no perception of light; PL, perception of light; RAPD, relative afferent pupillary defect.

(c) Affecting both eyes	
Bilateral arteritic ischaemic optic neuropathy (AION)	(*As above*)
Optic Neuritis	(*As above*)
Acute chiasmal lesion	May be infectious, inflammatory or vascular lesion. Pituitary apoplexy may complicate pituitary adenoma (Chapter 48). Typically results in bi-temporal hemianopia. III, IV or VI nerve palsies may be present if lesion extends into cavernous sinus.
Acute lesion affecting optic tract, the lateral geniculate body, the optic radiations, or the visual cortex	May be due to cerebral infarction or haemorrhage, or haemorrhage into brain tumour. Results in homonymous hemianopia.
Bilateral occipital lobe infarction	Due to posterior circulation stroke (see Chapter 56).
Reversible posterior leukoencephalopathy syndrome	Typically presents with seizures. Other features include headache, altered consciousness and visual abnormalities (e.g. blurred vision, homonymous hemianopia, cortical blindness).
Psychogenic	Diagnosis of exclusion.

Table 55.4 Differential diagnosis of transient visual loss.

Cause	Typical duration/characteristic features
Affecting one eye	
Amaurosis fugax	Typically 1–10 min
	Like a shutter coming down
	(Urgent referral to stroke team advised).
Ischaemia due to giant cell arteritis	Variable, may have preceding visual obscurations.
	May affect nerve (AION), retina (CRAO) or ocular circulation as a whole (ocular ischaemic syndrome).
	May also cause motility disturbance – cranial nerve palsies/extraocular muscles ischaemia.
Retinal vasospasm	Lasts 5–60 min
	Migrainous features such as aura and headache.
	Fortification spectra/scintillating scotoma are absent as they are cortical phenomena and relate to cephalic migraine.
Early retinal detachment	Variable – progressively worse, painless.
Uveitis	Variable – progressively worse and more painful.
Optic neuritis	Subacute visual loss with hyperaemic optic nerve and features of optic neuropathy: decreased colour vision, field loss and RAPD.
Intermittent angle-closure glaucoma	Brow ache and blurred vision – may get halos around lights and feel nauseous.
Affecting both eyes	
Migraine with visual aura	Lasts 10–30 min, migrainous features such as fortification spectra/scintillating scotoma and headache.
	Affects both eyes.
Raised intracranial pressure	Obscurations lasting seconds, which may be postural.
	Headache and other features of raised ICP.
	Bilateral disc swelling with preserved visual function (i.e. normal colour vision) in early stages.
	Enlarged blind spot in early stages.
Posterior circulation transient ischaemic attack affecting visual cortex	Lasts 1–10 min.
Epilepsy (ictal or post-ictal)	Ictal: 3–5 min.
	Post-ictal: 20 min.

Central versus peripheral visual field?

Central blurring or vision loss in one eye is typical of macular pathology (e.g. diabetic maculopathy).

Monocular peripheral visual loss may be due to retinal pathology (e.g. branch retinal vein/artery occlusion or retinal detachment) or optic nerve disease (e.g. ischaemic optic neuropathy, optic neuritis, glaucoma).

Painful versus painless?

Pain in the eye usually indicates anterior eye disease (e.g. keratitis, anterior uveitis, primary angle-closure glaucoma). Optic neuritis and giant cell arteritis can cause visual loss, which may or may not be associated with pain in the eye.

Painless loss of vision is typical of cataract, retinal disorders and disorders of the visual pathway.

Drug history

A careful drug history is essential as many drugs can cause transient or persistent visual loss (Table 55.5).

Further management

Visual loss due to suspected eye disease

Seek urgent advice from an ophthalmologist.

Suspected giant cell arteritis

If there is persistent visual loss, seek urgent advice from an ophthalmologist. IV methylprednisolone can be given.

If there has been transient visual loss in suspected GCA, prescribe prednisolone 60 mg PO. The patient should be reviewed by an ophthalmologist the same day. Consider starting aspirin 75 mg daily, unless there are contraindications such as active peptic ulceration or a bleeding disorder. Proton-pump inhibitors (PPI) should be provided for prophylaxis against peptic ulceration. Osteoporotic fracture risk should be assessed and bone protection therapy prescribed as appropriate.

Central and branch retinal artery occlusion

See urgent advice from an ophthalmologist.

Complete a full cardiovascular examination and record an ECG. Assess cardiovascular risk factors. Arrange an echocardiogram and carotid duplex scan to determine if there is an embolic source. Check full blood count, C-reactive protein ESR, blood glucose, biochemical profile and lipids. A referral to the stroke team should also be made and initiation of antiplatelet therapy should be considered.

Amaurosis fugax presents with transient visual loss, typically with a curtain appearing over the vision without pain. It should be managed as for CRAO and patients discussed with a stroke physician. See Chapter 56 for further management of amaurosis fugax/transient ischaemic attack.

GCA should always be considered in patients presenting with suspected CRAO or amaurosis fugax.

Central and branch retinal vein occlusion

Complete a full cardiovascular examination and record an ECG.

Consider diabetes and hyperviscosity syndromes (check full blood count and serum protein electrophoresis). In younger patients consider thrombophilia. Hypertension is the main risk factor but screen for other cardiovascular risk factors. Consider antiplatelet therapy if not contraindicated.

Arrange follow-up with an ophthalmologist.

Table 55.5 Drugs causing visual symptoms.

Drug	Comment
Amiodarone	Corneal verticillata – asymptomatic, optic neuropathy rarely.
Corticosteroids	Raised intraocular pressure/glaucoma. Cataract.
Ethambutol	Toxic optic neuropathy.
Hydroxychloroquine	Maculopathy.
Isotretinoin	Dry eye, IIH.
Phenothiazines	Blurred vision from anticholinergic effect, pigment deposition in skin, cornea and lens. Pigmented retinopathy.
Sildenafil	Blue vision/NAION
Tamoxifen	Crystalline maculopathy.
Topiramate	Angle closure glaucoma, periorbital oedema, acute onset myopia.
Vigabatrin	Visual field defects.

Optic neuritis

In most patients with optic neuritis complicating multiple sclerosis, symptoms resolve spontaneously, with recovery starting within 10 days and usually complete by six weeks. Corticosteroid therapy (methylprednisolone IV) may accelerate recovery but does not alter long-term outcomes.

Seek urgent advice from an ophthalmologist.

Further reading

Biousse V, Newman NJ. (2015) Ischemic optic neuropathies. *N Engl J Med* 372, 2428–2436. DOI: 10.1056/NEJMra1413352.

Lemos J, Eggenberger E. (2015) Neuro-ophthalmological emergencies. *The Neurohospitalist* 5, 223–233.

Sawaya R, El Ayoubi N, Hamam R. (2015) Acute neurological visual loss in young adults: causes, diagnosis and management. *Postgrad Med J* 91, 698–703. DOI: 10.1136/postgradmedj-2014-133071.

CHAPTER 56

Transient ischaemic attack and stroke

SOMA BANERJEE AND AJAY BHALLA

Transient ischaemic attack (TIA) is defined as a transient episode of neurological dysfunction caused by focal brain, spinal cord or retinal ischaemia, without evidence of acute infarction on brain imaging. The symptoms of confirmed TIA typically last only minutes. Any patient with a fully resolved acute onset neurological syndrome that might be due to cerebrovascular disease needs urgent specialist assessment (within 24 h) to determine whether the cause is vascular, given the substantial risk of subsequent stroke after a TIA (between 2 and 4% at 48 h post onset). Treatment for secondary prevention should be initiated as soon as the diagnosis is confirmed.

Priorities

Clinical assessment and investigation are directed at answering these questions:

1 Was it a TIA?

Establish if the symptoms were:

- Focal neurological or monocular rather than global (Table 56.1).
- Of sudden onset.
- Maximum at the onset, rather than spreading or stuttering (spreading of sensory symptoms over several seconds tends to indicate seizure activity, whereas spreading of sensory symptoms over several minutes indicates migraine).
- Negative (loss of function, e.g. weakness or numbness) rather than positive (e.g. jerking as a result of seizure or paraesthesia due to seizure or migraine).

If the answer is 'yes' to all four questions, then a diagnosis of TIA is highly likely. Other causes of transient neurological or visual symptoms to be considered when the diagnosis of TIA is less likely are given in Table 56.2.

2 Which arterial territory?

Carotid and vertebrobasilar territory TIA give rise to differing patterns of symptoms (Table 56.3). Establishing which territory was involved (or if TIAs have occurred in both territories) is important in the interpretation of the carotid duplex scan and further management.

Table 56.1 Focal neurological symptoms: attributable to a focal area of the brain and therefore more likely to represent TIA or stroke.

Weakness (hemiparesis) or incoordination of one side of body
Dysphagia
Ataxia

Dysphasia (receptive and/or expressive)
Dysarthria
Dyslexia
Dysgraphia
Dyscalculia

Hemisensory disturbance
Transient monocular blindness
Hemianopia or quadrantanopia
Bilateral blindness
Diplopia

Vertigo (only in association with other brain stem focal symptoms, unusual for vertigo as an isolated symptom to represent a TIA)

Dyspraxia
Visual-spatial dysfunction (visual neglect)
Amnesia (as an isolated symptom does not indicate TIA)

Note: if multiple stereotypical focal events occur over a period of time with the same symptoms, then a diagnosis of TIA is very unlikely: consider seizure activity. Rhythmic, involuntary jerky movements lasting a few minutes however can occur with TIA due to severe middle cerebral artery or internal carotid artery disease precipitated by changes in posture.

Table 56.2 Causes of transient neurological or monocular visual symptoms.

Cause	Comment
Migraine aura (with or without headache)	Stereotypical positive symptoms such as tingling and visual symptoms, spreading over several minutes and typically resolving within 60 min. Often positive family history for migraine.
Partial epileptic seizure	Positive symptoms (jerking or tingling, marching over several seconds). May have impaired awareness (partial complex seizure).
Transient global amnesia	Loss of anterograde memory usually accompanied by repetitive questioning. Resolves usually within 6 h. No language deficit. Able to recognize surroundings and familiar individuals.
Metabolic	Hypoglycaemia: consider if recurrent events associated with low blood glucose. See Chapter 46.
Structural lesion	For example brain tumour, chronic subdural haematoma.
Demyelination	Subacute onset in young adults. MRI clarifies diagnosis.
Mononeuropathy	Look for lower motor neuron signs.
Myasthenia gravis	Check for fatigability.
Monocular visual symptoms	Ocular or optic nerve disease. See Chapter 54.

Table 56.3 TIA: Which vascular territory was involved?

Symptom	Carotid territory	Vertebrobasilar territory
Dysphasia	Yes	No
Monocular visual loss	Yes	No
Unilateral weakness	Yes	Yes
Unilateral sensory loss	Yes	Yes
Dysarthria	Yes	Yes
Homonymous hemianopia	Yes	Yes
Ataxia/unsteadiness	Yes	Yes
Dysphagia	Yes	Yes
Diplopia	No	Yes
Vertigo	No	Yes

3 Does the TIA have a potentially treatable cause (Box 56.1)?

This is determined by clinical assessment and investigation (Table 56.4).

Always consider:

- Atherosclerotic carotid artery disease. Carotid duplex scan is indicated in patients who have had a carotid territory TIA (Table 56.3) and would be candidates for endarterectomy.

Box 56.1 Causes of transient ischaemic attack and ischaemic stroke.

Large arterial atherothromboembolism (45%)
Atherosclerotic disease of the aorta or extracranial carotid and vertebral arteries or ICAD (intracranial atherosclerotic disease).

Embolism from the heart (20%)
Atrial fibrillation (left atrial thrombus).
Infective endocarditis (see Chapter 15).
Prosthetic heart valve (see Chapter 20).
Recent myocardial infarction (left ventricular thrombus).
Dilated cardiomyopathy (left ventricular thrombus).
Rheumatic mitral stenosis.
Have a high index of suspicion of a cardiac embolic source if the clinical presentation of TIA suggests involvement of multiple cerebral arterial territories.

Small artery microatheroma (25%)

Internal carotid or vertebral artery dissection (5%)
Consider diagnosis if focal neurological symptoms preceded by headache (either frontal headache over the eye in carotid dissection or neck pain in vertebral dissection); look for Horner's syndrome in carotid dissection.

Others (5%)
Arteritis (consider if associated headache or systemic symptoms, raised C-reactive protein/ESR, headache; see Chapter 94).
Haematological (hyperviscosity syndrome, sickle cell disease, see Chapter 83).

ESR, erythrocyte sedimentation rate.

Table 56.4 Investigation after TIA and Stroke.

All patients

Full blood count

ESR or C-reactive protein (if raised, consider vasculitis, infective endocarditis, cardiac myxoma or systemic infection)

INR (if taking warfarin)

Sickle cell test (if sickle cell disease considered)

Antiphospholipid antibodies (unexplained TIA or ischaemic stroke)

Electrolytes and creatinine

Lipid profile

Blood glucose (exclude hypoglycaemia and diabetes mellitus)

Blood culture if febrile or infective endocarditis suspected (e.g. prosthetic heart valve)

ECG (atrial fibrillation, previous myocardial infarction and left ventricular hypertrophy)

Chest X-ray (exclude lung neoplasm and assess heart size)

Neuroimaging

First-line imaging for acute stroke is computed tomography (CT). For TIA the greater sensitivity of magnetic resonance imaging (MRI) to detect ischaemic lesions using diffusion-weighted imaging (DWI) makes it the modality of choice where the results are likely to influence management such as reducing diagnostic uncertainty, confirming the territory of ischaemia prior to making a decision about carotid artery surgery and prior to commencing dual antiplatelet therapy. When the exclusion of haemorrhage is the objective of imaging, early unenhanced (CT) remains the most sensitive investigation. CT/MR angiography should also be considered where a macrovascular cause for intracerebral haemorrhage is felt likely. When suspicious of cerebral venous sinus thrombosis consider CT/MR venogram.

Arterial imaging

- Patients with ischaemic stroke or TIA who after specialist assessment are considered candidates for carotid intervention should have carotid imaging performed within 24h of assessment.
- CT or MR angiography if carotid dissection or large-vessel vasculitis is suspected.

Echocardiography

- Transthoracic echocardiography (TTE) where a cardio-embolic cause for stroke is being considered.
- Bubble echocardiography where patent foramen ovale is suspected.
- Consider transoesophageal echocardiography (TOE) for patients with possible endocarditis, mechanical valve prosthesis and unexplained TIA/stroke in patients <50 years.

Ambulatory ECG monitoring

- Ambulatory monitoring beyond 24h if paroxysmal atrial fibrillation (AF) is suspected

---

- Embolism from the heart (e.g. atrial fibrillation and mechanical heart valve with INR < 2).
- Arteritis, suggested by headache or systemic symptoms, with elevated ESR and C-reactive protein.
- Haematological disease (e.g. erythrocytosis and thrombocythaemia).

Further management

Patients with minor ischaemic stroke or TIA should receive treatment for secondary prevention as soon as the diagnosis is confirmed, including

- Support to modify lifestyle factors (smoking, alcohol consumption, diet and exercise)
- Antiplatelet or anticoagulant therapy
- High-intensity statin therapy
- Blood pressure-lowering therapy with a thiazide-like diuretic, long-acting calcium channel blocker or angiotensin-converting enzyme inhibitor

Patients with suspected TIA should be given aspirin 300 mg immediately unless contraindicated and assessed urgently within 24 h by a stroke specialist clinician in a neurovascular clinic or an acute stroke unit.

Dual antiplatelet therapy with either aspirin and clopidogrel, or aspirin and ticagrelor, should be considered in patients presenting within 24 h of TIA and minor stroke for up to 21–30 days respectively followed by monotherapy.

For patients with recurrent TIA or stroke whilst taking clopidogrel, consideration should be given to clopidogrel resistance.

All patients with TIA should be informed that they must not drive for one month following onset.

Stroke

Stroke is defined as a rapidly developing clinical syndrome of presumed vascular origin, characterised by focal or global neurological symptoms and signs; with tissue injury confirmed on brain imaging.

Subtypes are as follows:

1 Ischaemic stroke, accounting for ~85% of all strokes.
2 Haemorrhagic stroke, accounting for ~15% of strokes, and which includes non-traumatic intracerebral haemorrhage (ICH) affecting the brain parenchyma, and subarachnoid haemorrhage (SAH) with bleeding into the arachnoid space. The latter will be covered in Chapter 53.

Immediate priorities

Acute stroke is a medical emergency. Treatments are time sensitive and always start with an ABCD approach for both ischaemic and haemorrhagic stroke. The initial workflow and management are summarised in Figure 56.1.

1 **If the patient is unconscious**, initial resuscitation is as for coma from any cause (Chapter 3). Check blood glucose to exclude hyper or hypoglycaemia.
2 **Is this a Stroke versus a Stroke Mimic?**
   - Differentiation of stroke from stroke-like presentations of other diseases can sometimes be difficult. The acute onset (or presence on waking from sleep) of asymmetric face, arm or leg weakness, speech disturbance or visual field defect supports a diagnosis of stroke. Fever at presentation, prominent headache, or neck stiffness should make you consider alternative diagnoses. Syncope or seizure activity may suggest an alternative diagnosis.
   - The disorders which are most commonly misdiagnosed as stroke are summarized in Table 56.5, and atypical presentations of stroke are in Table 56.6.
3 **If the working diagnosis is acute ischaemic stroke, is thrombolysis or thrombectomy indicated?**

Acute ischaemic stroke

Rapid assessment and accurate history taking is essential, including a collateral history when the patient is unable to communicate. Time of onset should be recorded, or if not known, the time 'last known well'. History should focus on indications and contra-indications for thrombolysis and thrombectomy. Examination should include doing a National Institutes of Health Stroke Scale (NIHSS) score (Table 56.8).

The aim of initial brain imaging is to exclude haemorrhage and assess eligibility for intravenous thrombolysis using non-contrast CT head (NCCT); MRI brain is acceptable, but typically less accessible as first-line imaging in most centres. Patients who are being considered for mechanical thrombectomy (see criteria below) will also require CT or MR angiography, looking for a large vessel occlusion (LVO).

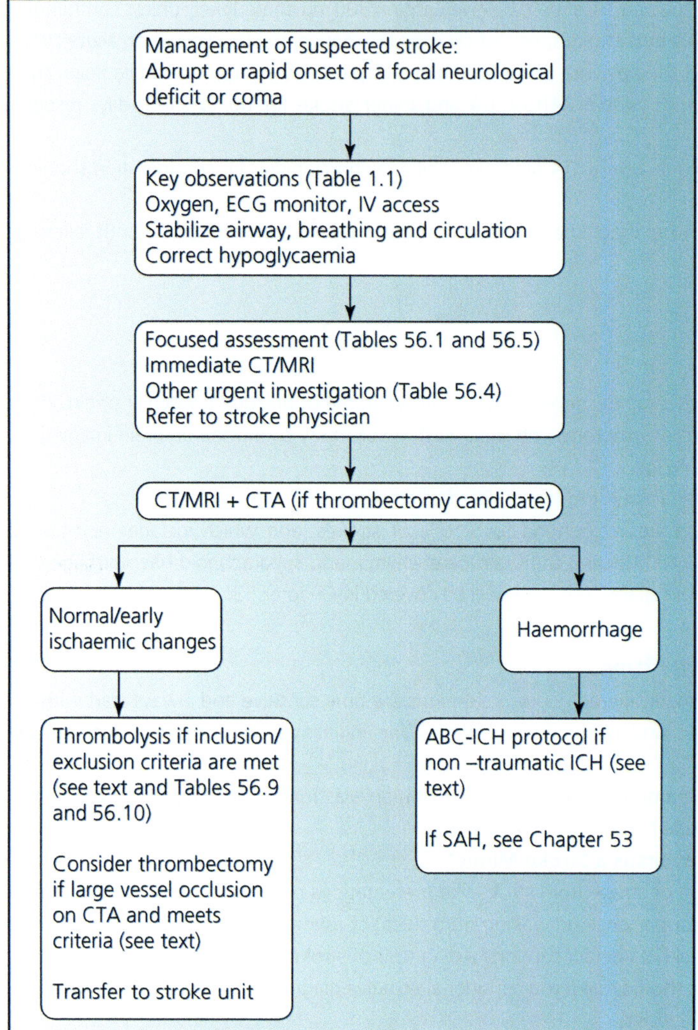

Figure 56.1 Management of suspected stroke.

Table 56.5 Conditions that may mimic stroke.

Disease	Comment
Subdural haematoma	May present with focal neurological deficits. Often no history of trauma. May have headache, fluctuating symptoms and signs. Diagnosis on brain imaging.
Subarachnoid haemorrhage	Classically presents with sudden onset headache with or without focal neurological signs. Diagnosis on brain imaging and lumbar puncture.
Brain tumour	Often progressive symptoms with or without symptoms of raised intracranial pressure. Diagnosis with contrast enhanced brain imaging.
Encephalitis	More often global signs such as clouding of consciousness, confusion, headache together with symptoms and signs of sepsis. Can have focal neurology. Diagnosis on lumbar puncture.

Table 56.5 (*Continued*)

Disease	Comment
Seizure with Todd's paresis	Collateral history important; tongue biting, incontinence, post-ictal phase, prior seizure history
Migraine with aura	'Positive' spreading symptoms, with or without headache, migraine history
Hypertensive encephalopathy and posterior reversible encephalopathy syndrome (PRES)	Usually generalized rather than focal symptoms such as headache, vomiting, clouding consciousness and seizures. May present with cortical blindness and other visual disturbance. Diagnosis on brain imaging and clinical picture. Patients often make good recovery with reversal of radiological abnormalities.
Cerebral vasculitis	Presents with focal neurological signs, sometimes in patients with known systemic vasculitis. Fluctuating course. Diagnosis on brain imaging, inflammatory and autoimmune markers and may need brain biopsy.

Table 56.6 Some atypical presentations of stroke.

Site of stroke	Clinical features
Brainstem	Isolated cranial nerve disorders, vertigo, crossed motor and sensory signs, ataxia
Frontal lobe	Change in behaviour/personality without focal neurological signs
Localized language area	Mobile aphasic patient often initially diagnosed as delirium/dementia
Bilateral thalamic infarction	Confusion and drowsiness
Pons	Locked in syndrome
Cortical lesions	Focal seizures
Basal ganglia	Abnormal movements, for example asterixis, hemifacial spasms
Visual cortex	Isolated visual symptoms, for example Anton's syndrome, Balint's syndrome
Frontal or posterolateral parietal lobe	Alien hand syndrome

The clinical assessment of the patient with suspected stroke is summarized in Tables 56.7 and 56.8, and investigations needed urgently are mentioned in Table 56.4.

Intravenous thrombolysis (IVT)

- This should only be considered when the patient is in a hospital with a well-organised stroke service, which has trained staff, immediate access to neuroimaging, protocols in place to manage complications and systems to audit outcomes.

Table 56.7 Focused assessment of the patient with suspected stroke.

History

Pattern of onset

Time of onset or time last known to be well

Medication and compliance (particularly anticoagulants)

Previous level of function and comorbidities

Examination

General – hydration, temperature

Cardiovascular – blood pressure, heart rate and rhythm, peripheral circulation

Respiratory – oxygenation, evidence of infection

Alimentary – swallowing

Skin – pressure areas

Urological – bladder, continence

Neurological assessment: see Table 56.1

Table 56.8 National Institute of Health Stroke Score (NIHSS). This should be completed on all patients with stroke to ensure that the stroke deficits are collected in a systematic way and the less-obvious signs of stroke are not missed.

Level of consciousness	Alert	0
	Not alert, but arousable with minor stimuli	1
	Not alert, needs repeated stimuli	2
	Coma	3
Level of consciousness questions	Answers both correctly	0
	Answers one correctly	1
	Answers both incorrectly	2
Level of consciousness commands	Performs both correctly	0
	Performs one correctly	1
	Performs neither correctly	2
Best gaze	Normal	0
	Partial gaze palsy	1
	Forced deviation	2
Visual field testing	No visual loss	0
	Partial hemianopia	1
	Complete hemianopia	2
	Bilateral hemianopia	3
Facial paresis	Normal facial movements	0
	Minor paralysis	1
	Partial paralysis	2
	Complete paralysis of one or both sides	3
Right arm motor function	No drift	0
	Drift	1
	Some effort against gravity	2
	No effort against gravity	3
	No movement	4
Left arm motor function	No drift	0
	Drift	1
	Some effort against gravity	2
	No effort against gravity	3
	No movement	4
Right leg motor function	No drift	0
	Drift	1
	Some effort against gravity	2
	No effort against gravity	3
	No movement	4
Left leg motor function	No drift	0
	Drift	1
	Some effort against gravity	2
	No effort against gravity	3
	No movement	4
Limb ataxia	Absent	0
	Present one limb	1
	Present two limbs	2
Sensory	Normal	0
	Mild-to-moderate loss	1
	Severe to total	2

Table 56.8 (*Continued*)

Best language	Normal	0
	Mild-to-moderate aphasia	1
	Severe aphasia	2
	Mute	3
Dysarthria	Normal	0
	Mild to moderate	1
	Severe/mute/anarthric	2
Extinction/inattention	No abnormality	0
	Visual, tactile, auditory or personal inattention	1
	Profound hemi inattention of extinction to more than one modality	2

For urgent investigations for acute stroke (see Table 56.4)

- Indications for thrombolysis are:
  - Patients with acute ischaemic stroke, regardless of age or stroke severity, in whom treatment can be started within 4.5h of known onset, should be considered for thrombolysis with alteplase or tenecteplase.
  - Patients with acute ischaemic stroke, regardless of age or stroke severity, who were last known to be well more than 4.5h earlier, should be considered for thrombolysis if:
    - Treatment can be started between 4.5 and 9h of onset, or within 9h of the midpoint of sleep if they woke with their symptoms AND they have evidence of CT perfusion mismatch.
    OR
    - MRI DWI-FLAIR mismatch of potential to salvage brain tissue.
- The final decision about thrombolysis is made if NO contraindications to thrombolysis treatment (Table 56.9).
- Risks and benefits of IVT should be explained to the patient (or next of kin, if they are unable to communicate) (Table 56.10).
- IVT is a time-sensitive treatment, and the aim should be to deliver this to appropriate patients **within 30min of arrival** to the emergency department.
- IVT is given to appropriate patients irrespective of whether they require mechanical thrombectomy. Table 56.10 summarizes how to administer intravenous thrombolysis.

Table 56.9 Contraindications to thrombolysis for cerebral infarction.

Evidence of intracerebral haemorrhage or previous intracerebral haemorrhage
Neurosurgery, head trauma or stroke in past 3 months
Uncontrolled hypertension (above 185/110mmHg) refractory to hyperacute antihypertensive treatment.
Symptoms suggestive of subarachnoid haemorrhage
Taking warfarin with INR >1.7, or a direct-acting oral anticoagulant taken within 48h
Bleeding diathesis
Active internal bleeding
Bacterial endocarditis or pericarditis
Rapidly improving symptoms
Arterial puncture or bleeding at non-compressible site within last 7 days
Witnessed seizure at stroke onset
Within 14 days of major surgery or within 21 days of GI/GU haemorrhage
Known intra-cranial aneurysm, arteriovenous malformation or neoplasm

Table 56.10 Intravenous Thrombolysis for ischaemic stroke.

Explain risks and benefits (2–5% symptomatic haemorrhage rate; improved chance of surviving with less disability. NNT of 7 treating within 3 h of symptom onset and NNT of 14 between 3 and 4.5 h).
Choice of IVT agent of either Alteplase **or** Tenecteplase.
Alteplase Dose: 0.9 mg/kg to a maximum of 90 mg with 10% of the bolus over 2 min intravenously and the remainder by an infusion over 60 min.
Tenecteplase Dose: 0.25 mg/kg (maximum total dose 25 mg). Give in a single intravenous bolus over 5 s
Check neurological signs and general observations:
- Every 15 min for 2 h
- Every 30 min for 6 h
- Every 60 min for 16 h
Repeat brain imaging after 24 h.
Keep blood pressure below 185/110 mmHg for first 24 h.
Do not give antiplatelet medication until 24 h after thrombolysis, and repeat brain imaging has excluded haemorrhage.

Mechanical thrombectomy (MT)

- Mechanical thrombectomy is an endovascular procedure that involves directly removing the clot in a large intracranial vessel (large vessel occlusion, LVO). An arterial catheter is passed through the groin (or wrist) up to the site of the occlusion, for selected patients with an LVO of the distal ICA (internal carotid artery), MCA (middle cerebral artery) or basilar artery (BA).
- MT should only be performed in a comprehensive stroke centre with access to a multi-disciplinary stroke team, neuro-interventionist team, anaesthetics, ITU and neurosurgery if required.
- Patients are eligible for this procedure if
  - LVO is demonstrated on CT or MR angiography
    AND
  - Pre-morbidly independent for their ADL's
    AND
  - The patient has a significant stroke syndrome. E.g. with NIHSS >/=6
- Patients may be eligible up to 24 h after the onset of symptoms or since 'last known well', however the greatest benefits are achieved if delivered as soon as possible within 6 h of onset.
- Advanced imaging (CT perfusion or hyperacute MRI) is required for delayed presentations beyond 12 h from onset (or last known well).
- Local protocols for eligibility and imaging should be reviewed for detailed criteria.

Early anti-platelet therapy

- Non contrast CT brain (or MRI) should be performed at 24 h after IVT or MT to exclude haemorrhage, and review size and location of infarct.
- Aspirin 300 mg once daily for 14 days should be started 24 h after thrombolysis (if no evidence of significant haemorrhage on 24-h scan), **or** as soon as possible in patients who do not receive thrombolysis.
- Patients with aspirin hypersensitivity, or those intolerant of aspirin despite co-administration of a proton pump inhibitor, should receive clopidogrel 75 mg once daily.
- In patients with minor stroke who did not receive thrombolysis or MT, dual antiplatelet therapy with either aspirin and clopidogrel, or aspirin and ticagrelor, can be considered for up to 21–30 days respectively followed by monotherapy.

Intracerebral haemorrhage

Non-traumatic intracerebral haemorrhage accounts for ~15% of stroke presentations, and is associated with a high early mortality (up to 50%) and morbidity, with only 20% of patients regaining independence long-term. The commonest cause is uncontrolled hypertension. Aetiology of ICH is summarised in Box 56.2.

Management of ICH is time sensitive. Expedited management with a structured approach using a care bundle has been shown to reduce mortality and improve functional outcomes.

The ABC-ICH care bundle (Box 56.3) is a protocol that is associated with reduced mortality in acute ICH management.

Box 56.2 Aetiology of haemorrhagic stroke.

Parenchymal haemorrhage (non-traumatic)
- Hypertensive arterial disease
- Cerebral amyloid angiopathy (CAA)
- Arteriovenous malformation, Aneurysm, Cavernoma
- Bleeding disorder (see Chapter 81)
- Haemorrhagic transformation of cerebral infarction (more commonly seen in infarction due to cerebral venous thrombosis)
- Reperfusion after carotid endarterectomy/angioplasty
- Mycotic aneurysm complicating infective endocarditis
- Underlying neoplasm/metastases

Venous stroke
Cerebral venous thrombosis (risk factors as for deep vein thrombosis plus local infection and trauma.

Subarachnoid haemorrhage (see Chapter 53)

Box 56.3 The ABC-ICH care bundle.

A – Rapid _A_nticoagulant reversing
Patients with ICH in context of warfarin treatment should have the anticoagulant urgently reversed with prothrombin complex concentrate (PCC) and intravenous vitamin K.

Patients with intracerebral haemorrhage in association with direct oral anticoagulant (DOAC) treatment should have the anticoagulant urgently reversed. For patients taking dabigatran, idarucizumab should be used. If idarucizumab is unavailable, 4-factor PCC may be considered. For those taking factor Xa inhibitors, 4-factor PCC should be considered and andexanet alfa may be considered.

B – Intensive _B_lood pressure lowering
Patients with acute spontaneous intracerebral haemorrhage with a systolic BP of 150–220 mmHg should be considered for urgent treatment within 6 h of symptom onset using a locally agreed protocol for BP lowering, aiming to achieve a systolic BP between 130 and 139 mmHg within 1 h and sustained for at least 7 days, unless:
- The Glasgow Coma Scale score is 5 or less;
- The haematoma is very large and death is expected;
- Macrovascular or structural cause for the haematoma is identified;

- Immediate surgery to evacuate the haematoma is planned, in which case BP should be managed according to a locally agreed protocol.

Note: For systolic BP>220 mmHg, caution should be exercised and systolic BP should not be lowered by more than 90 mmHg.

C – A *Care pathway for prompt neurosurgical referral*

Patients with intracranial haemorrhage who develop hydrocephalus should be considered for surgical intervention such as insertion of an external ventricular drain. Posterior fossa ICH may cause obstructive hydrocephalus or coma due to brainstem compression; urgent neurosurgical opinion should be sought for consideration of surgical decompression. The role of decompression in supra-tentorial ICH is not proven, though minimally invasive surgical techniques have shown emerging evidence of benefit. Early liaison with neurosurgery is therefore recommended.

Further management: stroke unit care

All stroke patients should be managed on a stroke unit unless other conditions requiring specialist care dominate (e.g. need for intensive care).

- Specialist interdisciplinary care is the most significant intervention that is available for the management of stroke patients.
- All stroke patients should have access to inpatient stroke-specific rehabilitation facilities, followed by early supported discharge to community stroke teams and longer-term rehabilitation.
- Cognitive and mood disturbance after stroke are common and should be screened for, with psychological support provided if needed.
- The underlying cause of the stroke needs to be established and appropriate secondary prevention provided.

Supportive care

- Maintain close observation and management of normal homeostasis, for example hydration, electrolytes, blood glucose, nutrition, oxygenation and temperature. Oxygen is only required if saturations <95% (and no contraindications). Aim blood glucose between 5 and 15 mmol/L.
- Patients with stroke should only receive blood pressure-lowering treatment acutely if there is an indication for emergency treatment, such as:
  - Prior to thrombolysis or thrombectomy (and up to 24 h after): aim systolic blood pressure below 185 mmHg or diastolic blood pressure below 110 mmHg
  - For ischaemic stroke patients who didn't receive thrombolysis or thrombectomy, no need to lower BP acutely unless systolic BP>220 mmHg; lower BP by 15% during the first 24 h after stroke onset in this scenario
  - Intracerebral haemorrhage (see ABC-ICH protocol, ICH section)
  - Hypertensive crisis
  - Aortic dissection
  - Pre-eclampsia or eclampsia
- Monitor cardiac rate and rhythm, looking in particular for atrial fibrillation

- Rehabilitation should start early, although intensive mobilisation within the first few hours of the stroke should be avoided.
- Screen for swallowing abnormalities before any food or fluid is given and certainly within 4h of admission. This should be done using a standardized screening protocol. If a patient is unable to swallow safely, consider feeding with a nasogastric tube within 24h of admission. If intravenous fluids are required then avoid the use of glucose solutions as hyperglycaemia may worsen outcomes.
- Venous thrombo-embolism is common. Evidence shows that intermittent pneumatic compression devices are safe and effective at preventing deep vein thrombosis. Thrombo-embolus deterrent stockings (both short and long) and prophylactic low molecular weight heparin are not used in this scenario.
- Patients should be carefully monitored for infection, which should be treated early. There is currently no evidence to support the use of prophylactic antibiotics after stroke.
- Urinary catheterisation should be avoided. Continence should be monitored.
- Constipation is common in immobile patients and should be monitored and treated appropriately.

Establishing the cause of the stroke: all patients

During stroke unit admission, comprehensive investigations are required to establish the aetiology of the stroke. See Box 56.2 and Box 56.4.

Box 56.4 Aetiological Classification of ischaemic stroke (TOAST classification).

Cardioembolic (~20%)
- Atrial fibrillation (thrombus in left atrium)
- Left ventricular mural thrombus
- Paradoxical embolism through a patent foramen ovale
- Embolism from infective endocarditis
- Atrial myxoma

Large vessel atherothromboembolic (~20%)
- Carotid atheroma (extra- or intra-cranial)
- Vertebro-basilar atheroma (extra- or intra-cranial)
- Cerebral artery occlusion (may complicate aortic dissection)
- Cervical artery dissection

Small vessel disease in Lacunar infarcts (~25%)
- Hypertensive arterial disease
- Diabetic vasculopathy

Others (~5%), including
- Antiphospholipid syndrome, acquired thrombophilia (malignancy)
- Cerebral vasculitis
- Genetic disorders: CADASIL syndrome (cerebral autosomal dominary arteriopathy with subcortical infarcts and leukoencephalopathy)
- MELAS syndrome (mitochondrial myopathy, encephalopathy, lactic acidosis and stroke-like episodes)

Undetermined aetiology in up to 30%

Preventing another stroke (secondary prevention): all patients

- Give advice and support for smoking cessation if indicated.
- Give personalised lifestyle advice on diet and exercise.
- Blood pressure management. Aim BP <130/80 long-term (unless contraindication).

Following ischaemic stroke (not related to AF)

- Give aspirin 300 mg daily for 2 weeks, followed by clopidogrel 75 mg thereafter.
- Treat lipids, aiming for LDL <1.8 mmol/L.
- Patients with non-disabling carotid artery territory stroke (or TIA) should be considered for carotid endarterectomy if the symptomatic extra-cranial ICA has a stenosis of greater than or equal to 50%.
- Patients with ischaemic stroke (or TIA) due to severe symptomatic intracranial atherosclerotic disease (ICAD) of the carotid or vertebrobasilar circulation should be considered for dual antiplatelet therapy with aspirin (75 mg) and clopidogrel (75 mg) for the first three months, followed by clopidogrel monotherapy thereafter.
- In patients with minor stroke, dual antiplatelet therapy with either aspirin and clopidogrel, or aspirin and ticagrelor, can be considered for up to 21–30 days respectively followed by monotherapy thereafter.

Following Ischaemic stroke related to atrial fibrillation (paroxysmal, persistent or permanent)

- Anticoagulate if no contra-indications. Choice of agents are DOAC (for non-valvular AF) or VKA (valvular AF, mechanical heart valve or end-stage renal failure). Timing of initiation of anticoagulation after the stroke will depend on the size of the infarct on brain imaging and should be discussed with the stroke team.
- Aspirin 300 mg daily should be used in interim, whilst waiting to be started on anticoagulation, as long as no significant haemorrhagic transformation on brain imaging.

Further reading

Intercollegiate Stroke Working Party. (2023) *National Clinical Guideline for Stroke for the UK and Ireland.* London: Intercollegiate Stroke Working Party. www.strokeguidelines.org.

Parry Jones A, Jarhult S, Kreitzer N, *et al.* (2024) Acute care bundles should be used for patients with intracerebral haemorrhage: an expert consensus statement. *Eur Stroke J*, 1–8. doi: 10.1177/23969873231220235.

Tunkl C, Mosconi MG, Thomalla G. (2024) *Hyperacute Essential Stroke Care Checklist.* World Stroke Organisation.

CHAPTER 57

Seizures and epilepsy

SHIVAM BHARGAVA

Box 57.1 Generalized tonic–clonic status epilepticus.

Defined as a generalized tonic–clonic seizure (GTCS) lasting more than 5 min or repeated seizures without recovery of normal alertness in between. As 98% of GTCS self-terminate in two minutes, any seizure lasting >5 min should be treated as status unless that patient is known habitually to have longer seizures.

Prompt treatment is needed to reduce cerebral damage and metabolic complications (hypoglycaemia, lactic acidosis and hyperpyrexia) and prevent mortality.

Mortality in status epilepticus occurs with both under and over-treatment.

Generalized tonic–clonic seizure

Priorities
Airway, breathing and circulation
- Clear the airway. Place a nasopharyngeal airway if needed to maintain a clear airway (Chapter 105).
- Put the patient in the lateral semi-prone position. Attach an electrocardiogram (ECG) monitor and oxygen saturation monitor.
- Give high-flow oxygen, obtain IV access and take bloods for urgent investigation (Table 57.1).

Exclude hypoglycaemia
Check blood glucose immediately by stick test. If blood glucose is <4.0 mmol/L:
- Give 100 mL of 20% glucose (or 200 mL of 10% glucose) over 15–30 min IV, or glucagon 1 mg IV/IM/SC.
- Recheck blood glucose after 10 min; if still <4.0 mmol/L, repeat the above IV glucose treatment.
- In patients with malnourishment or alcohol use disorder, there is a remote risk of precipitating Wernicke's encephalopathy by a glucose load; prevent this by giving thiamine 100 mg IV before or shortly after glucose administration.

See Chapter 46 for further management of hypoglycaemia.

CT scan can be delayed after first seizure, if recovered with no abnormal signs.

Acute Medicine: A Practical Guide to the Management of Medical Emergencies, Sixth Edition.
Edited by Mridula Rajwani, Leila Vaziri, and Ivie Gbinigie.

Table 57.1 Investigation in status epilepticus or after a first seizure.

Immediate
Blood glucose
Sodium, potassium, calcium, magnesium, urea and creatinine
Arterial blood gases and pH (not required after first seizure)

Later
Full blood count
Blood culture (×2) if febrile
Liver function tests
Anticonvulsant levels (if on therapy), consider toxic screen
Serum (10 mL) and urine sample (50 mL) at 4 °C for toxicology screen if poisoning suspected or cause of seizure unclear
ECG (NB A missed diagnosis of cardiac arrhythmia is more likely to lead to sudden death than a missed diagnosis of epilepsy. Look for long QT interval, conduction abnormality (e.g. left bundle branch block), Q waves indicative of previous myocardial infarction, evidence of left ventricular hypertrophy. If present, consider arrhythmia rather than seizure, arrange echocardiography and cardiology follow-up.)
Chest X-ray
Cranial CT scan*
Lumbar puncture (after CT) if suspected subarachnoid haemorrhage, meningitis or encephalitis
EEG (this test requires judgement as to when necessary: discuss with a neurologist)

* CT scan should be performed immediately after control of status epilepticus or after a first seizure if any of the following features is present:
- Focal neurological deficit
- Reduced conscious level
- Fever
- Recent head injury
- Persistent headache
- Known malignancy
- Warfarin or other anticoagulation
- HIV-AIDS

Give a benzodiazepine

Consider pre-hospital treatment. Give **lorazepam** 0.1 mg/kg (typically 4–8 mg) IV over 5–10 min, **midazolam** 10 mg buccally or **diazepam** 10–20 mg IV at a rate of <2.5 mg/min. (See Table 57.2 for more details.)

What is the likely cause of the seizure?

Obtain history from all available sources (emergency information, health app), do a systemic examination and check lab results (Table 57.3).
- Correct severe hyponatraemia (Serum Na < 120 mmol/L) with hypertonic saline (Chapter 52).
- Correct severe hypocalcaemia (Corrected Ca < 1.5 mmol/L) with calcium gluconate 1 g IV (10 mL of 10% solution) (Chapter 52).
- Correct hypomagnesaemia (Chapter 52)
- Give dexamethasone 10 mg IV if patient is known to have a brain tumour or active vasculitis.
- If patient is known to have epilepsy, restart any antiepileptic medication stopped within the last three weeks (via a nasogastric tube if IV or rectal preparations are not available).

Table 57.2 Drug therapy for generalized convulsive status epilepticus.

Drug	Dose	Comments
First line		
Lorazepam	0.1 mg/kg, give 4–8 mg IV	Dose can be repeated once after 20 min. Ampoules contain lorazepam 4 mg in 1 mL. Dilute 1 : 1 with water for injection. Longer duration of action and less likely to cause sudden hypotension or respiratory arrest than diazepam.
or Midazolam	10 mg in 1 or 2 mL (depends on manufacturer) buccally	In accord with NICE adult status guidelines but only licensed for those aged <18 years.
or Diazepam	10–20 mg IV at a rate of <2.5/min.	Risk of sudden apnoea with faster injection. Dose should not be repeated more than twice, or to a total dose >40 mg because of the risk of respiratory depression and hypotension.
Second line		
Phenobarbital	Loading dose: 10 mg/kg (max 1 g), given at 100 mg/min. Maintenance dose 1–4 mg/kg/day given IV, IM or PO	Contraindicated in acute intermittent porphyria. Hypotension. Respiratory impairment due to sedation.
or Phenytoin	Loading dose: 20 mg/kg IV (max 2 g). Infusion rate to not exceed 50 mg/min. Maintenance dose: 100 mg 6–8-hourly IV, adjusted according to plasma level. Give only one loading dose and do not load a patient who is taking oral phenytoin.	Monitor blood pressure and ECG (as risk of arrhythmia). Give through separate large-bore IV cannula, as alkaline and will precipitate other drugs. Valproate and levetiracetam are alternative second-line drugs
Third line		
Midazolam	0.1–0.2 mg/kg/h by IV infusion	
or Propofol	2 mg/kg IV bolus, repeat if necessary. Maintenance dose 5–10 mg/kg/h by IV infusion	
or Thiopentone	100–250 mg IV bolus, give 50 mg bolus every 3 min until burst suppression on EEG. Maintenance dose 2–5 mg/kg/h by IV infusion	

Further management
If fitting continues
- Transfer the patient to the ICU and discuss management with an anaesthetist and neurologist.
- Consider the possibility of psychogenic status epilepticus (Table 57.4). Definitive diagnosis may require EEG.
- Give either phenobarbital or phenytoin (Table 57.2) (please note the difference in time to treatment dose being given – many experts prefer phenobarbital for this reason).

If in refractory status epilepticus
If fitting continues despite phenytoin or phenobarbital IV:
- The patient should be intubated and ventilated.
- Midazolam, propofol or thiopentone should be given (Table 57.2), preferably with EEG monitoring.

Table 57.3 Causes of tonic–clonic status epilepticus.

In a patient known to have epilepsy
Poor compliance with therapy, therapy recently reduced or stopped or altered drug pharmacokinetics
Drug interaction causing alteration of their normal maintenance level
Intercurrent infection
Alcohol withdrawal
Alcohol or substance use

In a patient not known to have epilepsy
Stroke, especially haemorrhagic stroke
Meningitis or encephalitis
Brain tumour
Brain abscess (including toxoplasmosis)
Arteriovenous malformation
Acute head injury
Cerebral malaria
Metabolic disorder: cerebral anoxia from cardiac arrest, acute kidney injury, hyponatraemia, hypocalcaemia, hypomagnesaemia, hypoglycaemia
Hepatic encephalopathy
Poisoning: alcohol, tricyclics, phenothiazines, theophylline, cocaine, amphetamines, MDMA ('ecstasy'), heroin
Cerebral vasculitis
Hypertensive encephalopathy
Pre-eclampsia/eclampsia

Once fitting has stopped

Determine the cause (Table 57.3).

Consult neurologist on further management in complex patients with a history of epilepsy, speak to their usual consultant where possible.

After a first generalized tonic–clonic seizure

Was it a seizure?

Distinguishing between a seizure and syncope (Chapter 11) requires a detailed history taken from the patient and any eyewitnesses. Points to cover include the following (Tables 57.4 and 57.5):

Background

- Any previous similar attacks (including partial seizures such as déjà vu or myoclonic jerks in morning)
- Previous significant acquired brain injury (i.e. complicated or premature birth, trauma with skull fracture or loss of consciousness >1 h, meningitis or encephalitis, stroke)

Table 57.4 Characteristics of dissociative seizures (non-epileptic attack disorder).

Asynchronous bilateral movements of the limbs, asymmetrical clonic contractions, pelvic thrusting and side-to-side movements of head, often intensified by restraint
Gaze aversion, resistance to passive limb movement or eye-opening, focus on face if mirror used and eyes held open
Avoidance of the hand falling onto the face
Incontinence, tongue biting and injury rare (but can occur)
Normal or volitional pattern chest wall movements
Normal tendon reflexes, plantar responses, blink, corneal and eyelash reflexes
Absence of metabolic complications
No post-ictal confusion (drowsiness and dysarthria may be due to benzodiazepine given to treat suspected seizure)

Table 57.5 Features differentiating a generalized seizure from vasovagal and cardiac syncope (Stokes-Adams attack).

	Generalized seizure	Vasovagal syncope	Cardiac syncope (Stokes-Adams attack)
Occurrence when sitting or lying	Common	Rare	Common
Occurrence during sleep	Common	Does not occur	May occur
Prodromal symptoms	May occur with focal neurological symptom, automatisms or hallucinations	Typical with sweating, dizziness, nausea, blurring of vision, yawning	Often none; palpitation may occur
Focal neurology at onset	May occur (Possible cerebral lesion)	Never occurs	Never occurs
Tonic–clonic movements	Characteristic; occurs within 30s of onset	May occur after 30s of syncope (secondary anoxic seizure)	May occur after 30s of syncope (secondary anoxic seizure)
Facial colour	Flushing or cyanosis at onset	Pallor at onset	Pallor at onset; flushing afterwards
Tongue biting	Common	Rare	Rare
Urinary incontinence	Common	Uncommon	May occur
Injury	May occur	Uncommon	May occur
After the attack	Confusion common	Nauseated and 'groggy'	Usually well

- Febrile seizures in childhood (age six months to six years)
- Family history of epilepsy
- Cardiac disease (previous myocardial infarction, hypertrophic or dilated cardiomyopathy, long QT interval (at risk of ventricular tachycardia))
- Drug therapy
- Alcohol or substance use
- Sleep deprivation

Before the attack

- Prodromal symptoms: were these cardiovascular (e.g. dizziness, palpitation, chest pain) or focal neurological (aura)?
- Circumstances, for example exercising, standing, sitting or lying, asleep
- Precipitants, for example coughing, micturition, head-turning

During the attack

- Any focal neurological features at the onset: sustained deviation of the head or eyes or unilateral jerking of the limbs (bilateral 'twitching' is common in syncope)?
- Was there a cry (may occur in tonic phase of seizure)?
- Duration of seizure (must be assessed in relation to the reliability of the witness).
- Associated tongue biting, urinary or faecal incontinence or injury.
- Facial colour changes (pallor common in syncope, uncommon with a seizure).
- Abnormal pulse (must be assessed in relation to the reliability of the witness).
- Eyes rolled up consistent with syncope, eyes open and staring in any direction consistent with seizure.
- Waxing and waning over a long duration consistent with non-epileptic attack (dissociative seizure).

After the attack

Immediately well or delayed recovery with confusion or headache? (fatigue common after syncope, somnolence more common after seizure).

Is there evidence of an underlying cause of seizure?

* Are there any focal neurological signs? Like an aura preceding the seizure, these indicate a structural cause.
* Are there features of meningitis, encephalitis (Chapter 73) or subarachnoid haemorrhage (Chapter 53)?
* Does the patient have a systemic disease requiring urgent treatment, for example acute liver failure, hyperosmolar hyperglycaemic state?

If the patient is well

* Discharge if fully recovered and supervision by an adult for the next 24 h can be arranged.
* Advise the patient not to drive (in writing, as memory may be impaired after a seizure).
* Give first aid advice for seizure recurrence, also bathing and kitchen safety advice (see 'epilepsy app' from Epilepsy Action or National Society for Epilepsy).
* Outpatient investigation (CT if indicated) and follow-up by a neurologist should be arranged. EEG is not routine but is likely to be needed if seizure is suspected in a person <23 years.
* In general, anticonvulsant therapy should be started after a second seizure (not a first one) – local advice should be sought for choice of starting medication (which will be carbamazepine, lamotrigine or valproate).

After a generalized seizure in a patient with known epilepsy

* Take blood for anticonvulsant levels.
* If the current history deviates from the usual pattern of seizures, consider infection, alcohol use or poor compliance with therapy (an 'epilepsy app' can help with compliance).
* If the patient has had a typical seizure and is fully recovered, CT is not necessary.
* Discharge (with driving advice and outpatient follow-up arranged) if the patient is fully recovered and has no evidence of acute illness.

Alcohol withdrawal seizures

* Alcohol withdrawal seizures consist of 1–6 tonic–clonic seizures without focal features, which begin within 48 h of stopping drinking (although may occur up to seven days after stopping drinking if the patient has been taking a benzodiazepine). They are usually brief and self-limiting.
* Patients who have had withdrawal seizures once are highly likely to have a recurrence if they withdraw again.
* Patients with alcoholic hepatitis or chronic liver disease may have coagulation abnormalities, and if so, subdural haematoma should be excluded by CT.
* Cranial CT scan is not needed after suspected withdrawal seizures if:
  * A clear history of alcohol withdrawal is obtained.
  * The seizures have no focal features.
  * There is no evidence of head injury.
  * There are no more than six seizures.
  * The seizures do not occur over a period >6 h.
  * Post-ictal confusion is brief.
* Management of alcohol withdrawal.

Further reading

Betjemann JP, Lowenstein DH. (2015) Status epilepticus in adults. *Lancet Neurol* 14, 615–624.

Glauser T, Shinnar S, Gloss D, *et al.* (2016) Evidence-based guideline: treatment of convulsive status epilepticus in children and adults: report of the guideline Committee of the American Epilepsy Society. *Epilepsy Curr* 16, 48–61. doi: 10.5698/1535-7597-16.1.48.

Gov.UK Epilepsy and driving (DVLA guidance). https://www.gov.uk/epilepsy-and-driving.

National Institute for Health and Care Excellence Epilepsies in children, young people and adults. NICE guideline (NG217) Published: 27 April 2022. https://www.nice.org.uk/guidance/ng217.

CHAPTER 58

Peripheral neuropathy (acute and chronic)

SIMON RINALDI AND ROBERTO BELLANTI

Peripheral neuropathies result from damage and/or dysfunction of the peripheral nerves. This produces various combinations and patterns of motor weakness, large- and small-fibre sensory loss, ataxia, positive sensory symptoms, neuropathic pain, and autonomic, cranial or neuromuscular respiratory dysfunction.

Pathology may affect the axon, myelin and/or node of Ranvier (nodopathy). Pathology affecting the cell bodies (neuronopathy) is usually considered separately.

Priorities

Prompt identification of patients:
- With rapidly progressive, treatable neuropathies (Box 58.1)
- With or at risk of developing bulbar dysfunction or neuromuscular respiratory failure

The clinical assessment is summarized in Table 58.1. Features making certain aetiologies more likely are given in Table 58.2.

Box 58.1 Peripheral neuropathies – alerts.

- The most common peripheral neuropathies are late-onset, slowly progressive, length-dependent, symmetrical and sensory axonal in nature. The overwhelming majority of these will not produce significant disability, many will not have an identifiable cause, and only limited further investigation is typically appropriate.
- Red flags for more concerning pathology and/or a specific identifiable or modifiable cause include:
  - Acute onset and/or rapidly progressive (over days to weeks).
  - Prominent or proximal weakness (e.g. hip flexion and/or shoulder abduction).
  - Prominent ataxia
  - Asymmetric, non-length dependent, focal or multifocal pattern.
  - Neuropathy causing significant disability or impaired mobility.
  - Autonomic dysfunction (outside of diabetic neuropathy).
  - Global areflexia
  - Onset before 55 years old and/or a positive family history.

Table 58.1 Focused assessment of the patient with suspected peripheral neuropathy.

History

Age? Onset? Progression? Aggravating/relieving factors? Triggers?

Distribution? Length dependent? Focal? Multifocal? Symmetrical? Asymmetrical?

Weakness? Distal and/or proximal?

Sensory symptoms/dysfunction? Numbness? Paraesthesia? Pain? Burning? Sensory ataxia (worse in dark/eyes closed)?

Autonomic involvement? Postural light-headedness? Syncope? Dry mouth? Constipation/(nocturnal) diarrhoea?

Sweating abnormalities?

Cranial nerve involvement? Diplopia? Dysarthria? Dysphagia?

Neuromuscular respiratory involvement?

Functional impairment?

Prodromal illness or infection? Trauma? Compression? Arising from sleep?

Background

Systemic upset? Weight loss? Diet/malnutrition? Alcohol/drug/toxin exposure?

Past neurological or systemic disease?

Diabetes? Vascular risk factors? Family history?

Examination

Rapid assessment of ABC/vital signs/glucose. Check vital capacity if GBS possible

Assess visual function and cranial nerves

Assess for any weakness, and alteration of tone and reflexes (Chapter 54)

Check small (pain/temperature) and large fibre (vibration/proprioception/light touch) modalities

Look for other signs of proprioceptive loss. Rombergism? Pseudoathetosis?

Provocation tests if appropriate (Phalen's/Tinnel's/Spurling's). Assess for autonomic dysfunction (Lying and standing BP, heart rate variability)

Table 58.2 Clues to the pathology.

Characteristic	Potential causes
Acute (evolving over hours to days)	GBS, vasculitic, toxic, infectious, nutritional
Focal/multifocal	Vasculitic, compressive, amyloid, neoplastic, infectious, sarcoid, genetic (HNPP), inflammatory (MMN/MADSAM)
Autonomic involvement	Diabetes, amyloid, GBS/autoimmune
(Sensory) ataxia	Vitamin B12 deficiency, MFS/anti-MAG, dorsal root ganglionopathy (Sjogren's, lymphoma, paraneoplastic), vitamin B6 toxicity
Small fibre	Diabetes, amyloid, HIV

GBS; Guillain-Barré syndrome, HNPP; Hereditary Neuropathy with Pressure Palsies, MMN; Multifocal Motor Neuropathy, MADSAM; Multifocal Acquired Demyelinating Sensory and Motor Neuropathy, MFS; Miller Fisher Syndrome, anti-MAG; anti-myelin-associated glycoprotein.

Diagnostic tests are directed by the clinical picture. In the absence of any red flags, a simple set of screening bloods (FBC, U&Es, LFTs, TFTs, glucose/HbA1c, vitamin B12, paraprotein screen, erythrocyte sedimentation rate and fasting lipids) is typically sufficient and neurophysiology is not required.

Many polyneuropathies are sensory > motor, symmetric, length-dependent and slowly progressive.

Further management

- Further management is directed by the working diagnosis.
- Neuropathies may predispose to injury and falls, and these risks need to be evaluated and addressed.
- Neuropathic pain usually responds poorly to standard analgesic preparations, typically requiring neuropathic pain agents such as amitriptyline, gabapentin and/or pregabalin.

Further reading

Dyck PJ, Dyck PJ, Grant IA, Fealey RD. (1996) Ten steps in characterizing and diagnosing patients with peripheral neuropathy. *Neurology* 47(1), 10–17. doi: 10.1212/wnl.47.1.10.

CHAPTER 59

Guillain–Barré syndrome

Simon Rinaldi and Roberto Bellanti

Guillain–Barré syndrome (GBS) is an acute, immune-mediated neuropathy. Typical cases are characterized by largely symmetric, post-infectious, ascending weakness with arreflexia. Cranial nerve palsy (especially facial), pain and sensory symptoms are common, sensory signs less so. By definition, progression of weakness ceases within four weeks of onset. Nadir is reached earlier than this in most cases.

GBS has become the most common cause of acquired neuromuscular paralysis. GBS follows infection in approximately two-thirds of cases. Most often the infection is of upper respiratory tract, although *Campylobacter jejuni* (causing gastroenteritis) is the most frequently identified prodromal agent.

Miller–Fisher syndrome (MFS), characterized by a triad of ophthalmoplegia, ataxia and areflexia, is usually considered a regional variant of GBS, but is significantly less common. Other regional and overlap syndromes are also described.

The recovery phase in GBS can be extremely long, and at least 20% of patients fail to return to their premorbid baseline. Nevertheless, continuing improvement is possible even at two years from the initial presentation.

The risk of recurrent GBS is small but significant, at around 5%. Occasionally a further deterioration after initial improvement can represent a fluctuation related to the acute treatment 'wearing off', or indicate an alternative diagnosis such as chronic inflammatory demyelinating polyradiculoneuropathy (CIDP).

Consider GBS in patients with progressive symmetrical limb or facial weakness. Management of the patient with suspected GBS is summarized in Figure 59.1.

Priorities

The priorities are to establish the diagnosis in a timely manner (Tables 59.1 and 59.2; Box 59.1), exclude potential mimics (Table 59.3), and institute appropriate monitoring and therapy to manage or prevent potential complications.

Immediate management

- Promptly involve ICU if there is respiratory failure or autonomic dysfunction (the latter usually manifesting with labile blood pressure, refractory hypo/hypertension or cardiac arrhythmias).
- Monitoring cardiorespiratory function, including measurement of vital capacity with bedside spirometry, is an absolute requirement in the safe management of patients with GBS. Frequent monitoring is required during the initial phase, when the disease is still progressive.

Acute Medicine: A Practical Guide to the Management of Medical Emergencies, Sixth Edition.
Edited by Mridula Rajwani, Leila Vaziri, and Ivie Gbinigie.
© 2026 John Wiley & Sons Ltd. Published 2026 by John Wiley & Sons Ltd.

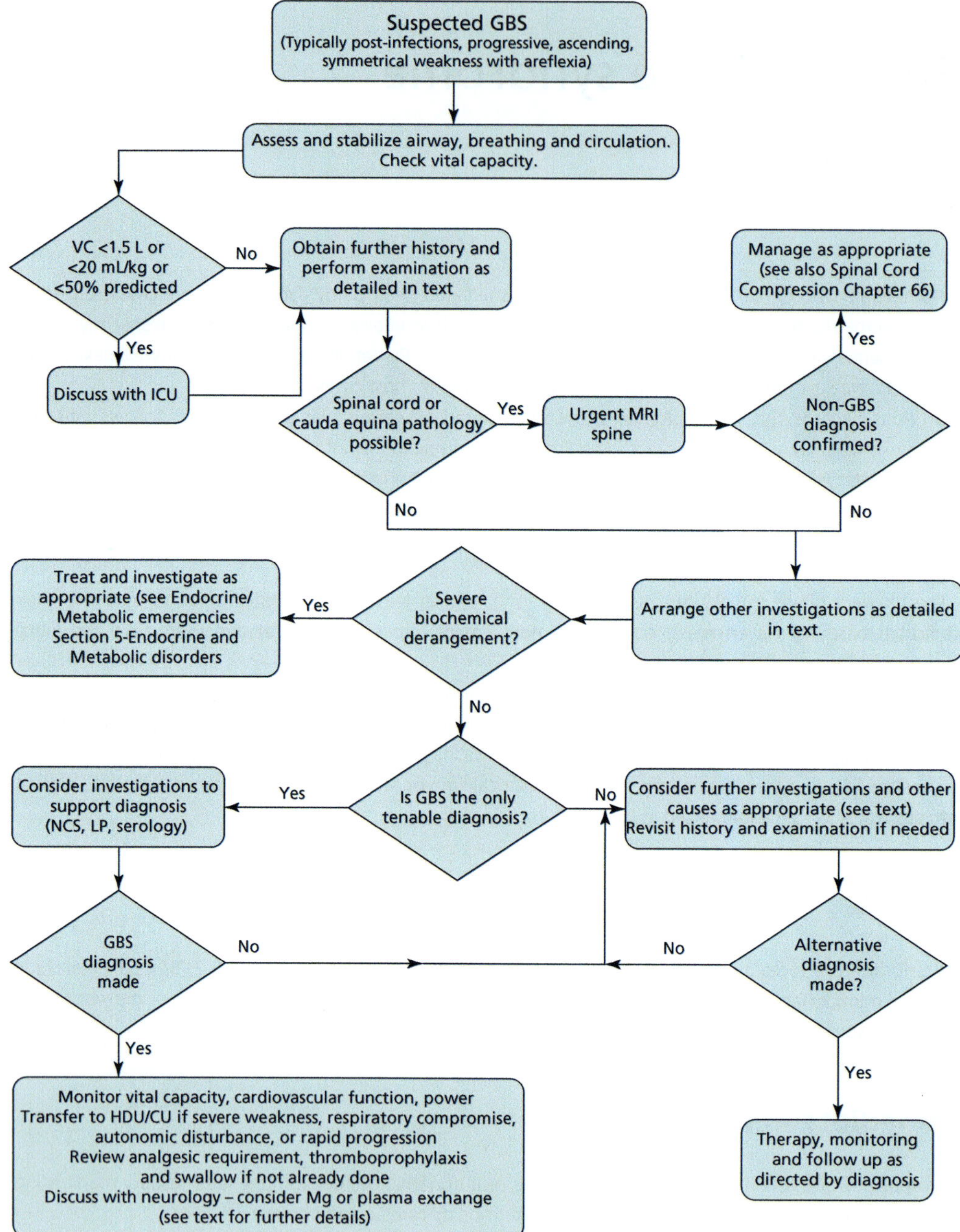

Figure 59.1 Management of suspected Guillain–Barré syndrome (GBS).

- An adult vital capacity of <1.5 L/<20 mL/kg is of immediate concern and warrants discussion with ICU.
- At <1 L/<15 mL/kg, or with a fall of 50% from baseline on serial testing, prompt ICU involvement is imperative, and intubation may be necessary.
- Peak expiratory flow or arterial blood gas measurements are inadequate for assessing neuromuscular respiratory compromise.

Table 59.1 Clinical assessment.

History

Prodromal illness (GI or respiratory)? Other potential trigger?

Backpain? Weakness? Sensory disturbance? Autonomic symptoms? Sphincter disturbance? Ataxia? Diplopia? Dysphagia? Dysarthria?

Onset? Progression? Fever? Rash? Ongoing systemic upset?

Prior episodes? Past history/comorbidities? HIV? Haematological malignancy? Tick bite? Alcohol excess? Poor diet?

Travel? Toxin/heavy metal exposure? Drugs?

Red flags for **alternative** diagnosis?

    Hyperacute onset, marked fluctuation/fatigability, sphincter disturbance at onset, persistent bowel/bladder dysfunction, progression greater than four weeks from onset, neurological dysfunction developing concurrently with systemic upset.

Examination

Supportive findings:

- Largely symmetrical, proximal *and* distal flaccid limb weakness.
- Areflexia: bilateral facial palsy +/− other cranial nerve palsies; autonomic dysfunction.

Examination red flags for **alternative** diagnosis: marked asymmetry; upper motor neuron signs; sensory level; rash; fever; fatigable weakness.

Table 59.2 Investigation in suspected Guillain–Barré syndrome (GBS).

Test	Comment
CSF analysis	CSF protein is usually elevated, but may be normal, especially early in the disease course. CSF lymphocyte count >10/mm^3 is unusual, and counts >50/mm^3 are 'never' seen in GBS, such that alternative diagnoses (haematological malignancy, HIV, Borrelia) must be strongly considered in this setting.
MRI spine	Mandatory if spinal cord/cauda equina compression is in the differential (see Figure 59.1).
Nerve conduction studies/electromyography (NCS/EMG)	Can support the diagnosis by demonstrating an (acute) neuropathy.
Blood tests	**All patients:** FBC, electrolytes (including calcium, phosphate and magnesium), LFTs, glucose, paraprotein screen, CK, TFTs, ESR. **In selected patients:** Anti-ganglioside antibodies, serological tests for prodromal infections, ANA/ANCA, anti-AChR, anti-VGCC, thiamine.

Table 59.3 Causes of acute weakness.

Site	Causes
Brain	Stroke, mass lesion, rhombencephalitis, central pontine myelinolysis
Spinal cord	Spinal cord/cauda equina/root compression (see Chapter 66), transverse myelitis, anterior spinal artery occlusion, Haematomyelia Poliomyelitis, rabies
Peripheral nerve	GBS, critical illness neuropathy, toxic (heavy metals, biological toxins or drug intoxication), nutritional (dry beriberi), acute intermittent porphyria, vasculitis (with mononeuritis multiplex), lymphomatous or carcinomatous (radiculo)neuropathy, diphtheria
Neuromuscular junction	Myasthenia gravis, Lambert–Eaton myasthenic syndrome, Botulism Biological or industrial toxins
Muscle	Hypokalaemia, hypophosphataemia, hypomagnesaemia, inflammatory myopathy, critical illness myopathy, acute rhabdomyolysis (see Chapter 86) Periodic paralyses

Box 59.1 Pitfalls in the diagnosis of Guillain–Barré syndrome (GBS).

The more common diagnostic pitfalls relate to distinguishing GBS from spinal cord or cauda equina syndromes. Acute (radiculo-) neuropathies related to nutritional deficiency, critical illness, haematological malignancy, infection or vasculitis are also occasional mimics.

Confusion also sometimes surrounds the concept of ascending weakness. Proximal weakness is usually found in an affected limb, and the typical progression is from legs to arms to cranial nerves and respiratory muscles – not from distal to proximal in individual limbs. Exceptions exist, but descending weakness (starting with the cranial musculature) should prompt thoughts of botulism, not GBS.

- Treat pain. Paracetamol and opioids can be used, but neuropathic pain agents (e.g. gabapentin, pregabalin and amitriptyline) are often required.
- Prevent complications: thromboprophylaxis, pressure area care, assess swallow and place nil by mouth (with feeding by nasogastric tube) if compromised.
- Consider disease-modifying treatment: IV immunoglobulin (IVIg) (0.4 g/kg × 5 days) or plasma exchange (PLEx), in discussion with a neurologist.

Monitoring

Close monitoring of cardiorespiratory function is required initially. As a minimum, two sets of observations an hour apart, including measurement of vital capacity, are suggested following the initial presentation. In the rapidly deteriorating patient, even more frequent assessment may be appropriate.

Selection of patients for ambulatory care, hospital admission and HDU/ICU admission

- All patients in the progressive phase of the disease will require admission for monitoring as a minimum.
- Non-ambulant patients and those with cardiovascular autonomic involvement should usually be monitored in a high-dependency setting at least.
- With evidence of neuromuscular respiratory compromise and/or pronounced cardiovascular autonomic instability involvement of ICU is recommended.

Risk-assessment models

Risk of mechanical ventilation can be assessed by the modified Erasmus GBS Respiratory Insufficiency Score (mEGRIS). Such risk is greater in patients with rapid disease progression in the first four weeks, bulbar palsy, and weakness of neck flexion and hip flexion. Overall, around one in four patients with GBS will require intubation.

Long-term prognosis (the probability of being unable to walk independently at four weeks, three months and six months) can be calculated by the modified Erasmus GBS Outcome Score (mEGOS). Both are available via https://gbsstudies.erasmusmc.nl/tools

Further management

- Patients who fail to improve after IVIg do not benefit from a second immunoglobulin dose, as this increases the risk of side effects (mainly thromboembolic) without improving neurological outcome. There is no evidence to support the use of plasma exchange after IVIg, or *vice versa*, in this situation. However, further therapy may be indicated in the context of a 'treatment-related fluctuation' (improvement then deterioration after treatment) or with ongoing progression beyond eight (and perhaps four) weeks (implying another, non-GBS diagnosis).
- For patients in the plateau or recovery phase of their disease, pain management, pressure area care and thromboprophylaxis remain important. Fatigue and low mood are also common problems which may require treatment. Input from physiotherapy is extremely valuable in maintaining and then improving mobility and functional ability. With the aid of occupational therapy, discharge home might be considered at this time, with or without an intermediate period spent in a specialist rehabilitation setting as appropriate.

Patient support groups

http://www.gaincharity.org.uk/
http://www.gbs-cidp.org/

Further reading

Bellanti R, Rinaldi S. (2024) Guillain-Barré syndrome: a comprehensive review. *Eur J Neurol* 31(8), e16365. doi: 10.1111/ene.16365.

van Doorn PA, Van den Bergh PYK, Hadden RDM, *et al.* (2023) European Academy of Neurology/Peripheral Nerve Society guideline on diagnosis and treatment of Guillain-Barré syndrome. *Eur J Neurol* 30(12), 3646–3674.

CHAPTER 60

Multiple sclerosis

GINA HADLEY AND GABRIELE C. DE LUCA

Introduction

Multiple sclerosis (MS) is the most common cause of non-traumatic central nervous system disease and long-term disability in young adults in Europe, Canada and the United States. According to MS society statistics, approximately 1 in every 500 people in the UK lives with MS with over 130 people a week being diagnosed with the condition. It is an immune-mediated disease of the central nervous system, first described by Charcot in 1868 as 'la sclèrose en plaques disseminées' whereby demyelination occurs in the brain and spinal cord.

Risk factors associated with developing MS are found in Box 60.1. At diagnosis, most patients have relapsing–remitting MS (RRMS) (85–90%). There is currently no cure. The aim of disease-modifying therapies is to prevent new demyelination from occurring. Natural history studies estimate that two-thirds would become secondary progressive (progressive neurological decline without relapses) however this is likely to be reduced with the emergence of disease-modifying therapies. A small subset of patients (10–15%) have primary progressive disease at onset.

Historically on the acute medical take, the general physician might see first presentations of demyelinating disease (transverse myelitis, brain stem syndrome and optic neuritis), a fresh bout of new inflammation (i.e. relapse) or managing the complications of progressive disease (urosepsis and the comorbidity of immobility).

Box 60.1 Risk factors for multiple sclerosis.

- Age (commonly affects individuals between 16 and 45 years with a peak onset in early thirties).
- Sex (Female : Male ratio > 2 : 1, but is variable).
- Certain infections (Epstein–Barr virus).
- Race
- Smoking
- Obesity
- Certain autoimmune diseases
- Climate (Increases with distance from equator (Orkney and Shetland – 300/100,000, England – 100+/100,000, Tropics – 2–5/100,000)).
- Vitamin D
- Family history of MS and other autoimmune conditions
- Genetics (HLA class II region (HLA-DRB1*15 haplotype with greatest odds ratio)) with many non-HLA loci implicated.

Acute Medicine: A Practical Guide to the Management of Medical Emergencies, Sixth Edition.
Edited by Mridula Rajwani, Leila Vaziri, and Ivie Gbinigie.
© 2026 John Wiley & Sons Ltd. Published 2026 by John Wiley & Sons Ltd.

A person with MS with infection or other systemic disturbance may present with worsening pre-existing symptoms (i.e. pseudo-relapse). Now the scope extends into complications of potentially highly immunosuppressive disease-modifying therapies and their sequalae. This chapter will cover diagnosis, relapse, treatment and complications.

Initial presentation and diagnosis

A diagnosis of MS requires demonstration that inflammatory demyelinating lesions are disseminated in space and time. (see Table 60.1 for Revised McDonald criteria 2017 for diagnosis of RRMS). The first clinical episode of CNS inflammatory demyelination is always isolated in time (monophasic) and usually isolated in space (monofocal). When examining the patient, supporting evidence localising to the central nervous system would be a relative afferent pupillary defect, upper motor neuron signs (e.g. a pyramidal distribution of weakness [upper limbs, extensors weaker than flexors and lower limbs flexors weaker than extensors], velocity-dependent increased tone, hyperreflexia and up going plantars), brainstem signs (e.g. internuclear ophthalmoplegia), cerebellar signs and gait impairment.

Clinical history can give dissemination in time and space. Dissemination in time can be ascertained by taking a history covering clinical symptoms localising to the central nervous system: optic neuritis, partial myelitis, sensory disturbance (limb, abdominal and chest), brainstem – intranuclear ophthalmoplegia, tinnitus/hearing loss, facial sensory disturbance (including trigeminal neuralgia), etc. lasting for at least 24h with a month between a previous bout of symptoms.

Patients must have an MRI scan of the brain and spinal cord with dissemination in space criteria being fulfilled if at least 2 of 4 MS-typical regions (periventricular, juxtacortical, infratentorial and spinal cord). Optic nerve pathology will likely soon be added as a space criterion. Dissemination in time can be ascertained on imaging if there are two scans taken at different time points with an increase in lesions consistent with inflammatory demyelination between them. Alternatively, if contrast is given and there is enhancement with background non-enhancing lesions, then one scan would be sufficient. Oligoclonal bands can also give dissemination in time.

Table 60.1 Revised McDonald criteria 2017 for diagnosis of RRMS.

Dissemination in time	Dissemination in space
i. ≥2 attacks separated by at least 1 month *or*	i. Objective clinical evidence of ≥2 lesions or objective clinical evidence of 1 lesion with reasonable historical evidence of a prior attack involving a different CNS site *or*
ii. Simultaneous presence of *asymptomatic* gadolinium-enhancing and non-enhancing lesions at any time *or*	
iii. A *new* T2 and/or gadolinium-enhancing lesion on follow-up MRI irrespective of its timing with reference to a baseline scan	ii. ≥1 T2 lesion in at least 2 of 4 MS-typical regions of the CNS (periventricular, juxtacortical, infratentorial and spinal cord)
iv. *Demonstration of CSF-specific OCBs (as a non-MRI method for DIT)*	

About 10–15% of people with MS do not have discreet attacks but rather an insidious accumulation of disability from the outset. This phenotype, primary progressive MS, typically presents in people over 40 years old when medical co-morbidities, such as vascular risk factors, are more common, which sometimes makes the diagnosis more challenging. Dissemination in space and time criteria also applies with slight alteration as outlined in Table 60.2. Source: Adapted from Thompson et al., 2018.

Table 60.2 Revised McDonald criteria 2017 for diagnosis of PPMS.

Required	AND any two of the following
Continued progression for >12 mo	One or more MRI detected brain lesions typical of MS OR Two or more MRI detected spinal lesions typical of MS OR Oligoclonal bands in the cerebrospinal fluid

It is important to consider mimics. Table 60.3 covers typical features of neurological symptoms associated with MS and atypical symptoms which should raise suspicion of an alternative diagnosis (Box 60.2).
Source: Adapted from Thompson et al., 2018.

Table 60.3 Neurological symptoms.

	Typical features	Atypical features
Optic nerve	• Optic neuritis in one eye • Mild pain on eye movement • Reduced visual acuity and reduced colour vision • Normal disc or mild disc swelling • Improvement begins within three weeks from onset • Afferent pupillary defect	• Optic neuritis in both eyes at the same time • Painless or very severe pain • No perception of light • Severe haemorrhages and exudates • Extended loss of vision • Vitritis and neuroretinitis • Photophobia
Brainstem or cerebellum	• Bilateral internuclear ophthalmoplegia • Ataxia and gaze-evoked nystagmus • Sixth nerve palsy (in patients aged 20–40 years) • Paroxysmal phenomena (occurring for at least 24 h) • Multifocal signs (e.g. facial sensory loss and vertigo) • Trigeminal neuralgia in a young person	• Complete external ophthalmoplegia • Vascular territory signs • Progressive trigeminal sensory neuropathy • Movement disorders • Fluctuating ocular or bulbar weakness or both
Spinal cord	• Incomplete transverse myelitis • Lhermitte's sign • Sphincter symptoms • Asymmetric limb weakness and sensory alteration • Deafferented hand • Progression to nadir between 4 h and 21 d	• Complete transverse myelitis • Complete Brown-Séquard syndrome • Cauda equina syndrome • Anterior spinal artery territory lesion • Localised or radicular spinal pain • Progressive and symmetrical spastic paraparesis or progressive sensory ataxia (from involvement of posterior columns) • Sharp level to all sensory modalities • Areflexia

Box 60.2 Multiple sclerosis mimics to consider.

Vascular – Strokes or cerebral small vessel disease (these can cause non-specific white matter changes on MRI).

Infection – Syphilis, human immunodeficiency virus 1, human T-cell lymphotropic virus 1 and 2 serology.

Nutritional and endocrine – vitamin B12, copper and thyroid function.

Other inflammatory – Neuro-Behçet's, sarcoid, systemic autoimmune disease (anti-nuclear antibody, ESR, Ro/La, SCL-70).

Other neurological – e.g. Neuromyelitis optica spectrum disorder (anti-aquaporin-4 and anti-myelin oligodendrocyte glycoprotein antibody screening).

Box 60.3 Common relapses.

- Optic neuritis (pain on eye movement, colour desaturation and visual loss).
- Brainstem syndrome (e.g. intranuclear ophthalmoplegia [INO], cranial nerve palsy and long-tract signs).
- Cerebellar syndrome (ataxia, slurred speech, nystagmus, dysmetria (intention tremor on finger to nose) and problems with heel to shin).
- Spinal cord syndrome (motor, sensory and sphincteric disturbance).

Box 60.4 Triggers for exacerbation of existing symptoms.

- Ambient heat (Uhthoff's phenomenon)
- Infection
- Stress (emotional or physical)
- Fatigue and sleep disturbance
- Biochemical/metabolic imbalance
- Constipation

Relapse

A relapse is defined as the emergence of new neurological symptoms (see Box 60.3) that last for more than 24 h that occur more than 30 d after a prior relapse. Symptoms reach maximal intensity approximately 24–60 h after onset but may progress slowly over 1–2 weeks. Exacerbation of existing symptoms are common and Box 60.4 covers triggers that can precipitate a 'pseudorelapse' – there is no new inflammatory demyelination but areas of existing damage have lower thresholds for unmasking prior symptoms.

An exacerbation of existing symptoms could include urinary problems, sensory issues, headaches and balance issues, visual, auditory or swallowing problems, limb weakness, neuropathic pain, a deterioration in walking distance and intractable vomiting. It is important to search for common triggers of pseudorelapse, which when addressed can improve symptoms. Patients with progressive MS may present with complications of bladder disturbance and immobility.

Treatment of an acute relapse

If a pseudorelapse has been excluded, NICE (2022) recommends a short course of high-dose methylprednisolone (500 mg daily for 5 days orally or 1 g daily for 3 days intravenously) within 14 days of onset for symptoms that are not spontaneously improving. It should be emphasised that steroids hasten recovery but their effect on outcomes is less certain. There are risks with high-dose steroids that depend on the age and comorbidities of the patient but include and are not limited to gastritis (a short course of proton pump inhibitors may be indicated), a metallic taste, insomnia, mood changes, psychosis, arrhythmias, femoral avascular necrosis and multiple courses may increase osteoporosis risk. Steroids also impair glucose intolerance and increase risk of infection.

Disease modifying therapy

An expanding number of disease-modifying therapies are for people with MS. Choice of disease-modifying therapy depends on disease activity (e.g. clinical relapses or new T2 lesions on MRI), patient co-morbidity and preference. The MS Trust has an excellent resource 'MS Decisions' that describes and compares each disease-modifying therapy. Table 60.4 describes the mechanism of action, route of administration, major side effects and 'expected' abnormal blood results to help the acute physician balance probabilities of diagnoses based on the known side effects of the drugs. Since these drugs are administered in hospital or delivered by a Home Care company, they are unlikely to appear on a list of medications from the GP's surgery and should specifically be asked for. The majority of disease-modifying therapies are available for RRMS, there are two options for secondary progressive multiple sclerosis (SPMS) with clinical or radiological activity and one option for primary progressive multiple sclerosis (PPMS).

Serious side effects

Side effects of these medications can come with a mortality risk. Progressive multifocal leukoencephalopathy (PML) becomes more common in patients on natalizumab (Tysabri) after two years of treatment if they have JC virus (John Cunningham virus [human polyomavirus 2]) in their blood, especially at high titres. Symptoms of PML include altered mental status, progressive motor deficits, limb and gait ataxia, visual symptoms (diplopia and hemianopia) and seizures. It is also a risk in patients with low lymphocytes on dimethylfumerate (Tecfidera) and rarely with Sphingosine-1-phosphate (S1P) receptor modulators (fingolimod, siponimod, posenimod and ozanimod).

Discontinuation of S1P receptor modulators has been associated with life-threatening rebound syndrome as lymphocytes are no longer sequestered in the lymph nodes. This occurs 2–26 weeks (median 9 weeks) after cessation of therapy with clinical symptoms including motor, brainstem or cerebellar and/or sensory symptoms. Radiographic activity can involve multiple enhancing (active) lesions and large, tumefactive lesions. Rebound syndrome can be fatal.

S1P receptor modulators can also be sight-threatening due to macula oedema and there should be a low threshold for ophthalmology review with visual symptoms.

Alemtuzumab is not widely used as serious side effects have emerged. Patients can be receiving infusions as day cases and hence may present overnight with infusion reactions including acute coronary syndrome, cerebrovascular events and pulmonary haemorrhage. Autoimmune thrombocytopenia can be an early complication (platelets measured on day 3 in the infusion protocol as a precaution). Later secondary autoimmunity can involve the liver and thyroid.

Multiple sclerosis in older adults

As people with MS age, they have an age-dependent propensity to develop co-morbidities (e.g. vascular disease) and other diseases (e.g. malignancy). Recent evidence points towards those with MS having a greater (1.5×) propensity to cardiovascular disease, which, in turn, is associated with greater disability. The first presentation of a band of sensory changes in the chest in a 65-year-old patient who smokes has high blood pressure, raised cholesterol and a family history of cardiovascular disease who has MS is having cardiac chest pain until proven otherwise. Sudden onset neurological symptoms in a patient with vascular co-morbidity should place stroke higher on the differential than a relapse. Pre-test probability is an important guide.

Table 60.4 Summary of disease-modifying therapies with serious side effects highlighted.

Drug name	Mechanism of action	Mode of delivery	Type of MS	Effectiveness	Side effects	Expected effect on normal blood values
Alemtuzumab (Lemtrada)	Monoclonal antibody against CD52, causing rapid elimination of CD52 immune cells in circulation, 'ordered' repopulation and thereby immune regulation.	Year 1, five consecutive days of infusions. Year 2, three consecutive days of infusions.	RRMS	High	Infusion reactions (>90%), usually mild but include acute coronary syndrome, cerebrovascular events, and pulmonary haemorrhage. Secondary autoimmunity: thyroid (36%), immune thrombocytopenia (1%), autoimmune haemolytic anaemia (1%), and anti-GBM disease (0.3%). Infections: upper respiratory tract infections, urinary tract infections, herpes, nocardia, listeria.	Low lymphocytes for few months post infusion (varies person to person).
Teriflunomide Aubagio	Dihydroorotate dehydrogenase inhibition inhibits de-novo pyrimidine synthesis and proliferation of activated lymphocytes.	Once daily tablet	RRMS	Moderate	Headache Nausea and diarrhoea Hair thinning Infections Increased levels of liver enzymes	
Beta-interferons (including Avonex, Extavia, Plegridy, Rebif)	Immunomodulator – shift from Th1 to Th2 response, reduce pro-inflammatory cytokines, reduce blood-brain barrier extravasation.	Injection, ranging from every other day to once every two weeks.	RRMS/active SPMS	Moderate	Flu-like symptoms Headache Injection site reaction Leukopenia Liver toxicity, development of anti-IFN antibodies	
Cladribine (Mavenclad)	Chlorinated analogue of the DNA building block deoxyadenosine, reduces both resting and dividing CD4+ T cells, CD8+ T cells and B cells.	Tablet, two treatment courses twelve months apart	RRMS	High		Low lymphocytes for few months post infusion (varies person to person).
Fumaric acid esters Dimethylfumerate (Tecfidera) and Diroximel fumarate (Vumerity)	Possibly modulation of cytokine expression, inhibition of immune cell proliferation, Nrf2 activation, lymphocyte apoptosis.	Twice daily tablet	RRMS	Moderate	Flushing Nausea Gastrointestinal upset Decrease in lymphocytes Rash Increased levels of liver enzymes	Expected lower lymphocytes than normal, $<0.8 \times 10^9$ increases risk of PML. Discontinue if $<0.5 \times 10^9$ for more than 6 mo due to PML risk.

(continued)

Table 60.4 (Continued)

Drug name	Mechanism of action	Mode of delivery	Type of MS	Effectiveness	Side effects	Expected effect on normal blood values
Glatiramer acetate (Copaxone and Brabio)	Immunomodulating drug comprising synthetic polypeptides.	Injection daily or three times a week	RRMS	Moderate	Injection site reactions Headache Feeling sick Lipoatrophy (indentations in the skin) A sensation of impending doom/palpitations, which occurs about 20–30 min after the injection and self-resolves within 30 min.	
Sphingosine-1-phosphate (S1P) receptor modulators (fingolimod, siponimod, posenimod, ozanimod)	Functional S1P modulator with retention of lymphocytes in lymphoid organs	Once daily tablet	RRMS/SPMS (siponimod)	Moderate	Increased infections (URTIs, UTIs, herpesvirus >>cryptococcal, PML) Impaired vaccine response (reduced T- and B-cell response to COVID-19). Slightly increased risk of PML and basal cell carcinoma Macular oedema Hypertension, hypercholesterolaemia, raised LFTs Cardiac conduction defects at first dosage Rebound syndrome (on discontinuation)	Expected lymphopenia (concern if serially below 0.15×10^9 with infection, <0.10 is problematic)
Natalizumab (Tysabri)	Monoclonal antibody against $\alpha4\beta1$ integrin, inhibits immune cells binding to endothelial cells via vascular cell adhesion protein (VCAM).	4–6 weekly infusion	RRMS	High	Increased risk of infection. Infusion reaction Development of antibodies Progressive multifocal leuko-encephalopathy (PML).	
Ofatunumab (Kesimpta)	Anti-CD20, causing depletion of immature and mature B cells. Early precursors of B cells, mature plasma cells are not eliminated	Monthly injection	RRMS	High	Injection-associated reactions Chest/gastro/viral infections Herpes infection (cold sore or shingles) Reduced response to vaccines	Decreased immature and mature B cells
Ocreclizumab (Ocrevus)	Anti-CD20, causing depletion of immature and mature B cells. Early precursors of B cells, mature plasma cells are not eliminated.	Six monthly infusion	RRMS/PPMS	High	Infusion-associated reactions Chest/gastro/viral infections Herpes infection (cold sore or shingles) Reduced response to vaccines.	Decreased immature and mature B cells.

Similarly, a change in bowel habits should be investigated as it would for any patient without MS. When one considers treatments in patients who are potentially older than the original trial populations with ageing immune systems – those on disease-modifying therapies may present with challenging side effects not least propensity to infection. Older patients on dimethylfumerate (Tecfidera) are at greater risk of developing lymphopenia putting this population at greater risk of PML.

Discharge planning

When encountering patients on the medical take, it isn't always primarily their MS that is the cause of their presentation – it may be related to side effects of their disease-modifying therapy or something entirely separate, such as infection or other medical problems entirely unrelated to their MS. Patients with MS relapses/diagnosis on admission should be discussed with the neurology registrar on-call and treated as per NICE guidelines if steroids are required. They can be referred as an outpatient to the MS clinic for diagnostic review and treatment consideration or to the relapse clinic to discern the presence of 'fresh' inflammation that may require treatment escalation. Escalation of disease-modifying therapy is rarely an emergency and the usual therapy assessments apply to ensure the patient is ready for discharge. In patients with complex symptom management again, this can be discussed with the neurology registrar on-call or the MS Nurses who can expedite specialist multidisciplinary team input as required.

Box 60.5 Key points for physicians on take.

- There are some typical neurological symptoms and/or signs that can suggest a first presentation in MS.
- In patients with known MS who present to hospital with neurological symptoms, it is necessary to distinguish relapse from pseudorelapse by exploring and addressing relevant triggers.
- Patients with progressive MS may present with complications of bladder disturbance and immobility.
- With the advent of disease-modifying therapy, patients may present with complications of treatment, especially infections.

Further reading

Galea I, Ward-Abel N, Heesen C. (2015 Apr). *Relapse in multiple sclerosis. Bmj.* 14, 350.

Graves JS, Krysko KM, Hua LH, *et al.* (2023) Ageing and multiple sclerosis. *Lancet Neurol* 22(1), 66–77.

McGinley MP, Goldschmidt CH, Rae-Grant AD. (2021) Diagnosis and treatment of multiple sclerosis: a review. *JAMA* 325(8), 765–779.

Miller DH, Chard DT, Ciccarelli O. (2012 Feb 1) Clinically isolated syndromes. *The Lancet Neurology.* 11(2), 157–169.

MS Society MS Society UK|information, research and support|MS Society. Last updated: 2 April 2024. https://www.mssociety.org.uk/.

MS Trust MS decisions aid|MS Trust. Last updated: 2 April 2024. https://mstrust.org.uk/information-support/ms-drugs-treatments/ms-decisions-aid.

NICE. (2022) *Multiple Sclerosis in Adults: Management.*

Thompson AJ, Banwell BL, Barkhof F, *et al.* (2018) Diagnosis of multiple sclerosis: 2017 revisions of the McDonald criteria. *Lancet Neurol* 17(2), 162–173.

CHAPTER 61

Myasthenia gravis

Samuel W. Mackrill, Bernard Liem, and M. Isabel Leite

Introduction

Myasthenia Gravis (MG) is an antibody-mediated disorder of the neuromuscular junction characterised by fatigable muscle weakness. This condition impacts the ocular, bulbar, axial, limb, and respiratory muscles. The hallmark of MG is the variability of symptoms, which classically worsen with muscle use and improve with rest. Such variability may confound clinical assessment resulting in misdiagnosis as a functional disorder.

In the majority of cases (approximately 85%), MG is associated with antibodies targeting the nicotinic acetylcholine receptor (AChR). Other patients may have antibodies against Muscle-Specific Kinase (MuSK) or Low-Density Lipoprotein Receptor-Related Protein 4 (LRP4), while a small number are seronegative (an entity that should be approached very carefully given the high risk of misdiagnosis). The presence of these antibodies can help guide diagnosis but are not directly used to guide treatment decisions. False positives can occur, and the detection of autoantibodies should always be assessed with clinical and electrophysiologic features to support a diagnosis of MG.

Clinical subtypes

MG can be grouped into various clinical subtypes, with ocular versus generalized involvement, early- versus late-onset groups, and by antibody status. Cases in the late-onset (>50 years) group are rising, and MG should be considered even in the elderly (>80 years). Thymic abnormalities, such as thymoma (seen in 15% of cases, with a peak at 50 years) and thymic hyperplasia, necessitate screening with CT thorax in all patients. Of note, thymoma is not associated with anti-MuSK antibodies.

Presenting features

Patients with symptoms due to new onset MG may present to acute hospital services. Ocular symptoms are the most common initial symptoms seen in up to 60% of patients. Patients may experience ptosis (drooping of one or both eyelids) and binocular diplopia, which tend to worsen with sustained gaze in a single direction or as the day progresses. Some degree of asymmetry can be expected. Notably, the pupils are unaffected in MG, unlike classical Horner syndrome or compressive oculomotor palsies.

Beyond ocular symptoms, MG may affect bulbar muscles, leading to dysarthria and dysphagia. Patients may exhibit fatigable speech difficulty with a nasal quality, and report nasal regurgitation of fluids due to palatal

Acute Medicine: A Practical Guide to the Management of Medical Emergencies, Sixth Edition.
Edited by Mridula Rajwani, Leila Vaziri, and Ivie Gbinigie.
© 2026 John Wiley & Sons Ltd. Published 2026 by John Wiley & Sons Ltd.

muscle weakness, difficulty moving food in the mouth due to tongue weakness, and fatigue when chewing indicative of jaw muscle involvement. Facial weakness may manifest as difficulty smiling, and in some cases patients may report facial motor weakness as a "numbness" around the mouth, such that MG is not initially considered. Axial weakness of neck flexion (more so than neck extension), and proximal limb weakness may also occur. Distal weakness, although less common, is seen in some cases. In the acute setting, severe isolated respiratory or bulbar presentations may require emergency admission to hospital and sometimes intensive care. In such cases, the underlying neurological disease may not be immediately apparent without a careful history and neurological examination.

Diagnosis

Antibody testing (with radioimmunoprecipitation assays, and/or more accurate cell-based assays) is now the mainstay of the diagnostic work up, supported by clinical neurophysiology including repetitive nerve stimulation (RNS) and single-fibre electromyography (sfEMG). CT thorax should be performed to look for thymic abnormalities in all patients. The edrophonium (Tensilon) is no longer recommended.

Management

The primary aim in managing MG is achieving symptom freedom with minimal side effects of therapy. Symptomatic therapy begins with pyridostigmine, an acetylcholinesterase inhibitor (AChEi), started at 30 mg three times daily. Any benefit is rapid and can then be up-titrated accordingly (typical doses 60 mg three to four times daily). Cholinergic side effects such as diarrhoea, abdominal cramping and increased secretions can be mitigated with mebeverine or glycopyrrolate. However, the effectiveness of AChEis is variable an insufficient, with most cases requiring some degree of immunosuppression.

Long-term management centres on corticosteroids and steroid-sparing agents like azathioprine, methotrexate, mycophenolate, and increasingly rituximab and complement factor inhibitors. Corticosteroids should be up-titrated gradually. Azathioprine is a good choice in women of childbearing age. These therapies can take several months to work, so are not effective acutely where intravenous immunoglobulin (IVIG) or plasma exchange (PLEX) are preferred. Minimally-invasive VATS (video-assisted thoracoscopic surgery) thymectomy should be considered in all patients with thymoma-associated MG and all patients up to 60 years in the absence of a surgical contraindications, and allow significant reduction of immunosuppression, and sometimes a sustained remission.

Acute decompensations and myasthenic crisis

Worsening of myasthenic symptoms is a common reason for patients with known MG to present to hospital acutely, and is more commonly encountered than new-onset MG. Worsening may occur for a number of reasons, including spontaneous fluctuations in disease activity, non-compliance with treatment, weaning of immunosuppression, intercurrent illness, medication interactions (see Box 61.1), pregnancy or post-operatively. Severe exacerbations characterised by acute respiratory insufficiency requiring either non-invasive ventilatory support or intubation are labelled myasthenic crisis. The lifetime risk of crisis is 10–20%, with an annual risk of 2–3%. Crises may occur due to worsening of the myasthenia itself or aspiration in patients with bulbar weakness.

Early recognition of impending respiratory failure due to myasthenic crisis improves management and helps avoid complications. Patients may be unable to complete full sentences and may describe a feeling of

Box 61.1 Medications associated with exacerbated myasthenic symptoms.

Aminoglycosides (gentamicin, streptomycin)

Quinolones (ciprofloxacin, levofloxacin, moxifloxacin, ofloxacin)

Tetracyclines (doxycycline, lymecycline, minocycline)

Macrolides (erythromycin, azithromycin, use of **telithromycin** has resulted in deaths)

Chloroquine and hydroxychloroquine

Magnesium, in particular if given intravenously

Lithium

Phenytoin

Various antipsychotics

Caution with beta-blockers, procainamide, quinidine

Possibly calcium channel blockers, gabapentin, pregabalin.

A complete list can be found on the Myaware website (www.myaware.org). In the event of a severe or life-threatening indication, the above medications can be considered with close monitoring and following discussion with neurology.

suffocation that worsens when lying flat (thought to be due to the facilitatory effect of gravity on the diaphragm when sat upright). Tachypnoea and a weak cough may be evident, associated with difficulty clearing secretions and risk of mucus plugging. In the elderly, confusion and agitation may signify impending respiratory failure.

Regular clinical reassessment and serial forced vital capacity (FVC) monitoring, at least 2 hourly at first, is advised as deterioration may be rapid. A handheld FVC device should be made available on all acute medical units. Patients should sit upright, inspire fully and blow steadily (not rapidly) for the duration of a full forced exhalation. A volume, typically measured in litres, is produced. In some cases, facial weakness may affect the ability to form a tight seal around the device mouthpiece, resulting in a falsely low reading – a mask can be used to mitigate this. Other measures including counting numbers in one breath, oxygen saturation (SaO_2), peak expiratory flow rate, and blood gas monitoring are insensitive and should not be relied upon. In particular, SaO_2 and blood gasses remain normal until respiratory failure is severe, providing false reassurance. Where swallow and aspiration are a concern, patients should be made nil-by-mouth pending a formal assessment.

An FVC threshold of 25–30 mL/kg ideal body weight is typically used for admission to intensive care and consideration of elective intubation (especially at <20 mL/kg), however the trend of serial measurements is of importance in understanding an individual patient's trajectory. MDT discussion, involving neurology, medicine and intensive care is advised. In patients who may not be candidates for intubation or in those with a less fulminant course, non-invasive ventilation can be considered.

In addition to ventilatory support, treatment with IVIg or PLEX alongside high dose corticosteroids (typically 40–60 mg prednisolone once daily) is usually indicated. Steroids alone do not act rapidly enough and are thought to drive a paradoxical worsening of motor weakness when started acutely at a high dose – an effect that is mitigated by ventilation and IVIg/PLEX. There is no appreciable difference in outcomes between the two acute treatments, although IVIg is safer in those with active infection, and PLEX may act more rapidly (and is favoured in anti-MuSK patients). IVIg is given at a dose of 2 g/kg ideal body weight spread over two to five days, with five days courses preferred if there is risk of fluid overload or VTE.

Chronic immunosuppressive therapies may be paused in the setting of acute infection, but otherwise can be continued until neurology review. Acetylcholinesterase inhibitors can be continued, but may worsen bronchorrhea and secretion burden, so dose reductions are often considered on this basis.

Finally, it is important to remember that not all acute neurological deteriorations in myasthenia patients are due to myasthenia. A wider differential diagnosis including stroke, tumours or bleeding should be considered, all of which can mimic worsening MG.

Prognosis

Prognosis varies widely, though those with frequent exacerbations/crises, severe bulbar symptoms, onset in older age, or thymoma-associated, appear to have a worse outcome. Inpatient mortality following acute myasthenic crisis approaches 10%.

Further reading

Gilhus and Verschuuren. (2015) Myasthenia gravis: subgroup classification and therapeutic strategies. *Lancet Neurol* 14(10), 1023–1036.

CHAPTER 62

Parkinson's disease and other movement disorders

Sanja Thompson

The most common movement and neurodegenerative disorder is Parkinson's disease (PD), affecting around 0.3% of people older than 40 years worldwide. PD diagnosis is based on clinical examination, as no final diagnostic radiologic, blood or physiologic test has yet been developed. The mean age of diagnosis is 70.5 years. PD is characterised by features of parkinsonism: bradykinesia, rigidity, resting tremor and postural instability. It is the only parkinsonism with a good and sustained response to antiparkinsonian drugs.

Priorities

Medical emergencies for patients with PD may be related to the disease itself, to the medication used for its treatment, or to another unrelated problem.

- If a previously stable PD patient presents with new symptoms or acute deterioration, a thorough history is needed, particularly the detailed drug history of any recent changes to the PD regime – increased, reduced, stopped or newly started drugs, with a work-up for metabolic or infectious disorders.
- Any elevation of body temperature in patients on antiparkinsonian drugs should raise suspicion of parkinsonism hyperpyrexia syndrome (PHS).
- If the history reveals previous diagnosis and treatment of a poorly levodopa-responsive parkinsonism, diagnosis of atypical parkinsonism is indicated.
- If a patient with parkinsonism is admitted to hospital, the admitting clinician should document immediately that dopamine antagonists are contraindicated (see drug-induced parkinsonism list below).
- If a patient with parkinsonism is admitted to hospital, the patient's individualized antiparkinsonian drug regime should continue in order to avoid serious complications.
- If swallowing tablets is difficult, crush normal-release L-dopa and dissolve in water prior to administration, or switch to equivalent dose of orodispersible L-dopa. In this situation, amantadine, COMT inhibitors (entacapone, tolcapone and opicapone) and MAO-B inhibitors (selegiline, rasagiline, safinamide) can be safely omitted. In case of combination L-dopa/entacapone tablets, switch only the equivalent dose of L-dopa to orodispersible form, and omit entacapone. Return to usual medication routine as soon as clinically possible.
- In patients who are nil-by-mouth (NBM) and for whom the enteral route is possible, a nasogastric tube (NGT) should be placed as soon as possible for administering PD medications. If the enteral route is not possible, commence rotigotine patch (see Tables 62.1 and 62.2).

Table 62.1 Conversion of oral dopamine agonists to rotigotine patch.

Pramipexole MR mg/day (expressed as base)	Pramipexole IR mg/dose – usually TDS dosing (expressed as base)	Ropinirole mg/day immediate release	Ropinirole MR mg/day	Rotigotine patch mg/24 h
0.26	0.088	Less 3 mg	2	2
0.52	0.18	3(1 md TDS)	4	4
1.05	0.35	6(2mg TDS)	6	6
1.57	0.53	9(3mg TDS)	8	8
2.1	0.7	12(4mg TDS)	12	10-12
2.62	0.88	18(6mg TDS)	16	14
3.15	1.05	24(8mg TDS)	24	16 (max)

Table 62.2 Conversion of oral levodopa preparations to rotigotine patch.

Current levodopa regime (mg/day)	Rotigotine patch equivalent/mg/24 h
50	1
100	2
150	4
200	4
300	6
400	8
600	12
800	16

- If a PD patient is admitted with hyperactivity and dyskinesia, but deliberately increases their own dopaminergic drug regime, a disorder of 'dopamine dysregulation syndrome' should be considered, resembling substance abuse pattern.
- Dopaminergic medications may cause impulse-control disorders such as compulsive buying or eating, hypersexuality, compulsive sexual behaviour and risk-seeking driving behaviour.
- Acute akinesia is the sudden onset of an akinetic state that is poorly responsive to treatment with antiparkinsonian medications and is a potentially fatal emergency condition that may last several days and requires hospitalization.

Further management

Attendance at emergency department (ED) by PD patients

Remember that only around 15% of PD patient admissions are related to motor symptoms.

The most common reason for PD patients to attend ED is infectious disease (21–32%) and falls. Looking for dysphagia in these patients is obligatory, as swallowing difficulty is highly prevalent particularly in advanced PD, thus increasing the risk of aspiration pneumonia. The other most common causes include cardiovascular/cerebrovascular (12–26%), gastrointestinal (8–11%) and metabolic (2–6%). Treatment of any of these conditions follows the usual guidelines.

Emergency attendance for PD-related issues are most commonly related to falls and trauma (13–27%). The most commonly implicated reasons are postural instability, freezing of gait and motor fluctuations/dyskinesia. In addition to examination, the usual investigations and assessments of patients presenting with falls, such as medication review or footwear review, it is important to look for significant postural hypotension (>20 mmHg). If postural hypotension is found, consider midodrine 2.5–10 mg up to 3 times daily and recommend an abdominal binder.

A specific problem to look for in patients presenting with falls is the presence of 'off periods', which are characterized by the re-emergence of poor mobility/parkinsonian symptoms at the end of the dose interval, i.e. usually 3–4 h after the last antiparkinsonian drug was taken. For such patients, seek advice from a movement disorder specialist.

If there is a history of multiple falls and worsening neurological symptoms, exclude subdural hematoma.

Common emergency psychiatric conditions in PD patients

Around 8% of PD patients present urgently with psychiatric conditions including delirium. As in other patients, investigations and treatment in PD patients includes multi-component interventions, e.g. looking for the cause, including recent introduction of a new drug, onset of new constipation or infection and treat these accordingly. If pharmacological treatment of delirium is needed (e.g. risk of injury to the patient or to others), quetiapine should be started (12.5 mg twice daily) and gradually increased if needed, to not more than 150 mg/day. With the improvement of delirium, prescription of quetiapine should be changed from regular to PRN, with the aim to discontinue when appropriate.

Psychosis in PD patients usually present with predominantly visual hallucinations and paranoid delusions. It could be triggered for example by infection. Apart from treating the underlying problem, the use of atypical antipsychotics may be indicated; quetiapine is recommended, starting with 12.5 mg twice daily. The use of clozapine, starting dose 6.25 mg a day, is better studied, but there is a risk of agranulocytosis.

Depression is one of the most common psychiatric conditions in PD. Therefore, patients should be assessed for suicidal ideation. Seek psychiatric help if indicated, and consider SSRI and cognitive behavioural therapy.

L-dopa-induced dyskinesia

LID may trigger emergency admission, if a patient presents with large-amplitude, abnormal involuntary movements. These are caused by L-dopa, but other drugs that enhance the effect of dopamine, for example dopamine agonists (DAs), may worsen it. In severe cases, it can cause rhabdomyolysis. Also, the respiratory muscles of some patients with LID may be affected, thus presenting with involuntary grunting, chest wall discomfort, dyspnoea and tachypnoea. The treatment is gradual reduction of L-dopa or removal of other dopaminergic drugs, like DAs. Refer to a movement disorder specialist for immediate advice.

Acute akinesia

Acute akinesia may last for several days and the patient may need hospitalization for supportive treatment. It can be provoked by for example bone fracture, medication changes, including starting antipsychotic drugs or errors in L-dopa administration. Refer to a movement disorder specialist for immediate advice.

Parkinsonism Hyperpyrexia Syndrome

A rare complication in PD patients is PHS, also known as neuroleptic malignant-like syndrome (NMLS), and is potentially fatal in around 4%. It occurs after sudden reduction/cessation of antiparkinsonian medications or sudden stoppage of deep brain stimulation (DBS). Symptoms are muscle rigidity, acute PD deterioration, agitation, sweating, tachycardia, fever and autonomic dysfunction such as uncontrollable hypertension. It resembles the clinical picture of neuroleptic malignant syndrome (NMS), although NMS is triggered by neuroleptic use. Treatment for PHS includes admission to intensive care, respiratory support, cooling down via ce packs, administration of antipyretics and cooled IV fluids, and the insertion of nasogastric tube (NGT) for additional doses of L-dopa. Treatment for NMS is discontinuation of antipsychotics. Refer to a movement disorder specialist for immediate advice.

The syndrome of dopamine dysregulation

For PD patients presenting with a freely chosen, self-elected increase of dopaminergic drugs and new onset hyperactivity, violent or repetitive behaviour, even dyskinesia, consider the syndrome of dopamine dysregulation (or levodopa misuse). It may be associated with hypomania or psychosis. The treatment is gradual reduction of dopaminergic drug doses and treatment of psychiatric complications. Refer to a movement disorder specialist for immediate advice.

Impulse control and related behavioural disorders

Impulse control and related behavioural disorders (ICBDs) may manifest with symptoms like compulsive cleaning, compulsive eating, compulsive spending or pathological eating and is associated more commonly with the use of DAs, younger age, male sex and depression. Treatment is the gradual discontinuation of DA therapy, with consideration given to quetiapine or SSRI. Refer to a movement disorder specialist for immediate advice.

Serotonin syndrome (SS) in PD patients

New onset tremor, muscle rigidity, confusion, agitation, myoclonus, autonomic instability with hyperthermia, hypertension, hypotension, leucocytosis and elevated creatine kinase (CK) in PD patients should be considered to be due to SS, particularly if the patients are taking the monoamine oxidase type B (MAO B) inhibitors (e.g. selegiline, rasagiline) with antidepressant with serotoninergic properties, such as SSRIs, SNRIs due to drug-drug interaction.

Emergency complications of device-assisted therapies

There are three device-assisted therapies for management of medically refractory motor complications: DBS (deep brain stimulation), continuous levodopa-carbidopa intestinal gel (LCIG), and continuous subcutaneous infusion (CSAI). All three therapies entail possible complications:
- DBS-related complications include infection, intracerebral haemorrhage, confusion, seizures, cerebrospinal fluid leak, the malfunction of implantable pulse generator, the fracture/migration of the wire, allergic reaction to the hardware.
- LCIG is delivered through a percutaneous gastrojejunostomy tube by battery-powered pump. Complications include blockage or displacement of the J-tube, abdominal pain, skin infection, peritonitis, pneumoperitoneum.
- CSAI complications include haemolytic anaemia, hypereosinophilia syndrome, confusion, severe postural hypotension and skin nodules at injection sites, which may undergo necrotic ulceration or cause eosinophilic panniculitis.

Emergency swallowing difficulty in PD patients

With any PD patient admitted to hospital, it is important to start the antiparkinsonian drug regime as soon as possible, considering that administration of antiparkinsonian drugs should be restored in less <24h. If the patient suffers with dysphagia, but can still swallow liquid, their immediate-release L-dopa tablets can be crushed, dissolved in water and given orally or via NGT, or the orodispersible form of L-dopa could be given instead. The total doses over 24h should be divided and administered equally throughout the waking day. Modified-release L-dopa tablets cannot be crushed, so calculate their total daily dose and administer as either crushed immediate-release tablets or as orodispersable tablets. A daily L-dopa dose reduction of about 30% may be required when converting from modified-release preparation to immediate release, along with more frequent administration.

If the patient is taking both immediate- and modified-release L-dopa, calculate the combined total daily dose and divide it equally throughout the waking day.

Immediate-release DA (pramipexole/ropinirole) can be crushed and dispersed in water for oral or via NGT administration, while modified-release DA should be switched to immediate-release equivalent and given in three divided doses via NGT (e.g. 24 mg MR ropinirole = 8 mg immediate-release ropinirole TDS) after being crushed and dispersed in water.

If any medication is given through NGT, flush the tube well to ensure complete administration and to prevent blockages.

If it is not possible to use NGT, e.g. due to gastro-intestinal system failure, convert each separate preparation of L-dopa or DA to equivalent rotigotine patch strength. NB: 100 mg levodopa is approximately equivalent to 2 mg/24 h rotigotine patch. If the total equivalent dose exceeds 16 mg (max dose of rotigotine), use it and contact a PD specialist immediately for further advice.

Rotigotine patch come in various strengths, and more than one patch may be used, but patches should not be cut. Rotigotine patch should be used with caution in patients with pre-existing dementia or if they suffer with delirium. Such patients may require dose reduction with a maximum recommended daily dose of 12 mg.

Remember that apart from PD, patients may have other forms of parkinsonism that usually mimic PD in the early phase, but respond poorly to L-dopa . If any such patient is on antiparkinsonian medications, approach the treatment of any complications or side effects in the way described above for PD patients. L-dopa in such patients should not be stopped suddenly, but if it contributes to the clinical problem (e.g. confusion, postural hypotension), it should be considered for tapering off gradually under the supervision of a movement disorder specialist.

Multiple system atrophy (MSA): parkinsonism + autonomic failure (e.g. orthostatic hypotension, urinary symptoms), and cerebellar signs. MSA has faster disease progression than PD. These patients could be taking 900 or 1000 mg of L-dopa (a recommended dose before it is declared a failed treatment). A complication that these patients sometimes present with is related to injurious actions to themselves and/or a bed partner due to rapid eye movement sleep behaviour disorder. If the behaviour is dangerous and repetitive, treatment includes changing the sleep environment and a trial of melatonin 3–18 mg, or clonazepam (to start from 0.25 mg at night). Some MSA patients may present with nocturnal laryngeal stridor, for which nocturnal positive pressure ventilation may be considered. However, there is an unpreventable risk of sudden death from disordered central respiration, suffocation by sputum and cardiac autonomic disturbance in some of these patients.

Dementia with Lewy bodies (DLB): parkinsonism + dementia with visual hallucinations, fluctuating cognition, delusions, and REM sleep behaviour disorder (RBD).

Corticobasal degeneration (CBD): parkinsonism + dystonia, focal myoclonus, alien limb phenomenon.

Progressive supranuclear palsy (PSP): parkinsonism + supranuclear vertical ophthalmoparesis, early onset of falls, urinary incontinence and in the majority of patients progressive cognitive impairment.

In **secondary parkinsonism**, the aetiology is known and treated accordingly:

- **Drug-induced**: Dopamine antagonists (antiemetics – metoclopramide and prochlorperazine; neuroleptics – haloperidol, risperidone and olanzapine). The diagnostic clue could be the presence of orofacial dyskinesia or other tardive movements. All patients presenting with parkinsonism must have current and past medication reviews, as parkinsonism may take up to a year to resolve after stopping the offending drug.
- **Neurogenetic disorders:** in younger patients presenting with parkinsonism, consider Wilson disease due to copper accumulation in the brain. However, there are reports of cases diagnosed in older age.
- **Infectious or autoimmune encephalitis**: Coxsackie virus, HIV, West Nile virus.
- **Toxic exposure**: cyanide, 1-methyl-4-phenyl-1,2,3,6-tetrahydropyridine (MPTP), manganese and some organic solvents.
- **Structural or traumatic**: brain tumours, trauma and cerebrovascular disease.

Further reading

Brennan KA, Genever RW. (2010) Managing Parkinson's disease during surgery. *Br Med J* 341, c5718.
Cosentino G, Avenali M, Schindler A, *et al.* (2021) A multinational consensus on dysphagia in Parkinson's disease: screening, diagnosis and prognostic value. *J Neurol.* 2022 269(3), 1335.
Peball M, Krismer F, Knaus HG, *et al.* (2020) Non-motor symptoms in Parkinson's disease are reduced by nabilone. *Ann Neurol* 88, 712.
Rizzo G, Copetti M, Arcuti S, *et al.* (2016) Accuracy of clinical diagnosis of Parkinson disease: A systematic review and meta-analysis. *Neurology* 86, 566.
Seppi K, Ray Chaudhuri K, Coelho M, *et al.* (2019) Update on treatments for nonmotor symptoms of Parkinson's disease-an evidence-based medicine review. *Mov Disord* 34, 180.
Stankovic I, Fanciulli A, Sidoroff V, Wenning GK. (2023) A review on the clinical diagnosis of multiple system atrophy. *Cerebellum* 22(5), 825–839. doi: 10.1007/s12311-022-01453-w.

CHAPTER 63

Motor neurone disease

Samuel W. Mackrill and Martin R. Turner

Introduction

Motor neurone disease (MND), also termed amyotrophic lateral sclerosis (ALS), is an adult-onset neurodegenerative disorder of the motor system. This is most obviously manifest clinically by *progressive* muscle weakness due to variable loss of brainstem bulbar and spinal cord anterior horn lower motor neurones, in combination with corticospinal tract (upper motor neurone) degeneration. Median survival is only 30 months from the first weakness, with death typically from the complications of neuromuscular respiratory failure.

The aetiology of MND is multifactorial, involving genetic and environmental factors. The histopathological hallmark is the presence of neuronal and glial cytoplasmic inclusions of TDP-43. ALS has an extra-motor cerebral pathology, involving a clinical and pathological continuum with frontotemporal dementia (FTD). Monogenetic forms of ALS are found in at least 10% of cases, and the absence of a family history cannot be relied upon to exclude this. The commonest monogenetic causes of ALS are an intronic hexanucleotide expansion in *C9orf72* (also linked to FTD), or pathogenic variants in *SOD1*. An aggressive form of ALS affecting young adults is associated with pathological variants in *FUS*.

Diagnosis

The diagnosis of MND can usually be made clinically with a history of 'progressive, painless, paralysis' (3 Ps) and mixed lower and upper motor neurone signs within individual body territories (arms, legs, bulbar). The diagnosis should be given by someone capable to then outline onward support (usually a neurologist), but it is essential for generalists to recognise MND when it presents acutely and refer appropriately.

MND symptoms most commonly appear in the 60s, but with a wide age range, including teenagers in rare cases. It affects both sexes, with a 3 : 2 male predominance overall. It can be classified based on the site of initial symptom onset, most often with focal weakness in one limb e.g. foot drop. Up to 30% present with dysarthria (bulbar onset), particularly in elderly women, often accompanied by sialorrhoea due to reduced swallowing frequency. Rarer presentations include cognitive and respiratory (see later).

Most cases exhibit Charcot's clinical hallmark of co-occurrence of upper and lower motor neurone signs (Table 63.1), but there may be a relative predominance of either within the spectrum of ALS, with the exception of a very rare (<3%) pure upper motor neurone syndrome primary lateral sclerosis (PLS) characterised by much slower progression. Features that should prompt consideration of an alternate diagnosis to MND include very prominent sensory or oculomotor dysfunction.

Patients with bulbar symptoms may exhibit explosive, short-lived episodes of crying (more rarely laughing) which they recognise as incongruous to their feelings. This emotional reflex hypersensitivity (historically termed

Acute Medicine: A Practical Guide to the Management of Medical Emergencies, Sixth Edition.
Edited by Mridula Rajwani, Leila Vaziri, and Ivie Gbinigie.

Table 63.1 Upper and lower motor neuron signs that may be observed in MND.

LMN signs	UMN signs
Fasciculation – this is a common *sign* in MND but only rarely the presenting *symptom*. It is neither essential nor diagnostic. It is often best seen in the first dorsal interosseous (FDI) muscles, upper arms, quadriceps or abdomen (therefore requiring exposure of the patient).	Hyperreflexia is common (sometimes also including jaw, trapezius, pectoral, finger and crossed knee adductor responses).
Limb muscle wasting (commonly seen in the FDIs, shoulder girdle, quadriceps and lower legs).	Spastic (velocity-dependent) hypertonia may be detected in the forearms with rapid supination at the elbow, or at the ankles with clonus.
Tongue signs e.g. lateral wasting, fasciculation or slowed movement, will not usually precede more obvious dysarthria and dysphagia (examine with the tongue resting in the mouth, not protruded to avoid false positive).	An upgoing (Babinski) response at big toe is often absent and so has limited independent diagnostic value.

'pseudobulbar affect') may cause significant social embarrassment. It is not a mood disorder but often responds to SSRI treatment.

MND may occur in association with variable degrees of frontotemporal cognitive and behavioural change, encompassing executive dysfunction and loss of social cognition, through to more frank dementia with loss of insight and marked apathy or disinhibition. In those severely affected with such pathology, FTD tends to occur as the initial feature in the months to years before motor dysfunction emerges. Close family may report significant personality change (sometimes with psychosis), problems at work, and loss of food repertoire with a strong preference for sweet items. MND with FTD is particularly linked to the repeat expansion in the gene *C9orf72*, and wider affected family members may have been diagnosed with FTD mislabelled as Alzheimer's disease or a primary psychiatric disorder.

Investigations

MND is often considered a diagnosis of exclusion. This is not justified. Specialised investigations may not be required to confirm an obvious clinical diagnosis and may contribute to avoidable delays in diagnosis and care.

Magnetic resonance imaging (MRI) is used to exclude structural lesions that might cause mixed upper and lower motor neurone signs, most commonly cervical spondylotic myeloradiculopathy, but such changes are usually incidental.

Electromyography (EMG) may provide evidence of LMN dysfunction in muscles where it is not already obvious clinically. It has limited sensitivity in the tongue, however. In patients with progressive dysarthria, the differential diagnosis of myasthenia is extremely unlikely without ocular involvement.

A mildly elevated creatine kinase (CK), up to 1000 U/L, is consistent with the denervation seen in established MND if other clinical features align, though significantly higher values should prompt consideration of rarer primary myopathies.

Genetic testing is now offered to all MND patients *after* diagnosis, regardless of the presence or absence of a family history, but it has *no* role in ruling in or ruling out the diagnosis. It must only be requested by those able to counsel the individual on potential outcomes and implications for other family members.

First presentation to acute services

Respiratory onset

Cases of MND with initial neuromuscular respiratory onset are rare (<5%) but more likely to present to the emergency department. The likely coincidence of respiratory infection means that a high index of suspicion is needed so that the implications of invasive ventilation can be considered fully. A potentially life-threatening hyperkalaemic response to depolarizing neuromuscular blockers may occur in those with generalised denervation (including Guillain–Barré as well as MND), and later it may not be possible to wean the patient from ventilator dependence.

Patients may report progressively worsening dyspnoea on exertion and characteristic orthopnoea due to the effect of gravity on diaphragm weakness. Nocturnal hypoventilation may disturb sleep and result in symptoms of morning hypercapnia such as headaches, fatigue and daytime somnolence. As the disease progresses, or with intercurrent illness, patients may decompensate resulting in more pervasive drowsiness.

Erect and supine bedside Forced Vital Capacity (FVC) measurements may detect diaphragmatic weakness with the greatest sensitivity, with a significant (>30%) fall in FVC on lying flat. Ventilatory failure is characterised by high pCO2 and low pO2 in arterial blood. If this occurs gradually it may be accompanied by a renally mediated compensatory elevation in the bicarbonate level to maintain a normal pH. The hallmark of decompensation is acidaemia due to respiratory acidosis, with an arterial pH < 7.35. Oxygen therapy alone in patients with chronic type II respiratory failure may worsen the retention of CO_2. Non-invasive intermittent positive pressure ventilation (NIPPV) is the method of choice in confirmed cases of MND, shown to lengthen survival as well as having marked symptomatic benefits. Careful history-taking from close family members and neurological examination may identify features suggesting MND as the cause of the respiratory failure, e.g. mobility decline and weight loss, to allow early consideration of NIPPV alongside treatment of any intercurrent infection. Once stable, EMG may help reveal the precise diagnosis.

Contemplation of *invasive* (tracheostomy) ventilation in MND requires prior discussion with the patient, focusing on what may be unrealistic expectations of the long-term outcome and outlining the significant benefits of NIPPV. This type of conversation may be very challenging in the acute setting when the patient is systemically unwell and needs close family support.

Other presentations

Cases of bulbar onset MND rarely present acutely as the symptoms are progressive over weeks to months. Nonetheless, elderly patients in particular may be erroneously referred to stroke services. MND patients, especially those living alone, may sometimes present to acute services in a state of advanced mobility decline associated with generalised weakness and weight loss. Without careful attention to the neurological examination, such patients may undergo extensive blood testing and cross-sectional imaging for the broad differential diagnoses of malignancy and systemic infection before a primary neurological disorder is considered.

Acute presentations in patients with established MND

Patients with established MND may present acutely with the complications of progressive motor dysfunction despite multi-disciplinary outpatient care that has dramatically reduced the frequency of hospital admission over the last 20 years.

Early in the disease course, there may be falls. Severe, even fatal head injury may occur as well as fractures. Progressive dysphagia in MND may lead to aspiration of food, liquids, and secretions resulting in pneumonia, though choking to death is not a feature of MND and patients should be reassured. Malnutrition and dehydration can also occur due to dysphagia and MND patients may benefit from percutaneous endoscopic gastrostomy (PEG) feeding to maintain nutrition and facilitate medication administration. Decision-making around PEG is highly individualised and requires careful discussions with the patient and their support network.

Dietary modification including thickened fluids, and timely insertion of a PEG reduce aspiration risk but do not eliminate it entirely. Aspiration events in isolation may cause a sterile pneumonitis and do not always require anti-microbial therapy unless there is evidence of secondary bacterial infection. Antibiotic and supplemental oxygen therapy form the mainstay of management along with an updated swallow assessment from a speech and language therapist.

Acute decompensation of progressive respiratory muscle weakness may occur despite timely intervention with NIPPV. Common triggers include acute intercurrent illness such as infection and occult venous thrombo-embolic disease, and during these periods of decompensation more continuous use of NIPPV may be required. Pulmonary embolism risk is significantly increased in MND though not more than for other chronic neurological disorders associated with reduced mobility. A high index of suspicion is needed when there is an abrupt change in respiratory function.

Significant depression is surprisingly uncommon in those with MND population, but the risk of self-harm and suicide, plus safeguarding issues in relation to care, need to be considered in those presenting to acute services and appropriate mental health and other professional input sought as necessary.

Unless specifically contraindicated the patient's long-term therapies should be continued during hospital admission. This is particularly important for symptomatic treatments for spasticity (though not routinely used in MND) and sialorrhoea, where abrupt withdrawal may cause rebound exacerbation.

Management at the end of life

Around the median survival of 30 months from the first weakness, there is a considerable variation between individuals. Importantly, the pace of deterioration in terms of physical disability tends to remain constant for an individual. Predictors of in-hospital mortality include established respiratory and bulbar involvement, and previously rapid disease progression. In those known to neurological services, advanced care planning and resuscitation discussions have often already taken place and referring to clinic letters can clarify any treatment escalation decisions and preferred place of care. Symptomatic dyspnoea may be palliated with small doses of opiates, anxiety and agitation managed with midazolam, and any secretion burden can be improved with hyoscine or glycopyrronium (including via a subcutaneous infusion).

Further reading

Hobson E, McDermott C. (2024) Advances in symptom management and in monitoring disease progression in motor neuron disease. *Int Rev Neurobiol* 176, 119–169.

NICE (2016) Motor neurone disease: assessment and management. NICE guideline (NG42) Last updated: 23 July 2019. https://www.nice.org.uk/guidance/ng42.

Turner MR, Talbot K. (2013) Mimics and chameleons in motor neurone disease. *Pract Neurol* 13, 153–164.

CHAPTER 64

Raised intracranial pressure

KAPIL MOHAN RAJWANI

Owing to its diverse causes (Table 64.1), raised intracranial pressure (ICP) can affect all ages and demographics. It can often present in an insidious manner with symptoms that may be difficult to differentiate from more benign pathologies. Recognition of raised ICP and urgent identification of the cause is crucial: because of the intracranial pressure–volume relationship (Box 64.1), even seemingly well, stable patients can deteriorate rapidly and without warning.

The importance of regular and reliable neurological observations should be emphasized to the nursing staff. In certain conditions, such as malignant middle cerebral artery (MCA) syndrome secondary to ischaemic stroke, even subtle changes to conscious level may be of critical importance and trigger urgent intervention.

Priorities

1 **If you suspect raised intracranial pressure (Table 64.2):**
   - Assess the airway, breathing and circulation and correct abnormal physiology.
   - Assess the conscious level: the Glasgow Coma Scale (GCS) is the most common tool healthcare providers use. A mental status change or depressed sensorium should be promptly evaluated. Seek urgent anaesthetic/intensive care opinion for patients flexing to painful stimuli or worse.
   - Assess pupillary light reflex and for papilloedema (fundoscopy).
   - Arrange brain CT. Emergent or urgent CT is required in almost all cases to determine the cause of raised ICP.
   - Seek urgent advice on management from neurology or neurosurgery. Lumbar puncture may be indicated, but should only be done on specialist advice (Box 64.2).
2 Prevent secondary brain injury
   - The cornerstone of preventing secondary brain injury is the maintenance of normal physiology. Arterial oxygen and carbon dioxide tensions should be kept within normal limits. Hypo- and hypertension should be avoided. Treat fever aggressively. Maintain normal blood glucose and treat electrolyte abnormalities.
   - Nurse the patient 30° head-up to optimize cerebral venous drainage. Keep the neck midline to facilitate venous drainage.
   - Adequate analgesia and sedation (if needed) as agitation and pain can increase the ICP.
   - Seizures are extremely deleterious in raised ICP and should be treated aggressively. Prophylaxis is often appropriate, especially in intracranial infection – seek specialist advice.
3 Consider therapy to reduce intracranial pressure
   - Give high dose **dexamethasone** (e.g. 4 mg 6-hourly IV/PO) to treat tumour-related vasogenic cerebral oedema. Steroids are contraindicated in trauma. They may be used sparingly in intracranial abscess or empyema if significant mass effect is present, but only on neurosurgical advice. Always co-prescribe a

Table 64.1 Causes of raised intracranial pressure.

Mechanism	Pathologies	Comment
Vascular	• Haemorrhagic stroke • Ischaemic stroke with mass effect ('malignant MCA syndrome') • Spontaneous subarachnoid haemorrhage • Cerebral venous sinus thrombosis	Vascular causes typically present suddenly, with headache, vomiting and neurological deficit. Patients with raised ICP secondary to ischaemic stroke present with pressure symptoms usually over 24h following the infarct, with severe headache and progressive reduction in conscious level.
Disorders of CSF hydrodynamics	• Obstructive hydrocephalus • Communicating hydrocephalus • Idiopathic intracranial hypertension	Obstructive hydrocephalus develops from a block in CSF pathways. It is due to a mass lesion, such as a tumour, and can present subacutely, but conscious level may deteriorate very rapidly. Such patients, particularly if young, may lose the ability to look upwards, due to dorsal midbrain compression. Communicating hydrocephalus usually occurs due to disruption of CSF reabsorption, such as following subarachnoid haemorrhage or meningitis. Head trauma is also a significant cause of hydrocephalus. Idiopathic intracranial hypertension (previously known as benign intracranial hypertension) occurs almost exclusively in young, obese females. It is characterized by headache, papilloedema and markedly raised CSF pressures on lumbar puncture.
Infection	• Brain abscess • Subdural empyema • Meningitis • Encephalitis	Brain abscess and empyema present with headache, confusion and seizures. There is usually a source such as sinusitis, dental abscess or infective endocarditis. Meningitis and encephalitis cause raised intracranial pressure secondary to cerebral inflammation, venous congestion and thrombosis and secondary hydrocephalus.
Trauma	• Severe head injury with traumatic haematoma (e.g. subdural or extradural haematoma) • Chronic subdural haematoma	Acutely raised intracranial pressure secondary to trauma presents with a clear history in a usually comatose patient. Chronic subdural haematoma is a common presentation to medicine, usually in elderly patients with a great variety of presentations. Most commonly it presents with deterioration in mobility, headache, confusion and occasionally focal deficit.
Neoplasia	• Primary brain tumour • Brain metastasis • Extra-axial tumour (e.g. meningioma)	Brain tumours present sub-acutely with headache, nausea, vomiting and focal deficits. There may be a history of previous cancer in patients presenting with brain metastasis. A small number of patients, usually with posterior fossa tumours, present in extremis with obstructive hydrocephalus.
Metabolic disorder	• Acute liver failure • Diabetic ketoacidosis • Hypoxic-ischaemic brain injury • Severe hyponatraemia • Acute mountain sickness	Metabolic presentations of raised ICP are varied, and the diagnosis is often suspected by the systemic condition of the patient, for example cerebral oedema in a young patient with diabetic ketoacidosis following fluid administration.

gastric protection (e.g. proton pump inhibitor or H2 receptor antagonist) to prevent steroid-induced gastritis and ulceration.
• Hyperosmolar therapy may be initiated to treat severely raised ICP secondary to cerebral oedema, and/or buy time prior to neurosurgical intervention in life-threatening situations. Seek specialist advice.
    • **Hypertonic Saline** 3% is commonly used and can be administered as a 3–5 ml/kg bolus or a continuous infusion; monitor sodium levels closely. Considered relatively safe while sodium is less than 160 mEq/L.

Box 64.1 Intracranial pressure–volume relationship.

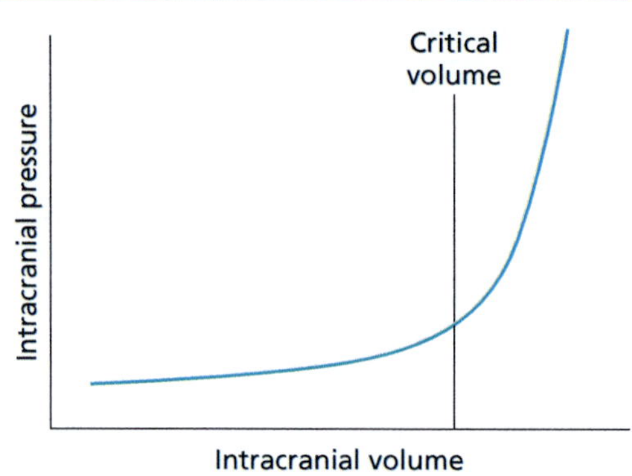

The relationship between intracranial pressure and volume is explained by the pressure-volume curve. The Monro-Kellie hypothesis states that in the rigid container of the skull, the volume of the intracranial constituents is constant (i.e. brain, blood and cerebrospinal fluid [CSF]). An increase in any component, or the addition of a component (i.e. a brain tumour), must be offset by a decrease in one or more of the others if intracranial pressure is to remain constant. Once this compensatory reserve is exhausted, ICP rises precipitously.

Table 64.2 Clinical features of raised intracranial pressure.

Feature	Comment
Headache	Classically wakes the patient from sleep in the early hours of the morning, due to recumbency and the vasodilating effect of hypercapnia while asleep. Also exacerbated by lying down or bending over, coughing, sneezing or laughing.
Vomiting	Vomiting is a late feature of raised ICP. It typically occurs after waking and is associated with morning headache.
Visual symptoms	These include a deterioration in visual acuity, field loss, blurring of vision and visual obscurations with episodic darkening of vision.
Reduced conscious level	As ICP increases, there is a progressive fall in conscious level (which is usually assessed by the GCS score) due to caudal displacement of the diencephalon and midbrain.
Papilloedema	Optic nerve head swelling suggests relatively long-standing raised ICP, as well as a threat to vision, and mandates urgent investigation. Retinal haemorrhages may also be present.
Focal neurological deficits	These include extraocular muscle palsy, facial nerve palsy, limb weakness or numbness, upper motor neuron signs such as extensor plantar response, ataxia, dysphasia and dysarthria. An abnormal neurological examination in the context of a suggestive history requires urgent investigation.

Box 64.2 Cautions before lumbar puncture.

Lumbar puncture is often an important investigation in certain suspected diagnoses, such as subarachnoid haemorrhage, meningitis and idiopathic intracranial hypertension. However, it has absolute and relative contraindications, many of which are encountered in raised ICP.

No patient should have a lumbar puncture without a CT scan of the brain. This is because lumbar puncture can cause a rapid decrease in ICP and the sudden change in volume can lead to herniation. Decreased conscious level is a relative contraindication, and if there are concerns about the safety of lumbar puncture, specialist advice should be sought before proceeding. In the absence of an obvious mass lesion, CT or MR imaging of the brain is poor at identifying raised intracranial pressure, and should not be relied on for this purpose.

- **Mannitol** 20% 0.25–1 g/kg IV. It must not be used in systemic hypotension. Check plasma osmolality, further doses may be given until osmolality reaches 320 mOsmol/kg. Beyond this, mannitol may cause rebound intracranial hypertension.

Further management

Further management is determined by the cause of raised ICP:
- Most cases of haemorrhagic or ischaemic stroke will be managed by stroke teams; only a small number will proceed to neurosurgical intervention.
- In general, hydrocephalus, raised ICP due to trauma and primary brain tumours will be managed by neurosurgical units, depending on the age and comorbidities of the patient. Patients with a new diagnosis of an intracranial tumour should be discussed with a neurosurgeon, but if stable generally require further investigations such as staging CT examination of the chest, abdomen and pelvis, and MRI of the brain.
- Patients with metabolic causes of raised ICP will often be managed by non-neuroscience clinical teams; however, advice on management should always be obtained.

Further reading

Bradley D, Rees J. (2013) Brain tumour: mimics and chameleons. *Pract Neurol* 13, 359–371.
Piper RJ, Kalyvas AV, Young AMH, *et al.* (2015) Interventions for idiopathic intracranial hypertension. *Cochrane Database Syst Rev* (8), CD003434. doi: 10.1002/14651858.CD003434.pub3. www.cochranelibrary.com.

CHAPTER 65

Acute spinal pain

Kapil Mohan Rajwani

Acute spinal pain can represent a significant diagnostic challenge. Possible causes can range from benign musculoskeletal pain requiring little treatment, to a first presentation of malignant disease. While serious causes of spinal pain are uncommon, recognizing them early and intervening appropriately requires careful assessment of all such patients. Lumbar spine, or low back pain, is the most common form of this presentation, and possibly the least likely to have a serious underlying cause. Low back pain will affect the majority of the population at some point during their lives, and is often short-lived. Cervical and thoracic spine pain are less common. They are more likely to have a sinister cause, although the majority of these patients again have a benign diagnosis.

Priorities

1 **Clinical assessment**

Look for 'red flag' features indicative of serious pathology (Table 65.1). Examine the spine and perform a full neurological examination, including assessment of perineal and perianal sensation (Box 65.1).

- Young patients rarely experience significant back pain and are unlikely to have established degenerative disease. Older patients will have conditions such as osteoporosis or primary cancers that predispose to serious spinal problems.
- Spinal pain following trauma may represent an unstable fracture, or vertebral body collapse in the presence of osteoporosis.
- A primary cancer and nocturnal spinal pain are predictors of secondary spinal malignancy.
- Thoracic spine pain is an unusual symptom and must always be taken seriously. In young patients it is particularly concerning and may be due to a sinister cause.
- Systemic features such as fever, sepsis, or weight loss suggest a generalized illness such as cancer or infection, which may have begun to involve the spine.
- Instability pain indicates a potential loss of spinal integrity, such as collapse, with resultant deformity secondary to malignancy, infection or benign fracture. It is characterized by pain present on mobilizing but usually absent at rest.
- Perineal/perianal or 'saddle' numbness, is a hallmark of cauda equina syndrome and must never be ignored.
- Bladder symptoms (especially inability to pass urine, or incontinence), and more rarely, bowel symptoms, may be due to cauda equina or spinal cord lesions.
- Progressive limb neurology suggests significant nerve or cord compression and urgent investigation is required.

2 **If malignant spinal cord or cauda equina compression is suspected, arrange emergency MRI imaging of the entire spine.**

Table 65.1 Focused assessment in acute spinal pain.

Red flags

While this term is overused and must be taken in context of the full assessment, the presence of one of these features may be the only indication of a significant underlying diagnosis.

History
Age younger than 20, or older than 55
Trauma
Known malignancy
Nocturnal pain
Thoracic pain
Systemic symptoms (fever, weight loss)
Significant pain on mobilizing that disappears at rest (may represent instability pain)
Perineal ('saddle') numbness
Bladder or bowel symptoms
Severe or progressive limb neurological deficit

Examination
Spinal deformity (e.g. kyphosis, 'step' in the posterior spine)
Bony spinal tenderness, particularly if thoracic
Significant weakness
Sensory level (i.e. a loss of sensation in all dermatomes below a certain level)
Upper motor neuron dysfunction (e.g. spasticity, brisk reflexes, extensor plantars)
Sacral dysfunction (e.g. absent anal tone, urinary retention, perineal/perianal numbness)

Box 65.1 Acute spinal pain – alerts.

Always consider potentially serious non-spinal causes of back or neck pain, including but not limited to ureteric colic, expanding abdominal aortic aneurysm, acute pancreatitis, aortic dissection and vertebral artery dissection.

A high index of suspicion and a low threshold for investigation should exist when considering spinal cord compression or cauda equina syndrome. The latter in particular is a clinical diagnosis. Emergency MRI imaging is needed and if delays are encountered, senior discussion should take place between the referring clinical specialty and Radiology immediately.

Always perform a perineal and perianal examination if you suspect spinal cord compression or cauda equina syndrome, for both clinical and medico-legal reasons. It is very useful and clinically prudent to document bladder motor function with a post-voiding bedside bladder scan.

In rectal examinations, references to 'reduced' anal tone are almost always extremely subjective and unhelpful; anal tone is better referred to as present or absent. It is also a very late sign of sacral nerve dysfunction. The absence of voluntary anal contraction is also unhelpful, as this occurs in many neurologically normal patients due to the unpleasant nature of the examination.

All patients requiring emergency MRI or CT scan may have a surgical diagnosis (e.g. cord compression, unstable spinal deformity) and should be kept nil by mouth pending their definitive imaging and discussion with a spinal surgeon. Keep the patient on bed rest; prescribe adequate analgesia; if there is significant sphincter involvement, particularly if in urinary retention, insert a bladder catheter.

If MRI imaging is unavailable, discuss with Neurosurgery or Oncology whether referral for imaging elsewhere is indicated. Consider CT scanning of the spine.

3 **If cauda equina syndrome is present, even if not thought to be malignant, arrange emergency MRI imaging of the lumbosacral spine**.

   If MRI imaging is unavailable, discuss with the relevant spinal regional centre whether transfer for imaging is indicated.

4 **If a significant traumatic injury is suspected, or a spinal deformity due to any cause is present, imaging with either CT or MRI will be required**.

   - Discuss choice of imaging with Radiology.
   - Plain X-rays may confirm the diagnosis and expedite cross-sectional imaging, but they are not definitive.
   - **If spinal infection is suspected**, obtain urgent bloods for full blood count, C-reactive protein, creatinine and electrolytes and bone profile. Take blood cultures.
   - Look carefully for a primary source.
   - Arrange urgent MRI imaging of the relevant area of the spine. Consider imaging the entire spine.

5 **If nerve or cord compression is suspected**, but not thought to be acute or malignant (e.g. lumbar radiculopathy without features of cauda equina syndrome; degenerative cervical myelopathy), routine inpatient MRI is usually appropriate.

Further management

Patients with a confirmed diagnosis of **malignant spinal cord or cauda equina compression** should be referred immediately to Neurosurgery and Oncology.

Cauda equina compression due to acute disc prolapse should also be referred immediately to Neurosurgery or the regional spinal service.

Traumatic spinal injuries and **spinal infections** should also be discussed with Neurosurgery or the regional spinal service, although many of these patients will be managed non-surgically and do not require transfer.

Patients with **lumbar radiculopathy** are usually managed on an outpatient basis by spinal surgeons. Discussion with the relevant specialty should take place if any uncertainty exists over the urgency of referral. **Cervical myelopathy** is also usually managed initially in outpatients, albeit on an expedited basis; it is prudent to discuss with the on-call specialty.

Osteoporotic collapse is managed by multiple modalities and specialties, but almost never by surgery. Vertebroplasty is advocated by some and may be appropriate in selected cases.

Patients without a significant diagnosis following investigation usually have musculoskeletal pain and are managed by adequate analgesia, mobilization and physiotherapy. Some patients will have an underlying rheumatological cause such as an inflammatory arthropathy and should be discussed with Rheumatology for further advice and management.

Further reading

Berbari EF, Kanj SS, Kowalski TJ, *et al*. (2015) Infectious diseases society of America: clinical practice guidelines for the diagnosis and treatment of native vertebral osteomyelitis in adults. *Clin Infect Dis* 61, e26–e46. http://cid.oxfordjournals.org/content/early/2015/07/22/cid.civ482.full.

Della-Giustina D. (2015) Evaluation and treatment of acute back pain in the emergency department. *Emerg Med Clin North Am* 33, 311–326.

CHAPTER 66

Spinal cord compression

KAPIL MOHAN RAJWANI

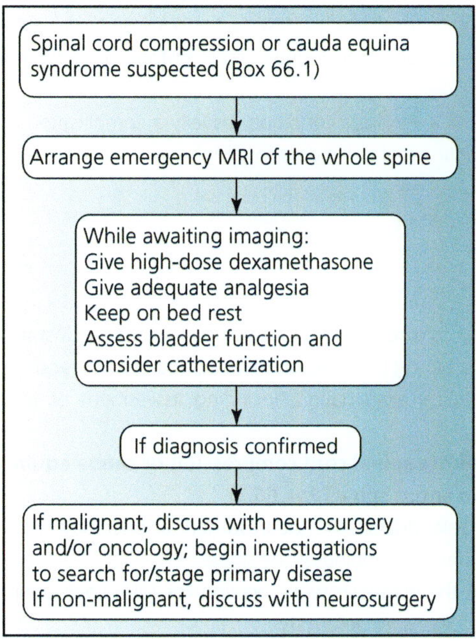

Figure 66.1 Management of suspected spinal cord compression or cauda equina syndrome.

Metastatic spinal cord compression

- The spine is the most common site of bony metastases in patients with cancer. Metastatic spinal cord or cauda equina compression will occur in 5–10% of patients with a malignancy. The thoracic region (70%) is the most common site of compression, followed by the lumbar (20%) and cervical (10%) spine.
- The most common primaries leading to spinal metastases are cancers of the lung, breast, and prostate, accounting for 70% of cases; however, cord or cauda equina compression may also occur secondary to myeloma, lymphoma, melanoma, renal, and gastrointestinal cancer.
- Metastases spread to the spine either directly, haematogenously, via arterial supply or venous drainage (e.g. prostate malignancy spreads from the pelvis via the valveless veins of Batson's plexus).
- Treatment rarely prolongs survival but can reduce pain and improve quality of life, especially in crucial areas such as mobility and continence.

Acute Medicine: A Practical Guide to the Management of Medical Emergencies, Sixth Edition.
Edited by Mridula Rajwani, Leila Vaziri, and Ivie Gbinigie.
© 2026 John Wiley & Sons Ltd. Published 2026 by John Wiley & Sons Ltd.

Other types of cord and cauda equina compression

- Degenerative disease, such as spondylosis and intervertebral disc disease, can cause an insidious onset of myelopathy in a variety of demographics and age groups. Cervical spondylosis is the most common cause of myelopathy in adults above the age of 55. With the exception of cauda equina syndrome secondary to acute lumbar disc prolapse, definitive management of this subgroup is rarely as urgent as in malignant disease, but investigation and referral should still occur promptly.
- Spinal epidural abscess is a rare entity, usually presenting with severe spinal pain and systemic upset. It most commonly results from haematogenous spread. It can also occur from the extension of soft tissue / bony infection, e.g. psoas abscess, spondylodiscitis. Risk factors include IV drug use, bacteraemia and immuno-suppression. In the presence of neurological signs and symptoms, investigation and management must be rapid.
- Spinal epidural haematoma is a very rare condition, usually a complication of anticoagulation. It tends to present suddenly with dramatic progressive deterioration.

Priorities

1 **Clinical assessment**

   General red flags of spinal cord compression include new onset gait instability; pain, weakness or numbness in limbs; sphincter disturbance; band-like trunk pain; age over 65; and midline pain. Examine the spine and perform a full neurological examination, including assessment of perineal and perianal sensation (Box 66.1).

2 **If the clinical features indicate spinal cord compression or cauda equina syndrome, arrange emergency MRI imaging of the entire spine (Box 66.2)**
   - If MRI imaging is unavailable, discuss with neurosurgery or oncology whether referral for imaging elsewhere is indicated. Consider CT scanning of the spine.
   - Plain X-rays may confirm the diagnosis while waiting for MRI. Look for bone loss, pedicle destruction (the 'winking owl' sign), collapse or deformity.
   - Arrange baseline blood tests and a chest X-ray.

3 **If malignancy is thought likely, give high dose dexamethasone,** typically 8–16 mg IV as a loading dose. Always co-prescribe a proton pump inhibitor or ranitidine.

Further management

Confirmed metastatic spinal cord or cauda equina compression

- Refer urgently to neurosurgery and oncology for consideration of surgery and/or radiotherapy, and to get advice on further management.
- Patients able to walk, but with a recent motor or sphincter deterioration, non-radiosensitive tumours, single-site compression, and with a prognosis of >six months, are good candidates for surgery. Surgery may also be required for tissue diagnosis in an unknown primary where CT-guided biopsy is not possible or unavailable.
- Patients with minimal deficit, or complete, established weakness, may be better managed by radiotherapy. Radiotherapy confers excellent pain relief.
- Surgery may also be indicated in patients with actual or impending instability, and good performance status. These patients should be maintained on strict bed rest. Seek advice from neurosurgery, or a spinal surgeon.

Box 66.1 Clinical features of spinal cord compression and cauda equina syndrome.

Clinical feature	Comment
Spinal pain	Almost all patients with cord compression due to malignant disease will have spinal pain, and pain is typically the first symptom. The pain is constant, classically worse at night, and with Valsalva manoeuvre (e.g. coughing). May be focal, radicular or referred.
Site of compression	Around 70% of metastatic spinal cord compression cases occur in the thoracic spine. The vast majority (>90%) are extradural; intramedullary (within the spinal cord) metastases are very rare. Thoracic pain following mild trauma may distract from the underlying diagnosis: trauma can precipitate a pathological fracture in pre-existing disease. 35–75% of patients have limb weakness at the time of diagnosis. Spasticity and hyperreflexia take time to develop, and may be absent in the acute setting. Patients with lumbosacral compression may present with cauda equina syndrome.

Motor system	Site of compression	Type of weakness
	Above C5	Spastic quadriparesis: upper motor neuron (UMN) distribution with spasticity and brisk reflexes in all four limbs and extensor plantars
	Between C5 and T1	Lower motor neuron (LMN) weakness at the level of the lesion (e.g. in the hands) and UMN weakness below
	Between T1 and L1	Spastic paraparesis: UMN weakness in the lower limbs; upper limbs unaffected
	Below L1	LMN weakness in the lower limbs

Sensory system	Site of compression	Sensory level
	Above C5	Neck
Sensory innervation of the skin	Between C5 and T1	Upper limbs
	Between T1 and T6	Thorax
	Between T7 and T12	Abdomen
	Below L1	Lower limbs

| **Sphincter disturbance** | Abnormalities of bladder function almost always precede those of bowel function.
Lesions at or above the conus medullaris (the termination of the spinal cord) lead to a reflex neurogenic, or 'automatic' bladder, with overactivity, urgency and incomplete emptying; this is an UMN lesion, best thought of as bladder spasticity. Bowel abnormalities present as constipation.
Lesions compressing the cauda equina cause overflow urinary incontinence due to a loss of bladder motor function, so that the bladder passively fills; this is a LMN lesion, best thought of as bladder flaccidity. Bowel abnormalities present as loss of anal sphincter tone and faecal incontinence. There is perineal sensory loss – the classic 'saddle anaesthesia'. |

Box 66.2 Spinal cord compression – alert.

All patients requiring emergency MRI or CT scan may have a surgical diagnosis (e.g. cord compression, unstable spinal deformity) and should be kept nil by mouth pending their definitive imaging and discussion with a spinal surgeon.

Keep the patient on bed rest; prescribe adequate analgesia. If there is significant sphincter involvement, particularly if in urinary retention, insert a bladder catheter.

- Surgery is also considered in radio-resistant tumours, such as melanoma, renal, or gastrointestinal carcinoma, or in patients that have progressed despite radiotherapy. However, infection and impaired tissue healing is a major concern in the latter group.

Arrange further investigations to seek a primary tumour, if none is known; or to re-stage known disease, depending on specialist advice. This is usually in the form of a CT scan of the chest, abdomen and pelvis; a myeloma screen; tumour markers; and a bone scan.

Confirmed non-malignant spinal cord or cauda equina compression

Stop steroids. Seek advice on further investigation and management from neurosurgery.

Further reading

Al-Qurainy R, Collis E. (2016) Metastatic spinal cord compression: diagnosis and management. *BMJ* 353, i2539. DOI: 10.1136/bmj.i2539.

Fehlings M, Nater A, Tetreault L, *et al.* (2016; 06-GO223) Survival and clinical outcomes in patients with metastatic epidural spinal cord compression: results from the AOSpine prospective multi-centre study of 142 patients. *Global Spine J.* DOI: 10.1055/s-0036-1582880.

Singleton JM, Hefner M. (2023) Spinal cord compression. In: StatPearls. Treasure Island (FL): StatPearls Publishing. Available from: https://www.ncbi.nlm.nih.gov/books/NBK557604/.

CHAPTER 67

Functional neurological disorder in the acute setting

ANNE-CATHERINE M.L. HUYS AND ABHIJIT DAS

Functional Neurological Disorder (FND) is a common cause of disabling neurological symptoms. Symptoms are varied and include amongst others abnormal control of movement (e.g. weakness, tremor, dystonic posturing), episodes of altered awareness resembling epileptic seizures (functional/dissociative seizures) and abnormal sensations. Fatigue, pain, and cognitive difficulties are common additional symptoms. FND cannot be explained by any structural, biochemical or genetic abnormality and instead is thought to be caused by a brain network dysfunction, predominantly involving areas of motor control, attention, emotions and agency. As such, the usual investigations are normal. Yet FND is not a diagnosis of exclusion, but largely diagnosed through positive signs.

In recent years, there has been increasing emphasis on the role of multidisciplinary management, involving neurology, general medicine, and if relevant psychiatry, physiotherapy, occupational therapy and speech and language therapy.

FND in A&E – Dos and Don'ts

- Suspect FND if the patient exhibits symptoms that are variable, improving with distraction or worsening with attention
- Avoid iatrogenic harm – avoid unnecessary and painful investigations, avoid giving unproven diagnoses before there is diagnostic certainty
- Avoid terminology such as 'pseudo-' (implies symptoms are fake), 'medically unexplained' (implies the condition is not understood), 'psychogenic', 'conversion', 'somatisation' (implies a psychogenic origin which in many cases is incorrect and frequently misunderstood as meaning it is not genuine, 'It's all in my head')
- Use terminology that is acceptable to patients: 'functional'

FND is among the most common conditions in neurology and the acute setting is no exception. The initial history taking, and examination is no different to other neurological conditions, with some additional components. The hallmark feature of FND is that symptoms worsen with attention and improve or disappear with distraction. In functional movement disorders, including in functional weakness, symptoms are present with wilful, explicit movements, and improve or disappear with automatic, implicit movements. Yet another way of looking at this phenomenon is apparent inconsistency – the ability to do or perceive something in one circumstance, but not in the other. Thus, in addition to the standard neurological examination, throughout the clinical encounter, one looks for signs of symptom improvement with distraction or under different circumstances.

Acute Medicine: A Practical Guide to the Management of Medical Emergencies, Sixth Edition.
Edited by Mridula Rajwani, Leila Vaziri, and Ivie Gbinigie.
© 2026 John Wiley & Sons Ltd. Published 2026 by John Wiley & Sons Ltd.

Diagnosis of FND

According to the DSM-5, the diagnosis of FND requires:

* **Criterion A**: One or more symptoms of altered voluntary motor or sensory function.
* **Criterion B**: Clinical findings provide evidence of incompatibility between the symptom and recognized neurological or medical conditions.

Demonstrating this incompatibility involves evaluating for positive signs during the physical examination, such as tremor entrainment and distractibility. These signs help confirm Criterion B, enabling a positive rule-in diagnosis, which differs from an exclusionary process. The DSM-5 has two more criteria:

* **Criterion C**: The symptom or deficit is not better explained by another medical or mental disorder.
* **Criterion D**: The symptom or deficit causes clinically significant distress or impairment in social, occupational, or other important areas of functioning or warrants medical evaluation.

Moreover, explaining to the patient how the diagnosis was reached by demonstrating positive physical examination signs can help them understand their condition better. There is strong evidence that early explanation and patient engagement improves the therapeutic outcome.

Common acute presentations

Functional symptoms often have a sudden onset and can be severe, so patients commonly present to acute care. The following are the most common acute presentations.

Functional/dissociative seizures

Functional/dissociative seizures can be difficult to differentiate from epileptic seizures by the non-experienced and indeed it is not infrequent for patients with functional/dissociative seizures to be misdiagnosed as treatment resistant epilepsy or in the acute setting as being in status epilepticus, be unnecessarily intubated and admitted to the intensive care unit. Table 67.1 summarizes the key differences. Home or inpatient video recordings often facilitate the diagnosis.

Table 67.1 Typical features of functional/dissociative and epileptic seizures.

		Functional/dissociative seizure	Epileptic seizure
Before	Trigger	Stress Other symptoms, e.g. migraine	Stress Sleep deprivation Strobe light – if photosensitive
	Prodrome	Not arising from EEG proven sleep Prodrome common May be prolonged Variable +/– other functional symptoms +/– autonomic arousal +/– anxiety, panic, hyperventilation or their associated symptoms +/– dizziness, light-headedness +/– dissociative symptoms +/– tension, pain +/– impending doom	May arise from EEG proven sleep Aura common in focal onset seizures – stereotyped Fear/panic may occur in temporal lobe epilepsy

Table 67.1 (*Continued*)

		Functional/dissociative seizure	**Epileptic seizure**
During	Movements	+/− flashback +/− gradual onset Occasionally, loss of consciousness is welcome, as it ends these distressing warning symptoms None (lying still) Asynchronous, erratic Thrashing, violent movements Side to side head / body movement Opisthotonos Typically no initial tonic phase Contraction followed by contraction of the antagonist muscles, may be tremor- or rigor-like	Frontal lobe seizures may be asynchronous, violent, thrashing, with retained awareness. Typically arise from sleep and short duration. Opisthotonus very rare Clonic movements (contraction followed by relaxation)
		Pelvic thrusting – Occasionally seen in functional/dissociative seizures and in frontal lobe epilepsy	
	Eyelids	Closed Eyelid flickering Resisting passive opening	Open Eyelid flickering in childhood absence
	Consciousness	May be retained despite inability to respond or control movements and whole-body abnormal movements	Generally lost in generalised seizures (may be retained in frontal lobe seizures)
	Tongue biting	Small, front of tongue	Large, side of tongue
	Respiration	Fast → Normal skin colour	Ceases → Cyanosis Frothing at mouth
	Grunting sound	Occasional	Common
	Duration	Long, >5 min	Mostly <5 min
	Variability	Fluctuating course, movements may vary widely throughout an individual seizure and between seizures	
	Injury	Typically milder (carpet burns, bruising), but may occasionally be more severe	More severe e.g. shoulder dislocation
	Urinary incontinence	Urinary incontinence	
After	Recollection	May remember the entire seizure	Largely only recollection of focal aware seizures or aura
	Confusion	No true postictal confusion	Postictal confusion
	Sleepy	Sleepy	
	Neurological symptoms persisting after the seizure	Functional neurological symptoms may persist for variable length (hours, days) following a seizure	Todd's paresis
	Emotions	Crying (may also occur interictally) Post-ictal relief	
	Breathing	Normal	Stertorous breathing
Investigations	Imaging	Normal	+/− abnormal
	Blood tests	Raised prolactin	
		Raised CK	
	EEG	Normal during a functional seizure	EEG typically abnormal during and shortly after an epileptic seizure +/− interictal epileptiform activity

Note that no single factor is absolute, nor diagnostic, but it is the combination of positive symptoms and signs that lead to the correct diagnosis.

Functional weakness

Functional weakness is a frequent stroke and cauda equina syndrome mimic and indeed often, especially initially, misdiagnosed as such. The onset can be sudden or gradual, yet the defining feature is that the weakness is variable. It typically improves with distraction, when implicit movement control takes over, or it may be present with some movements but not others.

In the case of leg weakness, test for Hoover's sign: weakness of voluntary hip extension that resolves when the contralateral unaffected hip is flexed against resistance. It can be tested in a sitting or lying position. (a video explanation can be found at: https://neurosymptoms.org/en/symptoms/fnd-symptoms/functional-limb-weakness/). In bilateral leg weakness resolution of weak hip extension may be demonstrated by asking the patient to lean forward against resistance in a sitting position. Table 67.2 summarizes the main features of functional weakness.

Table 67.2 Functional weakness.

Typical features and positive signs		Notes
General	Distractibility	
	Normal implicit movements	Get the patient to move implicitly, change the movement pattern, e.g. by asking them to skate, dance, walk sideways, backwards etc. A few normal steps can often be observed when the patient turns around (done implicitly), while the symptoms are more severe when the patient is focusing on walking. Note that non-functional dystonia improves when walking backwards or running
	Variability (extreme examples: maintain arm elevated, but unable to move it; unable to move leg when examined in the bed, but able to weight bear)	
	Co-contraction of agonist and antagonist muscle	Not frequently seen
	Give-way weakness	Also present in pain conditions and with unclear instructions
	Collapsing weakness (e.g. limb collapses from a normal position with light touch of the examiner, or normal muscle force can often be achieved transiently with encouragement but then suddenly gives way, collapses, or collapses after having been maintained for a fraction of a second)	
Functional arm weakness	Absent pronator drift – when asking to hold the arms outstretched in supination with eyes closed, the arm drifts downwards in supination, without the pronator drift typically seen in pyramidal weakness	
	The plegic arm may move implicitly, e.g. gesturing while talking	

Table 67.2 (*Continued*)

Typical features and positive signs		Notes
Functional leg weakness	Hoover's sign Dragging the leg behind 'like a log' when walking, typically with medial part of the foot in contact with the floor and leg externally rotated Knee buckling on walking Spinal Injuries Centre Test (leg with no tone nor power when directly examined stays in position when passively flexed at the knee in a supine position, with the heel resting on the bed)	The equivalent of the Hoover's sign can be demonstrated for many other movements, e.g. hip abduction of the weak leg when simultaneously abducting the normal hip; grip strength, when pulling the examiner towards them; arm strength when holding on to the examiner while walking, etc. Knee buckling also seen in cataplexy, negative myoclonus, drop attacks
Functional cranial nerve weakness	Functional ptosis is typically accompanied by depression of the ipsilateral eyebrow Wrong way tongue – the tongue deviates away from the side of the functional hemiparesis Ipsilateral weakness of the sternocleidomastoid accompanying functional hemiparesis	In non-functional ptosis there is typically frontalis overactivity in an attempt to overcome the ptosis Weakness of this bilaterally innervated muscle is rare in non-functional hemiparesis

Note that no single factor is absolute, nor diagnostic, but it is the combination of positive symptoms and signs that lead to the correct diagnosis.

Functional movements disorders

Functional movement disorders can be of any type: tremor, dystonia, myoclonus, tics, gait disorder and others. The key factor is to look for, again, is distractibility, the improvement of the abnormal movement with distraction. Note, that stress or anxiety will worsen all movement disorders, functional and non-functional. Table 67.3 summarizes the key.

Table 67.3 Functional movement disorders.

	Typical features and positive signs	Notes
Functional tremor	Distractibility Variability – frequency and direction are better measures than amplitude since amplitude also varies moderately in non-functional tremors. Entrainment (functional tremor takes on the frequency (or a harmonic) of another body movement's tapping frequency, or sometimes even of music). Alternatively, there may be difficulties in copying a tapping movement with an unaffected limb. Worsening of the tremor when the tremoring limb is restrained, or appearance of the tremor elsewhere in the body when the tremoring limb is restrained by the examiner	Non-functional tremors may vary – Action tremors such as essential or dystonic tremor largely disappear at rest – Parkinsonian tremor disappears, or tends to become milder on action – Dystonic tremor worsens in certain positions – Stress worsens any type of tremor Amplitude may vary in non-functional tremors
	Stops transiently with ballistic movements Increases with weight loading Co-contraction tremor (co-activation sign: tremor appears with co-activation of the agonist and antagonist muscles) Most common hand and arm tremor, finger tremor is less common	Non-functional tremor typically improves with weight loading

(*continued*)

Table 67.3 (*Continued*)

	Typical features and positive signs	Notes
	Can also affect head, legs or palate Clonus of the ankle – ankle clonus when putting weight onto toes	
Functional dystonia	Typically, fixed dystonia, right from the start Often triggered by physical injury Often painful – note possible overlap with complex regional pain syndrome Distractibility/variability/inconsistency (often hard to demonstrate in fixed dystonia) Adult-onset foot dystonia Mostly limbs, but can also affect neck or jaw Typical patterns – Foot inversion and plantar flexion – Flexion of the 3rd to 5th fingers with sparing of thumb and index	Non-functional dystonia is typically mobile and worsens with activity in other body parts With the exception of cervical dystonia, non-functional dystonia is typically pain-free Watch out for painful torticollis due to trauma causing atlanto-axial subluxation Improve with sensory tricks (geste antagoniste) Non-functional lower limb dystonia typically presents in childhood, it rarely presents in adulthood and if so, it is typically exercise/action induced
Functional myoclonus	Functional myoclonus is most often proximal or axial Distractibility, variability Entrainment Strong stimulus sensitivity (much more than in non-functional myoclonus) Often more complex than non-functional myoclonus with multiple components over time Increased startle or startle like movements are frequent Anticipatory myoclonus (elicit 'stimulus' or 'reflex' myoclonus even when stop just before touching the patient)	The most common non-functional myoclonus is cortical myoclonus, which affects the distal limbs and is stimulus sensitive
Functional tics	Can be difficult to differentiate from non-functional tics Blocking – the tick stops the ongoing action/sentence Usually not preceded by an urge Inability to suppress Limbs and trunk more often involved Further factors that are more typical in functional rather than non-functional tics: • Abrupt onset in adulthood • No childhood tics • Female predominance • No family history • precipitating event • No OCD nor ADHD • No waxing and waning, instead rapidly deteriorating or severe at onset • Multiple movements and vocalisations, dramatic, frequently changing • Vocalisation of long variable phrases • Tick attack may resemble functional seizures – thrashing mov, not individual tics	Non-functional tics are also distractible In non-functional tics, the action/sentence that is interrupted by the tic is typically continued after the tick Typically preceded by an urge to perform the tic Ability to suppress for short periods Cranio-cervical predominance Typical factors in favour of non-functional tics – childhood onset simple tics – Male predominance – Family history – no precipitating event – Associated with OCD, ADHD – Waxing and waning course – Stereotyped – Pali-, echo- and copro-phenomena

Table 67.3 (*Continued*)

	Typical features and positive signs	**Notes**
Functional gait disorder	Typically associated with other functional movement disorders Common patterns: – Dragging behind of the weak leg, 'like a log', typically with medial part of the foot in contact with the floor and leg externally rotated – Subjective poor balance, with swaying but no or only minor falls, prolonged one-legged stance, actually demonstrating good balance – Walking on ice pattern – Veering to either side – Sudden knee buckling – Scissoring gait increasing on tandem walking – Excessive slowness of gait – Absent arm swing when walking with normal arm swing when trunk passively rotated Patients do not seem to compensate for the gait problem they complain of in an optimal way – e.g. complaining of unsteadiness, but walking with a narrow base – Uneconomic postures – Shifting centre of gravity by pivoting from side to side at the waist on a narrow base	Non-functional gait disorders can fluctuate/be variable, e.g. dystonia improved when walking backwards, biphasic dyskinesias in Parkinson's disease Walking on ice pattern also seen in sensory ataxia Knee buckling also seen in cataplexy, negative myoclonus, drop attacks Scissoring also seen in non-functional gait disorders, but without increase on tandem gait Watch out: 'bizarre' gait also seen in non-functional disorders – Huntington's disease and other choreas – Biphasic dyskinesia in Parkinson's disease – Neuroacanthocytosis – Dystonia – Status cataplecticus ('limp man syndrome')
Functional facial spasm/weakness	Corner of the mouth is typically pulled downwards (increased muscular contraction) and the jaw may also be pulled laterally Platysma muscle is typically contracted (and indeed contributing to the downward pull). In addition to orbicularis oculi contraction there is typically depression of the ipsilateral eyebrow, plus minus elevation of the contralateral eyebrow (known as the 'false other Babinski sign'). The tongue may also be affected, deviating to the ipsilateral side on protrusion, something not typically be seen in hemifacial spasm. Mostly intermittent	Patients typically report facial weakness, when in fact there is increased muscular contraction. Functional facial spasm can sometimes be mistaken for a lower facial upper motor neuron lesion such as a stroke or a peripheral facial nerve palsy such as Bell's palsy. In upper and lower motor neuron lesions, there is weakness of the affected face muscles. The other main non-functional differential diagnosis is hemifacial spasm. In this condition the movements are irregular in rhythm and degree, but synchronous in all affected muscles. As such, the 'other Babinski sign' is often seen, in which there is unilateral contraction of the frontalis muscle, causing eyebrow elevation with simultaneous contraction of the ipsilateral orbicularis oculi muscle, causing eyelid closure.

Note that no single factor is absolute, nor diagnostic, but it is the combination of positive symptoms and signs that lead to the correct diagnosis.

Table 67.4 Functional visual symptoms.

	Typical features and positive signs	Notes
Visual loss	May be variable, improved with distraction +/– discrepancy with day-to-day functioning or during the clinical encounter Occasionally the same line on the visual acuity chart may be readable from different distances	In unilateral visual loss, test for stereopsis (depth perception) as it requires good vision and good binocular fusion Further ophthalmological testing may confirm unilateral functional visual loss: preserved vision may be demonstrated by testing monocular vision with rapidly changing blurring lenses leading to an inability to differentiate which eye is being tested; by subtly fogging the lens in front of the 'good' eye; or with the use of coloured lenses while reading alternating coloured letters.
Visual field	Tunnel vision (concentric loss of peripheral vision, with visual fields of identical diameter when viewed from different distances)	Contradicts laws of physics Other visual field loss patterns that can be detected by formal visual field testing are: – spiral visual field loss – jagged, inconsistent star pattern visual field
Convergence spasm	Unilateral or bilateral persistence of convergence after initial voluntary convergence Normal eye movements often observed outside of the neurological examination	

Note that no single factor is absolute, nor diagnostic, but it is the combination of positive symptoms and signs that lead to the correct diagnosis.

Functional sensory symptoms

Functional sensory symptoms are inherently more difficult to diagnose than movement disorders, due to the lack of visible signs. Factors that point towards a functional origin are sensory distributions that do not correspond to known anatomy, or symptoms that are present in one situation, but not another. A good example is absent lower limb proprioception on joint position testing, with a normal Romberg's test.

Functional visual symptoms

Table 67.4 summarizes functional visual symptoms.

Functional speech disorders

As with all functional neurological symptoms, an important factor to look out for is worsening of the functional speech disorder with attention, which includes its discussion and examination. Conversely, there is improvement with distraction or when performed implicitly. The main patterns are summarized in Table 67.5.

Note that functional dizziness as part of persistent postural-perceptual disorder (PPPD) generally develops following an initial triggering event that causes vestibular symptoms or disrupts balance. In addition, symptoms need to be present for at least three months prior to diagnosis. As such it does not generally present in the acute setting.

Management

FND symptoms and their impact on quality of life are just as severe as equivalent neurological conditions and the prognosis, particularly without adequate management, can be poor. Early intervention, including referral to the necessary services, improves prognosis, and this starts with the communication of the diagnosis and

Table 67.5 Functional speech disorders.

Prosodic abnormalities	Functional foreign accent syndrome – Appearance of a foreign accent in the patient's native language, combined with grammatical errors typically made by native speakers of the foreign accent's language – +/– modifiability - may be able to imitate another accent if asked to do so – Note that foreign accent syndrome can be of non-functional origin, but is not associated with the above-mentioned grammatical errors Infantile/childlike prosody
Dysfluent speech	Functional stammering – high variability with periods of fluent speech and periods of significant stammering – excessive consistency – stammering on every word, syllable or sound – +/– effortful physical struggle while speaking
Dysphonia	Complete aphonia may present acutely

Note that no single factor is absolute, nor diagnostic, but it is the combination of positive symptoms and signs that lead to the correct diagnosis.

its explanation. When giving the diagnosis, stress the positive signs that led to the diagnosis, show the examination findings to the patient and validate their symptoms.

Approximately two thirds of people with FND have had a previous or current adverse event and addressing any psychological difficulties associated with this is often crucial for symptom improvement. However, a third of people have not had any such adverse event and one needs to be very tactful in enquiring about it. If it is obvious that there has been psychological trauma, then early referral to psychology/psychiatry is indicated.

Priorities in acute management

1 Immediate assessment

- Obtain a full set of physiological observations
- Review the patient's medical history
- Conduct a full clinical assessment, additionally looking for distractibility and variability under different circumstances
- Arrange urgent investigations or urgent neurology referral to rule out concomitant structural or other non-functional causes

2 Reassurance and explanation

- Clearly explain the diagnosis to the patient
- Focus on explaining and demonstrating the 'rule-in' positive clinical signs (e.g. Hoover's sign) that led to the diagnosis. Focusing on the absence of abnormal investigations may make the patient feel that the diagnosis is unknown, that more specialised investigations are missing, and that the diagnosis was given because no better cause could be thought of. The latter may lead to rejection of the diagnosis, further presentations in the acute setting and most importantly, impaired outcome for the patient.
- Provide reassurance that FND is a well-recognized, common and treatable condition

3 Symptom management

- Arrange for neurology referral and follow-up
- Specialized physiotherapy techniques for motor symptoms
- Distraction techniques for symptom improvement
- Relaxation techniques such as meditation or box breathing
- Grounding techniques for functional/dissociative seizures
- Occupational therapy for functional limitations
- Speech and language therapy for speech disorders
- Treat comorbidities such as migraine, depression, anxiety

- Refer to psychology/psychiatry if indicated
- Signpost useful information for patients and their families:
  - Websites
    - www.neurosymptoms.org
    - www.nonepilepticattacks.info
  - Books
    - **CBT self-help**: 'Overcoming Functional Neurological Symptoms' by Chris Williams
    - **FND stories**: 'Personal and Professional Experiences of Functional Neurological Disorder', by Gregg H. Rawlings
  - Patient organizations
    - www.fndhope.org
    - www.fndaction.org.uk

Specialist physiotherapy is recommended for this group of patients as the approach involves primarily distraction and implicit movement and hence differs from standard physiotherapy.

Table 67.6 details simple distraction/grounding techniques that can be used:

Table 67.6 Sensory grounding, box breathing and progressive muscle relaxation.

Technique	Description
1 Sensory grounding	The 1-2-3-Safe method can help stop, or at least delay, functional/dissociative seizures, dissociation, anxiety, and panic. Practice this method when you're feeling okay, so it comes automatically when you need it. Just like you wouldn't wait to practice first aid until someone was in trouble! **1 Feel**: Find one thing with an interesting texture (e.g., keys, pine cone) and touch it with your fingers and thumbs. Focus your thoughts on how it feels, and how the sensations change as you rub harder or softer in different directions. **2 Look**: Find two objects around you and describe them in detail to yourself, either silently or out loud. **3 Listen**: Listen to your surroundings and identify three different sounds, such as birds singing, a washing machine, or traffic. **4 Remind**: Remind yourself that you are safe. **5 Distraction**: Engage in a simple but absorbing distraction to fully occupy your mind. Examples include: • Count backwards from 100 to 0, subtracting 7 each time: 100, 93, 86, 79. . . • Count forwards, alternating letters and numbers: A, 1, B, 2, C, 3. . . • Try to spell 'supercalifragilisticexpialidocious'. • Name all the players in your favorite sports team.
2 Box Breathing	Box breathing, also known as square breathing, is a powerful technique for managing stress and anxiety. **1 Inhale**: Sit comfortably with your feet flat on the floor. Close your eyes if you feel comfortable doing so. Breathe in slowly and deeply through your nose for a count of four. Focus on filling your lungs completely and expanding your belly. **2 Hold**: Hold your breath for a count of four. During this pause, try to keep your body relaxed. Feel the fullness of your lungs and the stillness of the moment. **3 Exhale**: Slowly exhale through your mouth for a count of four. Focus on emptying your lungs completely and allowing your belly to contract.

Table 67.6 (*Continued*)

Technique	Description
	4 Hold: After exhaling, hold your breath for another count of four. Use this time to relax and prepare for the next breath.
	5 Repeat: Continue this cycle for several minutes. You can start with one to two minutes and gradually increase the duration as you become more comfortable
3 Progressive Muscle Relaxation	Progressive Muscle Relaxation is a technique designed to reduce stress and anxiety by tensing and then relaxing different muscle groups in the body. (You can also search for recordings online)

1 **Prepare your environment**:
- Find a quiet place free from distractions.
- Lie on the floor or recline in a comfortable chair.
- Loosen any tight clothing and remove glasses
- Rest your hands comfortably in your lap or on the arms of the chair.
- Slow your breathing. Spend a few minutes practicing box breathing

2 **Focus on each muscle group**:
- Concentrate on one area at a time, ensuring the rest of your body remains relaxed.

3 **Forehead**:
- Squeeze the muscles in your forehead as if you are frowning. Hold this tension for five seconds, feeling the muscles become tighter. Slowly release the tension while counting to five. Notice the contrast in how your muscles feel when relaxed. Continue breathing slowly and evenly. (This applies for all muscle groups)

4 **Jaw**:
- Clench your jaw muscles tightly. Hold for five seconds and release the tension slowly while counting to five.

5 **Neck and shoulders**:
- Raise your shoulders toward your ears, increasing the tension in your neck and shoulders. Hold for five seconds and gradually release.

6 **Hands**:
- Make fists with your hands and squeeze tightly for five seconds. Hold for five seconds and gradually release

7 **Arms**:
- Curl your biceps as if trying to crush an apple between your lower and upper arms. Hold for five seconds and gradually release

8 **Feet**:
- Point your feet like a ballet dancer, creating as much tension as possible in your insteps. Hold for five seconds and gradually release

9 **Experiment with other muscle groups**:
- Feel free to apply the same technique to other muscle groups such as your thighs, abdomen, and chest. Hold for five seconds and gradually release

10 **Visualize relaxation**:
- Some people find it helpful to visualize the feeling of relaxation flowing through their body like water or white light.

Further reading

Aybek S, Perez DL. (2022) Diagnosis and management of functional neurological disorder. *BMJ* 376, 64.

Finkelstein SA, Cortel-LeBlanc MA, Cortel-LeBlanc A, Stone J. (2021) Functional neurological disorder in the emergency department. *Acad Emerg Med* 28(6), 685–696.

Gilmour GS, Nielsen G, Teodoro T, *et al.* (2020) Management of functional neurological disorder. *J Neurol* 267(7), 2164–2172.

Nielsen G, Stone J, Matthews A, *et al.* (2015) Physiotherapy for functional motor disorders: a consensus recommendation. *J Neurol Neurosurg Psychiatry* 86(10), 1113–1119.

Geriatric Medicine

CHAPTER 68
Comprehensive geriatric assessment

Ojaswini Pathak

Comprehensive geriatric assessment (CGA) is the specialist intervention provided by geriatricians and those who specialise in care of the older adult. CGA delivers a multidisciplinary (MDT), multidimensional assessment of any older adult deemed to benefit from it.

CGA is time and person intensive and not synergistic with the ethos of the acute floor. Frail patients are likely to come to harm in the acute care environment. An MDT-led CGA must be targeted to the 'frailest frail' to deliver maximum impact.

Numbers needed to treat (NNT) to prevent admission into 24-h care and progressive frailty from CGA is 20. Compare this to the NNT for most medical interventions and the benefit is clear.

The CGA domains lead to a stratified problem list that can be addressed in order of urgency to modify and delay the frailty syndromes. These actions can be completed within primary or secondary care. Various models of service have been used to provide geriatrician input at the front door: dedicated units, in reach liaison services: this will vary according to local resources but regardless of the model, a specialist MDT delivering CGA is key.

The 2021 UK census demonstrated that the number of centenarians living in England and Wales has increased by 24.5% since 2011. The older demographic is increasing faster than the number of geriatricians and those practicing on the acute floor must have competencies and confidence in managing the frail older adult.

Not all older adults are frail. It is important to consistently identify the frailest to target disease-modifying specialist intervention.

> *The Rockwood clinical frailty scale (CFS) has been adopted by most due to its simplicity. It is important to score at patient baseline (2 weeks prior to admission).*
>
> *The score runs 1–9 with the higher score indicating the frailest phenotype.*

A CFS > 6 (the need for care prior to admission: care package or placement) is when hospital-related harm increases exponentially (increased lengths of stay, readmission rates and mortality).

Acute Medicine: A Practical Guide to the Management of Medical Emergencies, Sixth Edition.
Edited by Mridula Rajwani, Leila Vaziri, and Ivie Gbinigie.
© 2026 John Wiley & Sons Ltd. Published 2026 by John Wiley & Sons Ltd.

The frailty phenotype is a medical term but has negative stigma with patients and carers. Care providers favour terms like 'care of the older adult' or positive acronyms like 'FIT, RACE, OPAL' when branding their service for the patient facing population. Whatever the name: service-delivery remains via an MDT-driven CGA for our frailest populations.

> *CGA is not a 'one stop' assessment but a dynamic, 'living' assessment that reflects the evolving patient journey. Acute floor CGA should focus on urgent medical issues and risk stratify other issues to be addressed by the most appropriate primary or secondary care teams post discharge.*
>
> *Succinct discharge documentation including CFS, cognitive screening, and onward recommendations is essential. It may be the only handover document at the secondary/ primary care interface.*
>
> *Aim to communicate- what was found – what was done and what needs doing.*

CGA can be initiated by any member of the MDT. Your local MDT may vary as per resource but may include physio and occupational therapists, links to social workers, specialist nurses, advanced care practitioners, pharmacists and liaison mental health colleagues.

CGA on acute care wards and in the community have different priorities. Community CGA may focus on chronic cognitive impairment, mood disorder, nutrition, weight loss, falls prevention and advance care planning over a period of months. This chapter focuses on CGA on the acute floor.

> *The acute frailty syndromes conveniently spell the word itself to serve as an aide memoire and are common presentations to the acute take. Patients presenting with a CFS>6 and an acute frailty syndrome with no requirement for specialist intervention should be highlighted to your local CGA MDT.*

Consider CGA MDT when CFS>6 (prior care needs) AND

F   Falls
R   Reduced mobility
A   Acute confusion (delirium)
I   Incontinence (recurrent UTI/ constipation/urinary retention)
L   Lots of medications (polypharmacy: number of medication and susceptibility to side effects)
       NOT requiring a speciality team (e.g. MI, stroke haemorrhage)
       Surgical or trauma issues should be triaged by the emergency department and addressed prior to referral to the acute medical take.

Medical

It is important to complete a thorough medical clerking with a collateral history.

Any acute illness can cause deconditioning in the frail adult.

Older physiology is not represented in medical textbooks: do not be misled by normal bloods; use clinical examination, bedside tests (ECG, bladder scan and postural BP readings) and simple imaging (chest radiograph) to consider atypical presentations which are common with increasing frailty.

Falls

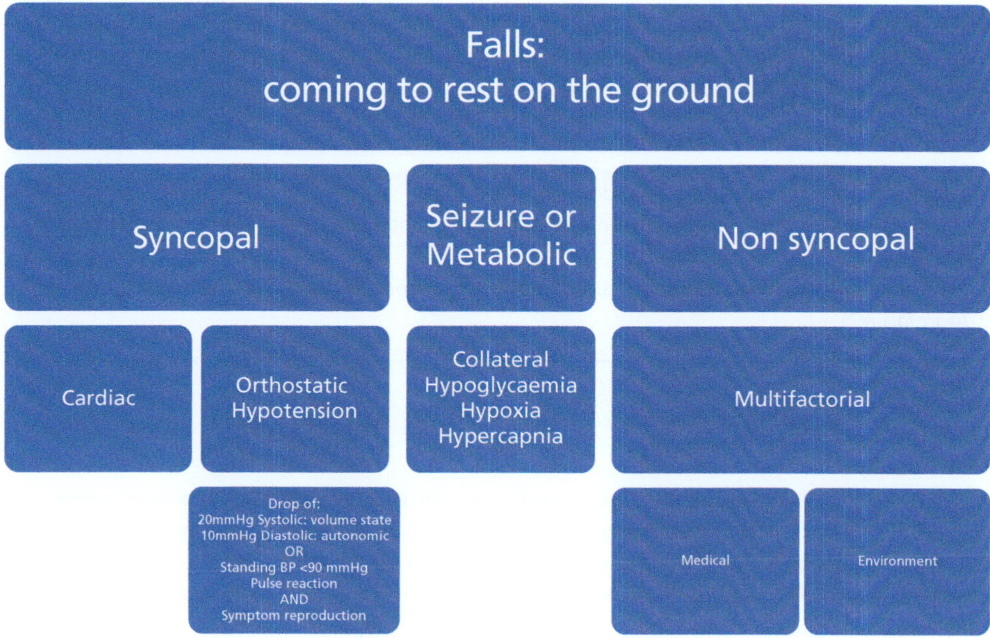

Postural blood pressure readings are rarely performed accurately on the acute floor. If a drop is recognised it is important to note heart rate variability and if index symptoms are reproduced.

The systolic drop suggests hypovolaemia (consider a fluid challenge and repeat: beware the iatrogenic hypovolaemia from prolonged waits for assessment). Consider stopping antihypertensive medications prior to the initiation of fludrocortisone (which has a poor evidence base).

The diastolic drop suggests autonomic dysfunction (diabetes, MS, Parkinson's and alcohol) and is harder to manage but may respond better to alpha agents like midodrine.

Normal physiological response to standing is an increased heart rate. If this does not happen it may indicate autonomic dysfunction, bradyarrhythmia or tight rate control.

Non-syncopal

Likely to be multifactorial due to cognition, impaired sensorium (hearing or visual impairment), acute infection, polypharmacy or environmental (loose carpet or ill-fitting slipper).

> *Differential: cardiac disease or arrhythmia, seizure activity, metabolic (hypoglycaemia)*

Injury sustained during a fall should be assessed by your triaging trauma/ED colleagues. 'Silver' trauma is a specialist area.

A new fracture should prompt a review of bone health. If you do not have an established fracture liaison service locally: this can be done with the FRAX NOGG tool and recommendations forwarded to primary care.

Reduced mobility (e.g. unable to get out of bed)

Frailty reflects a reduced resilience to stressors like illness and may present as a fall or reduced mobility. Look for the underlying acute illness, if not present this may reflect care strain (inadequate support in community to meet current care needs) and prompt OT review.

> *Differential: vestibular or cerebellar syndromes.*
>
> *Limb/musculoskeletal injury with pain affecting mobility (atraumatic? think gout, haemarthroses, bursitis)*
>
> *Peripheral oedema: heavy legs are hard to move (think dependent oedema, medication related or heart failure?)*

Acute confusion

Delirium may be superimposed on dementia or present on its own. It can affect 30% of hospitalised patients. It is important to consider metabolic, infectious and medication causes. Delirium can take up to 6 months to settle. Most hospitals have delirium care bundles and pathways to guide management and acronyms to help work through potential triggers, e.g. PINCH ME (pain, infection, nutrition, constipation, hydration, medication and environment).

4AT is used to screen for delirium with the 6CIT for chronic/mild cognitive impairment.

Collateral history will clarify chronicity.

Cognitive Screening			
Diagnosis of Dementia? Yes / No Memory affected in the last 12 months? Yes / No Mood disturbances? Yes / No			
Confusion Screen Results:			

4AT Assessment Test for Delirium & Cognitive Impairment		Six-item Cognitive Impairment Test (6CIT)		
		Question	Score Range	Score
1	ALERTNESS attempt to wake with speech or gentle touch on shoulder.	What year is it?	Correct: 0 points Incorrect: 4 points	
Normal (0) Mild sleepiness (0) Clearly abnormal (4)		What month is it?	Correct: 0 points Incorrect: 3 points	
2	AMT4 Age, date of birth, place (name of hospital or building), current year.	Give memory phrase	**John/Smith/42/ West Street / Bedford**	
No mistakes (0) One mistake (1) Two or more mistakes (2)		What time is it?	Correct: 0 points Incorrect: 3 points	
3	ATTENTION "Please tell me the months of the year in backwards order starting at December."	Count back from 20–1	Correct: 0 points One error: 2 points Over one error: 4 points	
More than seven (0) Scores less than seven or refuses (1) Untestable or refuses to start (2)		Say the months in reverse	Correct: 0 points Incorrect: 4 points	
4	ACUTE CHANGE OR FLUCTUATING Over the last 2 weeks and still evident in the last 24hrs.	Repeat the memory phrase	Correct: 0 points 2 points per error (Max 10)	
No (0) Yes (4)				
4 or above: possible delirium +/- cognitive impairment 1-3: possible cognitive impairment 0: delirium or severe cognitive impairment unlikely	Score	0–7 Normal 8–9 Mild cognitive impairment 10–28 Significant cognitive impairment		Score

CT brain imaging can be overutilized in the confused patient, but it is an important investigation to consider if bedside tests, bloods and plain radiographs are inconclusive.

Any cognitive impairment identified during acute admission should be highlighted to primary care to monitor or refer to memory services.

> *Differential: Stroke (do not mistake dysphasia with confusion), post ictal states (these can last longer in older adults), encephalitis (infective or autoimmune), hypercalcaemia, hypoglycaemia, thyroid dysfunction, B12 and folate deficiencies.*

Incontinence

Urinary incontinence may result from intercurrent urinary tract infections. Urine dipsticks are likely to be positive in the care home and catheterised population, so it is important to make this diagnosis with enough corroborating evidence from blood work, symptomology and microscopy results.

Urinary tract infections are over-diagnosed and is important to consider mimics: urinary retention or diuresis. Recurrent UTIs are not normal and onward urological investigation should be considered to identify the underlying cause.

Faecal incontinence can be due to overflow diarrhoea (constipation) or common prescriptions (metformin, nutritional and mineral supplements and antibiotics). Once addressed, consider red flag symptoms that warrant onward bowel investigation.

General incontinence may be functional (i.e. the person is not mobile enough to get to the toilet) and be a result of the environment or clothing. Occupational therapy input will address this.

> *Differential: acute neurological issues, malignancy (frail patients may not tolerate or benefit from invasive investigations or therapies; this needs to be mutually considered with the patient or advocates)*

Lots of medications (polypharmacy)

The multimorbidity and significant polypharmacy seen with increasing age, brings with it an increased risk of adverse drug reactions which is implicated in 6% of emergency hospital admissions.

Physiology changes with age, affecting drug pharmacokinetics and excretion. The accumulation of drugs and side effects can trigger an acute frailty syndrome. This opportunity for medication review should not be missed.

Polypharmacy not only implicates the number of medications but also the increasing susceptibility to adverse side effects.

Many drugs have anti-cholinergic properties with an accumulative effect. These can cause falls, cognitive impairment, constipation and urinary retention (acute frailty syndromes) and deprescribing should be considered.

Online tools (STOPP START) and calculators (ACBcalc.com) are available to aid in deprescribing decisions with patient and carer discussion.

Deprescribing saves money from the fewer medications dispensed and from the prevention of adverse drug reactions. The cost implication is underestimated but patient experience, journey and outcome are improved.

Full medication reviews do not have to be done on the acute floor. Identifying and signposting on to an appropriate service (pharmacist, GP or geriatrician) is sufficient for the acute physician.

Medication reviews may lead to addition of prescriptions including pain relief, laxatives, bone protection or supplements.

Overview of the MDT

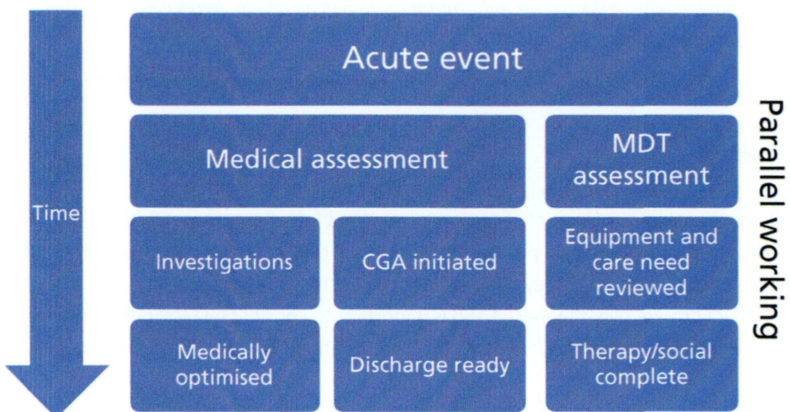

People over the age of 85 account for 25% of inpatient hospital bed days. CGA and MDT working encourages the consideration of wider issues that may impact patient well-being and promote safe, sustainable discharges.

The acute floor CGA includes the functional, psychological, social and environmental factors which are assessed by the MDT whilst medical assessment continues. Barriers to discharge are identified and addressed enabling discharge when medically optimised. This reduces lengths of stay and hospital delay-related harm.

Physiotherapists focus on mobility assessments and the need for walking aids, onward community therapy or falls programme referrals.

OT will review equipment and formal care needs. Patients admitted from 24-h placements may be better assessed by community teams as returning to a place of safety may prevent hospital delay-related harm and deconditioning.

Social workers source care packages and placements based on recommendations of the MDT. Safeguarding concerns raised must be reviewed by the social work team prior to discharge.

> *The acute physician must competently identify the frailty phenotype and syndromes and initiate management, including the CGA. Once urgent issues have been addressed pending domains can be handed over to a secondary (CGA MDT) or primary care (virtual ward, GP) team for ongoing management.*

Further reading

NHS Acute Frailty Network (2017) Acute care for frail older people toolkit. NHS Elect AFN Toolkit October 2017 edition.pdf. https://www.nhselect.nhs.uk/uploads/files/1/NHS%20Elect%20AFN%20Toolkit%20 October%202017%20edition.pdf.

Royal Pharmaceutical Society Medicines optimisation. Rpharms.com

The Health Foundation Frailsafe: a safety checklist for frail older patients entering acute hospital care. https://www.health.org.uk/improvement-project/frailsafea-safety-checklistfor-frail-olderpatients-enteringacute-hospital.

CHAPTER 69

Delirium, dementia and cognitive disorders

ALEXANDRA MONTAGU AND CHRISTOPHER AMBROSE

Consider delirium in patients with:
- Abnormal cognitive function (confusion, impaired concentration, slow responses to questions – the patient described as a 'poor historian').
- Abnormal mood (new onset 'depression').
- Abnormal perception (visual or auditory hallucinations).
- Abnormal behaviour (restlessness, agitation or reluctance to mobilize; unwillingness to eat or drink; abnormal sleep–wake cycle).
- Abnormal social behaviour (withdrawal from social contact; unwillingness to cooperate with care – the patient described as 'uncooperative' or 'difficult').

Introduction

Delirium is a disorder characterized by disturbance of consciousness, attention and cognition, not accounted for by pre-existing dementia. The term 'acute confusional state' is often used synonymously with delirium, although delirium is preferred, as confusion (uncertainty about what is happening, intended or required) is not specific to delirium and its medical definition is imprecise.

It can reflect a primary neurological disorder, substance intoxication or withdrawal, an adverse effect of drugs (especially those with an anti-cholinergic effect) or a systemic disorder such as sepsis. Often it is multifactorial, e.g. infection, hyponatraemia and side effects of medications. Causes of delirium are given in Appendix 69.1.

Distinguishing delirium from dementia is often a diagnostic challenge (see Table 69.1). Dementia and delirium often co-exist and dementia is a major risk factor for delirium. It is also worth bearing in mind that delirium is also a risk factor for the development of long-term cognitive decline. Several neuropsychiatric disorders may give rise to abnormal consciousness, language, memory or behaviour, and should be considered in the differential diagnosis of delirium (Table 69.2).

Delirium is a clinical diagnosis; criteria are given in Table 69.2. History including a good collateral is key to this.

Initial assessment of the patient with delirium is summarized in Figure 69.1.

Acute Medicine: A Practical Guide to the Management of Medical Emergencies, Sixth Edition.
Edited by Mridula Rajwani, Leila Vaziri, and Ivie Gbinigie.
© 2026 John Wiley & Sons Ltd. Published 2026 by John Wiley & Sons Ltd.

Appendix 69.1 Causes of delirium.

Category of disorder	Examples/comment
Primary neurological disorders	Head injury
	Post-ictal state
	Non-dominant parietal lobe stroke
	Subdural haematoma
	Subarachnoid haemorrhage
	NCSE
	Meningitis
	Encephalitis – infective or autoimmune
	Raised intracranial pressure
Substance intoxication or withdrawal	Alcohol intoxication or withdrawal
	Wernicke's encephalopathy
	Intoxication with amphetamine and amphetamine-type drugs, benzodiazepines, cannabis, cocaine, opioids and other psychoactive substances
	Withdrawal of opioids
Adverse effect of drugs	Side effects of medications: Benzodiazepines, tricyclics, analgesics (especially opiates), lithium, high-dose corticosteroids, and drugs for parkinsonism
	Neuroleptic malignant syndrome (Appendix 73.2)
Infection	Urinary or respiratory tract infections are the commonest causes.
	Bacterial meningitis (Chapter 73), infective endocarditis (Chapter 15) and intra-abdominal sepsis, e.g. cholangitis (Chapter 5), cellulitis should also be considered in patients with delirium and signs of sepsis.
	Exclude tropical diseases if there has been recent travel (Chapter 75).
Others	Constipation
	Urinary retention
	Hypoglycaemia
	Hyperglycaemic states
	Any organ failure
	Severe electrolyte disorders
	Severe endocrine disorders, e.g. hypothyroidism
	Other metabolic disorders
	Hypothermia

Table 69.1 Differentiating delirium from dementia.

	Delirium	Dementia
Conscious level	Can often be low (hypoactive) or agitated (hyperactive)	Normal until late in disease
Onset	Acute onset	Gradual onset
Course of disease	Fluctuations in symptoms are typical. Can resolve in days to weeks, a proportion develop into chronic delirium	Usual gradual decline, although fluctuation in severity can sometimes suggest Lewy body dementia
Attention	Deficits common	Deficits usually occur much later in the progression of dementia
Reversibility	Reversibility with correction of the underlying cause	Usually permanent and progressive

Table 69.2 Differential diagnosis of acutely disturbed behaviour or language.

Diagnosis	Comment
Delirium	Diagnostic criteria: • There is a disturbance of attention and awareness. • There is a change in cognition, such as memory deficit, disorientation, language disturbance or the development of a perceptual disturbance that is not better accounted for by a pre-existing dementia. • The disturbance has developed over a short period of time (usually hours to days) and tends to fluctuate during the course of the day. • There is evidence from the history, examination or laboratory findings that the disturbance is caused either by the direct physiological consequences of a general medical condition, or by substance intoxication/withdrawal or by medication.
Acute psychosis (mania or schizophrenic)	Typical features of acute psychosis include: • Hallucinations • Delusions • Confused and disturbed thoughts • Lack of insight and self-awareness A diagnosis of delirium rather than acute psychosis is more likely if: • The patient is older than 40 with no previous psychiatric history • There are major medical comorbidities • There is disorientation, clouding of consciousness or decreased alertness that fluctuates throughout the day, or • Physiological observations are abnormal
Other psychiatric disorders	Agitated depression, anxiety disorder, borderline and anti-social personality disorders may result in acutely disturbed behaviour.
Non-convulsive status epilepticus (NCSE)	In NCSE, there are often mild clonic movements of the eyelids, face or hands, or simple automatisms. The EEG is abnormal.
Transient global amnesia	Abrupt onset of antegrade amnesia without clouding of consciousness or loss of personal identity. Cognitive impairment is limited to amnesia, and there are no focal neurological or epileptic signs. Symptoms resolve within 24 h.
Fluent aphasia	Speech is fluent but with meaningless words, unnecessary phrases and nonsensical grammar. There is no clouding of consciousness. Caused by an acute stroke or brain injury to Wernicke's area

Source: Adapted from American Psychiatric Association (2013).

Priorities

1 Make a rapid assessment to ensure that airway, breathing and circulation are not compromised. Check blood glucose and correct hypoglycaemia (Chapter 46).

2 Assess the mental state. This can be done using the ten-item abbreviated mental test score (Table 69.3) or similar screening test, e.g. 4 A's Test (4AT) or Confusional Assessment method (CAM).
- The diagnosis of delirium is based on the criteria shown in Table 69.2. Delirium is characterized by a change in the mental state (occurring over hours or days, often fluctuating over the course of the day), associated with a causative factor (Appendix 69.1).

3 What is causing delirium?
- Establish current symptoms, context and past history by talking to family members, carers, or hospital staff and reviewing relevant medical records. Documentation from the ambulance worker's initial assessment is often a very helpful source of information.

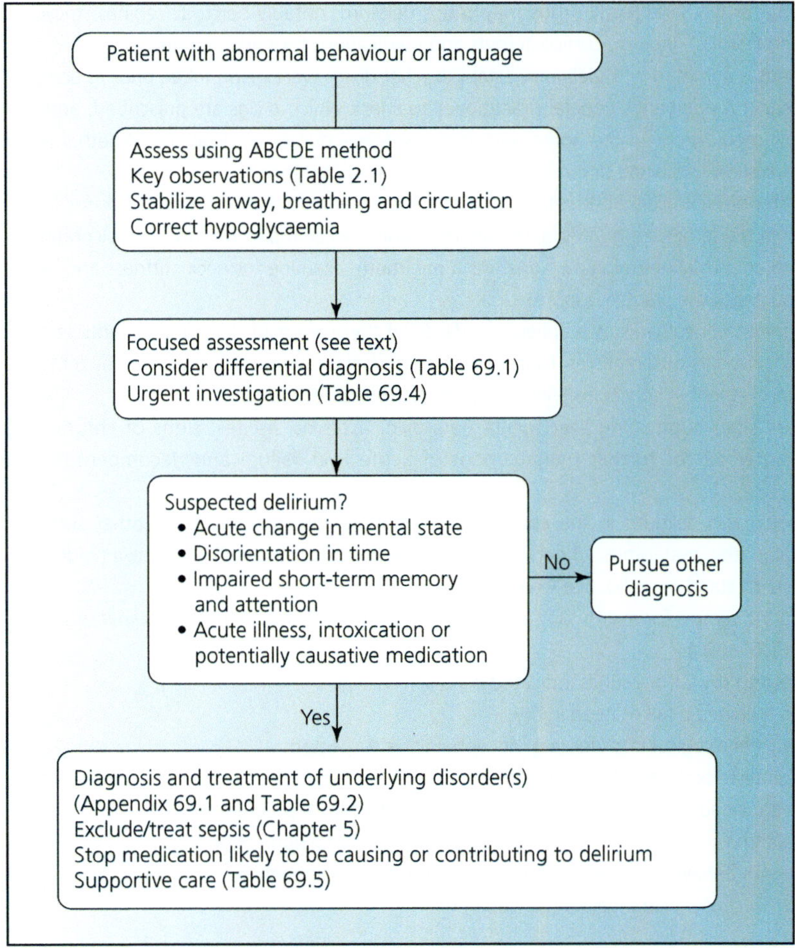

Figure 69.1 Assessment of the patient with delirium.

Table 69.3 Abbreviated mental test score.

- Age
- Time (to nearest hour)
- Address for recall at end of test – this should be repeated by the patient to ensure it has been heard correctly: 42 West Street
- Year
- Name of hospital
- Recognition of two people (e.g. doctor and nurse)
- Date of birth (day and month sufficient)
- Year of the Second World War
- Name of present monarch
- Count backwards 20–1

Each correct answer scores one mark. The healthy elderly score 8–10.

- Check the drug chart. Many drugs may cause delirium, notably benzodiazepines, tricyclics, analgesics (including NSAIDs), lithium, corticosteroids and medications for parkinsonism.
- If a patient is admitted with delirium, establish what drugs were being taken prior to admission: if necessary, contact the patient's general practitioner to check which drugs are prescribed, and ask relatives to collect all medications in the home, including over-the-counter medications. Whether any medications have been recently started or changed is of particular importance.
- Review the physiological observations and make a systematic examination. Check for focal chest signs, abdominal tenderness or guarding, urinary retention, faecal impaction, pressure ulceration and cellulitis. Are there abnormal neurological signs? As a minimum, examine for neck stiffness and lateralized weakness, and check the plantar responses.
- Consider non-convulsive status epilepticus (NCSE) if there are mild clonic movements of the eyelids, face or hands or simple automatisms. Diazepam (10 mg IV, at a rate of <2.5 mg/min) may terminate the status with improvement in conscious level. Seek advice from a neurologist.
- Are there signs suggesting liver failure (jaundice, asterixis, ascites, signs of chronic liver disease)? See Chapter 42 for further management of acute liver failure and decompensated chronic liver disease.
- In patients with delirium in the context of alcohol-use disorder, check for other signs of Wernicke's encephalopathy: nystagmus, VI nerve palsy (unable to abduct the eye) and ataxia (wide-based gait; may be unable to stand or walk). See Chapter 106 for management.
- Send a urine sample for microscopy and culture. Undertake a chest X-ray. Other investigations needed are given in Table 69.4.

4 **Neuroimaging** (by CT or MRI) is indicated if
- Delirium followed a fall or head injury.
- A primary neurological disorder (e.g. encephalitis) is suspected.
- There are new focal neurological signs.
- There is papilloedema or other evidence of raised intracranial pressure.
- The patient has cancer, HIV-AIDS or other cause of immunosuppression.
- The patient's behaviour prevents adequate neurological examination.
- No systemic cause for the delirium is apparent.

Table 69.4 Urgent investigation in delirium.

Blood glucose
Plasma sodium, potassium, urea and creatinine
Liver function tests, albumin and calcium
Full blood count
Prothrombin time or international normalized ratio (INR)
C-reactive protein
Blood culture if temperature <36 or >38 °C
Urine culture
ECG
Chest X-ray
Arterial blood gases
Neuroimaging, if indicated: see text (point 4)
Lumbar puncture, if indicated: see text (point 5)
EEG, if indicated: see text

Source: Reference: Oxford Clinical Diagnosis and Treatment eds Davey & Sprigings, OUP 2018. Reproduced with permission.

Table 69.5 Supportive care of the patient with delirium.

Exclude/treat sepsis
Stop medications likely to be causing or contributing to delirium
Prevent dehydration: ensure adequate fluid intake
Exclude/relieve urinary retention
Exclude/prevent constipation
Exclude/prevent pressure ulceration
Assess for/relieve pain
Prevent DVT: give thromboprophylaxis if indicated
Prevent sleep disturbance
Ensure spectacles and hearing aid are worn if needed
Reality orientation: give the patient information about time, place and person, repeated at regular intervals

5 **Lumbar puncture** with examination of the cerebrospinal fluid should be done (assuming no contraindication to lumbar puncture) if
   - Suspicion of meningitis or encephalitis – consider autoimmune or infective.
   - The patient is febrile and no systemic focus of infection is found.
   - The cause of delirium remains unclear.
6 **Electroencephalography (EEG)** is indicated if
   - NCSE or encephalitis is suspected.
   - It is unclear if the diagnosis is delirium or psychosis.
   - No cause for delirium is apparent, despite investigation.

Further management

Identify and treat the underlying cause (Appendix 69.1; Table 69.2).

Ensure comprehensive supportive care (Table 69.5), with avoidance of physical restraint, and anticipation and prevention of complications of delirium (e.g. dehydration, constipation and pressure ulceration).

- In the United Kingdom, Mental Capacity Act and Deprivation of Liberty Safeguards should be utilised as needed.
- Review the drug chart. Avoid unnecessary medications, especially those with an anti-cholinergic effect.
- If needed, to relieve severe distress or prevent injury, give short-term therapy (one week or less) of haloperidol (in a dose of <3 mg daily) or olanzapine (the latter is contraindicated in patients with dementia). If the patient has Parkinson's disease/parkinsonism or Lewy Body Dementia then benzodiazepines are the drug of choice. Seizures and alcohol withdrawal should also be treated with benzodiazepines.

Further reading

Fong TG, Davis D, Growdon ME, *et al*. (2015) The interface between delirium and dementia in elderly adults. *Lancet Neurol* 14, 823–832.

Inouye SK, Westendorp RGJ, Saczynski JS. (2013) Delirium in elderly people. *Lancet* 383, 911–922.

National Institute for Health and Care Excellence. (2023) *Delirium: Prevention, Diagnosis and Management in Hospital and Long-Term Care*. London: National Institute for Health and Care Excellence (NICE). https://www.nice.org.uk/guidance/cg103www.nice.org.uk/guidance/cg103.

Woodford HJ, George J, Jackson M. (2015) Non-convulsive status epilepticus: a practical approach to diagnosis in confused older people. *Postgrad Med J* 91, 655–661.

CHAPTER 70
Perioperative medicine

SHVAITA RALHAN AND MUSTAFA ALSAHAB

Perioperative medicine is a rapidly growing medical specialty that focuses on the care of patients prior, during, and after surgery in a multidisciplinary, patient-centred and integrated fashion. It includes assessment and optimisation of patient's health status prior to surgery, shared decision making regarding surgical options, management of medical issues that may arise during the perioperative period, as well as guide rehabilitation. The average age of surgical patients is increasing with one-third of people having surgery being 75 years or older; these patients are at higher risk of postoperative mortality, more likely to experience medical rather than surgical postoperative complications, have longer hospital stays and are at increased risk of discharge to a care facility. The National Emergency Laparotomy Audit (NELA) reported that 30-day mortality was doubled in patients aged over 65 years living with frailty (18% versus 9.3%). These changes require novel challenges to our healthcare system and hence the increased importance and development of perioperative medicine services. Depending on the hospital, the perioperative medicine team may cover a range of elective and emergency surgical areas such as trauma, elective orthopaedics, general and vascular surgery.

There are several national databases such as the NHFD (National Hip Fracture Database), TARN (Trauma Audit and Research Network) and NELA which are set up to monitor and improve surgical patients' outcomes in different surgical specialties in the NHS.

Orthogeriatrics

Orthogeriatricians provide the comprehensive perioperative care which is relevant to orthopaedic patients, working closely with surgeons, anaesthetists and allied healthcare professionals. It originated in the UK in 1960s. A neck of femur (NOF) fracture is the most common serious fragility fracture among the elderly accounting for 76,000 factures a year and an annual cost of approximately £2 billion. It is associated with significant morbidity and mortality;10–20% of those admitted from home move to institutional care, 10% of people die within first month, and about one third die within 12 months.

Hip fracture care is the area where the evidence for perioperative medicine is strongest, and the principles for hip fracture care have led the way in the development of perioperative services in other surgical areas. Benefits of this integrated care include higher functional outcomes, fewer postoperative complications, reduced length of stay, and reduced mortality.

Much of the orthogeriatric model is based on Comprehensive Geriatric Assessment (CGA): a multidisciplinary diagnostic process which focuses on older patients undergoing surgery. There is emerging evidence that CGA is beneficial to older elective and emergency surgical patients. Please refer to Chapter 68 for further information on CGA.

Acute Medicine: A Practical Guide to the Management of Medical Emergencies, Sixth Edition.
Edited by Mridula Rajwani, Leila Vaziri, and Ivie Gbinigie.
© 2026 John Wiley & Sons Ltd. Published 2026 by John Wiley & Sons Ltd.

Orthogeriatric assessment includes

- Identification and management of medical conditions (both pre-existing and new)
- Medications review
- Identification and management of frailty
- Consideration of ceilings of care and DNACPR status
- Assessment of cognition and delirium risk
- Decisions around capacity to consent to surgery
- Liaison with patients and their next of kin to articulate benefits and risks of surgery
- Discharge planning
- Falls assessments
- Review of bone health

Major trauma geriatrics

Major trauma was previously considered a disease of young men with the predominant mechanism of injury being road traffic accidents. However, what constitutes major trauma in the western world has changed. The combination of an ageing population, rising incidence of osteoporosis and improved road safety means that over 50% of major trauma occurs in those above the age of 65 falling from standing height. The commonest injuries sustained in this age group are head, spinal and thoracic injuries. Trauma in this age group is often termed 'stealth trauma' as it is harder to identify for the following reasons:

- lower mechanism of injury
- pre-existing cognitive impairment and brain atrophy making traumatic brain injury less obvious
- comorbidities or their treatment make haemodynamic compromise due to blood loss harder to identify e.g. beta blocker treatment for arrythmias masking the expected tachycardia

The acute physician must therefore have a high index of suspicion for trauma in this age group to avoid missing injuries given the differing routes of referral of these patients into the hospital. Furthermore, many of these injuries are managed conservatively, or a cohort of these patients may be deemed unsuitable for invasive surgical treatment due to their frailty or comorbidities so may well be under the care of medical specialties rather than the surgeons. Rib fractures, in particular, have been deemed a Cinderella condition in this group where standardisation of care and outcomes for patients are poor. Chest X-rays are inadequate and early CT is the gold standard allowing accurate identification of injuries that usually carry high risk of morbidity and mortality. Analgesia (including involvement of pain teams to consider regional anaesthetic blocks) is the cornerstone of treatment, coupled with chest physiotherapy and a low threshold for antibiotics as many develop pneumonia as a complication. Since the introduction of the best practice tariff uplift for clinical frailty assessment in major trauma geriatric patients in 2019 in England, many major trauma centres have developed perioperative medicine services for major trauma providing much needed expert knowledge in this growing patient group.

Aspects of perioperative medicine that acute physicians are commonly asked to advise on are covered in more detail below.

Cognition and delirium management

Post-operative delirium is the commonest complication in the older surgical population and has significant implications. It increases hospital stay by 2–3 days, has a 30-day mortality of 7–10%, and also increases healthcare resource expenditure. It is most prevalent in those with preoperative cognitive disorders, those undergoing complex or emergency surgery and those undergoing orthopaedic surgery where the risk can be as high as

60%. Those with hypoactive delirium have poorer outcomes. Delirium assessment includes cognitive screening (most commonly AMTS & 4AT score) pre and postoperatively. Perioperative measures that can be taken to prevent or reduce severity of delirium include:

- Avoidance of hypotension (usually defined as a 20% reduction in BP from baseline or a BP below 100 mmHg)
- Avoidance of hypoxia
- Limit length and depth of anaesthesia when delirium risk is high
- Limit the use of delirium inducing drugs e.g. opiates, benzodiazepines
- Taking a thorough drug and alcohol history to avoid withdrawal symptoms
- Perioperative treatment with antipsychotics before delirium develops. This is not widespread practice as studies were small and limited to elective hip, elective knee and hip fracture surgery. However, it is worth considering in some patients with a significant risk of florid delirium. A typical regime is haloperidol 0.5 mg BD for three days starting preoperatively.

All perioperative delirium should be documented and discussed with the patient or their relatives, with repeat cognitive testing after recovery from surgery in the community. Assessment of cognition in the perioperative period will also contribute to the assessment of capacity with respect to consent for surgery. Please refer to Chapter 69 for further information on general management of delirium.

Analgesia

It is estimated that at least 80% of patients experience acute postoperative pain. Poorly controlled post operative pain can cause various adverse outcomes such as delirium, prolong admission, increase morbidity, delay rehabilitation and contribute to the development of chronic pain syndrome. Multimodal analgesia (MMA) is the use of multiple pain management medications during the perioperative period. The goal is to optimise pain control and minimise using high dose opioids. MMA includes paracetamol, ketamine, NSAIDs, regional analgesia, and opioids. An individualised approach is needed for every patient and should consider:

- Severity of pain
- Preoperative opiate use
- Renal impairment
- Variable absorption e.g. in surgical conditions that involve pathology of the GI tract
- Side effects e.g. co-prescription of laxatives & naloxone with all opiates

Non-opioid analgesia such as paracetamol is rarely problematic but NSAIDs should be used more cautiously, particularly in the elderly and patients with other comorbidities due to their potential side effects on the renal tract, upper GI tract and cardiovascular system. Weak opioids such as codeine are commonly used in the perioperative period but it is important to recognise that these are prodrugs and their effectiveness is influenced by the individual patient's ability to metabolise the drug. 5–10% of the population are poor metabolisers of codeine, and get little therapeutic benefit from these medications and 10% of the Caucasian and 30% of the African population are ultrarapid metabolisers leading to a higher risk of opiate toxicity. Strong opioid analgesics such as morphine and oxycodone are often needed in the perioperative period but require vigilant monitoring due to the risk of respiratory depression particularly in those with renal impairment.

Regional anaesthesia techniques (usually delivered by specialist pain teams or the emergency department) such as a fascia iliaca block in femoral fractures and erector spinae blocks in rib fractures, enhance perioperative pain control and reduce opioid use, and are therefore an important aspect to consider when managing perioperative pain.

Frailty and surgical outcomes

Frailty is a state of increased vulnerability to stressors due to a decline in physiological function and reserve in organ systems, resulting in adverse outcomes. Preoperative frailty independently predicts:

- higher frequency and severity of postoperative complications
- increased length of stay and rehabilitation period
- discharge to an assisted-living facility
- higher delirium risk
- poor wound healing and tissue damage
- higher mortality

The ageing process reduces physiological reserve making frailty more common in the elderly. However, frailty is not exclusively a syndrome of the elderly and is distinct to comorbidity. A study on emergency laparotomy showed greater mortality hazard ratios for those with higher Clinical Frailty Scale grades: 4 (3.93, 95% CI 1.89–8.20), 5 (5.86, 95% CI 2.87–11.97), and 6–7 (14.17, 95% CI 7.33–27.40). These findings were not confounded by the indication for surgery, sepsis, intraperitoneal soiling or malignancy status.

Recognising and managing frailty in surgical patients is important to try to improve outcomes, set appropriate expectations, and to frame discussions around appropriate treatment escalation plans and decisions about resuscitation when perioperative risks are high. The most commonly used frailty screening tool in preoperative assessment is the Clinical Frailty Scale (CFS) due to its simplicity and speed of completion. Once frailty has been identified a frailty assessment tool such as the Edmonton Frail Scale can provide more in-depth information regarding domains/targets for managing frailty prior to the operation. Please refer to Chapter 68 on frailty for further information.

Treatment escalation plans

It is important to establish as soon as possible whether the patient has an existing advanced care plan, a lasting power of attorney or any specific wishes about resuscitation in the event of a cardiac or respiratory arrest. When the risk of surgery is high it is vital to establish the patients premorbid functional and cognitive status so decisions about treatment escalation including appropriateness of HDU, ITU and multiorgan support can be made, ideally prior to going to theatre.

Perioperative nutrition and hydration

Nutritional status is a known determinant of surgical outcomes. Perioperative nutritional support, especially in malnourished surgical patients and those at risk of it improves surgical outcomes. The first step is nutritional screening using a validated screening tool such as the Malnutrition Universal Screening Tool (MUST) and to ensure nutritional team support for those at high risk. Metabolic optimisation through preoperative carbohydrate loading and postoperative glycaemic control are commonly adopted strategies in elective surgery; carbohydrate loading using isotonic carbohydrate solutions the night prior to surgery and 2 h before surgery. Postoperative hyperglycaemia can be avoided by reducing preoperative fasting, early postoperative feeding, and a glucose-insulin infusion if required. Please refer to The ERAS (Enhanced Recovery After Surgery) society guidelines for further details.

Preoperatively: ensure adequate hydration and allow clear fluid until 2 h prior to surgery. Ensure extra fluid replacement for those with high stoma output and enterocutaneous fistula. Some local protocols allow ensure juices up to 2 h before theatre; these are considered a clear fluid.

Intraoperatively: maintain fluid balance and avoid excessive IV fluid. Fluid replacement should be guided by monitoring parameters using Hartmann's as it is more physiological, reducing the risk of hyperchloremia which is more common with normal saline. Blood transfusion is guided by blood loss and transfusion thresholds should be adjusted in patients with a history of ischaemic heart disease to prevent perioperative cardiac events.

Postoperatively: encourage early oral intake and supplemental IV fluid if inadequate oral intake, early removal of NG tube and maintaining fluid balance. Consider enteral or parental nutrition when oral intake delayed.

Perioperative medication management in emergency surgery

Decisions about stopping or continuing medications perioperatively are based on risks of withdrawal, risks of disease progression if therapy is discontinued, risks of drug interactions with anaesthetic medications and the patient's short-term quality of life. Table 70.1 below summarises common medications that should be suspended, those that should be continued, and some where careful clinical judgement may be required.

Table 70.1 Perioperative Medication Management (1, 2).

Medications to be suspended:
- ACE inhibitors and ARBs (risk of AKI and hypotension outweighs the harm of a moderately high blood pressure).
- Calcium channel blockers: risk of hypotension and urinary retention.
- Diuretics: risk of hypovolemia and electrolytes depletion.
- Metformin: omit on the day of the procedure, and for 48 h when having contrast injection or if eGFR less than 60 mL/min/1.73 m^2.
- SGLT-3 inhibitors: risk of euglycemic ketoacidosis, Ideally stop before surgery and only restart on discharge.
- NSAIDs: risk of AKI and GI bleeding.
- Warfarin: reverse anticoagulant effects, aim INR = <1.5 on day of surgery. Warfarin can be reversed with prothrombin complex (PCC) or IV vitamin K 5–10 mg. For patients with high thrombotic risk, seek an opinion from a Haematologist regarding bridging therapy.
- DOAC: hold 24–96 h, based on DOAC type, bleeding risks, and renal function. Reversal agents such as idarucizumab can be used for dabigatran, and andexanet for apixaban and rivaroxaban in certain clinical scenarios. For patients with high thrombotic risk, seek opinion from a Haematologist.

Medications to be continued:
- Parkinson's Disease medications: time critical medication that must be given even if NBM for theatre. Consider a Rotigotine patch or NG route if the patient's swallow is unsafe or the patient cannot tolerate oral route.
- Antiepileptics: time critical medication that must be converted to the IV route where possible. Levetiracetam, phenobarbital, phenytoin and sodium valproate can all be converted to IV with a 1 : 1 conversion rate. Carbamazepine can be converted to rectal administration with a 25% increase in the dose.
- Tricyclic antidepressants: risk of delirium, confusion and depressive symptoms.
- Benzodiazepines: risk of benzodiazepine withdrawal.
- Long term steroids: double the dose orally or give IV hydrocortisone if oral route unavailable for three days minimum.
- Long-acting insulin.
- B-blocker (unless bradycardic or hypotensive).
- Digoxin (unless bradycardic or AKI).
- Alpha 2 agonist: Clonidine, Methyldopa (risk of rebound hypertension).
- Levothyroxine and Anti-thyroid drugs.
- Statins.
- DPP-4 inhibitor (e.g., sitagliptin).
- SSRIs (risks of exacerbation of mood disorders).
- Antipsychotics (risks of psychotic crisis).

Medications where clinical judgment is exercised:
- Aspirin and/or Clopidogrel: depends on indications of the antiplatelets, bleeding risks of the surgery and its urgency. In general, Aspirin and/or Clopidogrel can be continued unless spinal anaesthesia is the safest option and in high bleeding risk operations. Seek opinions from a Perioperative Medicine Consultant/Anaesthetist/ Cardiologist.

References

1 Johnson S, Haywood C. (2022) Perioperative medication management for older people. *J Pharm Pract Res* 52, 391–401. Available at: https://doi.org/10.1002/jppr.1834 (accessed 20 July 2024).
2 Whinney C. (2009) Perioperative medication management: general principles and practical applications. *Cleve Clin J Med.* 76(Suppl 4), S126–S132. 10.3949/ccjm.76.s4.20. PMID: 19880829 (accessed 20 July 2024).

Further reading

Abebe MM, Arefayne NR, Temesgen MM, Admass BA. (2022) Evidence-based perioperative pain management protocol for day case surgery in a resource limited setting: systematic review. *Ann Med Surg* 80, 104322. DOI: 10.1016/j.amsu.2022.104322 (accessed 28 July 2024).

British Orthopaedic Association, British Geriatrics Society (2007) The blue book: the care of patients with fragility fracture. www.fractures.com/pdf/BOA-BGS-Blue-Book.pdf (accessed 1 August 2024).

Isand KG, Hussain SF, Sadiqi M, *et al.* (2024) Impact of frailty on outcomes following emergency laparotomy: a retrospective analysis across diverse clinical conditions. *Eur J Trauma Emerg Surg*: DOI: 10.1007/s00068-024-02632-6 (accessed 27 August 2024).

Jin Z, Hu J, Ma D. (2020) Postoperative delirium: perioperative assessment, risk reduction, and management. *Br J Anaesth* 125(4), 492–504. DOI: 10.1016/j.bja.2020.06.063 (accessed 28 July 2024).

Miller RL, Barnes JD, Mouton R, *et al.* (2022) Comprehensive geriatric assessment (CGA) in perioperative care: a systematic review of a complex intervention. *BMJ Open* 12, e062729. Available at: https://bmjopen.bmj.com/content/12/10/e062729 (accessed 28 July 2024).

Infectious Diseases

CHAPTER 71

Cellulitis and necrotising fasciitis

DAVID SPRIGINGS AND JOHN L. KLEIN

Assessment of suspected cellulitis is given in Figure 71.1.

Box 71.1 Cellulitis, erysipelas and necrotising fasciitis

Cellulitis is an acute spreading bacterial infection of the deeper dermis and subcutaneous tissue, typically of the lower leg, which may complicate a wound, ulcer, interdigital fungal infection or primary skin disorder. Predisposing factors include previous episodes of cellulitis, limb oedema and lymphoedema. *Streptococcus pyogenes* (Group A streptococcus) and *Staphylococcus aureus* are the most common causative organisms.

Erysipelas is an acute bacterial infection of the upper dermis and epidermis, which may be clinically distinguished from cellulitis by a more clearly demarcated border between infected and healthy skin. Assessment and management are the same as for cellulitis.

Necrotising fasciitis is a rapidly progressive infection of the deep fascia and muscle, and should be suspected in an ill patient with severe pain and marked local tenderness. In the later stages, the skin may show blue-black discolouration and blistering. The majority of cases are polymicrobial and caused by anaerobes, Gram-negative bacilli and streptococci (not *S. pyogenes*). Most other cases are caused by *S. pyogenes* or *Clostridium perfringens* (gas gangrene). Management requires resuscitation, antibiotic therapy and debridement.

Priorities

Make a focused assessment and consider the differential diagnosis (Figure 71.1, Table 71.1). Bilateral cellulitis is very rare. Mark the margin of affected skin with a single-use surgical skin marker. Investigation required urgently is given in Table 71.2.

If cellulitis is the likely diagnosis, assess the severity of the illness, on the basis of the clinical features and comorbidities, and manage the patient accordingly (Tables 71.3 and 71.4).

If necrotising fasciitis is suspected, give IV fluid, start antibiotic therapy after blood cultures have been drawn (Table 71.4), and seek urgent advice from a plastic surgeon and an Infection specialist.

Acute Medicine: A Practical Guide to the Management of Medical Emergencies, Sixth Edition.
Edited by Mridula Rajwani, Leila Vaziri, and Ivie Gbinigie.
© 2026 John Wiley & Sons Ltd. Published 2026 by John Wiley & Sons Ltd.

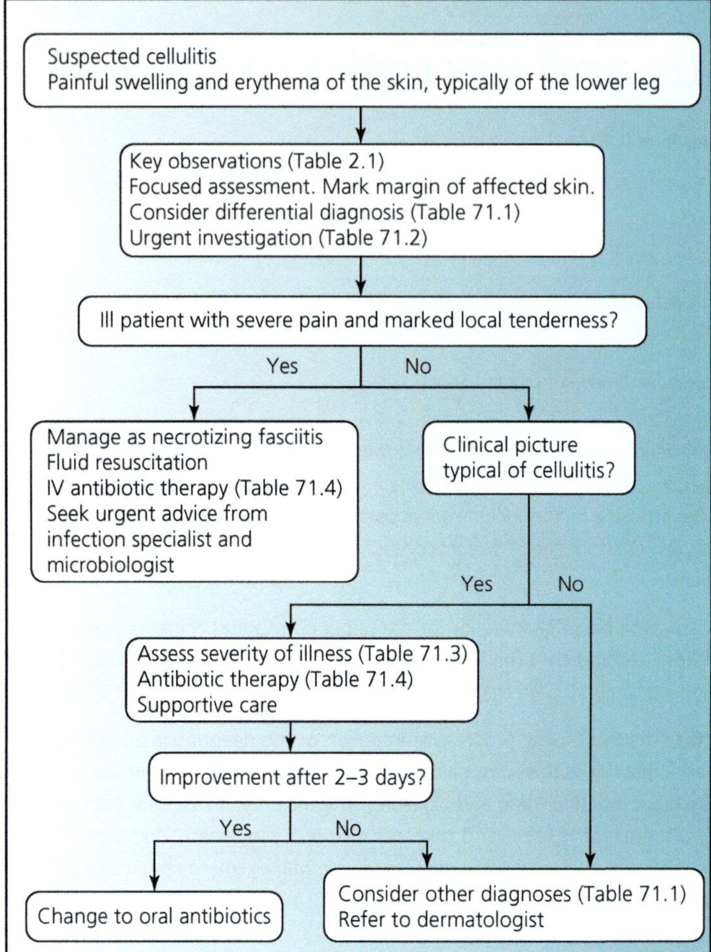

Figure 71.1 Assessment of suspected cellulitis.

Further management

Any underlying skin disorder should be treated. Seek advice from a dermatologist.

Supportive care of the patient with cellulitis of the lower leg includes:

- Elevation of the limb
- Use of a bed cradle
- Analgesia
- DVT prophylaxis
- Adequate hydration
- Treatment of comorbidities, for example diabetes

Clinical improvement is usually seen after 2–3 days, and with this, patients treated initially with IV antibiotic therapy can be switched to oral therapy, to complete a 5 – 7 day course. If there is no improvement at this time, other diagnoses should be considered and a dermatological opinion obtained.

Table 71.1 Disorders that may be mistaken for cellulitis.

Disorder	Distinguishing features
Necrotising fasciitis	Ill patient. Severe pain disproportionate to physical signs. Soft tissue may be very tender, with blue-black discolouration, blistering and (less commonly) crepitus. Rapid clinical progression (over hours)
Leg eczema (venous eczema or contact dermatitis) (*NB cellulitis may complicate eczema*)	Longer history May be bilateral No fever or systemic symptoms Itching rather than tenderness of the skin History of varicose veins or deep vein thrombosis (DVT) Crusting or scaling (in cellulitis the skin is typically smooth and shiny)
DVT (*NB DVT may complicate cellulitis*)	Proximal margin of erythema usually not well demarcated. If clinical setting suggests DVT (Chapter 31), duplex scan of leg veins is needed to exclude this.
Allergic reaction to insect sting or bite	No ascending lymphangitis, itching, may be urticaria
Chronic oedema/lymphoedema (*NB cellulitis may complicate chronic oedema or lymphoedema*)	Usually bilateral. Erythema may be feature. No fever
Gouty arthritis	Arthritis prominent. Typically involves first metatarsophalangeal joint (Chapter 92).
Pyoderma gangrenosum	Rapidly enlarging painful ulcer. Associated systemic disease (most often inflammatory bowel disease) in 50%.

Table 71.2 Urgent investigation in suspected cellulitis or necrotising fasciitis.

Full blood count
C-reactive protein
Electrolytes and renal function
Blood culture (in class 3 or 4 illness – see Table 71.3)
Microscopy and culture of blister fluid if present
Urgent imaging (e.g. CT or MRI scan) may be useful in suspected necrotising fasciitis
Urgent Gram stain of debrided tissue (in necrotising fasciitis)
Duplex scan if deep venous thrombosis is possible (Chapter 31)

Table 71.3 Cellulitis: assessment of severity of illness and management.

Class	Features	Management
1	No significant systemic illness No uncontrolled comorbidities	Oral antibiotic therapy (Table 71.4) Outpatient management
2	Significant systemic illness or comorbidity (e.g. peripheral arterial disease, morbid obesity)	IV antibiotic therapy (Table 71.4) Outpatient/inpatient management*
3	Haemodynamic instability or delirium. Limb-threatening infection due to vascular compromise Comorbidities that may interfere with response to therapy	IV antibiotic therapy (Table 71.4) Inpatient management: level 1/HDU
4	Sepsis syndrome and/or Suspected necrotising fasciitis	IV antibiotic therapy (Table 71.4) Inpatient management: HDU/ITU

*Contraindications to outpatient management of patients with class 2 cellulitis:

- Penicillin/cephalosporin allergy
- Chronic liver or renal (CKD 4 or 5) disease
- Immunosuppression
- Facial or orbital cellulitis
- Non-compliance with outpatient management likely
- Unable to cope at home.

Source: Eron LJ (2000) Infections of skin and soft tissue: outcomes of a classification scheme. *Clinical Infectious Diseases* 31, 287 (A432). Reproduced with permission of Oxford University Press.

Table 71.4 Initial antibiotic therapy in cellulitis and necrotising fasciitis.

Setting	Organisms to be covered in addition to *Streptococcus pyogenes* and *Staphylococcus aureus*	Antibiotic therapy	
		Not allergic to penicillin	Penicillin allergy
Otherwise well	Nil	Flucloxacillin	Clarithromycin or clindamycin
Known or suspected to be methicillin-resistant *S. aureus* (MRSA) colonised	MRSA	Vancomycin or teicoplanin	Vancomycin or teicoplanin
Diabetes with foot ulcer	Gram-negative and anaerobic bacteria	Co-amoxiclav	Clindamycin
Human/animal bite	Mixed oral flora including anaerobes	Co-amoxiclav	Doxycycline + metronidazole
Suspected necrotising fasciitis*	Streptococci, Gram-negative bacilli and anaerobic bacteria	Piperacillin/ tazobactam	Vancomycin or teicoplanin + gentamicin + metronidazole

* If strong microbiologic or clinical evidence of *S. pyogenes* infection, consider adding clindamycin and administration of intravenous immunoglobulin (discuss with Infection specialist)

Patients who have recurrent episodes of cellulitis should be considered for prophylactic antibiotic therapy: seek advice from a dermatologist or infection specialist.

Further reading

Hua C, Urbina T, Bosc R, *et al.* (2023) Necrotising soft-tissue infections. *Lancet Infect Dis*, e81–e94.

Sartelli M, Coccolini F, Kluger Y, *et al.* (2022) WSES/GAIS/WSIS/SIS-E/AAST global clinical pathways for patients with skin and soft tissue infections. *World J Emerg Surg* 17, 3.

CHAPTER 72

Urinary tract infection

CAROLYN HEMSLEY, CLAIRE VAN NISPEN TOT PANNERDEN, AND NICOLA JONES

Consider urinary tract infection (UTI) when the patient has symptoms directly referable to the urinary tract:

- Dysuria, frequency, sensation of incomplete voiding
- Haematuria
- Lower abdominal, suprapubic or loin pain
- Abdominal pain and/or fever in pregnancy

UTI is in the differential diagnosis of non-specific presentations:

- Unwell after urological intervention or catheterization
- General malaise or fever in patients with long-term urinary catheter
- Delirium or vomiting, with or without fever (especially in children or the elderly)
- Frailty syndromes including falls, confusion, functional decline
- Septic shock, without localizing signs (Chapter 5).

Point-of-care (POC) urinary testing by urinary dipstick in those with symptoms suggestive of UTI, assessing for pyuria, is sensitive and specific in the non-immunosuppressed population, and can support or deter the diagnosis at the patient's bedside. POC urine tests are not reliable in frail patients or in catheterized patients where asymptomatic bacteriuria is common.

Priorities

1 Determine whether the infection is uncomplicated or complicated (Table 72.1) by clinical assessment (Table 72.2), review of previous microbiology results and previous investigations (Tables 72.3 and 72.4). This will guide the need for further investigation, the choice of empirical antibiotic therapy, the length of treatment, and the requirement for follow-up.

It is not always apparent at the time of acute presentation whether the infection is complicated or not, but this may become obvious later in the course of treatment.

- **Uncomplicated**: simple lower urinary tract infection in an otherwise healthy, non-pregnant woman.
- **Complicated**: UTI in the presence of an underlying condition that increases the risk of infection or the chance of failing therapy (Table 72.1).

Acute Medicine: A Practical Guide to the Management of Medical Emergencies, Sixth Edition.
Edited by Mridula Rajwani, Leila Vaziri, and Ivie Gbinigie.
© 2026 John Wiley & Sons Ltd. Published 2026 by John Wiley & Sons Ltd.

Table 72.1 Factors suggestive of complicated urinary tract infection.

Patient demographics
 Very young or advanced age
 Pregnancy
 Male sex
Comorbidities
 Diabetes mellitus
 Immunosuppression
 Renal transplant
 Chronic kidney disease
Anatomical abnormalities
 Urinary tract instrumentation, including urethral catheter, ureteric stent, nephrostomy
 Prostatic pathology
 Urethral stricture
 Renal or bladder stones
Other factors
 Health-care-associated infection
 Failure of recent antimicrobial therapy

Table 72.2 Focused assessment of the patient with suspected urinary tract infection.

History
- Major symptoms and time course – differentiate between lower urinary tract symptoms, upper tract symptoms and systemic features
- Previous history of urinary tract infections
- Antibiotic history
- Presence/absence of urinary catheter, recent catheterization, blocked catheter, catheter change
- History of recent urinary tract intervention or urological intervention
- Previous history of renal tract pathology such as chronic kidney disease, renal stones, single kidney, structural abnormality
- Pregnancy?
- Diabetes?
- Sexual history
- If primarily urethritis or penile discharge, consider sexually transmitted infections (*Neisseria gonorrhoea*, *Chlamydia trachomatis*, *Herpes simplex*, *Trichomonas vaginalis*)
- Symptoms of sexually transmitted infections and PID or epididymo-orchitis?
- Review any recent GP or hospital microbiology results
- Consider points relevant to differential diagnosis – gastrointestinal symptoms

Examination
- Vital signs and key observations if critically ill and resuscitate as appropriate
- Assessment of presence/absence of loin tenderness
- Presence or absence of catheter and quality of catheter urine
- Consider alternative source of sepsis

Note: Gram-negative sepsis secondary to a urinary focus can be difficult to distinguish from suspected acute respiratory tract infection in the elderly.

Table 72.3 Urgent investigations in suspected urinary tract infection.

Suspected simple uncomplicated UTI
- Urine for dipstick as a point-of-care test to detect presence/absence of nitrites and leucocyte esterase
- Urine dipstick for glucose
- Send urine for microscopy, culture and sensitivities – before antibiotics are started (may not be needed if first presentation of lower urinary tract infection in a woman) (Box 72.1)

Suspected complicated UTI
- Urine dipstick and culture as above
- Full blood count
- C-reactive protein
- Electrolytes, urea and creatinine, liver function tests
- Venous blood gas for lactate
- Blood glucose
- Pregnancy test in women of childbearing age with lower abdominal symptoms
- CT KUB – if history of renal stones or features of renal colic
- Renal/urinary tract ultrasonography – urgent in the setting of acute kidney injury
- Blood cultures

Box 72.1 Definitions.

A urinary tract infection (UTI) is defined by the presence of $\geq 10^3$–10^4 organisms per mL urine, associated with clinical symptoms. Causative organisms are given in Appendix 72.1.

UTI encompasses simple lower urinary tract infection (cystitis), upper urinary tract infection (pyelonephritis, pyonephrosis) and infection resulting in bacteraemia and septic shock.

Table 72.4 Indications for renal/urinary tract imaging.

Urgent
Features of renal colic or suspicion of renal stones +/ renal tract obstruction (plain X-ray and CT KUB)

As soon as possible (renal ultrasound is the usual initial investigation):
- Acute kidney injury
- Pyelonephritis in men or children
- Recurrent episode of pyelonephritis in women
- History of renal pathology
- Persistent fever despite 48–72 h of appropriate antibiotic
- Uncertain diagnosis, for example considering genitourinary pathology or appendicitis

Referral for renal tract imaging post treatment of acute infection
- Urinary infection in boys and men with no known risk factors for UTI
- Recurrent urinary tract infections (>three/year)
- Haematuria

Not indicated
- Uncomplicated lower tract infection in women
- First episode of pyelonephritis in women with no AKI and rapid treatment response (within defervescence within 48–72 h)

2 If the patient is febrile or has significant systemic upset send peripheral blood as well as urine for culture before starting appropriate empirical antibiotics (Tables 72.5 and 72.6).
- The choice of agent depends on local epidemiology and resistance rates of common urinary pathogens and is usually indicated by local and national guidelines, e.g. NICE guidelines Ng 109–113.
- Consider recent antibiotic history, especially if considering treatment failure.

Table 72.5 Empirical antibiotic therapy in suspected urinary tract infection.

Always refer to any local guidelines as resistance rates vary, and consider community versus health-care associated infection (HAI). HAIs are commonly more resistant than community acquired UTIs. Examples of standard recommendations are given below.

Consider also adverse effects associated with some antibiotics (e.g. fluoroquinolones) and risks of Clostridium difficile infection. Agents with higher risk of CDI include the '4 Cs' – amoxicillin-clavulanate (co-amoxiclav), ceftriaxone, clindamycin and ciprofloxacin. Agents with lower risk of CDI include trimethoprim, cefalexin, nitrofurantoin, sulphamethoxazole-trimethoprim (co-trimoxazole), amoxicllin, doxycyline and gentamicin.

Simple community-acquired lower urinary tract infection
Refer to NICE guideline 109
Trimethoprim 200 mg 12-hourly PO PO or nitrofurantoin 100 mg 12-hourly PO
Women - three days;   Men - seven days treatment
(Nitrofurantoin is not appropriate if upper renal tract or prostatitis is possible as it does not achieve reliable prostatic or renal parenchymal tissue concentrations. Nitrofurantoin is also not appropriate if eGFR is <45 mL/min.)

Simple health-care-associated acquired lower urinary tract infection
1st line: Nitrofurantoin 100 mg 12-hourly PO or trimethoprim 200 mg 12-hourly
2nd line: Pivmecillinam 400 mg initial dose then 200 mg 8-hourly or fosfomycin 3 g single dose
Women - three days;   Men - seven days treatment

Suspected pyelonephritis
Refer to NICE guideline 111
Aminoglycoside (e.g. gentamicin* 5 mg/kg) OD IV **plus** IV amoxicillin 1–2 g 8 hourly IV
or
Aminoglycoside (e.g. gentamicin* 5 mg/kg) OD IV **plus** a first or second-generation cephalosporin IV (e.g. cefazolin or cefuroxime)
or Ambulatory care options for pyelonephritis include
Cefalexin 500 mg twice or three times a day (up to 1 to 1.5 g three or four times a day for severe infections) for 7 to 10 days
Or, Trimethoprim-sulfamethoxazole 960 mg 12-hourly PO for 7-10 days
Or, trimethoprim 200 mg twice a day for 14 days (only if known susceptible organism)
Or, Co-amoxiclav 500/125 mg three times a day for 7 to 10 days (only if known susceptible organism)
Or, Oral quinolone (e.g. ciprofloxacin 500 mg po 12 hourly for 7 days) if other options are not possible and mild illness in a patient in whom the likelihood of quinolone resistance is <10% (based on local epidemiology) and there has been no quinolone exposure in the last three to six months.
Or Gentamicin * 5 mg/kg OD IV
In all cases, subsequent antibiotic therapy post 48 h should be tailored to an appropriate single agent on receipt of susceptibility data and consider IV to oral switch depending on defervescence and clinical improvement.

*gentamicin can be given on a daily basis for treatment of UTI; therapeutic drug monitoring is recommended, gentamicin levels should be measured 6–14 h after administration so that dosing interval can be calculated from nomogram [*BMJ* 2012;345, e6354. DOI: 10.1136/bmj.e6354]. Possible adverse effects are nephrotoxicity and vestibular toxicity.

- Consider recent microbiological culture results if available.
- Mode of delivery of the antibiotic (intravenous versus oral) will depend on the acuity of the illness and ability of the patient to tolerate oral antibiotics.
- Review choice of antibiotic in light of pregnancy, allergy history and potential interactions with concomitant regular medication.

3 If suspected uncomplicated urinary tract infection (i.e. only lower urinary tract symptoms in a young woman with no features of systemic upset and no previous antimicrobial therapy) then treatment with empirical antibiotic without the need for urine culture is appropriate (Table 72.5). The patient should be advised to return if treatment fails to resolve symptoms, at which point urinary culture is indicated to guide further correct antimicrobial selection. Uncomplicated UTI or pyelonephritis in a young woman with complete symptom resolution does not need follow-up.

Table 72.6 Common antimicrobials in the treatment of urinary tract infection.

Drug	Absorption (bioavailability following oral admin)	Amount excreted unchanged in urine	Dosing in renal impairment
Amoxicillin	89%	60%	Oral – high dose amoxicillin reduce dose if eGFR <10 mL/min IV – high dose amoxicillin reduce dose if eGFR <30 mL/min (risk of crystalluria with high doses)
Co-amoxiclav	75%	60% amoxicillin 40% clavulanic acid	Oral – no dose adjustment required IV – reduce dose if eGFRl <30 mL/min
Cefalexin	>90%	>90%	Reduce dose if eGFR <50 mL/min
Ciprofloxacin	70–80%	40–70%	Oral – reduce dose if eGFR <20 mL/min IV – reduce dose if eGFR <20 mL/min
Trimethoprim	>90%	40–60%	Reduce dose if eGFR <30 mL/min
Nitrofurantoin	94% (lower if administered without food)	30–40%	**Contraindicated** if eGFR <45 mL/min
Fosfomycin	40%	>70%	Avoid if eGFR <10 mL/min
Gentamicin	N/A	95%	Reduce dose if eGFR <20 mL/min
Amikacin	N/A	95%	Reduce dose if eGFR <20 mL/min

4 Relieve acute urinary retention. UTI is a common precipitant for acute on chronic retention in older men with prostatic enlargement and partial bladder outflow obstruction. Constipation can be a precipitant of Retention and UTI in older females.
- Catheterize if in acute urinary retention.
- Unblock or replace blocked infected urinary catheters with appropriate antibiotic cover if long-term catheter in situ.
- Treat constipation

5 If there is an associated acute kidney injury, manage this along standard lines (Chapter 86).
- Ensure appropriate fluid management including input/output chart.
- Arrange ultrasonography of the kidneys and urinary tract to exclude obstruction requiring intervention.

6 Consider the need for urinary tract imaging (Table 72.4).

Further management

1 Review urinary culture results and change antimicrobial therapy as guided by susceptibility data. Urine culture results will usually be available at 24–48 h. Antibiotic course length depends on the clinical picture and whether it is uncomplicated or complicated UTI (Tables 72.1, 72.5 and 72.6).

2 If persisting fever at 72 h or ongoing symptoms or sepsis despite antimicrobial therapy:
- Consider wrong diagnosis. If dysuria, consider perineal candidiasis, vaginitis, urethritis or sexually transmitted infection.
- If suprapubic or abdominal discomfort, review the need for abdominal imaging to exclude an alternative diagnosis, for example salpingitis, diverticulitis, appendicitis. Is the patient on the appropriate antimicrobial therapy?
- Review microbiology results and discuss antibiotic therapy with microbiologist or infection specialist.
- Has renal tract imaging been performed (Table 72.4)? Consider the presence of underlying complete or partial upper renal tract obstruction needing decompression. Consider the presence of a collection requiring drainage (radiologically guided or surgical).

3 Decide if you should refer to a urologist, either acutely or for follow-up (Table 72.7):
- Decompression of upper renal tract if ureteric obstruction is present, for example by nephrostomy.
- Drainage of perinephric collections or renal abscess.
- Men with recurrent cystitis should be evaluated for prostatitis.

Table 72.7 Indications for referral to urology.

Urgent
Septic shock with associated ureteric obstruction/hydronephrosis with suspicion or pyonephrosis
Fever and features of renal colic

As soon as possible
Hydronephrosis/ureteric obstruction on imaging +/− AKI OR persisting fever after 72 h on appropriate antibiotic therapy
Renal abscess detected on renal tract imaging
Emphysematous cystitis or pyelonephritis detected on imaging
Non-obstructing stones found on imaging
Acute on chronic retention requiring catheterization

Routine follow-up through clinic
Unexplained recurrent urinary tract infection
Recurrent urinary tract infections in children

4 Change long-term urinary catheters. In catheter-associated urinary tract infections (CAUTIs), urinary catheter colonization with bacteria is inevitable and hard to eradicate. Replacement of urinary catheters whilst on antibiotic treatment is advisable.

5 Presentation with recurrent symptoms within a few weeks of treatment should have further evaluation for complicated UTI:
   * Have they had renal/urinary tract imaging?
   * Repeat a urine culture for resistant bacteria.
   * Consider performing urodynamics. Is there bladder dysfunction or incomplete emptying or uterine prolapse/cystocele.
   * Consider referral to urologist for cystoscopy.
   * Post menopausal woman – atrophic vulvitis? Consider oestrogen topical therapy and referral for urodynamics.

Appendix 72.1 Causative agents of urinary tract infection (UTI) and urethritis.

Organism	Comment
Typical	
Escherischia coli	Responsible for >80% of urinary tract infections. Increasing resistance amongst urinary isolates both in hospital acquired UTI and community settings since 2000.
Klebsiella species	As with *E coli* increasingly resistant isolates seen in UTI.
Proteus species	Often associated with stone formation and therefore indication for renal tract imaging. Intrinsically resistant to nitrofurantoin.
Staphylococcus saphrophyticus	Common cause of UTI in young women.
Less common	
Other enterobacteriacae (*Enterobacter* spp, *Serratia* spp, *Citrobacter* spp) *Enterococcus* spp	More common in health-care associated infection. Typically more resistant to standard antibiotics. Often harbour ESBLs (extended spectrum beta lactamases) conferring resistance to penicillins and third-generation cephalosporins.
Unusual	
Pseudomonas aeruginosa	Unusual community pathogen. More commonly seen in CAUTIs, history of renal tract intervention, renal stones or health-care exposure.
Candida	When seen in culture often reflects perineal organisms or genital mucosal candidiasis as a cause of dysuria as opposed to true UTI. However, can (rarely) be isolated as a genuine urinary pathogen, and isolation in true UTI would be an indication for renal tract imaging to exclude micro-abscesses or Candida balls.
Staphylococcus aureus	Atypical urinary pathogen outside the setting of urinary tract instrumentation. Bacteriuria can be seen in the setting of *S. aureus* bacteraemia from a non-urinary focus and UTI should not automatically be attributed as primary focus. Blood cultures are indicated.

Further reading

MHRA Fluoroquinolone adverse effects. https://www.gov.uk/drug-safety-update/fluoroquinolone-antibiotics-must-now-only-be-prescribed-when-other-commonly-recommended-antibiotics-are-inappropriate.

Hooton TM. (2012) Uncomplicated urinary tract infection. *N Engl J Med* 366, 1028–1037.

NICE. (2012) How to monitor aminoglycosides (nomograms). *BMJ* 345, e6354. DOI: 10.1136/bmj.e6354.

NICE guidelines: NG109-113. https://www.nice.org.uk/.

Shaeffer AJ, Nicolle LE. (2016) Urinary tract infections in older men. *N Engl J Med* 374, 562–571.

CHAPTER 73

Central nervous system infection

JOHN L. KLEIN

Central nervous system (CNS) infections, usually manifesting as meningitis or encephalitis, are rare but potentially devastating diseases that require prompt assessment, diagnostic tests and often empirical antimicrobial therapy. The incidence of these infections varies widely by country and over time. In the UK, for example, the incidence of invasive meningococcal infection (including meningitis) has approximately halved over the last 10 years, mainly due to the sequential introduction of meningococcal vaccines targeted at serogroups A, C, W, Y and B.

Most patients presenting with fever with headache and/or decreased conscious level will not have CNS infection, which can lead to diagnostic uncertainty if a careful history, examination and (in most cases) a lumbar puncture is not undertaken. Patients with suspected or confirmed meningitis (without encephalitis) should not receive aciclovir: herpes simplex meningitis (usually HSV-2) is a benign disease that does not normally require anti-viral therapy.

Meningitis

Acute bacterial meningitis is a medical emergency and should be considered in any patient with fever, headache, neck stiffness or a reduced conscious level: 95% of patients with bacterial meningitis will have at least two of these four features. Bacterial meningitis can also present as sepsis or septic shock. Management of suspected bacterial meningitis is summarized in Figure 73.1. Most cases in the developed world are caused by *Neisseria meningitidis* or *Streptococcus pneumoniae*. In the context of immunosuppression, alcohol-use disorder or age >60 years, *Listeria monocytogenes* should also be considered. In resource-poor settings, *M. tuberculosis* or *Cryptococcus neoformans* may predominate (Appendix 73.1).

A viral aetiology is more common than bacterial in many settings. The commonest causes are enteroviruses, herpes simplex virus (mainly HSV-2) and varicella-zoster virus (VZV). Presentation may mimic bacterial infection, although patients appear less systemically unwell and are less likely to be febrile. A rash may be present (e.g. a vesicular rash in shingles or enteroviral infection). Inflammatory markers (white cell count and C-reactive protein) are often normal or mildly elevated and the CSF findings are usually distinctive (Table 73.5).

Disorders which can mimic meningitis include subarachnoid haemorrhage (Chapter 53) viral encephalitis, brain abscess, subdural empyema and cerebral malaria.

Priorities

1 Review the physiological observations, make a focused clinical assessment (Table 73.1) and arrange urgent investigations (Table 73.2).

Acute Medicine: A Practical Guide to the Management of Medical Emergencies, Sixth Edition.
Edited by Mridula Rajwani, Leila Vaziri, and Ivie Gbinigie.
© 2026 John Wiley & Sons Ltd. Published 2026 by John Wiley & Sons Ltd.

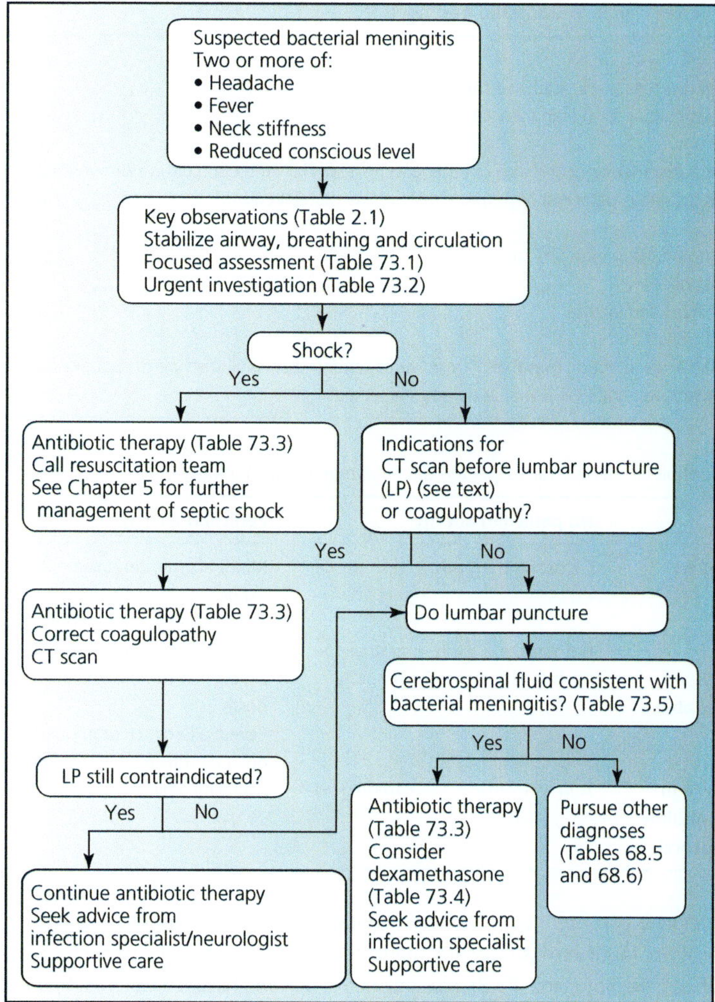

Figure 73.1 Management of suspected bacterial meningitis.

Table 73.1 Clinical findings in bacterial meningitis.

Prodromal illness for one to two days

Fever

Purpuric/petechial rash (especially meningococcal infection)

Features of meningeal irritation: headache, neck stiffness, vomiting, photophobia

Reduced conscious level

Seizures

Cranial nerve palsies

Focal neurological signs (if bacterial meningitis is complicated by cerebral venous sinus thrombosis or arteritis)

General examination may show signs of predisposing disorders:

• Ear infection

• Sinusitis

• Pneumonia

Table 73.2 Urgent investigation in suspected meningitis.

Blood culture (×2)
Lumbar puncture (if not contraindicated: see text)
Throat swab (request culture for meningococci)
Full blood count
EDTA sample for PCR (for meningococci and pneumococci) – especially if blood cultures drawn after antibiotic therapy
Coagulation screen if there is petechial or purpuric rash or low platelet count
C-reactive protein
Blood glucose (for comparison with CSF glucose)
Creatinine and electrolytes
Arterial blood gases, pH and lactate
Chest X-ray (?pneumonia)
CT head if suspected sinus infection (nasal discharge, sinus tenderness), skull fracture or space occupying lesion
Throat and rectal swabs for viral PCR if viral aetiology suspected

Table 73.3 Initial antibiotic therapy for suspected bacterial meningitis in adults.

Setting	No penicillin allergy	Penicillin allergy
Adult aged under 60	Cefotaxime 2 g qds or ceftriaxone 2 g bd	Minor allergy: cefotaxime 2 g qds or ceftriaxone 2 g bd Severe allergy: chloramphenicol 25 mg/kg qds
Age over 60, Immunocompromised or chronic alcohol abuse	Cefotaxime 2 g qds or ceftriaxone 2 g bd + amoxicillin 2 g 4 hourly	Minor allergy: cefotaxime 2 g qds or ceftriaxone 2 g bd + co-trimoxazole 90 mg/kg/day in 2–4 doses Severe allergy: chloramphenicol 25 mg/kg qds + co-trimoxazole 90 mg/kg/day in 2–4 doses
In regions with a high prevalence of penicillin-resistant pneumococci	Add vancomycin 15–20 mg/kg bd	Add vancomycin 15–20 mg/kg bd

2 If the clinical picture is consistent with bacterial meningitis, and the patient has shock, a reduced conscious level or a petechial/purpuric rash (suggesting meningococcal infection), take blood for culture and immediately start antibiotic therapy (Table 73.3), plus adjunctive dexamethasone (Table 73.4), if indicated.

3 In patients with suspected meningitis without signs of sepsis or septic shock, lumbar puncture (LP) should ideally be performed within 1 h of arrival at hospital, provided there is no contraindication to LP. Antibiotic therapy (Table 73.3) should be started immediately after LP, and within the first hour.

Table 73.4 Adjunctive dexamethasone in suspected bacterial meningitis.

Indications
Strong clinical suspicion of bacterial meningitis, especially if CSF is turbid

Situations where dexamethasone not advised
Antibiotic therapy already begun (although consider using up to 12 h after antibiotics in pneumococcal meningitis)
Septic shock
Suspected meningococcal disease (petechial/purpuric rash)
Immunosuppressed patient

Regimen
Give dexamethasone 10 mg IV before or with the first dose of antibiotic therapy (Table 73.3)
Continue dexamethasone 10 mg 6-hourly IV for four days if CSF shows Gram-positive diplococci, or if blood/CSF cultures are positive for *Streptococcus pneumoniae*

If LP cannot be done within 1 h (e.g. because of the need for CT or the presence of a coagulopathy), take blood for culture and immediately start antibiotic therapy (Table 73.3).

4 CT should be done before LP if there are risk factors for an intracranial mass lesion, or signs of raised intracranial pressure:
* Immunosuppression (e.g. HIV/AIDS, immunosuppressive therapy)
* History of brain tumour or focal infection
* Uncontrolled seizures
* Papilloedema
* Reduced conscious level (Glasgow Coma Scale score <13)
* Focal neurological signs (not including cranial nerve palsies)

5 If the patient is taking antiplatelet or anticoagulant therapy, or has thrombocytopenia or a coagulopathy, discuss management with a haematologist before LP. See also Chapters 81 and 85.

6 Perform a Lumbar Puncture
* Measure and record the opening pressure. If the opening pressure is >40 cm CSF, indicating severe cerebral oedema, give mannitol 0.5 g/kg IV over 10 min plus dexamethasone 12 mg IV. Discuss further management with a neurologist.
* Send CSF for cell count, protein concentration, glucose (fluoride tube), Gram stain and culture. PCR for meningococcus and pneumococcus should be undertaken if blood/CSF cultures are negative. Viral PCR should be undertaken in patients with lymphocytic CSF findings. Consider requesting microscopy and culture for acid-fast bacilli (5–10 mL is required) +/− TB PCR if tuberculosis is suspected (Appendix 73.1); in immunosuppressed patients (especially those with HIV infection), request an India ink stain and a cryptococcal antigen test (Appendix 73.2).

7 Patients with suspected bacterial meningitis should be isolated (contact precautions) until at least 24 h into treatment.

8 Blood-stained CSF may be due to a traumatic tap or subarachnoid haemorrhage. The presence of bilirubin in the CSF (detected by spectrophotometry) indicates red cell breakdown products and confirms subarachnoid haemorrhage (Chapter 53).

Further management

1 If organisms are seen on Gram stain of the CSF, bacterial meningitis is confirmed. The cell count will usually be high, with a polymorphonuclear leucocytosis, but may be low in overwhelming infection or immunosuppression. Modify or start antibiotic therapy (Table 73.3). Ask advice from an infection specialist on the best antibiotic regimen and duration of treatment.

2 If no organisms are seen on Gram stain, management is directed by the clinical picture and CSF findings (Table 73.5):

Normal cell count: that is, bacterial meningitis highly unlikely. Consider other infectious diseases which may give rise to meningism (e.g. bacterial tonsillitis).

Table 73.5 Typical CSF findings in meningitis.

Element	Pyogenic meningitis	Viral meningitis	Tuberculous meningitis	Cryptococcal meningitis
White cell count/mm³	>1000	<500	<500	<150
Predominant cell type	Polymorphs	Lymphocytes	Lymphocytes	Lymphocytes
Protein concentration (g/L)	>1.5	0.5–1.0	1.0–5.0	0.5–1.0
CSF: blood glucose	<50%	>50%	<50%	<50%

Table 73.6 Causes of meningitis with a high CSF lymphocyte count.*

Viral meningitis
Partially treated pyogenic bacterial meningitis
Other bacterial infections – tuberculosis (Appendix 73.1), leptospirosis, brucellosis, syphilis, listeriosis
Fungal (especially cryptococcal) infection (Appendix 73.2)
Parameningeal infection – brain abscess or subdural empyema
Neoplastic infiltration

*Viral encephalitis may give a similar CSF picture.

High polymorph count: this is typical of pyogenic bacterial meningitis, although may occur early in the course of viral meningitis. Modify or start antibiotic therapy (Table 73.3). Ask advice from an infection specialist on the best antibiotic regimen and duration of treatment.

High lymphocyte count: this may be seen in many diseases (Table 73.6). Distinguishing between viral and partially treated pyogenic bacterial meningitis can be difficult. If in doubt, start antibiotic therapy, awaiting the results of culture of blood and CSF. If viral meningitis is suspected, request CSF PCR for HSV-1&2, VZV and enteroviruses. If tuberculous or cryptococcal meningitis is possible on clinical grounds (see Appendices 73.1 and 73.2), or on the results of CSF examination, ask for microscopy and culture for acid-fast bacilli (consider TB PCR) and an India ink stain/cryptococcal antigen test.

- The values given are typical, but exceptions occur.
- Antibiotic therapy substantially changes the CSF findings in pyogenic bacterial meningitis, leading to a fall in cell count, increased proportion of lymphocytes and fall in protein level. However, the low CSF glucose level usually persists.

3 Supportive care of the patient with bacterial meningitis includes:
- Analgesia as required (e.g. paracetamol, NSAID or codeine).
- Control of seizures (see Chapter 57).
- Attention to fluid balance. Losses are increased due to fever. Aim for an intake of 2–3 L/day, supplementing oral intake with IV normal saline/5% glucose if needed. Check creatinine and electrolytes initially daily. Hyponatraemia may occur due to inappropriate ADH secretion.

4 Contacts of patients with confirmed or suspected meningococcal meningitis should be identified. Ciprofloxacin (500 mg stat PO for adults) should be offered to household contacts and other close contacts (e.g. sexual partners). Rifampicin (600 mg twice daily PO in adults for two days) is an alternative.

5 Viral meningitis (ensuring encephalitis has been excluded) does not need specific anti-viral therapy and usually has a benign prognosis.

6 The district community medicine specialist should be informed promptly about confirmed cases of meningitis.

Encephalitis

Consider encephalitis in any febrile patient with abnormal behaviour or reduced conscious level. These clinical features have a broad differential diagnosis (Table 73.7), which must be considered. As prompt treatment of herpes simplex encephalitis (Appendix 73.3) minimizes brain injury and dramatically improves outcomes, aciclovir should be given to all patients with possible encephalitis, until the results of diagnostic tests are known.

- Empirical antibiotic therapy for bacterial meningitis should also be given if the patient has features of both meningitis and encephalitis.
- Tuberculous and cryptococcal meningo-encephalitis should considered in at-risk groups (see Appendices 73.1 and 73.2). Meningism may be absent or mild in these diseases.

Table 73.7 Causes of fever with abnormal behaviour and/or reduced conscious level.

Intracranial infection
Viral encephalitis
Other infectious causes of encephalitis
Bacterial meningitis
Tuberculous meningitis (Appendix 73.1)
Cryptococcal meningitis (Appendix 73.2)
Subdural empyema
Brain abscess

Systemic infection
Septic encephalopathy
Infective endocarditis
Mycoplasma pneumoniae infection
Syphilis, Lyme disease, leptospirosis
Cerebral malaria

Non-infectious
Poisoning (e.g. with amphetamine or cocaine)
Alcohol withdrawal syndrome (Chapter 41)
Cerebral vasculitis
Cerebral venous thrombosis
Acute disseminated encephalomyelitis (seen in young adults; usually follows infection)
Auto-immune encephalitis (sub-acute history, fever often absent, abnormal movements common, more frequently female, CSF WCC usually <50/mm^3)
Neuroleptic malignant syndrome (Appendix 73.4)
Acute intermittent porphyria
Heatstroke

- A broad array of infectious agents must be considered in patients with the relevant travel or exposure history (Chapter 75) e.g. West Nile Virus, rabies, tick-borne encephalitis, malaria – seek the advice of an infection specialist in these circumstances
- Advice from an infection specialist should also be sought in the immunocompromised in whom encephalitis may be caused by a broad array of opportunistic infections (e.g. *Toxoplasma gondii*, cytomegalovirus, JC virus).

Priorities

1 Review the physiological observations and make a focused clinical assessment (Table 73.8).
2 If you suspect encephalitis, start aciclovir 10 mg/kg 8-hourly IV (dose adjustment may be required in renal impairment). If meningism is present, or there are other reasons to suspect bacterial meningitis, take blood cultures and start appropriate antibiotic therapy.
3 Arrange CT head, LP and other urgent investigations (Table 73.9). In high-resource countries, the ready availability of CT makes it reasonable to do CT before LP in every case. CT should definitely be done before LP if there are risk factors for an intracranial mass lesion, or signs of raised intracranial pressure:
   - Immunosuppression (e.g. HIV-AIDS, immunosuppressive therapy)
   - History of brain tumour or focal infection
   - Uncontrolled seizures
   - Papilloedema
   - Reduced conscious level (Glasgow Coma Scale score <13)
   - Focal neurological signs (not including cranial nerve palsies)

Table 73.8 Focused assessment in suspected encephalitis.

Current major symptoms and their time course (confirm with family or friends)
Recent foreign travel (Chapter 75)
Insect or animal exposure (occupational/recreational)
Contact with infectious disease
Sexual history
Immunization history
Immunosuppression? Consider immunosuppressive therapy, HIV-AIDS, active cancer, advanced chronic kidney disease, liver failure, diabetes, malnutrition, splenectomy, IV drug use
Drug history (if treated with neuroleptic in preceding two weeks, consider neuroleptic malignant syndrome (Appendix 73.4))
Alcohol/substance use

Table 73.9 Urgent investigation in suspected encephalitis.

Blood culture (×2)
CT head
LP if not contraindicated (send CSF for PCR for HSV-1/2, VZV, enteroviruses and parechovirus in addition to other tests)
Nose/throat swab for enterovirus, *Mycoplasma pneumoniae*, influenza and adenovirus
Rectal swab for enteroviruses
Full blood count and film
Blood film for malaria if indicated
Coagulation screen
C-reactive protein
Blood glucose
Sodium, potassium, urea and creatinine
Liver function tests
Creatine kinase
Urinalysis
Toxicology screen if poisoning is possible (send serum (10 mL) + urine (50 mL))
Arterial blood gases and pH
Chest X-ray
Save serum (for targeted serological tests as indicated)
Immunological tests if suspected autoimmune encephalitis

Further management

1 Management is directed by the clinical picture, neuroimaging and CSF findings (see Tables 73.5 and 73.6).
2 If viral encephalitis is probable or cannot be excluded, continue aciclovir and seek advice from an infection specialist and neurologist.
3 Supportive treatment of viral encephalitis includes:
   - Analgesia as required (e.g. paracetamol, NSAID or codeine).
   - Control of seizures (see Chapter 57).
   - Attention to fluid balance. Losses are increased due to fever. Aim for an intake of 2–3 L/day, supplementing oral with IV normal saline if needed. Check electrolytes and creatinine, initially daily. Hyponatraemia may occur due to inappropriate ADH secretion.

Appendix 73.1 Tuberculous meningitis.

Element	Comment
At risk	Birth in a region with a high incidence of tuberculosis (TB) (e.g. Indian sub-continent, and Africa)
	Recent contact with TB
	Previous pulmonary TB
	Alcohol- or substance-use disorder
	Immunosuppression (organ transplant, lymphoma, steroid therapy, anti-TNF therapy, HIV/AIDS)
Suggestive clinical features	Subacute onset
	Cranial nerve palsies
	Retinal tubercles (pathognomonic but rarely seen)
	Evidence of extra-meningeal TB (e.g. miliary change on CXR)
	Hyponatraemia
CSF findings	Raised opening pressure
	High lymphocyte count
	High protein level
	Rare for acid-fast bacilli to be seen on microscopy, but PCR for *M. tuberculosis* DNA has a higher sensitivity
CT brain	Hydrocephalus common
	Cerebral infarction due to arteritis may be seen
	Tuberculomas may be seen
Treatment	Combination chemotherapy with isoniazid (plus pyridoxine to avoid neuropathy), rifampicin, pyrazinamide and ethambutol
	Consider adjunctive dexamethasone (seek expert advice)

Appendix 73.2 Cryptococcal meningitis.

Element	Comment
At risk	Immunosuppression (organ transplant, lymphoma, steroid therapy, HIV/AIDS)
Suggestive clinical features	Insidious onset
	Neck stiffness absent or mild
	Papular or nodular skin lesions
CSF findings	Raised opening pressure
	High lymphocyte count (20–200/mm^3)
	Protein and glucose levels usually only mildly abnormal
	Cryptococci may be seen on Gram stain
	India ink preparation positive in 60%
	CSF culture positive
	Cryptococcal antigen test positive (highly sensitive)
CT brain	Usually normal
	May show hydrocephalus
	May show mass lesions (~10%)
Treatment	Amphotericin B plus flucytosine: seek expert advice

Appendix 73.3 Herpes simplex encephalitis.

Element	Comment
Clinical features	Acute onset (symptoms usually <one week)
	Fever
	Personality change/abnormal behaviour
	Alteration in conscious level
	Seizures
	Focal neurological abnormalities (cranial nerve palsies, dysphasia, hemiparesis, ataxia)
CT brain	May be normal
	May show generalized brain swelling with loss of cortical sulci and small ventricles
	May show areas of low attenuation in the temporal and/or frontal lobes
CSF findings	High lymphocyte count (50–500/mm^3), with predominance of polymorphs in early phase, and red cells often present
	Protein concentration increased, up to 2.5 g/L
	Glucose is usually normal
	Herpes simplex DNA is usually detected in CSF by PCR (>95% sensitive)
Electroencephalography	Abnormal in two-thirds of cases, with a spike and slow wave pattern localized to the area of brain involved.
Management	Aciclovir 10 mg/kg 8-hourly IV
	Seek expert advice from an infection specialist and a neurologist

Appendix 73.4 Neuroleptic malignant syndrome.

Element	Comment
Clinical features	Preceding use of neuroleptic (usually develops within two weeks of starting medication)
	Agitated delirium progressing to stupor and coma
	Generalized 'lead-pipe' muscular rigidity, often accompanied by tremor
	Temperature >38 °C (may be >40 °C)
	Autonomic instability: tachycardia, labile or high blood pressure, tachypnoea, sweating
CT brain	Typically normal
CSF findings	Typically normal
	May show raised protein
Electroencephalography	Generalized slow wave activity
Blood tests	High creatine kinase (typically >1000 units/L, and proportionate to rigidity)
	High white cell count (10–40 × 10^9/L)
	Electrolyte derangements and raised creatinine common
	Low serum iron level
Management	Stop neuroleptic
	Supportive care
	Use benzodiazepine if needed to control agitation
	Consider use of dantrolene, bromocriptine or amantadine
	Seek expert advice from a neurologist

Further reading

Brouwer MC, Tunkel AR, McKhann GM II, van de Beek D. (2014) Brain abscess. *N Engl J Med* 371, 447–456.

Defres S, Tharmaratnam K, Michael BD, *et al.* (2023) Clinical predictors of encephalitis in UK adults – A multi-centre prospective observational cohort study. *PLoS One* 18(8), e0282645. DOI: 10.1371/journal.pone.0282645.

Graus F, Titulaer MJ, Balu R. (2016) A clinical approach to diagnosis of autoimmune encephalitis. *Lancet Neurol* 4, 391–404.

Jarrin I, Sellier P, Lopes A. (2016) Etiologies and management of aseptic meningitis in patients admitted to an internal medicine department. *Medicine* 95, e2372. Open access.

McGill F, Heyderman RS, Michael BD, *et al.* (2016) The UK joint specialist societies guideline on the diagnosis and management of acute meningitis and meningococcal sepsis in immunocompetent adults. *J Infect* 72, 405–438. Open access. http://www.journalofinfection.com/article/S0163-4453(16)00024-4/pdf.

Solomon T, Michael BD, Smith PE, *et al.* (2012) Management of suspected viral encephalitis in adults. *J Infect* 64, 347–373.

CHAPTER 74

Pancytopenia and febrile neutropenia

EDMUND WATSON

Pancytopenia describes the combination of neutropenia, anaemia and thrombocytopenia. It may be due to reduced synthesis (i.e. bone marrow failure: the inadequate or defective production of blood cells), increased destruction or complex mechanisms (see Table 74.1).

Table 74.1 Causes of pancytopenia (non-exhaustive).

Mechanism	Causative diseases

Reduced synthesis	Therapeutic agents
	• Chemotherapy/radiotherapy
	• Other drugs – e.g.
	  • Rheumatologic agents, NSAIDs
	  • Anti-microbials
	  • Anti-epileptics
	  • Anti-psychotics.
	Marrow infiltration
	• Bony metastases from solid organ malignancy
	• Haematological malignancy
	  • Any, but acute leukaemia especially
	  • History/examination often unremarkable, but:
	    • Lymphadenopathy and splenomegaly in high-grade lymphoma
	    • Splenomegaly in myelofibrosis
	Megaloblastic anaemia (B12 and/or folate deficiency)
	• Consider dietary or absorptive features
	• Look for associated symptoms – e.g. neuropathy and glossitis
	Panhypopituitarism
	• Perhaps following history of critical illness
	• Exclude symptoms of hormone deficiency
	Aplastic anaemia, incl. hepatitis-associated
	• Often without aetiological clues
	• Jaundice suggests hepatitis-associated form (need not be specific hepatitis virus *per se*)
	Congenital causes
	• Presentation in childhood
	• Clinical characteristics include:
	  • skeletal abnormalities and short stature
	  • changes in skin pigmentation

Table 74.1 (*Continued*)

Mechanism	Causative diseases

Increased destruction	Splenic sequestration
	• Due to splenomegaly of any aetiology
	Immune destruction
	• Acute infection – e.g. acute CMV; EBV
	  • Can be complicated by haemolysis, ITP and immune neutropenia, with circulating atypical lymphocytes in peripheral blood concerning for acute leukaemia
	• Evans syndrome
	  • Usually ITP with autoimmune haemolytic anaemia (AIHA), but can have pancytopenia
	Macrophage activating syndrome (MAS)
	• Incl. haemophagocytic lymphohistiocytosis syndrome
	• Umbrella term: persistent fevers, cytopaenias, consumptive coagulopathy, deranged liver function, gross hyperferritinaemia and hypertriglyceridaemia
	• Congenital and acquired forms, incl. triggered by HIV, EBV and CMV; malignancies (e.g. lymphoma); CTD

Complex pathology	HIV infection Hepatitis B and C Paroxysmal nocturnal haemoglobinuria (PNH) • Complement-mediated haemolysis occurring in context of disturbed bone marrow (e.g. aplastic anaemia and myelodysplastic syndrome) • Patients suffer thrombotic events and symptoms of intravascular haemolysis incl. haemoglobinuria Systemic immune disorders (e.g. SLE) Storage disorders

An approach to pancytopenia is suggested in Figure 74.1, where the basic sequence is:

1 Contact the haematologist-on-call, and urgently assess the patient:
   a Are they sick? Is the FBC result in-keeping?
   b Do they have neutropenic fever or neutropenic sepsis (see Figure 74.2)?
   c Consider transfusion:
       i Are they haemorrhagic (n.b. avoid PR exam in neutropenia)?
       ii Have they significant anaemia symptoms?
       iii Recall that some patients require irradiated blood products because they are at risk of transfusion-associated graft vs host disease, a very rare but invariably fatal condition, so any products potentially carrying viable lymphocytes (whole blood, red cells, platelets, granulocytes) must be subject to gamma or X-irradiation (see Table 74.2).

2 Urgently send a targeted group of blood tests, and either in parallel or after stabilisation, comprehensively work up the patient for the cause of their pancytopenia (see Table 74.3).
   a The commonest cause of pancytopenia presenting to acute medical teams is the expected and transient consequence of recently delivered chemotherapy. While this is unlikely to be a diagnostic challenge, there is a significant potential risk to the patient from neutropenic sepsis, which requires prompt recognition and treatment.

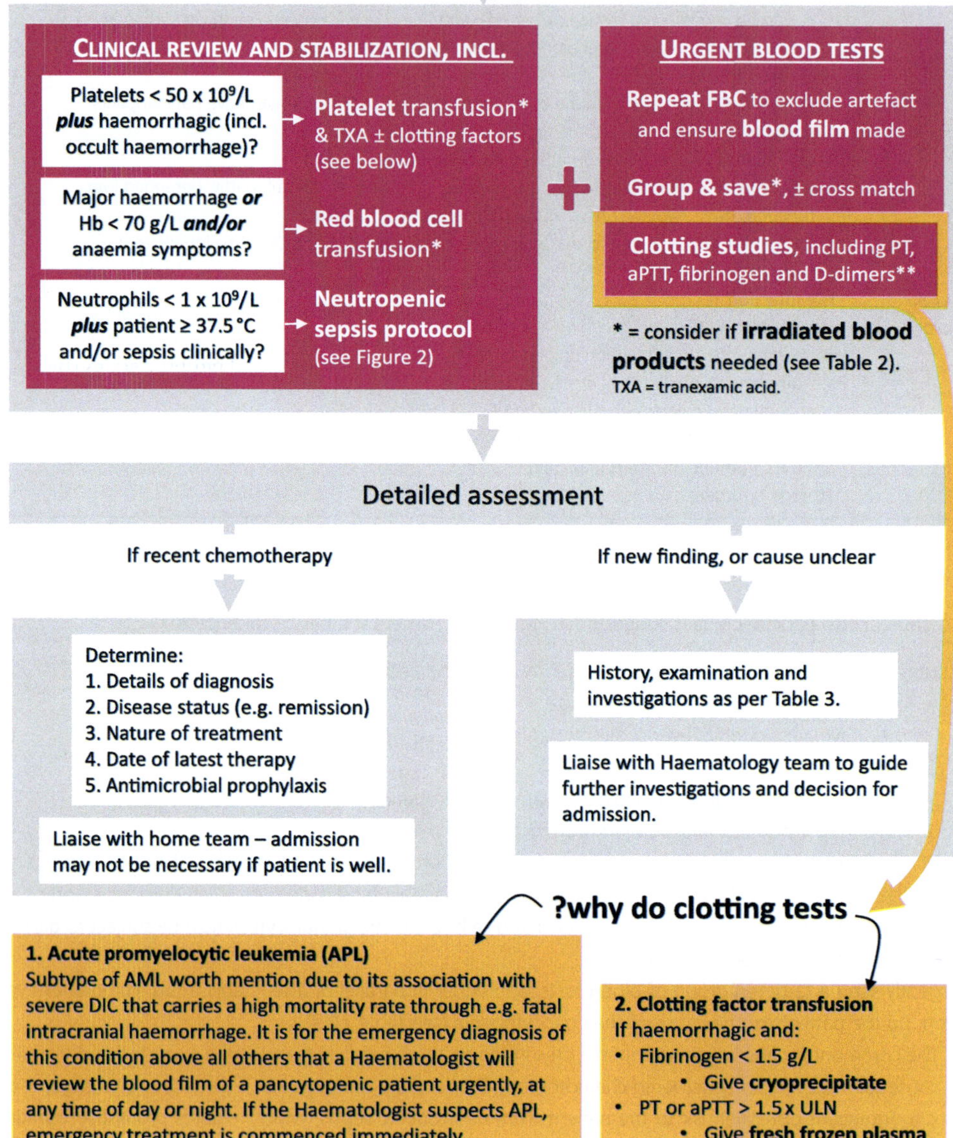

Figure 74.1 Suggested approach to pancytopenia.

Neutropenic sepsis
(see box below)

⬇

Stabilisation with sepsis six

1	Administer oxygen to keep saturations > 94% *Or* 88-92% if at risk of CO_2 retention
2	Take blood cultures • At least peripheral set • CXR and urinalysis for all adults
3	Give IV antibiotics • According to Trust protocol • Beware of allergies
4	Give IV fluids • If low BP/lactate > 2 mmol/L, 500 mL stat
5	Check serial lactates • Corroborate high VBG lactate with arterial sample
6	Measure urine output • Ensure fluid balance chart completed hourly

Liaise with Critical Care where formal organ support deemed likely. Prognosis will be required to inform this discussion, so ensure Haematology or home team involved.

Patients may have PICC or other central lines for chemotherapy administration/ongoing vascular access; all lumens of this line should be cultured, and the line inspected as a possible source of infection.

While searching for sources, recall that *per rectum* examinations are relatively contra-indicated in neutropenic patients.

Neutropenic patients are at risk of **atypical** infections, including *Pseudomanas*. If neutropenia particularly prolonged or profound, **fungal** infections can intercede. Similarly, immunosuppressed patients are at risk of **PCP** and opportunistic **viral** (re)activation.

Take note if a patient is on prophylactic antimicrobial therapy.

Neutropenic sepsis or febrile neutropenia?

Sepsis – *"life-threatening organ dysfunction (e.g. low GCS; high respiratory rate; low systolic BP) caused by a dysregulated host response to infection" (from Sepsis-3) – in the context of neutrophils $<1 \times 10^9$/L. Sepsis need not present with clear infective symptoms, and it should be suspected in all neutropenic patients who are unwell.*

Neutropenic patients may present with fever only (no evidence of organ dysfunction). In the Acute Medical setting, where the trajectory of the acute illness is not yet clear and where neutropenia means these patients are at high risk for deterioration, it is usually preferable to treat as if they had neutropenic sepsis until it is deemed safe to de-escalate therapy.

Figure 74.2 Approach to neutropenic sepsis. Adapted from sepsistrust.org.

Table 74.2 Indications for irradiated blood products. Liaise with haematology and blood bank for advice.

Disorders

Hodgkin lymphoma (even if long-term remission)

T lymphocyte immunodeficiency syndromes

Autologous bone marrow transplant recipients require irradiated products:

• For 7 days prior to harvest

• For 3 months post Day 0 (transplant date) or 6 months if total body irradiation

CAR-T recipients require irradiated products:

• In the 7 days prior to harvest

• For 3 months post CAR-T

(continued)

Table 74.2 (*Continued*)

Allogeneic bone marrow transplant recipients require irradiated products until all of:
- > 6 months have elapsed since Day 0
- Lymphocyte count is >1 × 10^9/L
- Patient does not suffer with active chronic graft vs host disease
- They are not on active immunosuppression

Chemotherapy and immunosuppressive agents

Purine analogues – fludarabine, cladribine, bendamustine, pentostatin, clofarabine

Deoxycoformicin

Alemtuzumab (Campath)

Anti-thymocyte globulin

Table 74.3 Detailed work-up to determine the cause of pancytopenia.

History

Any recent ill-health, especially suggestive of conditions described in Table 74.1

Features of (occult) malignancy – weight loss, fevers, night sweats, focal symptoms

Current and recent medications, incl. over the counter

Past medical history, incl. previous chemotherapy

Occupational history and exposure to toxins (e.g. solvents and pesticides)

Family history of bone marrow failure, anaemia or malignancy

Examination

Features of pancytopenia, incl. pallor; petechiae, bruising and mucosal blood blisters

Features to suggest underlying aetiology (with reference to Table 74.1)
- Palpate for spleen
- Examine for lymphadenopathy in neck, axillae and inguinal regions
- Breast examination

Investigations from peripheral blood

Repeat FBC	• To exclude artefact (e.g. drip, clotted sample)
Reticulocyte count	• Low reticulocyte (marrow failure > consumption)
Blood film	• For morphological diagnostic clues
Group and save	• In case transfusion is required
Direct antiglobulin test	• Positive in AIHA (e.g. Evans syndrome)
Serum B12 and folate	• To exclude remediable deficiencies
Serum ferritin	• Likely elevated in acute infection/inflammation
	• Grossly elevated in haemophagocytic syndrome
LFTs	• For acute hepatitis, EBV and CMV infection
	• Unconjugated hyperbilirubinaemia in haemolysis
LDH	• Typically elevated in:
	• Haemolysis
	• B12 and folate deficiency
	• High-grade lymphoma
	• Hepatitis
PT, APTT, fibrinogen	• To assess for DIC (incl. in APL)
Acute viral serology (EBV, CMV IgM and IgG)	• Potential causes of acute onset pancytopenia
	• Monospot (EBV) quick, but false neg/pos
Chronic viral serology (HIV, Hepatitis B/C)	• Each can cause pancytopenia; recognized association between hepatitis and marrow aplasia
Autoimmune profile	• Rare presentation of SLE, and other CTDs
Lipid profile	• Elevated triglycerides in MAS

Table 74.3 *(Continued)*

Specialty investigations (Liaise with/ performed by haematology)

Bone marrow aspirate	• Morphological assessment (rapid)
	  • Frequently diagnostic but not always
	• Flow cytometry (same day/next day)
	  • Diagnostic, or confirmatory of morphology
	  • Critical for distinguishing, e.g. ALL from AML
	• Genomic (days/weeks)
	  • Molecular and chromosomal studies
	  • Diagnostic and often prognostic

Bone marrow trephine	• Morphological assessment (days)
	  • Information on structure – often critical for lymphoma, fibrosis
	• Immunostaining (days +)
	  • For diagnosis

LFTs, liver function tests; LDH, lactate dehydrogenase; PT, prothrombin time; APTT, activated partial thromboplastin time; EBV, Epstein–Barr virus; CMV, cytomegalovirus; HIV, human immunodeficiency virus; AIHA, autoimmune haemolytic anaemia; DIC, disseminated intravascular coagulation; APL, acute promyelocytic leukaemia; SLE, systemic lupus erythematosus; CTD, connective tissue disorder; ALL, acute lymphoblastic leukaemia; AML, acute myeloid leukaemia.

Further reading

Foukaneli T, Kerr P, PHB B-M, *et al.* (2020) Guideline on the use of irradiated blood components. *Br J Haematol* 191(5), 704–724. *A discussion of the evidence and advice for irradiation of blood products.*

NICE Clinical guideline CG151: neutropenic sepsis: prevention and management in people with cancer. https://www.nice.org.uk/guidance/cg151. *A detailed approach to the managing neutropenic sepsis, including at the system level.*

CHAPTER 75

Fever on return from abroad

NICK BEECHING, MIKE BEADSWORTH, AND STEVE WOOLLEY

The management of the patient with a febrile illness within two months of travel abroad is summarized in Figure 75.1. See Box 75.1 for sources of advice on the diagnosis and management of infectious diseases acquired abroad.

- Malaria must be excluded if there has been travel through an endemic area (most of Africa, Asia, Central and South America). Malaria is the most common single cause of fever requiring admission to hospital after travel to the tropics, accounting for 40–60% of cases from sub-Saharan and West Africa and about 10% from Southeast Asia. Its clinical features are non-specific, and diagnosis requires examination of blood films for parasites, supplemented by rapid diagnostic tests and/or polymerase chain reaction (PCR). Chemoprophylaxis against malaria does not ensure full protection and may prolong the incubation period.
- Other common causes of fever in travellers include respiratory and gastrointestinal infections. Arboviruses such as dengue, chikungunya and Zika virus infections are widespread, and enteric fevers (typhoid and paratyphoid) are common, particularly in Asia and the Indian subcontinent. Tick typhus is common in visitors to Africa.
- For travellers who have returned within 21 days from rural west Africa and central Eurasia (especially Afghanistan and rural Pakistan), a viral haemorrhagic fever must be considered. Isolate the patient and follow local and national protocols for investigation. Seek advice from local infection and public health specialists and consult the national Imported Fever Service in the United Kingdom.
- Consider other causes of febrile illness unrelated to travel, such as influenza, prevailing respiratory infections such as COVID-19, community-acquired pneumonia (Chapter 25) and urinary tract infection (Chapter 72).

Priorities

- Admit to a single room and nurse with standard isolation technique until the diagnosis is established.
- The focused assessment of the patient with fever on return from abroad is given in Table 75.1, and typical incubation periods for selected tropical infections are in Table 75.2.
- Investigations needed urgently are given in Table 75.3.
- Clinical features of malaria and enteric fever are summarized in Tables 75.4 and 75.5.

Further management

This will depend on the clinical syndrome and likely pathogens.

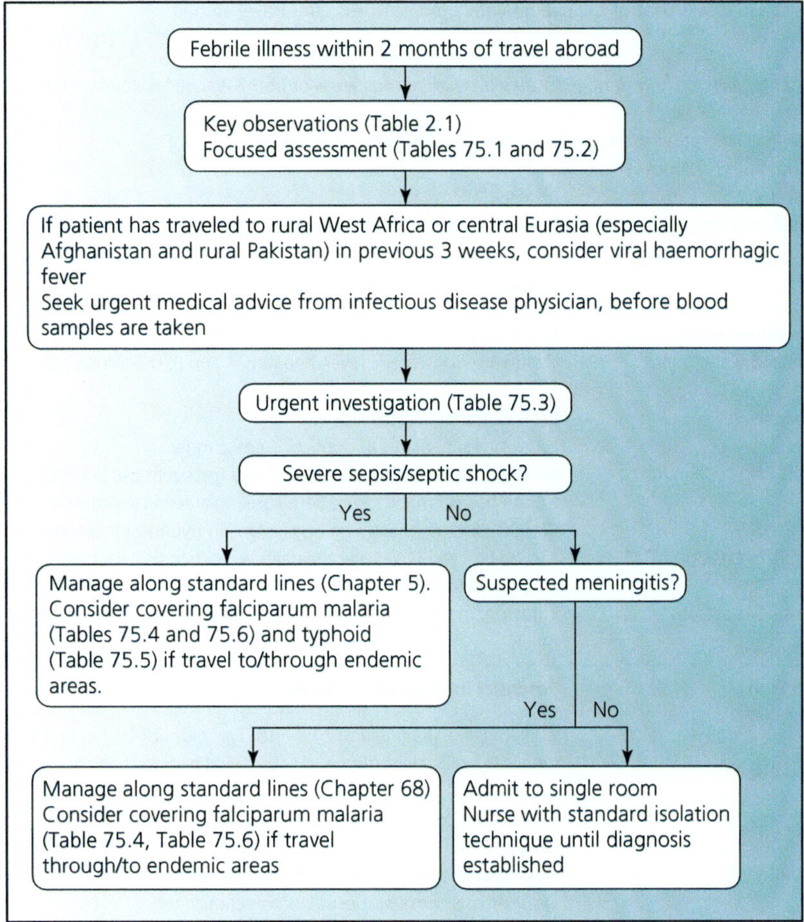

Figure 75.1 Management of the patient with a febrile illness within two months of travel abroad.

Box 75.1 Advice on management of infectious diseases acquired abroad.

Imported Fever Service: 24-h advice on clinical management, diagnostic tests and public health aspects of imported infection. Call the service on 0844 778 8990 after first obtaining advice from local infection specialists (infectious diseases or microbiology). Provides all VHF screening for England and Wales https://www.gov.uk/guidance/imported-fever-service-ifs

National Travel Health Network and Centre (NaTHNaC): detailed pre-travel advice and frequent intelligence reports on outbreaks overseas that may be imported to the United Kingdom http://travelhealthpro.org.uk/

Malaria Guidelines: UK Government website providing access to current UK standards of diagnosis, treatment and prevention of malaria https://www.gov.uk/government/collections/malaria-guidance-data-and-analysis

British Infection Association: publishes numerous guidelines on infection, including imported diseases, with free access to these from https://www.britishinfection.org/guidance/published-guidelines

Table 75.1 Focused assessment of the patient with a febrile illness after travel abroad.

History

Which countries travelled to and through? Travel in urban or rural areas or both? Precise localities and dates essential.

Immunizations before travel

Malaria prophylaxis taken as prescribed? Insect bite avoidance measures taken?

When did symptoms first appear (Table 75.2)?

Treatments taken?

Known or possible occupational or recreational exposure to infection (including sexually transmitted diseases)?

Exposure	Potential infection or disease
Raw or undercooked foods	Enteric infections, hepatitis A and E, trichinosis
Drinking untreated water; milk, cheese	Gastroenteritis, enteric fever, hepatitis A and E, brucellosis, tularaemia
Freshwater swimming	Schistosomiasis, leptospirosis
Sexual contact	HIV, syphilis, hepatitis B, gonococcaemia, mpox
Insect bites	Malaria, chikungunya, dengue and Zika (mosquitoes); tick typhus, Crimean-Congo haemorrhagic fever, borreliosis, tularaemia (ticks); scrub typhus (mites); Chagas' disease (triatomine bugs); African trypanosomiasis (tse tse flies)
Animal exposure or bites	Rabies, brucellosis, Q fever, tularaemia, borreliosis, viral haemorrhagic fevers, plague, MERS CoV
Exposure to infected persons	Influenza, measles, viral hepatitis, viral haemorrhagic fevers, meningococcaemia, mpox

Examination Sign	Potential infection or disease
Rash	Chikungunya, dengue and Zika virus, typhoid, tick-borne, endemic or scrub typhus, syphilis, gonorrhoea, measles, viral haemorrhagic fever, mpox
Jaundice	Hepatitis A, B and E (patients usually afebrile when jaundice appears), malaria, yellow fever, leptospirosis, relapsing fever, cytomegalovirus and Epstein–Barr virus infection
Lymphadenopathy	Rickettsial infections, brucellosis, dengue fever, HIV, tuberculosis, visceral leishmaniasis, toxoplasmosis, EBV infection
Hepatomegaly	Amoebiasis, malaria, typhoid, hepatitis, leptospirosis, most arboviruses
Splenomegaly	Malaria, relapsing fever, trypanosomiasis, typhoid, brucellosis, kala-azar, typhus, chikungunya, dengue and Zika
Eschar (crusted ulcer with black centre and erythematous margin)	Typhus (tick-borne or scrub), borreliosis, Crimean-Congo haemorrhagic fever, cutaneous anthrax (relatively painless oedema as well)
Haemorrhage	Severe dengue; meningococcaemia; epidemic louse-borne typhus; Rocky Mountain spotted fever, viral haemorrhagic fevers

Septic shock

- Initial antimicrobial therapy for patients from endemic regions may need to cover falciparum malaria (Tables 75.4 and 75.6) and enteric fever (Table 75.5). Typhoid, paratyphoid and many other bacterial infections acquired in the tropics are increasingly resistant to many antimicrobials, particularly if the traveller has been in the Middle East or Asia and/or in contact with healthcare settings while travelling. Fluoroquinolone resistance is common in Gram-negative organisms and resistance to cephalosporins and carbapenems is rapidly increasing, so local sepsis treatment policies may not be appropriate and infection specialists should be consulted to advise on empirical treatment until results of cultures and sensitivity patterns become available.

Table 75.2 Indicative incubation periods for selected tropical infections.

Short (<10 days)
Arboviral infections (including chikungunya, dengue and Zika virus)
Enteric bacterial infections
Malaria (minimum six days)
Plague
Scrub typhus, Q fever, spotted fever group, for example tick typhus (louse-borne and flea-borne)
Typhoid and paratyphoid
Viral haemorrhagic fever (VHF) (Lassa, Marburg, Crimean-Congo haemorrhagic fever, Ebola, Rift Valley)

Medium (10–21 days)
African trypanosomiasis
Brucellosis
Leptospirosis
Malaria
Scrub typhus, Q fever, spotted fever group, for example tick typhus
Typhoid and paratyphoid

Long (>21 days)
Amoebic liver abscess
Filariasis
HIV
Malaria
Schistosomiasis (Katayama fever)
Tuberculosis
Viral hepatitis
Visceral leishmaniasis

Table 75.3 Urgent investigation of the patient with a febrile illness after travel abroad.

Full blood count and differential white count
Blood films and rapid diagnostic tests for malarial parasites if travel to or through an endemic area; the intensity of the parasitaemia is variable in malaria. If the diagnosis is suspected but the film and rapid diagnostic test (RDT) or PCR are negative, repeat blood films three times over 24–48 h
Blood culture × 2
C-reactive protein
Blood glucose
Sodium, potassium, urea and creatinine
Liver function tests
Throat swab
Urine stick test, microscopy and culture
Stool microscopy and culture
Serology as appropriate, for example for suspected viral hepatitis, Legionella pneumonia, typhoid, amoebic liver abscess, leptospirosis (save serum initially if diagnosis uncertain)
Chest X-ray and ultrasound liver if clinical suspicion
Lumbar puncture if neck stiffness present (preceded by CT only if indicated) (Chapter 73)

Table 75.4 Falciparum malaria.

Element	Comment
Clinical features	Prodromal symptoms of malaise, headache, myalgia, anorexia and mild fever
	Paroxysms of fever lasting 8–12 h but classical cyclical fever patterns rarely present in early infection
	Dry cough, abdominal discomfort, diarrhoea and vomiting common
	Moderate tender hepatosplenomegaly (without lymphadenopathy)
	Jaundice may occur
Cerebral malaria	Reduced conscious level
	Focal or generalized fits
	Abnormal neurological signs may be present (including opisthotonos, extensor posturing of decorticate or decerebrate pattern, sustained posturing of limbs, conjugate deviation of the eyes, nystagmus, dysconjugate eye movements, bruxism, extensor plantar responses and generalized flaccidity)
	Retinal haemorrhages common (papilloedema may be present but is unusual)
	Abnormal patterns of breathing common (including irregular periods of apnoea and hyperventilation). Tachypnoea may be due to acidosis or adult respiratory distress syndrome
Blood results	Neutropenia
	Thrombocytopenia
	Low pH, raised lactate
	Haemolysis and anaemia
	Hypoxaemia
	Hypoglycaemia
	Renal failure
	Disseminated intravascular coagulation
	Abnormal transaminases
	Hyperbilirubinaemia and sometimes hyperbilirubinuria
Diagnosis	Microscopy of Giemsa-stained thick and thin blood films and rapid diagnostic tests (RDT and/or PCR) for malaria. RDT, PCR and thick films are more sensitive for detection of malaria and the thin film allows species identification and quantification of the percentage of parasitized red cells
Treatment	Supportive management as for severe sepsis; early admission to high dependency or intensive care facility.
	Chemotherapy: see Table 75.6
	Seek advice from an infectious disease or tropical physician
Management of complications	See Table 75.7

Table 75.5 Enteric fever (typhoid and paratyphoid).

Element	Comment
Clinical features	Insidious onset with malaise, headache, myalgia, dry cough, anorexia and fever
	Abdominal pain, distension and tenderness
	Sustained high fever
	Diarrhoea early and late, constipation in mid course of illness. Ileal perforation (due to necrosis of Peyer patch in bowel wall) resulting in peritonitis in ~2%
	Gastrointestinal bleeding (due to erosion of Peyer patch into vessel) in ~15%
	Encephalopathy in ~10%
	Liver and spleen often palpable after the first week
	Erythematous macular rash (rose spots) on upper abdomen and anterior chest (may occur during the second week) in ~25%

Table 75.5 (*Continued*)

Element	Comment
Blood results	Raised white cell count
	Mild thrombocytopenia
	Abnormal liver function tests
Diagnosis	Blood culture positive in 40–80%
	Stool and urine culture positive after the first week
	Laboratory should test isolates for fluoroquinolone resistance (common)
Treatment	Supportive management as for severe sepsis
	Antibiotic therapy with azithromycin or ceftriaxone

Table 75.6 Chemotherapy of falciparum malaria.

Patient seriously ill or unable to take tablets

IV artesunate is treatment of choice, but if not immediately available start with IV quinine. There is no added benefit from giving both agents, but the WHO suggests giving both if there is concern about delayed blood film clearance with artemisinin alone.

Artesunate regimen: 2.4 mg/kg given as an intravenous injection at 0, 12 and 24 h, then daily thereafter. After completion of a minimum of 24 h therapy (maximum five days), a full course of an oral ACT should be taken when the patient can tolerate oral medication.

All patients receiving artesunate or ACT in hospital should have a follow-up full blood count two weeks later for possible anaemia.

OR

IV quinine: loading dose of 20 mg/kg quinine dihydrochloride in 5% dextrose or dextrose saline over 4 h (usual maximum dose 1.4 g), followed by 10 mg/kg (usual maximum 700 mg) every 8 h for first 48 h (or until patient can swallow). Frequency of dosing should be reduced to 12 hourly if intravenous quinine continues for more than 48 h. Omit high loading dose if quinine, quinidine or mefloquine is given within the previous 12 h.

Parenteral quinine therapy should be continued until the patient can take oral therapy, when quinine sulphate 600 mg should be given three times a day to complete five to seven days of quinine in total.

Quinine treatment should always be accompanied by a second drug: doxycycline 200 mg daily (or clindamycin 450 mg three times a day for children or pregnant women), given orally for total of seven days from when the patient can swallow.

Patient not seriously ill and able to swallow tablets

Artemether with lumefantrine (Riamet): if weight is over 35 kg, give four tablets initially, followed by five further doses of four tablets at 8, 24, 36, 48 and 60 h (total 24 tablets over 60 h).

or

Dihydroartemisinin-piperaquine (DHA-PPQ) is another co-artem combination that may be used: if 36–60 kg, 3 tablets daily for 3 days; if >60 kg 4 tablets daily for 3 days. See product literature cautions, especially in patients with cardiac conditions and/or taking agents that prolong QT interval.

or

Atovaquone with proguanil (Malarone) four tablets once daily for three days.

or

Quinine 600 mg of quinine salt 8-hourly PO for 5–7 days, PLUS doxycycline 200 mg daily PO (or clindamycin 450 mg 8-hourly) for 7 days (start these as soon as possible with the quinine).

It is not necessary to give doxycycline or clindamycin with or after treatment with agents other than quinine.

Source: see guidelines in Further References and *British National Formulary*.

Table 75.7 Management of complications of falciparum malaria.

Complication	Management
Hypotension	Transfer to high dependency unit Give IV fluids (weight based) to maintain blood pressure but caution against fluid overload. Maintain adequate oxygenation Start inotropic vasopressor therapy if systolic BP remains <90 mmHg despite fluids (Chapter 2) Start antibiotic therapy for possible coexistent Gram-negative sepsis after taking blood cultures (Chapter 5)
Hypoglycaemia	This is a common complication Blood glucose should be checked 4-hourly, or 2-hourly while on IV quinine, or whenever conscious level deteriorates or if seizures occur If blood glucose is <4 mmol/L, give 100 mL of glucose 20% IV and start an IV infusion of glucose 10% (initially 1 L 12-hourly) via a large peripheral or central vein
Seizures	Recheck blood glucose Manage along standard lines (Chapter 57) Exclude coexistent bacterial meningitis by CSF examination (NB lumbar puncture should not be done within 1 h of a major seizure)
Pulmonary oedema	May occur from excessive IV fluid or ARDS Manage along standard lines (Chapter 14)
Renal failure and acidosis	Haemofiltration may be needed for renal failure or control of acidosis or fluid/electrolyte imbalance
Anaemia and thrombocytopenia	Both improve after several days of malaria chemotherapy. Anaemia is haemolytic and transfusion is only required for severe symptomatic anaemia. Thrombocytopenia is common and may be profound but platelet transfusions are not usually indicated

ARDS, acute respiratory distress syndrome; CSF, cerebrospinal fluid.

- Empirical treatment for suspected enteric fever or gastroenteritis severe enough to merit antimicrobials is currently with azithromycin or ceftriaxone for severe enteric fever.
- Patients with severe falciparum malaria and hypotension should also receive antimicrobial therapy to cover Gram-negative infection, as mixed infections may occur. See Chapter 5 for the management of sepsis and septic shock.
- If malaria has been excluded and leptospirosis and/or rickettsial infection are possible diagnoses, doxycycline should be included early in empirical therapy.

Chest X-ray shadowing

Consider pulmonary tuberculosis, COVID-19, SARS, MERS CoV, and Legionnaires' disease, in addition to the common causes of community-acquired pneumonia (Chapter 25).

Meningism

- See Chapter 73 for the management of suspected bacterial meningitis and encephalitis.
- Perform a lumbar puncture, preceded by CT only if indicated.
- If the CSF shows no organisms but a high lymphocyte count, consider tuberculous meningitis (Appendix 73.1), leptospirosis or brucellosis.
- If there are other features suggesting leptospirosis (haemorrhagic rash, conjunctivitis, renal failure and jaundice), give ceftriaxone, benzyl penicillin or doxycycline.

Jaundice

- See Chapter 35 for the assessment of the patient with acute jaundice.
- Always consider falciparum malaria. Others causes are viral hepatitis A, B and E (but with these infections patients are usually afebrile when jaundice appears), leptospirosis, cytomegalovirus and Epstein–Barr virus infection, in addition to non-infectious causes, including drug and alcohol toxicity.

Diarrhoea

- See Chapter 34 for the management of the patient with acute diarrhoea.
- Causes to consider following recent travel abroad are given in Table 34.5.

Eosinophilia

The presence of eosinophilia in association with fever in returned travellers usually indicates an invasive helminth infection, but exclude other causes, especially atopy and drug reactions. Causes include filariasis (clues nocturnal or diurnal fever pattern); early phase of strongyloides and hookworm infections (abdominal pain and diarrhoea); hookworm and roundworm pneumonitis (cough and wheeze); early schistosomiasis (freshwater exposure especially in Africa/Middle East, urticarial rash, wheeze and altered semen); and loiasis (travel to Africa, transient peripheral skin swellings). Seek expert advice on special investigations needed.

Further reading

Centers for Disease Control and Prevention Traveler's health. https://www.cdc.gov/.

Eckerle I, Briciu VT, Ergönül Ö, *et al.* (2018) Emerging souvenirs – clinical presentation of the returning traveller with imported arbovirus infections in Europe. *Clin Microbiol Infect* 24, 240–245.

Fink D, Wano RD, Johnston V. (2018) Fever in the returning traveller. *BMJ* 360, 158–161.

Johnston V, Stockley JM, Dockrell D, *et al.* (2009) Fever in returned travellers presenting in the United Kingdom: recommendations for investigation and initial management. *J Infect* 59, 1–18.

Lalloo DG, Shingadia D, Bell DJ, *et al.* (2016) UK malaria treatment guidelines. *J Infect* 72, 635–649.

Nabarro LE, McCann N, Herdman MT, *et al.* (2022) British Infection Association guidelines for the diagnosis and management of enteric fever in England. *J Infect* 84, 469–489.

Thakker C, Warrell C, Barrett J, *et al.* (2024) UK guidelines for the investigation and management of eosinophilia in returning travellers and migrants. *J Infect, on-line ahead of print, article* 106328.

Thwaites GE, Day NP. (2017) Approach to fever in the returning traveler. *N Engl J Med* 376, 548–560.

CHAPTER 76

Pyrexia of unknown origin

STEPHEN WOOLLEY, MIKE BEADSWORTH, AND NICK BEECHING

Pyrexia of unknown origin (PUO) was defined over 60 years ago as an illness lasting for three weeks or more, with fever greater than 38.3 °C (101 °F) on several occasions, the cause of which remained uncertain after a week of investigation in hospital. The investigation period has been reduced to three days in hospital or 3 clinic appointments. Subgroups have been suggested according to patient status or situation, including nosocomial, neutropenic, HIV-related and children or seniors (65 or over). Over 200 causes of PUO have been described, broadly categorized as infectious, inflammatory, neoplastic or miscellaneous (Tables 76.1 and 76.2). The prominence of each aetiological category varies with host status, geography, and access to sophisticated investigations; no cause is found in 25–50% of cases despite extensive investigation.

A structured, stepwise approach to diagnosis is mandatory. Patients should be involved early in related decision-making so that they understand that this aims to minimise unnecessary investigations and reduce the likelihood of following diagnostic 'red herrings'. A thorough history and physical examination should be repeated at regular intervals. Irrespective of age, the history should include possible occupational, recreational or other exposures to potential pathogens, animals and toxins; illness in family or contacts; sexual history; and health care contacts (operations, IV lines etc) in the preceding 6 months. A detailed drug history should cover prescribed and over the counter medications, traditional and 'natural' remedies and recreational drugs. A full travel history should be obtained (see Chapter 75).

A detailed multi-system examination should cover often neglected areas such as the ears, throat, mouth including dentition, temporal arteries and fundoscopy. It is important to exclude back tenderness and to consider pelvic and rectal examinations including the prostate in men. If the patient has implanted material such as prosthetic joints, pacemakers, in-dwelling vascular devices, shunts, grafts or meshes, possible implant infection should be considered. Body temperature should be measured and recorded by health care workers rather than by the patient, using the same method each time.

All patients should have a standard set of basic investigations, some of which might be repeated to observe trends (Table 76.3). In addition, focal symptoms and/or physical signs may provide clues to prompt focussed organ- or system-oriented investigations. These can broadly be aimed at detection of infection (Table 76.4) or other causes (Table 76.5). If this first round of investigation yields a likely cause, this can be investigated and managed in detail.

However, if there is no obvious focus or cause identified after reviewing the above and repeated history taking and physical examination, whole body imaging should be considered. Over the past decade 2-deoxy-2-^{18}F-fluoro-D-glucose (^{18}F-FDG) positron emission tomography with CT (PET-CT) scans have become more accessible. These have better positive and negative diagnostic yields than most other scan combinations to identify physical targets for further investigation by e.g. biopsy, or generalized conditions such as large vessel inflammation. Early use of PET-CT, rather than delaying it until after whole body CT with contrast, is likely to reduce the length of hospital stay and/or number of clinic visits, the number of investigations and the

Acute Medicine: A Practical Guide to the Management of Medical Emergencies, Sixth Edition.
Edited by Mridula Rajwani, Leila Vaziri, and Ivie Gbinigie.
© 2026 John Wiley & Sons Ltd. Published 2026 by John Wiley & Sons Ltd.

Table 76.1 Infective causes of PUO in alphabetical order within each category.

Immunocompetent	Immunocompromised
Atypical bacterial infections such as bartonellosis, brucellosis, Q fever	• **Bacterial** including non-typhoidal salmonellosis, melioidosis, syphilis, non-tuberculous mycobacteria, tuberculosis.
Infective endocarditis	• **Viral-** arboviruses, CMV, EBV, HIV seroconversion, parvovirus.
Discitis	• **Fungal-** aspergillosis, candidiasis, cryptococcosis, endemic dimorphic mycoses and histoplasmosis.
Infected implantable devices/prosthetic material	• **Parasitic-** visceral leishmaniasis
Malaria	• Immune reconstitution inflammatory syndromes (IRIS).
Occult abscesses	
Osteomyelitis	
Prostatitis	
Syphilis	
Tuberculosis	
Viral e.g. prolonged primary CMV	

CMV, Cytomegalovirus; EBV, Epstein-Barr virus.

Table 76.2 Non-infective causes of PUO in alphabetical order within each category.

Rheumatological/Inflammatory
Behçet's disease
Familial Mediterranean fever
Felty's syndrome
Giant cell arteritis and temporal arteritis
Gout and pseudogout
Granulomatosis with polyangiitis
Polyarteritis nodosa
Polymyositis
Rheumatoid arthritis
Sarcoidosis
Still's disease
Systemic lupus erythematosus
Takayasu's arteritis

Solid Organ Malignancies
Atrial myxoma
Colonic cancer
Hepatic carcinoma
Metastatic disease
Pancreatic cancer
Renal cell carcinoma

Haematological malignancies
Leukaemia
Lymphoma
Multiple myeloma
Myeloproliferative disorders

Miscellaneous
Drug fever
Factitious fever
Hypoadrenalism
Hypothalamic dysfunction
Inflammatory bowel disease
Thyroiditis

Table 76.3 Baseline investigations for PUO in all patients.

Urinalysis (and culture if any abnormality)
Full blood count with white cell differential
C-reactive protein (CRP)
Erythrocyte sedimentation rate (ESR)
Serum biochemistry: renal, liver and bone profiles, creatinine kinase
Serum ferritin
Chest imaging (CXR or CT)
Ultrasound of abdomen
At least 2 peripheral blood cultures
HIV test
Tuberculin test or IGRA

Table 76.4 Second line investigations for possible infective aetiology.

Infective cause diagnostics	
Microbiology	**Radiology/other imaging modalities**
Blood cultures (including paired peripheral and line cultures if an intravascular device is in situ)	CT-neck/thorax/abdomen and pelvis
	Echocardiogram including TOE
Lumbar puncture- opening pressure, CSF protein, CSF glucose [paired with serum], CSF lactate, microbiological culture and virology PCRs	MRI head and/or spine
	OGD +/− biopsies
Malaria screen (RDT and 3 malaria films over 3 consecutive days and if negative consider malaria PCR)	PET-CT
Lymph node biopsy (culture including mycobacterial culture and histology)	
Serology and molecular tests dependent on risk factors and travel history- all should have HIV serology, consider HBV and HCV	
Sputum for culture- fungal, mycobacterial and virology testing as required	
Stool samples for culture, PCR and OCP	
Urine culture +/− 3 consecutive early morning urines to exclude tuberculosis	
Wound cultures	

CSF, cerebrospinal fluid; CT, computed tomography; MRI, magnetic resonance imaging; OCP, ova, cysts and parasites; OGD, oesophago-gastro-duodenoscopy; PCR-polymerase chain reaction; PET-CT, positron emission tomography-computed tomography; RDT, rapid detection test; TOE, transoesophageal echocardiogram.

amount of radiation exposure for patients. Disadvantages include the need for pre imaging fasting, loss of diagnostic sensitivity if the patient is taking steroids, and inequity of access to scans in different hospitals or regions.

If the above sequence does not provide an obvious cause, a pause for observation is usually appropriate. Revisit the history often and rule out factitious (self-induced) fever and drug induced fever. Drug-fever typically starts 7–10 days after commencing a new therapeutic. It is unlikely to be a cause if the fever persists 96-hours after stopping the drug; typical culprits include antimicrobials, non-steroidal anti-inflammatory agents, anti-arrhythmics, anti-convulsants and anti-depressants. If no diagnosis can be made, the patient can be reassured that the outcome is likely to be benign, even if minor symptoms persist for some months. Patients with a normal PET-CT are six times more likely to have a benign outcome.

Avoid the temptation to prescribe empirical antimicrobials, non-steroidal anti-inflammatories or steroids unless there is a strong suspicion of immediate threat to life by conditions such as large vessel vasculitis, miliary tuberculosis, infective endocarditis or sepsis. Common pitfalls and good practice points are summarised in Table 76.6.

Table 76.5 Second line investigations for possible non-infective aetiology.

Non-infective causes	
Rheumatological/Inflammatory/Other	**Neoplastic/Other**
Antibodies- ANA (+/− anti-Ro/La/Sm, dsDNA, histone, SCL-70, centromere), ACA, ANCA, anti-CCP, autoimmune thyroid antibodies (thyroglobulin, peroxidase, TSH-receptor stimulating Ab), rheumatoid factor Biochemistry- complement C3/C4 levels, cryoglobulins, ferritin, immunoglobulins, joint aspiration for crystals, LDH, pituitary screen, serum ACE, serum electrophoresis, serum urate, synacthen test, thyroid function tests, urine for BJP Histology- temporal artery biopsy Radiology- angiography (CT or MRI), CT-neck/thorax/abdomen/pelvis, CT-PET	Biochemistry- calcium, electrophoresis, LDH, urine for BJP Histology- bone marrow trephine, lymph node tissue Imaging- colonoscopy, CT-neck/thorax/abdomen/pelvis, echocardiogram, OGD, PET/CT

ACA, anti-cardiolipin antibody; ACE, angiotensin converting-enzyme; ANA, antinuclear antibody; ANCA, antineutrophil cytoplasmic antibody; BJP, Bence-Jones protein; CCP, cyclic citrullinated peptide; CT, computed tomography; dsDNA, double-stranded deoxyribonucleic acid; LDH, lactose dehydrogenate; MRI, magnetic resonance imaging; OGD, oesophago-gastro-duodenoscopy; PET-CT, positron emission tomography-computed tomography; TSH, thyroid-stimulating hormone.

Table 76.6 Common pitfalls and good practice points.

Take an adequate history and examine the patient fully.
Return to the patient's history and examination at regular intervals.
Consider non-infectious causes of fever early in the patient's journey.
Consider:
- discitis in a patient with back pain/tenderness
- empyema in slowly resolving pneumonia
- peritonitis in a patient with ascites
- tuberculosis in a patient with sterile pyuria
- endocarditis in patients with 'skin commensals' in blood cultures (including coagulase negative staphylococci)
- chronic prostatitis in men with lower urinary tract symptoms

All patients should have an HIV test.
Do not perform multiple serological testing if there is no history of exposure to the pathogen you are testing for, or other related diagnostic clues.
Malaria can present up to 2 years after leaving an endemic area.
Tuberculin skin test and TB IGRA tests are often negative in disseminated mycobacterial disease. A negative result does not rule out the diagnosis; a positive test is not diagnostic for TB – microbiological confirmation is required.
Avoid inappropriately enthusiastic investigation. Treat the individual rather than the symptoms.
Avoid early initiation of empirical antimicrobials or steroids.
Look for a further diagnosis if fever persists after treatment for the first diagnosis considered.

Further reading

Fernandez C, Beeching NJ. (2018) Pyrexia of unknown origin. *Clin Med (Lond)* 18(2), 170–174.
Haidar G, Singh N. (2022) Fever of unknown origin. *NEJM* 386(5), 463–477.
Wright WF, Kandish S, Brady R, *et al.* (2024) Nuclear medicine imaging tools in fever of unknown origin: time for a revisit and appropriate use criteria. *Clin Infect Dis* 78, 1148–1153.
Yates GP, Feldman MD. (2016) Factitious disorder: a systematic review of 455 cases in the professional literature. *Gen Hosp Psychiatry* 41, 20–28.

CHAPTER 77

HIV infection

MAS CHAPONDA AND NICK BEECHING

People living with human immunodeficiency virus (PLHIV) get common diseases as well as those that reflect their immune deficiency. The spectrum of HIV infection is summarized in Box 77.1.

Box 77.1 Spectrum of HIV infection.

Group 1	Acute infection or primary HIV infection (a mononucleosis-like syndrome associated with sero-conversion)
Group 2	Asymptomatic infection
Group 3	Symptomatic disease
Group 4	Advanced disease: CD4+T cell count <200 × 10⁶/L

Constitutional disease (e.g. fever, weight loss, diarrhoea)
Neurological disease (HIV encephalopathy, progressive multifocal leucoencephalopathy)
Other conditions (thrombocytopenia, non-specific interstitial pneumonitis)
Opportunistic infections:
- Pneumocystis: pneumonia
- Cytomegalovirus: chorioretinitis, colitis, pneumonitis or oesophagitis
- *Candida albicans*: oral thrush, oesophagitis
- *Mycobacterium avium* complex: localized or disseminated infection
- *Mycobacterium tuberculosis:* localized or disseminated infection
- *Cryptococcus neoformans*: meningitis or disseminated infection
- *Toxoplasma gondii*: encephalitis or intracerebral mass lesions
- Herpes simplex virus: severe mucocutaneous lesions, oesophagitis
- *Cryptosporidium* spp.: diarrhoea
- *Cystoisospora belli*: diarrhoea
- EBV: oral hairy leukoplakia

Neoplasms:
- Kaposi's sarcoma (cutaneous and visceral)
- Lymphoma (brain, bone marrow, pleura, lung and gut).

Acute Medicine: A Practical Guide to the Management of Medical Emergencies, Sixth Edition.
Edited by Mridula Rajwani, Leila Vaziri, and Ivie Gbinigie.

- Establish from the patient who else knows about the HIV diagnosis among the patient's relatives and friends: be sensitive to their needs and respect the patient's right to confidentiality.
- Take appropriate safety precautions when handling body fluids and label specimens according to local policies.
- The management of acute medical problems in the patient with HIV/AIDS is often complex, and you should seek advice from an infectious disease (ID) physician early on.

Breathlessness

Pulmonary infection (especially *Pneumocystis jirovecii* pneumonia) remains the most common acute presentation in HIV-positive patients. Other causes to consider are given in Table 77.1. Management is summarized in Figure 77.1.

1 Attach a pulse oximeter and check arterial blood gases: the patient may be severely hypoxaemic with minimal lung signs. Give oxygen to maintain arterial oxygen saturation >90%. Investigations needed urgently are given in Table 77.2.
2 Your clinical assessment and the chest X-ray appearance may provide clues to the likely diagnosis (Table 77.3).
   - Dual pathology is relatively frequent, and definitive diagnosis depends on microbiological findings.
   - A high-resolution CT of the thorax may be helpful in establishing a diagnosis.
   - Examination of induced sputum and/or bronchoscopic alveolar lavage fluid is often helpful in making a diagnosis.
   - Initial treatment for suspected *P. jirovecii* pneumonia (PCP) is given in Table 77.4.
   - Seek advice from a chest physician and ID physician on further management.

Table 77.1 Respiratory symptoms in the HIV-positive patient.

CD4 cell count (×10⁶/L)		
>500	**200–500**	**<200**
Usual causes	Usual causes especially pneumococcal pneumonia	Usual causes
Mycobacterium tuberculosis infection	*M. tuberculosis* infection	*Pneumocystis jirovecii* pneumonia
		M. tuberculosis infection
		Mycobacterium avium complex infection
		Cytomegalovirus pneumonitis
		Fungal pneumonia
		Kaposi's sarcoma

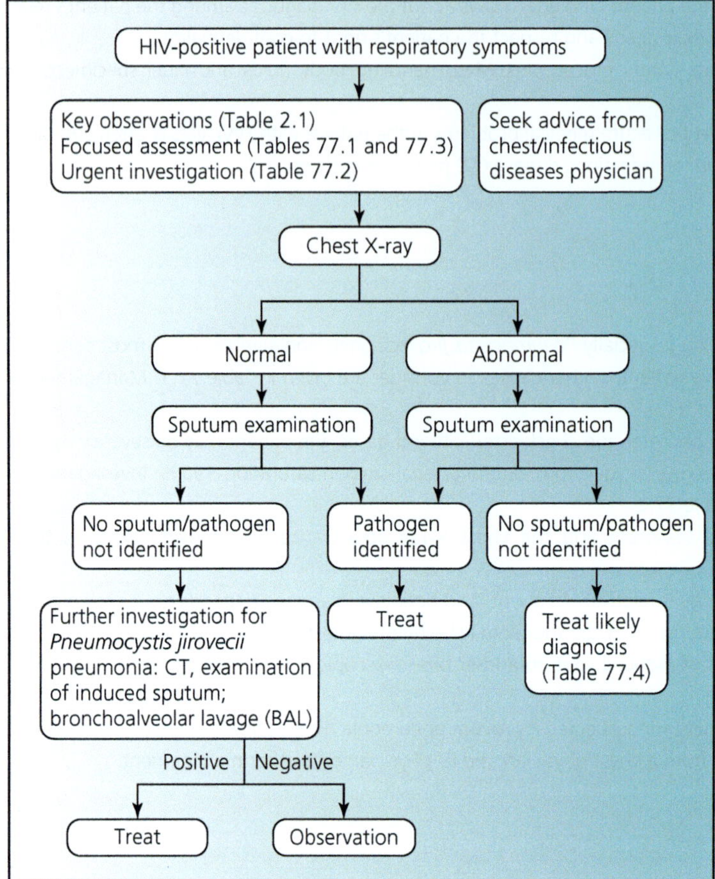

Figure 77.1 Assessment and management of the HIV-positive patient with respiratory symptoms.

Table 77.2 Urgent investigation of the HIV-positive patient with respiratory symptoms.

Chest X-ray

Arterial blood gases and pH and lactate

Full blood count and differential white count

CD4 cell count and HIV viral load

Blood culture (positive in most patients with *M. avium* complex infection: use specific mycobacterial culture bottles)

Blood G6PD level

Sodium and potassium, urea and creatinine

Liver function tests

Lactate dehydrogenase (raised in *P. jirovecii* pneumonia and lymphoma)

Expectorated sputum if available for Gram and Ziehl–Neelsen stains, TB PCR and culture

Induced sputum (using hypertonic saline via nebulizer) for staining or PCR for *P. jirovecii* and mycobacterial stains and culture

High-resolution CT scan of thorax

Consider fibreoptic bronchoscopy (for bronchoalveolar lavage or transbronchial biopsy)

Table 77.3 Diagnostic clues in the HIV-positive patient with respiratory symptoms.

Diagnosis	Clinical features	Chest X-ray features
Pneumocystis jirovecii pneumonia (PCP)	Dyspnoea, often of slow onset Dry cough Lungs clear, or sparse basal crackles Fever See Table 77.4	Perihilar haze: diffuse bilateral interstitial or alveolar shadowing Lobar consolidation rare Pleural effusion rare Pneumothorax may occur See Table 77.4
M. tuberculosis infection	Cough, fever, haemoptysis, weight loss, night sweats	More often typical of tuberculosis if CD4 cell count is >200 × 10^6/L: multiple areas of consolidation, often with cavitation, in one or both upper lobes
M. avium complex infection	Cough, dyspnoea, fever	Often normal, fibro-cavitary or nodular bronchiectatic changes
Bacterial pneumonia (Chapter 25)	Commoner in smokers Productive cough Focal signs, fever	Focal consolidation
Cytomegalovirus pneumonitis	Clinically indistinguishable from PCP (dual infection may occur)	Diffuse bilateral interstitial shadowing
Fungal pneumonia	Fever, cough, weight loss Systemic features of fungal infection may be present (skin lesions, lymphadenopathy and hepatosplenomegaly)	Diffuse bilateral interstitial shadowing in ~50% Focal shadowing, nodules, cavities, pleural effusion and hilar adenopathy may be seen
Kaposi's sarcoma	No fever Dyspnoea May be associated with cutaneous Kaposi's sarcoma	Diffuse bilateral interstitial shadowing, more nodular than PCP May be unilateral and associated with hilar adenopathy Pleural effusion strongly suggestive

Neuro-ophthalmic problems

With improved PCP prophylaxis, HIV-positive patients are presenting more frequently with neuro-ophthalmic problems (Table 77.5).

Delirium with or without headache (see also Chapters 53 and 69)

Consider toxoplasmosis, cryptococcal meningitis (Chapter 73), cerebral lymphoma and progressive multifocal leucoencephalopathy. HIV encephalopathy is diagnosed by exclusion of other causes.

- Arrange an urgent CT scan of the brain with contrast or MRI.
- Perform a lumbar puncture (LP) if the scan is normal. Send CSF for cell count and differential; protein concentration; glucose (together with blood glucose taken at same time); Gram, Ziehl–Neelsen and India ink stains; TB PCR, culture and syphilis tests. Request specific tests for *Cryptococcus* spp., *Toxoplasma gondii* and mycobacteria.
- If no specific diagnosis can be made, consider giving empirical treatment for toxoplasmosis with pyrimethamine and sulphadiazine, and repeat the scan after 2–3 weeks.
- Seek advice from an ID physician and neurologist.

Table 77.4 *Pneumocystis jirovecii* pneumonia (PCP): diagnosis and management.

Element	Comment
Patients at risk	Newly diagnosed HIV infection with advanced disease (CD4 cell count $<200 \times 10^6$/L) Patients with previous PCP or CD4 cell count $<200 \times 10^6$/L, who are not taking prophylaxis
Clinical features	Subacute onset Fever ($\sim$90%) Cough ($\sim$95%), usually non-productive Progressive breathlessness ($\sim$95%) Tachypnoea ($\sim$60%) Chest examination normal in $\sim$50%
Chest X-ray features	Initially normal in up to 25% Commonest abnormalities are diffuse bilateral interstitial or alveolar shadowing Lobar consolidation and pleural effusion: rare. Pneumothorax may occur
CT scan features	Extensive ground glass infiltrates. Spontaneous pneumothorax and an upper lobe distribution of parenchymal opacities
Induced sputum	Staining of induced sputum for *P. jirovecii* trophic forms and cysts Specificity $\sim$100%, sensitivity 50–90% PCR Sensitivity 98%, specificity 80–98%
Bronchoscopy with bronchoalveolar lavage	Indicated if PCP or TB is suspected if induced sputum is non-diagnostic or cannot be done Specificity $\sim$100%, sensitivity $\sim$80–90%
Antimicrobial therapy	First choice: co-trimoxazole PO or IV for 21 days. Causes haemolysis in some G6PD-deficient patients (African/Mediterranean). Other side effects include nausea, vomiting, fever, rash, marrow suppression and raised transaminases Alternative regimens: primaquine + clindamycin; atovaquone; pentamidine
Adjuvant steroid therapy	Start immediately if severe PCP (breathless at rest; PaO_2 breathing air <8 kPa; extensive interstitial shadowing on chest X-ray) Give prednisolone 40 mg twice daily PO for 5 days, followed by prednisolone 40 mg daily PO for 5 days, then prednisolone 20 mg daily PO for 11 days

Table 77.5 Headache/delirium/focal neurological signs in the HIV-positive patient.

CD4 cell count ($\times 10^6$/L)		
>500	**200–500**	**<200**
Usual causes (see also Chapters 53 and 69)	Usual causes HIV encephalopathy Tuberculous meningitis (Chapter 73)	Usual causes Primary CNS lymphoma Tuberculous meningitis (Chapter 73) Toxoplasmosis Cryptococcal meningitis (Chapter 73) Progressive multifocal leucoencephalopathy

Focal upper motor neurone signs

- Consider toxoplasmosis or lymphoma.
- Arrange an urgent cranial CT scan of the brain with contrast or MR scan.
- Perform an LP if the scan is normal and send CSF for investigation as above.

- If focal lesions (ring-enhancing, with surrounding oedema on CT), treat as toxoplasmosis.
- Seek advice from an ID physician and neurologist.
- Consider stereotactic biopsy.

Impaired vision (see also Chapter 54)

Ophthalmic complications are more likely in advanced HIV and CD4 cell count $<50 \times 10^6$/L, particularly cytomegalovirus (CMV) retinitis and toxoplasmosis. Syphilis and tuberculosis may also affect the eye and can occur at any CD4 cell count.

Suspect CMV retinitis: fundoscopy shows characteristic infiltrates, similar in appearance to soft exudates; or confluent areas of retinal necrosis with haemorrhages in posterior pole ('pizza' or 'cottage cheese with ketchup' appearance); or marked vascular sheathing ('frosted branch angiitis').
- Seek advice from an ophthalmologist.
- Treatment is with ganciclovir (or cidofovir or foscarnet if ganciclovir is contraindicated; both are nephrotoxic). Ganciclovir and its oral form valganciclovir can cause severe marrow depression which must be monitored.

Acute diarrhoea

See Chapter 34 for the assessment and management of the patient with acute diarrhoea.

Establish the differential diagnosis from the history and examination (Table 34.1). Strict infection control protocols must be followed (including barrier nursing and handwashing). Investigations needed urgently are given in Table 34.2.
- Features of community-acquired infective diarrhoea are given in Table 34.3 and hospital-acquired diarrhoea in Table 34.4.
- Pathogens to consider in the patient with a low CD4 cell count are given in Table 77.6.
- Seek advice from an ID physician and gastroenterologist.

Table 77.6 Chronic diarrhoea in the HIV-positive patient: specific pathogens to consider.

Cause	Clinical features	Diagnosis/treatment
Cryptosporidiosis (*Cryptosporidium* species)	Subacute onset Associated abdominal pain Severe diarrhoea	Identification of oocysts in stool Seek expert advice on treatment
Cystoisosporiasis (*Cystoisospora belli*)	Incubation period one week Associated fever, abdominal pain, diarrhoea with fatty stools	Identification of oocysts in stool, duodenal aspirate or jejunal biopsy Seek expert advice on treatment
Cytomegalovirus (CMV)	Diarrhoea may be accompanied by systemic illness and hepatitis	Serology and/or blood PCR for CMV; consider large bowel endoscopy and biopsy Seek expert advice on management
Mycobacterium avium complex (MAC)	Chronic diarrhoea, abdominal pain, persistent fever, weight loss and progressive wasting	Endoscopic biopsy and culture; blood culture also useful as MAC often grows within 10 days Seek expert advice on treatment

Source: in addition to other causes: see Chapter 34.

Further reading

British Association for Sexual Health and HIV Guidelines. https://www.bashh.org/guidelines.
British HIV Association (BHIVA) Guidelines. http://www.bhiva.org/guidelines.aspx.
European AIDS Clinical Society Guidelines. Version 12.1. November 2024. www.eacs.sanfordguide.com.
Maartens G, Celum C, Lewin SR. (2014) HIV infection: epidemiology, pathogenesis, treatment and prevention. *Lancet* 384, 258–271.
Panel on Guidelines for the Prevention and Treatment of Opportunistic Infections in Adults and Adolescents with HIV. Guidelines for the prevention and treatment of opportunistic infections in adults and adolescents with HIV. National Institutes of Health, Centers for Disease Control and Prevention, HIV Medicine Association, and Infectious Diseases Society of America. https://clinicalinfo.hiv.gov/en/guidelines/adult-and-adolescent-opportunistic-infection. [updated regularly in real time].
World Health Organization Consolidated guidelines on HIV, viral hepatitis and STI prevention, diagnosis, treatment and care for key populations. Last Updated: July 2022. https://www.who.int/publications/i/item/9789240052390.

CHAPTER 78

COVID-19 and future pandemics

ROBERT H. SHAW AND MAHESHI N. RAMASAMY

The management of severe acute respiratory syndrome coronavirus 2 (SARS-CoV2) infection, in terms of intervention, supportive measures and infection control measures has changed hugely since the start of the coronavirus infectious diseases 2019 (COVID-19) pandemic in December 2019 and continues to change still. Many of the lessons learnt during the pandemic will be applicable to similar situations in the future.

SARS-CoV2 is a novel coronavirus that causes a spectrum of disease from asymptomatic infection to mild symptomatic upper respiratory tract infection through to severe inflammatory lung disease (COVID-19). Estimates for the infection fatality rate vary, but in the setting of a high-income country, such as the United Kingdom, this was about 1% in an unvaccinated population. The high levels of transmission meant that this mortality rate translated into large absolute numbers requiring hospital care, either overwhelming or threatening to overwhelm healthcare services. The possibility of healthcare services saturation risked an increase in preventable mortality and so public health measures were employed to 'flatten the pandemic curve'.

Throughout the pandemic, there were waves of infection, which appeared to be driven mostly by a change in the predominant circulating variant. The changes in variant affected transmission rates, severity of disease as well as the syndrome that people experienced. However, all these were confounded by changes in public health measures and social distancing as well as the fact that progressively more of the population had developed immunity against the virus either through natural exposure or through immunization, once it become available.

The challenge with writing about SARS-CoV2 management is that it has changed radically and will continue to do so. Some of the public health and infection prevention and control (IPC) measures were specific to certain points in the pandemic, driven by transmission rates, healthcare capacity, new variants, seropositivity rates in the population and immunization roll out.

The next pandemic, when it arrives, will be different. We will need to take the general principles learned from this pandemic and apply them to the next.

History

History	Detail expansion
Symptoms	See below
Duration of symptoms	Timing of inflammatory deterioration
SARS-CoV2 exposure history	Pre-test likelihood of being positive and therefore cohorting decisions
Vaccination/Previous SARS-CoV2 infection history	Serostatus and the risk of developing inflammation in the lungs
Immunocompromise	Risk of deterioration despite vaccination
	Which immunomodulatory treatments may be of benefit

Acute Medicine: A Practical Guide to the Management of Medical Emergencies, Sixth Edition.
Edited by Mridula Rajwani, Leila Vaziri, and Ivie Gbinigie.

SARS-CoV2 syndrome

Cardinal symptoms*	Continuous cough, fever and change/reduction in sense of smell/taste (often in the absence of nasal congestion or rhinorrhoea)
Other associated symptoms and signs	Shortness of breath, fatigue, myalgia, headache, sore throat, nasal congestion, rhinorrhoea, diarrhoea, nausea, low oxygen saturations

*Different variants appear to have slight differences in prominence of different symptoms and this may further change in the future.

The illness in an unvaccinated population was frequently biphasic, with the initial illness appearing as an upper respiratory tract infection that would last a few days, often with near-complete recovery, followed by a respiratory deterioration 7–10 days after the initial onset of symptoms. This second phase of illness is regarded predominantly to be immune-mediated. During this second phase, there was often disparity between level of hypoxia and severity of symptoms, with some patients appearing relatively comfortable despite very low oxygen saturations.

It is important to distinguish the COVID-19 syndrome that was frequently observed in the early part of the pandemic (biphasic illness due to SARS-CoV2 infection resulting in bilateral peripheral ground glass changes on radiological imaging with hypoxia) from symptomatic SARS-CoV2 infection in a frail patient with underlying comorbidity. The former typically occurs in an unvaccinated, infection-naïve population, but it can occur in those vaccinated, if they have other risk factors such as immunocompromise or increased BMI. The latter is typically a relatively mild infective syndrome which can significantly destabilise an underlying comorbidity – such as heart failure or chronic obstructive pulmonary disease. This can result in severe illness with hospitalization and even death, but the pathophysiology of SARS-CoV2 infection in the lungs is distinctly different from the COVID-19 syndrome.

Diagnosis

Syndromic	Initially, in the absence of molecular tests, diagnosis was made on epidemiological risk and symptoms. This was a prudent initial approach, but epidemiological risk by defined exposure quickly became difficult to judge as virus transmission became widespread and asymptomatic transmission was recognised. Subsequently, NHS contact-tracing apps gave some limited help in assessing epidemiological risk, but by this point molecular diagnostics were available. The impact of contact-tracing on overall national transmission, clinical outcomes and mortality was difficult to assess due to limited uptake and compliance.
Polymerase chain reaction (PCR)	Although highly sensitive, PCR diagnostic assays pose several issues. Firstly, inadequately administered tests (either by the patient or healthcare professionals) result in reduced sensitivity. Secondly, sensitivity is dependent on timing of testing according to the syndrome, with peak sensitivity occurring with the first phase of illness. Thirdly, viral RNA was discovered, in some cases to be present for prolonged periods following recovery from infection – up to three months in some cases. Many PCR platforms had more than one target (e.g. Spike (S), Nucleocapsid (N) and ORF1). As viral variants emerged, the primers targeting the most mutable proteins (S) were less effective at binding viral nucleic acid templates, and so automated laboratory diagnosis algorithms had to change (e.g. 'S-gene drop-outs' were used as a correlate to diagnose some new variants).
Whole genome sequencing (WGS)	An additional molecular diagnostic, where available, which did not suffer from the problems of mutability of primer target.
Lateral flow antigen test (LFA)	These were point-of-care tests used for diagnosis. They were commercially available with differences in sensitivity between brands. Additionally, there appeared to be a loss in sensitivity against more recent variants. Similar molecular mutation caveats affected LFAs as they did PCR, although there appeared to be a closer correlation with active viral replication (and therefore an inference of transmission risk) with a positive LFA than a positive PCR test.
Imaging	Plain film chest radiographs and chest CT/CTPA were the mainstay of radiological diagnosis, but used alone, are non-specific and lack sensitivity. COVID-19 lung findings included bilateral peripheral ground glass changes and/or consolidation.

Infection prevention and control

In the absence of vaccination and effective treatments, prevention of transmission was of the utmost importance. SARS-CoV2 was predominantly spread by droplet, although transmission via fomites and aerosol was also described. Regular hand-washing alongside surgical masks for those with a confirmed or suspected diagnosis if tolerated, as well as adequate PPE including gloves, aprons and surgical masks for staff (or FFP3 masks and face shields if performing aerosolizing procedures) was essential.

Hospital practices

Consideration of modification of hospital practices and patient flows based on careful risk assessments with available evidence may be required to minimize transmission, to protect both staff and patients:

Social distancing of staff to reduce transmission

Staff PPE requirements – some of these may be centrally mandated by UKHSA, some may be local policy

Risk assessment of procedures that may produce aerosols/transmission events and therefore necessitate a higher level of PPE

Regular staff testing to minimize staff-to-patient transmission in hospital

Risk assessment of staff vulnerability to infection and reallocation of role as appropriate

Reallocation of staff from elective or low-footfall areas to accommodate increased burden of care in acute units

Cohorting of patients and judicious use of side rooms – this may be helped through the implementation of a traffic light system of risk to aid decision-making

Restriction of visitor footfall within the hospital. This needs to be counter-balanced with measures to ensure communication between patients and their carers/next of kin in order to minimize emotional distress (e.g. video calling facilities)

Care needs to be taken not to cause secondary injury by delaying the diagnosis of non-COVID illnesses due to changes in hospital processes. There was evidence of preventable death by cardiac causes.

Medication policies may be adjusted to allow for reduced patient contact, e.g. using medications that are administered OD or by infusion rather than TDS. If this policy extends to antibiotic usage, care needs to be taken to consider the use of as narrow a spectrum alternative antibiotic as possible – there was a spike in *Clostridiodes difficile* cases post-pandemic that was temporally in keeping with antibiotic prescribing changes.

Distinct team shift working may be implemented (e.g. red and blue teams) such that if one member of a team is taken ill, the rest of their team would be contacts and perhaps advised to self-isolate, but the other team would remain free to continue work. A situation without separated teams more easily results in everyone being classified as contacts.

Vaccination

During the COVID-19 pandemic, several vaccines were developed at incredible speeds by both industry and academia. Some received emergency use authorization under regulation 174 including the Oxford/AstraZeneca vaccine (Vaxzervria, ChAdOx1 nCoV-19) and Pfizer/BioNTech (Comirnaty, BNT162b2) which were both widely used in the United Kingdom. Vaccination was highly effective at preventing severe disease (the COVID-19 syndrome of inflammatory lung changes) and there is very limited evidence that this protection wanes over time or with different variants. Protection against symptomatic infection varied more between vaccines and waned relatively quickly after 3–6 months. Several studies, including randomised control trials and national observational studies showed the feasibility of using heterologous schedules (different vaccine platforms for first and second doses) and a permissive approach to the interval between these doses.

Vaccination is the single biggest intervention that protects individuals from severe SARS-CoV2 infection. It reduces healthcare burden and has allowed the easing of national and international social restrictions.

Vaccines, as any new medication, carry the risk of adverse reactions. There may be some serious adverse reactions that are so rare that they are not picked up in clinical trials and therefore physicians need to be mindful of any significant and unusual pathologies.

Vaccine-induced thrombocytopaenic thrombosis (VITT) or thrombosis with thrombocytopaenia syndrome (TTS)	Venous or arterial thrombosis (often cerebral or abdominal) in the context of thrombocytopenia, the presence of anti-PF4 antibodies and a raised D-dimer. Seen predominantly after adenoviral-vectored COVID vaccines and typically occur within 42 d (more commonly a) after the first dose, b) in under 65 s, c) in females). Approximate incidence 1/100,000 doses
Myocarditis/Pericarditis	Seen with mRNA vaccines. Usually mild/self-limiting. Approximate incidence 6–14/1,000,000 first doses (8/1,000,000 second doses), more commonly in younger patients.

Treatments

When considering treatments for the management of COVID-19, there was guidance from central governing bodies, which were then enacted at local hospitals depending on availability of medication and local policy. These were regulated by various criteria, such as whether there was an oxygen requirement and whether the infection was community or hospital acquired. Many of these rules came either directly or by inference from the inclusion and exclusion criteria of the clinical trials that showed efficacy or from subgroup analyses.

There are broadly two categories of intervention – anti-viral and immunomodulatory. The principles underlying the timing of their administration are that antivirals should be administered early in the course of disease, whilst there is still active viral replication, whereas immunomodulatory treatments affect the second 'immune' phase of illness, where immunopathology is causing most of the damage. Below is a list of the more commonly used medications. The indications and contraindications may change depending on the most up-to-date information. **Always refer to specific local guidance for indications, contraindications, duration and dose**. Always consult specialist infection services in complex cases. Indications and exclusions may change after the publication of this text and clinicians should always seek the most up-to-date information regarding these medications.

It should be noted that the clinical trials which showed efficacy of many of these treatments occurred at certain points in time during the pandemic. This means that their effect was measured during the presence of a particular circulating variant in a population that may have been completely naïve or may have been partially or fully vaccinated. It is impossible to say with certainty what the benefit for some of these treatments are, with the current and future circulating variants and in a fully immunised population. New evaluations would have to be undertaken to understand this and would be unfeasibly large and expensive to perform. It is, however, likely that the benefit of many of the immunomodulatory interventions will not be as great in a seropositive population and those who do not have evidence of inflamed lung (COVID-19) during their SARS-CoV2 infection.

Anti-viral treatments

Medication	Comments
Remdesivir (Veklury)	Adenosine nucleotide prodrug Treatment of adults and children with **COVID-19 with pneumonia requiring** supplemental oxygen **or** who are at increased risk of progressing to severe COVID-19. Also used in non-hospitalised patients. Check for hepatic and renal impairment prior to and during use. Care when prescribing to pregnant or breast-feeding patients.
Nirmatrelvir plus ritonavir (Paxlovid)	Treatment of adults and children with **symptomatic COVID-19 not requiring** supplemental oxygen **and** who are at increased risk of progressing to severe COVID-19. Also used in non-hospitalised patients. Check for hepatic and renal impairment prior to and during use. Check for drug–drug interactions. Do not administer during pregnancy. Use with caution in breastfeeding.

Medication	Comments
Sotrovimab (Xevudy)	Recombinant human IgG1 monoclonal antibody (mAb) targeting the receptor binding domain (RBD) of the SARS-CoV2 spike protein. For patients >12 who do not require supplemental oxygen Monoclonal antibody efficacy is often dependent on the circulating strain. Sufficient mutation in the binding region (the RBD) can result in loss of efficacy, which has been the case for several previous mAbs used alone or in combination. Also used in non-hospitalised patients.
Molnupiravir (Lageviro)	Only used in the community in the United Kingdom. Originally shown to be efficacious in an unvaccinated population, the PANORAMIC trial then failed to show superiority above standard of care in a vaccinated population.

Immunomodulatory treatments

Dexamethasone	Low dose 6 mg (base) daily for 10 days or until discharge, whichever is sooner, was shown to have a dramatic effect on outcome. Using higher dose steroid resulted in relatively increased mortality. Equivalent doses of Prednisolone 40 mg or hydrocortisone can be considered in special situations including where dexamethasone is contraindicated
Tocilizumab	Anti-IL-6 monoclonal antibody For patients with COVID-19 requiring Oxygen Check for hepatic and renal impairment prior and during. Dose adjustment in obesity. Care in those already immunosuppressed. Blunts CRP response for up to 3 months after administration.
Baricitinib	Selective and reversible inhibitor of Janus kinase 1 and 2 (JAK1/JAK2) Do not administer during pregnancy or in those breastfeeding.
Inhaled Budesonide	Shown by the PRINCIPLE trial to shorten time to recovery in those at risk of severe illness, but results were not implemented in the United Kingdom.

Supportive/adjunctive treatments

Oxygen therapy	Extrapolation from wider data in hypoxia (not specific to COVID-19) has informed the convention of supplemental O_2 to achieve 94–98% in hypoxic patients with T1RF. It is unclear whether supplemental oxygen therapy is beneficial to those with SARS-CoV2 infection and low oxygen saturations, in terms of mortality or progression to intubation. However, it is a challenging decision not to give oxygen to patients who are overtly hypoxic. In those for whom there is symptomatic relief of breathlessness, it may be beneficial as well as for those in whom other comorbidity (cardiac and respiratory) may be destabilized by low oxygen saturations.
Pressure support	CPAP was used empirically, in part, to maintain critical care capacity. There is some limited evidence that CPAP may reduce progression to intubation and is reasonably used as first-line supportive therapy in those for whom supplemental oxygen alone was insufficient. However, a clear mortality benefit has not yet been established. Patients with pre-existing conditions and T2RF should still be considered for bi-level pressure support.
Thromboprophylaxis	The most recent reviews suggest that routinely increasing standard prophylactic anticoagulation doses does not confer a survival benefit in hospitalised patients, however UK practice still varies due to variability in results from a number of randomised control trials.
Community management Follow-up	Some patients may be able to be managed in the community on a 'virtual ward' if safety criteria are met and suitable hospital infrastructure is in place. Chest imaging follow-up may be of benefit as part of a holistic system to identify those who may require further follow-up in a post-COVID or 'Long COVID' service.

Complications of SARS-CoV2 infection

Venous thromboembolism	Imaging (CTPA/USS Dopler) to diagnose and anticoagulation to treat. Use prophylactic anticoagulation in all inpatients and consider selected high-risk outpatients.
Myocardial injury	Frequently self-limiting if mild. Seek specialist advice if severe.
Secondary infection, including bacterial pneumonia	Relatively rare, but treatment with antibiotics where clinically indicated according to local guidelines.
Dermatological manifestations	Several described phenomena (vesicular eruptions, maculopapular eruptions, urticarial lesions, livedo or necrosis and pseudo-chilblain). Generally non-severe and self-limiting. The different manifestations occur at varying timepoints through the disease course.
Long COVID	Characterised commonly by extreme tiredness, shortness of breath, loss of smell and muscle aches. However, there are many other symptoms patients can experience post-COVID-19 including brain fog, chest pain/tightness, insomnia, palpitations, dizziness, paraesthesia, arthralgia, depression, anxiety, tinnitus, ear ache, nausea, diarrhoea, abdominal pain, anorexia, cough, headache and sore throat. Recognition of the syndrome and referral to appropriate local services when criteria are met is an important aspect of management of this condition.

Secondary pandemic injuries

Missed diagnoses	Care must be taken to ensure that other diagnoses are not missed through increased infection prevention precautions – such as malaria in the returning traveller and myocardial infarction.
Delayed non-COVID emergency care	Routine emergency and urgent care should not be compromised. Adequate mitigating measures should be taken such as PPE and managing hospital flows.
Delayed elective/routine care	Planning at a local and national level needs to happen to mitigate this.
Mental/psychological health	Data are still coming through regarding suicide and reported attempted suicide rates during the pandemic. It is not currently clear exactly what effect the pandemic had. There were certainly impacts on psychiatric presentations to secondary care and physicians need to be aware of the impact that such pandemics have on psycho-social wellbeing. In 2022, the number of mental health referrals remained above pre-pandemic levels.
Financial/Educational	Many people and businesses were affected by the pandemic and experienced financial hardship. Children were also heavily impacted by massive interruption to education.

Special cases

Immunocompromised and other 'at risk' patients may not respond as well or at all to vaccination and therefore may still be at risk of severe COVID-19. Additionally, their immune system is weakened, either by their underlying disease or iatrogenically. Depending on the nature of immunosuppression, there may be an increased risk of prolonged viral replication or failure of viral clearance. Alternatively, there may be detrimental consequences to further immunosuppression as part of therapy for the immunopathological stage of COVID-19. Evidence is generally lacking surrounding this, and discussion with specialists is advised. This group in particular may benefit from repeated COVID-19 vaccination doses.

Research

Rapidly enacted descriptive research studies such as ISARIC were key to describing the illness when little was known about it. Pivotal interventional trials such as RECOVERY and REMAP-CAP successfully defined successful interventions and importantly excluded ineffective and potentially harmful interventions. In future pandemics, the maintenance of such studies that are 'ready to go' will be key to a rapid response. Awareness of clinicians to recruit to such studies enables successful interventions to be rapidly identified. Clinicians need also to be careful of posited treatments without evidence, which have the potential to cause harm both directly and indirectly through individuals increasing their risk-taking behaviour and not seeking timely medical attention.

The next pandemic

The future of SARS-CoV2 is that it will likely become a part of our daily life as other seasonal human coronaviruses have done in the past. The threat of a resurgence of a more pathogenic variant is still present, but may not be very high. We are now in a better situation to mitigate the impacts of any future pandemics through experiences and established systems that can hopefully rapidly be resurrected if required.

CHAPTER 79

Septic arthritis

KEHINDE SUNMBOYE AND JOHN L. KLEIN

Consider this diagnosis in any patient who has fever with joint pain and swelling, particularly if only one large joint is involved.

- Septic arthritis is typically mono-articular but can be poly-articular (15% of cases).
- The knee is the joint most commonly involved, followed by the elbow, shoulder and hip.
- *Staphylococcus aureus* is the causative organism in 50% of cases of native joint infection; other causative organisms include streptococci, gonococci and Gram-negative bacilli.
- Prosthetic joint infection is caused by a wider range of pathogens.

Priorities

Your clinical assessment should address the following points:

- Does the patient have arthritis or periarticular inflammation (bursitis, tendinitis or cellulitis)? Painful limitation of movement of the joint suggests arthritis. Causes of acute mono- or oligo-arthritis are given in Table 79.1.

Table 79.1 Comparison of gonococcal and non-gonococcal septic arthritis.

	Gonococcal septic arthritis	Non-gonococcal septic arthritis
Organisms	*Neisseria gonorrhoeae*	*Staphylococcus aureus* Beta-haemolytic streptococci *Streptococcus pneumoniae* Gram-negative rods
Patient profile	Young, healthy and sexually active	Elderly, rheumatoid arthritis, prosthetic joint, IV drug use, bacteraemia, immunosuppression
Initial presentation	Migratory polyarthralgia, tenosynovitis and dermatitis	Typically with a single hot, swollen, painful joint, but can be poly-articular (15% of cases)
Joints involved	Often poly-articular, especially knee and wrist	Knee joint is most commonly involved, followed by the elbow, shoulder and hip
Other signs	Tenosynovitis, rash	Source of bacteraemia
Gram stain of synovial fluid	<25% positive	50–75% positive
Culture of synovial fluid	25% positive	85–95% positive
Blood culture	<10% positive	50% positive
Genitourinary culture (swab of urethra, cervix and anorectum)	80% positive	Not indicated

Table 79.2 Investigation in suspected septic arthritis.

Joint aspiration (Chapter 111)
X-ray joint for baseline
Blood glucose
Creatinine and electrolytes
Liver function tests
Full blood count
Erythrocyte sedimentation rate and C-reactive protein
Blood culture (×2)
Urine stick test, microscopy and culture
Swab of urethra, cervix and anorectum for culture and nucleic acid amplification test if gonococcal infection is possible

- Is the patient at risk of septic arthritis? Septic arthritis usually follows an overt or occult bacteraemia (e.g. from infective endocarditis, pneumonia or IV drug use) in a patient at risk because of rheumatoid arthritis, the presence of a prosthetic joint or immunosuppression from disease or use of medication such as biologic therapies for active autoimmune rheumatic disease Examples of biologic therapies include, but are not limited to, tumor necrosis factor inhibitors, Rituximab, Tocilizumab to name a few.
- Could this be crystal arthritis (gout or pseudogout; Chapter 92): is there a history of previous similar attacks of arthritis?
- Could this be reactive arthritis: is there an associated rash, diarrhoea, urethritis or uveitis?
- Could this be gonococcal arthritis (Table 79.1)?

  Aspirate the joint (Chapter 111) and send synovial fluid for cell count (in an ethylenediaminetetraacetic acid (EDTA) tube; normal cell count is <180/mm^3, most mononuclear), Gram stain, culture and microscopy under polarized light for crystals. Other investigations needed urgently are given in Table 79.2.

- If you are not familiar with joint aspiration, ask the help of a rheumatologist or orthopaedic surgeon.
- Both crystal and septic arthritis give rise to a purulent effusion, although the white cell count is usually higher in septic arthritis (50,000–200,000/mm^3), with a polymorphonuclear cell count of >90%.
- Bloodstaining of the effusion is common in pseudogout but rare in sepsis.

Further management

Organisms on Gram stain of synovial fluid, or high probability of septic arthritis

Start antibiotic therapy IV (Table 79.3).

- Intra-articular administration is not needed.
- The antibiotic regimen may need modification in the light of blood and synovial fluid culture results: discuss this with a microbiologist.
- Antibiotic therapy for non-gonococcal septic arthritis usually needs to be given for two to four weeks, initially IV, but may be switched to an appropriate oral agent in uncomplicated cases.
- Gonococcal arthritis may be cured with just one to two weeks of therapy.

  If septic arthritis is confirmed, seek advice on further management from a rheumatologist or orthopaedic surgeon.

- Daily aspiration of the joint until an effusion no longer re-accumulates is an acceptable approach where access to the joint is easy (e.g. the knee).
- Other larger joints (e.g. hip or shoulder) may be more effectively drained by arthroscopic washout.
- While the infection is resolving, the joint should be immobilized using a splint or cast.

Table 79.3 Initial antibiotic therapy for suspected native joint septic arthritis.

	Antibiotic therapy (IV, high dose)	
Organisms on gram stain	**Not allergic to penicillin**	**Allergic to penicillin**
Gram-positive cocci	Flucloxacillin Vancomycin if Methicillin resistant *Staphylococcus aureus* (MRSA) suspected	Clindamycin
Gram-negative cocci	Ceftriaxone	Ceftriaxone (mild allergy) Seek expert advice if severe allergy
Gram-negative rods	Piperacillin-tazobactam	Ciprofloxacin
None seen	Flucloxacillin Vancomycin if MRSA suspected	Clindamycin

- Physiotherapy should be started early.
- Give a non-steroidal anti-inflammatory drug (NSAID) for pain relief (e.g. Naproxen or Etoricoxib).
- In patients with gonococcal arthritis, a sexual health screen of the patient and his/her sexual partners should be offered.

No organisms on Gram stain of synovial fluid and low probability of septic arthritis

Consider the other causes of acute arthritis (Table 79.1).

- Pseudogout is a common cause of acute mono- or oligo-arthritis in the elderly. Hold off antibiotic therapy (pending the results of blood and synovial fluid culture for definite exclusion of infection).
- Treat with an NSAID, covered with a proton-pump inhibitor in the elderly or patients with previous peptic ulceration.
- If gout is confirmed (also check plasma urate) and fails to respond to an NSAID, use colchicine. Allopurinol should not be started until the acute attack has completely resolved.

Further reading

Brusch JL (2023) Septic arthritis treatment & management: approach considerations, antibiotic therapy, Joint Immobilization and Physical Therapy. Available from: https://emedicine.medscape.com/article/236299-treatment. [Accessed: 8 May 2024].

Momodu II, Savaliya V. (2025) Septic arthritis. [Updated 2023 Jul 3]. In: StatPearls [Internet]. Treasure Island (FL): StatPearls Publishing. Available from: https://www.ncbi.nlm.nih.gov/books/NBK538176/.

Sharff KA, Richards EP, Townes JM. (2013) Clinical management of septic arthritis. *Curr Rheumatol Rep* 15, 332. DOI: 10.1007/s11926-013-0332-4.

Haematology

CHAPTER 80

Anaemia: blood transfusion and alternatives

EDMUND WATSON

Anaemia is of interest to the Acute Physician. It is an easily diagnosed and relatively unambiguous entity, defined by a haemoglobin below the reference age for the patient (with different ranges for children, women and men and for the pregnant state). It may provide an explanation for a patient's attendance to secondary care – for instance, with fatigue, breathlessness or dizziness, or decompensation of some other chronic illness – and therefore offers an opportunity for a valuable therapeutic intervention. Additionally, or alternatively, its presence may suggest an important underlying diagnosis whose work-up should occur during admission or be handed over to community services on discharge.

Diagnostic approach to anaemia

Individual patient trends in mean cell volume (MCV) can be more sensitive than absolute numbers

The well-practised categorisation of anaemia by red cell volume into microcytic (MCV<80 fL), normocytic (MCV 80–100 fL) and macrocytic (MCV>100 fL) is a helpful conceptualisation of the aetiology of anaemia (see Table 80.1).

However, these useful absolute definitions are not personalised, and **the physician must look for trends over time in individual patients**. For instance, in a case of iron-deficiency anaemia, a patient's MCV may never become formally microcytic but nonetheless may drop over several months from 97 to 82 fL. This same statement is widely applicable across laboratory values, including haemoglobin itself.

Co-existing chronic diseases can make diagnosis difficult

Often, even when the MCV is duly considered, the diagnostic process stalls at the entity of anaemia of chronic disease (ACD). **ACD is the most frequent cause of anaemia in hospitalised patients**. It is believed to result from hepcidin-mediated sequestering of iron away from erythroid precursor cells and into reticuloendothelial and gut cells, in combination with reduced erythropoietic activity and shortened red cell lifespan. It was classically described in malignancy and chronic infectious and inflammatory conditions but is now also believed to occur in heart and renal failure, obesity and acutely in critical illness.

ACD represents a significant challenge. No laboratory test can currently diagnose ACD, meaning it remains a clinical diagnosis. Furthermore, it often co-exists with other forms of anaemia, especially iron deficiency – but

Acute Medicine: A Practical Guide to the Management of Medical Emergencies, Sixth Edition.
Edited by Mridula Rajwani, Leila Vaziri, and Ivie Gbinigie.
© 2026 John Wiley & Sons Ltd. Published 2026 by John Wiley & Sons Ltd.

Table 80.1 Differential diagnosis of anaemia.

Aetiology	Suggestive, first/early-line laboratory findings
MCV <80 fL	

Iron deficiency	• FBC parameters –
	   • Decreasing MCV and MCH over time
	   • Rising red cell distribution width (RDW)
	   • Dropping red cell count
	   • Increasing platelet count
	 • Blood film – anisocytosis; elliptocytes; pencil cells
	 • Iron profile –
	   • **Low ferritin is diagnostic** – i.e. <15–30 µg/L
	   • Transferrin saturations <20%
	   • High transferrin
	   • (Iron levels too variable to be useful)
	 • *Possible follow-on laboratory tests:* Coeliac screen

Thalassemia	• FBC parameters –
	   • Stable red cell parameters over time
	   • Elevated red cell count
	 • *Possible follow-on laboratory tests:* Hb HPLC

Sideroblastic anaemia	• Blood film – siderocytes, with basophilic stippling • Iron profile – elevated ferritin
Lead poisoning	• Blood film – siderocytes, with basophilic stippling
MCV 80–100 fL	
ACD only	• Elevated CRP or ESR • Iron profile – elevated ferritin, suppressed transferrin • eGFR often <30 if renal anaemia

ACD plus iron deficiency	• FBC – no specific signature
	 • Blood film – no specific pattern
	 • Iron profile
	   • Ferritin ≤100 µg/L
	   • Transferrin saturation <20%, but may be spuriously normal (owing to low TF levels in ACD)

Bleeding (recent)	• Blood film – polychromasia

Haemolysis	• Raised reticulocytes
	 • Blood film –
	   • Polychromasia
	   • Spherocytes
	   • Bite cells (if oxidant damage)
	   • Schistocytes (if MAHA)
	 • Biochemistry –
	   • raised (unconjugated) bilirubin
	   • increased LDH
	   • reduced haptoglobins (esp if intravascular)
	 • *Possible follow-on laboratory tests:* Coombs test

BM infiltration, incl.
 • Myeloma
 • Myelodysplasia
 • Acute leukaemia
 • Myelofibrosis
	• FBC – neutropenia and/or thrombocytopenia
	 • Blood film –
	   • Rouleaux (in myeloma)
	   • Leucoerythroblastic (in myelofibrosis)
	   • Blasts (in acute leukaemia)
	 • Immunology (in myeloma) –
	   • M protein by protein electrophoresis
	   • Reduced non-affected Igs
	   • Abnormal kappa:lambda ratio

Table 80.1 (*Continued*)

Aetiology	Suggestive, first/early-line laboratory findings
MCV >100 fL	
Many drugs, e.g.	• FBC – may see additional cytopenias with some drugs
• Chemotherapy	• Blood film – no specific clues
• ACEi/AR2B	
• Anti-retrovirals	
Alcohol excess	• FBC – may see lymphopenia, thrombocytopenia
	• Biochemistry – elevated AST (>ALT), γGT
B12 and folate deficiency	• FBC – neutropenia and/or pancytopenia
	• Blood film – hypersegmented neutrophils
	• Biochemistry – low B12, low folate
Haemolysis	• If marked reticulocytosis (reticulocytes are large cells)
	• As with haemolysis in MCV 80–100, above
Liver disease	• FBC – thrombocytopenia (if portal hypertension)
	• Biochemistry – LFT derangements, low albumin
Hypothyroidism	• TSH elevated

Table 80.2 A suggested approach to anaemia.

History
- Blood loss, incl. non-visible – e.g. dyspepsia; bowel habit change
- Dietary issues and malabsorption symptoms
- Co-morbidity – malignancy; inflammatory or infective; heart, liver or renal failure
- Drug history
- Alcohol use
- Family history of thalassemia

Suggested screening panel
- FBC
- Blood film
- Reticulocytes
- Iron profile
- B12 and folate levels
- LFTs, eGFR and CRP
- Protein electrophoresis, immunoglobulins, light chains

where diagnosis of low iron stores is difficult as the superimposed ACD leads to a spurious normalisation of the ferritin level (and transferrin saturation).

Consequently, a **pragmatic approach might be to screen for a selection of common and/or actionable causes of anaemia** (see Table 80.2), investigate and manage these as necessary, and make a judgement as to whether the persisting anaemia is reasonably explained by ACD. Outside of ACD, employing a screening approach will also help to detect other instances of co-existing contributors – for instance, iron deficiency with folate deficiency in an undiagnosed case of coeliac disease.

Never hesitate to talk with haematology

We would always recommend that a haematologist is consulted where the cause of anaemia is not certain, and where haemolysis or a bone marrow pathology is suspected.

Red blood cell transfusion and alternatives

Wherever appropriate, the underlying cause of anaemia should be fully investigated and addressed. The Hb may then spontaneously recover, but in the meantime, the Physician must decide whether – and if so, how – to intervene to accelerate Hb normalisation. There is no simple algorithm for this. Ultimately, the approach will be informed to varying degrees by the anaemia's aetiology, trajectory and severity – where severity can be described numerically (the Hb level), and more importantly, in terms of patient symptomatology.

Red blood cell transfusion is a blunt but effective tool in anaemia correction

There are two main indications for transfusion:

1 Where rapid anaemia correction is required (e.g. haemorrhage; unstable patient).

2 Where anaemia is/will become severe, and there is no other strategy available.

There are risks and benefits with transfusion as with any treatment, but there is additionally an onus on Physicians to safeguard a resource that has been donated selflessly by the public. NHS Blood and Transplant provides a framework for good transfusion practice to ensure good stewardship and patient safety (see Table 80.3).

Alternatives to transfusion to correct anaemia are limited

Iron replacement, for iron deficiency (incl. following acute blood loss)

Oral iron is available in multiple formulations, where a single dose should contain roughly 50–100 mg of elemental iron. Gastrointestinal disturbance secondary to iron supplementation is a substantial cause of non-compliance, with no head-to-head data suggesting which formulation is best tolerated.

The current consensus from the British Society of Gastroenterology suggests it should be taken once daily in the fasted state (with concomitant ascorbic acid in e.g. orange juice potentially enhancing absorption), and the patient's FBC should be repeated two to four weeks after starting with an expected Hb rise of 10 g/L per fortnight. Once the Hb has normalised, oral iron should be continued for three months to ensure replenishment of total iron stores. A failure to respond to oral iron could be due to many factors, including non-compliance, ongoing bleeding or co-existing pathology.

For most patients with iron deficiency anaemia, oral iron is sufficient. However, intravenous iron replenishes total body iron more rapidly and circumvents enteral absorption issues and side effects. It therefore offers an important alternative for cases such as concomitant ACD; where Hb recovery is needed more promptly (though the difference is small, being <10 g/L at four weeks post-treatment in one post-operative cohort) (5); menorrhagia; and where oral iron is poorly tolerated and/or has been ineffective within two weeks. Normalisation of anaemia should be confirmed following treatment, as with oral iron.

Erythropoietin stimulating agents (ESAs), for specialist indications

Erythropoietin (EPO), the endogenous hormone responsible for driving erythropoiesis, can be given in recombinant forms in different parenteral preparations. This is a valuable intervention where endogenous EPO signal is pathologically low – such as end-stage renal failure – or inappropriately low – such as myelodysplastic syndrome. However, the indications for ESAs are limited and all require involvement of specialist teams, not least because of a signal for harm with the use of ESAs in the form of arterial events.

Table 80.3 The ten commandments of transfusion.

1 Transfusion should only be used when the benefits outweigh the risks and there are no appropriate alternatives.

2 Results of laboratory tests are not the sole deciding factor for transfusion.

3 Transfusion decisions should be based on clinical assessment underpinned by evidence-based clinical guidelines.

4 Not all anaemic patients need transfusion (there is no universal 'transfusion trigger').

Outside of major haemorrhage and patients on a chronic transfusion programme, **NICE Guidance NG24** suggests a threshold of 70g/L or 80g/L in acute coronary syndrome.

This should be applied in a patient-dependent context: a patient who is light-headed and breathless, or suffers angina, with an Hb of 82g/L may well benefit from transfusion.

Equally, a patient with very mild symptoms and an Hb of 67g/L secondary to iron deficiency could wait for a response to iron therapy.

The practice of **restrictive transfusion**, also suggested in NG24, is a logical extension of these first four recommendations. A single unit prescription (approximately 280mL, which should increment Hb by 10g/L in a 70kg person) followed by clinical and laboratory reassessment prior to the next unit of blood ensures the patient is not exposed to unnecessary risk. Consider transfusions of less than one unit in patients with low weight: a dose of 4mL/kg typically lifts Hb by 10g/L, so a 50kg patient may only require 200mL.

5 Discuss the risks, benefits and alternatives to transfusion with the patient and gain their consent.

Patients should consent prior to transfusion or pre-emptively if transfusion is deemed likely. If consent was not possible at the time owing to a temporary lack of capacity, the patient should be advised of the transfusion after the event.

Approximately 2 million units of blood products are transfused each year in the United Kingdom, and the **Serious Hazards of Transfusion (SHOT)** organisation collects reports from across the country to provide annual reports of the risks associated with transfusion. There were 35 deaths attributed to blood transfusion in 2022.

Patients should be advised of the following **risks**:

- Febrile non-haemolytic reaction – *mild reactions common; severe rare*
  - Temperature rise, occasionally with SIRS response
- Allergic reaction – *mild reactions common; severe rare*
  - Ranging from mild events (e.g. urticaria) to true anaphylaxis
- Antibody formation – *quite common*
  - Asymptomatic process, but important for future transfusions
- **Transfusion-associated circulatory overload (TACO)** – *rare, but under-reported*
  - Second-most common cause of transfusion-related death in 2022 ($n = 8$)
  - Caution needed in fluid overload states; ensure fluid balance assessments before each unit and consider role of diuresis.
- Haemolytic transfusion reaction – *rare*
  - Patient's antibodies react with incoming blood cells; acute or delayed forms.
- Wrong blood, wrong patient – *very rare*
  - Including potentially fatal ABO incompatibility
- Transfusion-associated lung injury (TRALI) – *very rare*
  - Breathlessness and hypoxia secondary to ARDS-type picture
- Transfusion-associated infection – extremely rare (<1/million units)
  - An understandably sensitive topic given the Contaminated Blood scandal
- Not a risk *per se*, but a clear impact of receiving blood is that a patient can never themselves be a blood donor.

(continued)

Table 80.3 (*Continued*)

6   The reason for transfusion should be documented in the patient's clinical record.

7   Timely provision in major haemorrhage can improve outcome – good communication and teamwork are essential.
The most common cause of death associated with transfusion as per the SHOT 2022 report was delay to transfusion.

8   Patient identifiers on the ID band and blood pack must be identical. Any discrepancy, DO NOT TRANSFUSE.

9   The patient must be monitored during the transfusion.
The most recent British Society for Haematology guidance on the investigation and management of acute transfusion reactions includes the following algorithm:

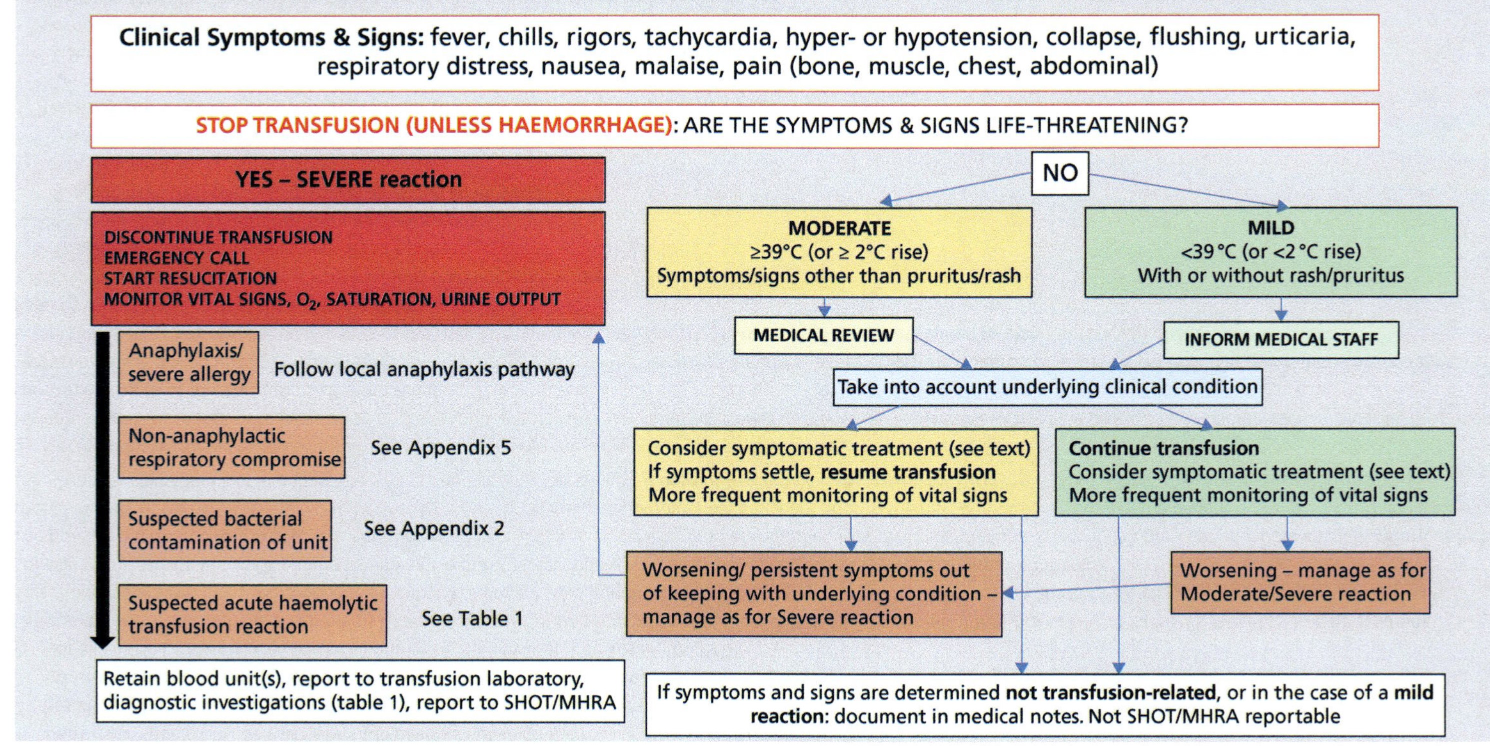

10   Education and training underpin safe transfusion practice.

Sources: Adapted from (1–4).

References

1 Joint United Kingdom (UK) Blood Transfusion and Tissue Transplantation Services Professional Advisory Committee. Transfusion ten commandments. Last updated: 11 January 2024. https://www.transfusionguidelines.org/transfusion-handbook/1-transfusion-ten-commandments.

2 Joint United Kingdom (UK) Blood Transfusion and Tissue Transplantation Services Professional Advisory Committee. Consent for blood transfusion – guidance for healthcare practitioners in the UK. Last updated: 11 January 2024. https://www.transfusionguidelines.org/transfusion-practice/consent-for-blood-transfusion/guidance-for-healthcare-practitioners-involved-in-this-role.

3 Serious Hazards of Transfusion. 2022 annual SHOT report – individual chapters. Last updated: 11 January 2024. https://www.shotuk.org/shot-reports/report-summary-and-supplement-2022/2022-annual-shot-report-individual-chapters/.

4 Soutar R, McSporran W, Tomlinson T, *et al*. (2023) British Society of Haematology guideline on the investigation and management of acute transfusion reactions. *B J Haem* **201**(5), 832–844. *A practically-oriented approach for physicians responding to transfusion reactions*.

5 Bisbe E, Moltó L, Arroyo R, *et al*. (2014) Randomized trial comparing ferric carboxymaltose vs oral ferrous glycine sulphate for postoperative anaemia after total knee arthroplasty. *Br J Anaesth* 113, 402–409.

Further reading

Snook J, Bhala N, Beales ILP, *et al*. (2021) British Society of Gastroenterology guidelines for the management of iron deficiency anaemia in adults. *Gut* 70, 1–22. *Guidelines for investigating and managing iron deficiency*.

Soutar R, McSporran W, Tomlinson T, *et al*. (2023) Guideline on the investigation and management of acute transfusion reactions. *Br J Haematol* 201, 832–844.

Website of JPAC, the Joint United Kingdom (UK) Blood Transfusion and Tissue Transplantation Services Professional Advisory Committee. Extensive resources regarding theory and practice of blood transfusion. transfusionguidelines.org.

Weiss G, Ganz T, Goodnough LT. (2019) Anaemia of inflammation. *Blood* 133(1), 40–50. *A review article discussing ACD, with some diagnostic protocols including ACD with concomitant iron deficiency*.

CHAPTER 81

Bleeding disorders

SUSAN SHAPIRO

Consider a bleeding disorder (Table 81.1) in the patient with spontaneous, prolonged or disproportionate bleeding.

Bleeding disorders may be caused by:

- Coagulation factor deficiency
- Reduced platelet function (too few or dysfunctional platelets)
- Microvascular abnormalities

The commonest causes of acquired bleeding disorders are:

- Medications (anticoagulants/antiplatelets)
- Liver disease

Table 81.1 Causes of abnormal bleeding.

Cause	Comment
Direct effect of drugs	
Warfarin	Inhibits vitamin K-dependent gamma-carboxylation of coagulation factors II, VII, IX and X
Direct-acting oral anticoagulants (e.g. dabigatran, rivaroxaban, apixaban and edoxaban)	These drugs are direct inhibitors of factor IIa (dabigatran) or Xa (rivaroxaban, apixaban and edoxaban)
Unfractionated heparin	Inhibits thrombin
Low-molecular-weight heparins	Inhibit factor Xa and thrombin
Thrombolytic agents (e.g. alteplase)	Activate plasminogen and thus the fibrinolytic system
Antiplatelet agents (e.g. aspirin, clopidogrel, ticagrelor)	Inhibits platelet function/aggregation
Platelet glycoprotein IIb/IIIa-receptor antagonists	Inhibit platelet function/aggregation
Acquired coagulation factor deficiency or inhibitor	Includes liver disease, vitamin K deficiency and DIC. See Table 81.2. Acquired inhibitors are antibodies to coagulation factors, which may be idiopathic or associated with malignancy, autoimmune disorders, pregnancy and clonal lymphoma proliferative disorders (e.g. Waldenstrom macroglobulinaemia) Typically presents with bleeding into muscles or large ecchymoses
Acquired thrombocytopenia	Platelet count: • $<50 \times 10^9$/L: excessive bleeding is seen after surgery or trauma • $<20 \times 10^9$/L: spontaneous bleeding is common • $<10 \times 10^9$/L: spontaneous bleeding is usual

Acute Medicine: A Practical Guide to the Management of Medical Emergencies, Sixth Edition.
Edited by Mridula Rajwani, Leila Vaziri, and Ivie Gbinigie.
© 2026 John Wiley & Sons Ltd. Published 2026 by John Wiley & Sons Ltd.

Table 81.1 (*Continued*)

Cause	Comment
Acquired platelet dysfunction	Most often due to drugs, notably antiplatelet agents, but also non-steroidal anti-inflammatory drugs (NSAIDs). Also seen in advanced renal failure and myelodysplasia
Acquired microvascular abnormality	Corticosteroid therapy, scurvy
Inherited disorders of coagulation factors or platelets (number/ function)	These are rare in acute medicine. If the patient has had previous significant injury, surgery, tooth extraction or childbirth without abnormal bleeding, an inherited disorder of haemostasis is unlikely. If the person is known to have an inherited bleeding disorder, then call the haematology team immediately.

- Vitamin K deficiency (malnutrition, obstructive jaundice and small bowel disease)
- Disseminated intravascular coagulation (DIC)

Priorities

1 Make a clinical assessment and take a detailed drug history. Is there a known inherited disorder or family history of abnormal bleeding?
2 If the patient has had previous significant injury, surgery, tooth extraction or childbirth without abnormal bleeding, an inherited disorder of haemostasis is unlikely.
3 Check a full blood count, blood film and coagulation screen (including fibrinogen level): interpretation of the coagulation screen is summarized in Table 81.2. Check renal and liver function. Other investigations will be determined by the clinical context.

Table 81.2 Causes of prolonged prothrombin time (PT) and activated partial thromboplastin time (APTT).

PT	APTT	Cause
Prolonged	Normal	Warfarin or other vitamin K antagonist therapy Vitamin K deficiency Liver disease Low fibrinogen Inherited factor VII deficiency (rare)
Normal	Prolonged	Heparin therapy Lupus anticoagulant (not associated with bleeding) Haemophilia A/B, von Willebrand disease Acquired inhibitors to factor VIII (acquired haemophilia A)
Prolonged	Prolonged	Liver disease Disseminated intravascular coagulation (associated with low fibrinogen and high D-dimers) Excess warfarin or other vitamin K antagonist therapy Heparin + warfarin therapy Deficiencies of factors II, V, X (rare)
Variable	Variable	The direct-acting oral anticoagulants (dabigatran, rivaroxaban apixaban, edoxaban) have variable effects on the PT and APTT, depending on the drug, its concentration (the dose–response is not always linear) and the particular laboratory assay. Normal PT and APTT do not exclude therapeutic Direct Oral AntiCoagulant (DOAC). If you have a patient taking one of these drugs who is bleeding, always consult local major bleeding guidelines and consider calling a haematologist. See Chapter 85.

Further management

1 Further management is directed at the underlying disorder. Seek expert advice from a haematologist on management and haemostatic support, particularly in the event of unexplained bleeding, positive family history, prior bleeding; and for help with blood product support.
2 Clinical features and management of disseminated intravascular coagulation are summarised in Appendix 81.1.

Appendix 81.1 Disseminated intravascular coagulation (DIC).

Element	Comment
Description	Inappropriate activation of the coagulation pathways leads to widespread thrombin activation with microthrombus formation, depletion of clotting factors and consumption of platelets
Causes	Sepsis
	Malignancy (e.g. mucinous adenocarcinomas and acute myeloid leukaemia)
	Obstetric complication (amniotic fluid embolism and placental abruption)
	Trauma (major injury, head injury and fat embolism)
	Rarer: anaphylaxis, haemolytic transfusion reaction, transplant rejection and giant haemangioma
Clinical features	Bleeding from skin and mucosae (nose and gums)
	Bleeding from surgical incisions, wounds, venepuncture sites
	End-organ damage from microthrombi
Full blood count and film	Thrombocytopenia
	Fragmented red cells (schistocytes) may be present (but this is not sensitive or specific to DIC)
Blood results	Prolonged prothrombin and activated partial thromboplastin times
	Low fibrinogen concentration
	Raised concentration of fibrin degradation products/D-dimer
Differential diagnosis	Thrombotic thrombocytopenic purpura (Appendix 82.2)
	Acute liver failure
	Decompensated chronic liver disease
	HELLP syndrome of pregnancy (haemolysis, elevated liver enzymes and low platelet count)
Management	Treatment is of the underlying disorder.
	Consider blood product replacement therapy if the patient is actively bleeding or requires an intervention.
	Seek urgent advice from a haematologist

CHAPTER 82

Thrombocytopenia and thrombosis

Susan Shapiro

Clinical features and management of heparin-induced thrombocytopenia and thrombotic thrombocytopenic purpura are summarised in Table 82.1 and Appendices 82.1 and 82.2.

Table 82.1 Diagnosis of heparin-induced thrombocytopenia (HIT): the 4T score.

Category	2 points	1 point	0 points
Thrombocytopenia	Platelet count fall >50% and platelet nadir $\geq 20 \times 10^9$/L	Platelet count fall 30–50% or platelet nadir 10–19×10^9/L	Platelet count fall <30% or platelet nadir $<10 \times 10^9$/L
Timing of platelet count fall	Clear onset between days 5 and 10 or platelet fall ≤ 1 d (prior heparin exposure within 30 d)	Consistent with days 5–10 fall, but not clear (e.g. missing platelet counts) or onset after day 10 or fall ≤ 1 d (prior heparin exposure 30–100 d ago)	Platelet count fall <4 d without recent heparin exposure
Thrombosis or other sequelae	New thrombosis (confirmed) or skin necrosis at heparin injection sites or acute systemic reaction after intravenous heparin bolus	Progressive or recurrent thrombosis or non-necrotizing (erythematous) skin lesions or suspected thrombosis (not proven)	None
Other causes for thrombocytopenia	None apparent	Possible	Definite

Total points:
≤ 3 = low probability of HIT
4–5 = intermediate probability of HIT
≥ 6 = high probability of HIT.
Source: Lo GK, Juhl D, Warkentin TE, Sigouin CS, Eichler P, Greinacher A (2006) Evaluation of pretest clinical score (4Ts) for the diagnosis of heparin-induced thrombocytopenia in two clinical settings. *J Thromb Haemost* 4, 759–65. Reproduced with permission of John Wiley & Sons.

Appendix 82.1 Heparin-induced thrombocytopenia.

Element	Comment
Cause	Formation of Immunoglobulin G (IgG) autoantibody to heparin, results in platelet activation, thrombocytopaenia and thrombosis.
Clinical features	Recognized by a falling platelet count (platelet count falls by >50% to <150 × 10^9/L) in a patient receiving unfractionated or (much more rarely) low-molecular-weight heparin, with or without previous exposure to heparin; classically onset is 4–10 d after starting heparin. Thrombotic complications (venous and arterial) occur in 20–50%. Bleeding is rare. Probability of diagnosis can be assessed by 4T score (Table 102.3). Diagnosis proved by the presence of heparin-dependent antibodies.
Differential diagnosis	Sepsis Thrombocytopenia caused by other drugs Post-transfusion purpura
Management	Seek urgent advice from a haematologist Stop heparin Use alternative anticoagulant therapy such as fondaparinux, direct-acting thrombin inhibitor (e.g. bivalirudin) or heparinoid (danaparoid) if needed. Direct Oral AntiCoagulants (DOACs) may be considered if the patient has had a venous thrombosis, but should not be used for new arterial thrombosis associated with heparin-induced thrombocytopenia (HIT). Do not transfuse platelets for thrombocytopaenia as this can result in further platelet activation and thrombosis. The platelet count typically recovers within 4–14 d after stopping heparin. The risk of thrombosis persists for several weeks after stopping the heparin. Give the patient an ALERT card: HIT will reoccur if the individual is re-exposed to heparin.

Appendix 82.2 Thrombotic thrombocytopenic purpura.

Element	Comment
Description	This is a haematological emergency. It is crucial to recognise early and refer to haematology as mortality without urgent treatment is very high. It is caused by autoantibodies to ADAMTS13. This prevents the usual cleavage of von Willebrand factor, resulting in large strings of von Willebrand factor binding platelets and causing microthrombosis. It is a rare disorder (incidence ~1 per 100,000 per year). Onset is typically in adults and women are more commonly affected than men. TTP may be associated with other autoimmune disorders (Systemic Lupus Erythematosus [SLE], antiphospholipid antibody syndrome and scleroderma), pregnancy, and with drugs (e.g. quinine, clopidogrel and cancer chemotherapy)
Clinical features	Fever Anaemia (haemolytic anaemia: jaundice and haemoglobinuria) Thrombocytopaenia (purpura, bleeding) Neurological abnormalities (fits and fluctuating focal deficits) (present in ~50%) Acute kidney injury (in ~30%)
Full blood count and film	Anaemia Thrombocytopenia Fragmented red cells (schistocytes) characteristic Increased reticulocyte count
Blood results	Normal prothrombin and activated partial thromboplastin times Increased LDH and unconjugated bilirubin (reflecting haemolysis) Raised creatinine in ~30%

Appendix 82.2 (*Continued*)

Element	Comment
Differential diagnosis	Disseminated intravascular coagulation (Appendix 81.1)
	In pregnant women, pre-eclampsia/eclampsia and HELLP syndrome, Evans syndrome
	Autoimmune haemolysis
	Immune thrombocytopenic purpura
Management	Seek urgent advice from a haematologist
	Do not transfuse platelets
	High dose corticosteroids, plasma exchange until platelet count normal

CHAPTER 83

Acute painful sickle cell crisis

Noor Al-Zubaidi and Rachel Kesse-Adu

Pain due to vaso-occlusion, also referred to as sickle cell pain crises, accounts for more than 80% of acute presentations by individuals with sickle cell disease (SCD).

Establishing the diagnosis

Most individuals with SCD are aware of their diagnoses and hence sickle pain crises are straightforward to diagnose. It is however also an important differential diagnosis in people of Afro-Caribbean, Arab or Indian origin who present with acute pain with no clear cause.

For patients presenting with acute sickle cell pain rapid investigation and pain management is the primary aim.

Essential history and examination

It is important to undertake a detailed history with focus on potential triggers of sickle cell crises. Common triggers include infection, dehydration, stress and cold exposure. A full systems examination should be undertaken and note any limb or joint abnormalities indicating inflammation, any evidence of abnormal neurology and documentation of hepatosplenomegaly especially in paediatric patients in whom this may indicate a sequestration crisis.

Baseline investigations

- FBC, blood film, reticulocyte count
- Group & save
- CRP, U+Es, LFT, LDH
- ABG if hypoxic; $SO_2 < 94\%$ on room air
- Septic screen if indicated (blood, urine, sputum cultures and viral respiratory swabs)
- Chest X-ray if febrile or signs of acute chest syndrome
- Urine pregnancy test (if female of child-bearing age)
- To consider: Electrocardiogram, imaging as required guided by symptoms/signs
  To diagnose SCD in patients without a known diagnosis in whom a sickle crisis is queried confirm diagnosis with:
- Sickle cell solubility and high-pressure liquid chromatography (or haemoglobin electrophoresis).

Acute Medicine: A Practical Guide to the Management of Medical Emergencies, Sixth Edition.
Edited by Mridula Rajwani, Leila Vaziri, and Ivie Gbinigie.
© 2026 John Wiley & Sons Ltd. Published 2026 by John Wiley & Sons Ltd.

Pain management

Individuals with SCD presenting to health care settings with pain encounter multiple challenges: their pain is often underestimated. There are no pathognomonic signs or laboratory markers for SCD pain crisis other than the patient's report of pain. It is important to listen to SCD patients and treat them as experts in their condition, as per the National Institute for Health and Care Excellence guidance on managing SCD pain. Treat SCD pain as a medical emergency:

- Refer to patient's individualised pain plan, if available.
- Find out what analgesia has been taken prior to presentation, for severe pain, offer strong opioids, and for mild to moderate pain offer weak opioids.
- Offer analgesia within 30 min of presentation (as per NICE guidelines) then assess their response to pain every 30 min until pain is controlled, then 4 hourly.
- Prescribe analgesia as per WHO ladder: paracetamol, NSAID (if no contraindications), dihydrocodeine.
- Consider patient-controlled analgesia if no relief despite repeated doses of strong opioids.
- Wean down analgesia and switch to oral once appropriate.

General measures

Inform the haematology team of all SCD admissions even if the differential diagnosis is unrelated to the SCD. All SCD patients receiving opioid must be monitored for opioid toxicity. For all admissions consider:

- Appropriate initiation of antibiotics. SCD patients are hyposplenic and infection is a common trigger of crises – refer to local microbiology advice. Hyposplenic patients are at particular risk of infection with encapsulated bacteria: pneumococcus, meningococcus and *Haemophilus influenzae* type B.
- Offer VTE prophylaxis as there is a high risk of thrombosis.
- Hydration: aim for an intake of 3 L/day in adults. IV fluids if unable to maintain adequate hydration (e.g. vomiting).
- Oxygen: some patients find comfort in oxygen therapy (ensure oxygen saturations are routinely checked off oxygen to detect early signs of acute chest syndrome).
- Others: folic acid, prophylactic antibiotics (hold while on antibiotics for infection), offer incentive spirometry to prevent acute chest crisis. While on opioids: laxatives, antiemetics, antipruritic agents.

Transfusion support

Transfusion is usually not indicated in the management of a simple sickle cell pain crisis.

Unless immediately life- or organ-saving individuals with SCD should not be transfused without involvement of their Haematology teams.

Transfusion is usually part of management of these SCD complications:

A decreased haemoglobin (20 g/L below the patient's baseline haemoglobin) that may be due to:

- Increased haemolysis
- Sequestration both splenic or hepatic (raised reticulocyte count)
- Aplastic crisis (parvovirus infection and decreased reticulocyte count)

Blood transfused to SCD patients must be matched for full Rh and Kell type (liaise with the transfusion lab).

Exchange transfusion, which combines venesection and transfusion aiming to replace SCD blood with non-SCD blood may be indicated in certain severe complications including acute stroke and acute chest syndrome.

Other acute sickle complications

- Acute chest syndrome
  - Fever +/– respiratory symptoms with new lung infiltrates on CXR.
  - Around 30% of people with SCD will have one episode of acute chest syndrome in their lifetime.
  - Needs urgent haematology and intensive care input if suspected.
  - Likely to require blood transfusion if hypoxic.
- Acute stroke
  - Acute neurological symptoms may indicate ischaemic or haemorrhagic stroke.
  - Urgent brain imaging.
  - Will require emergency exchange transfusion.
- Priapism
  - Painful and persistent penile erection.
  - Initial treatment includes gentle exercise, encourage urination, hydration and pain relief. Oral etilefrine may be of help.
  - Patients are advised to present with episodes lasting >2hours, they will require penile aspiration if episode becomes fulminant, lasts >4hours.
- Splenic (and or hepatic) sequestration
  - Common in children. Rapid enlargement of spleen (and or liver) and fall in haemoglobin. Treated supportively with blood transfusion.
- Aplastic crisis
  - Acute anaemia due to parvovirus B19 infection. Characterized by low reticulocyte count. Treated supportively with blood transfusion.

Further reading

Howard J, Hart N, Roberts-Harewood M, *et al*. (2015) Guideline on the management of acute chest syndrome in sickle cell disease. *Br J Haematol* 169, 492–505. http://onlinelibrary.wiley.com/doi/10.1111/bjh.13348/epdf.

National Institute for Care and Health Excellence (2012) Sickle cell disease: managing acute painful episodes in hospital. Clinical guideline (CG143). https://www.nice.org.uk/guidance/cg143.

NICE. (2021) *Sickle Cell Disease*. NICE.

NICE Sickle cell disease|health topics A to Z|CKS|NICE. https://www.nice.org.uk/cks-uk-only.

CHAPTER 84

Common haematological malignancies

CONNOR SWEENEY AND SUE ANNE NG

Acute leukaemias

Acute myeloid leukaemia
Rapidly progressive cancer of the myeloid lineage of blood cells, characterised by proliferation of haematopoietic progenitor cells in the bone marrow and maturation arrest.

Aetiology
- Idiopathic.
- Previous chemotherapy (e.g. alkylating agents and topoisomerase II inhibitors) and radiotherapy.
- Preceding chronic myeloid malignancy – myelodysplastic syndrome (MDS) and myeloproliferative neoplasm (MPN).
- Genetics – Down syndrome, Fanconi syndrome and Li-Fraumeni syndrome.

Acute lymphoblastic leukaemia
Rapidly progressive cancer of the lymphoid lineage of blood cells, characterised by accumulation of immature lymphoblasts.

Aetiology
- Idiopathic.
- Previous chemotherapy (e.g. alkylating agents and topoisomerase II inhibitors) and radiotherapy.
- Genetics – Down's syndrome, Fanconi syndrome and Li-Fraumeni syndrome.

Common to both AML and ALL
Clinical features
Rapid onset of symptoms over days/weeks
  Signs and symptoms are due to bone marrow failure, catabolic state and organ infiltration
- Anaemia – fatigue, breathlessness and pallor.
- Neutropenia – recurrent infections, opportunistic infections and mouth ulcers.
- Thrombocytopenia – bleeding, bruising and purpura.
- Tissue infiltration – gum hypertrophy, skin infiltration, lymphadenopathy (monocytic leukaemia) and bone pain.
- Fevers, sweats, weight loss and malaise.

Acute Medicine: A Practical Guide to the Management of Medical Emergencies, Sixth Edition.
Edited by Mridula Rajwani, Leila Vaziri, and Ivie Gbinigie.
© 2026 John Wiley & Sons Ltd. Published 2026 by John Wiley & Sons Ltd.

- Leukostasis due to high white cell count ($>100 \times 10^9$/L) – pulmonary infiltration, confusion, retinal haemorrhage (commoner with acute myeloid leukaemia [AML]).
- Central nervous system involvement (commoner with acute lymphoblastic leukaemia [ALL]).

Classification

- French-American-British (FAB) classification, based on morphology.
- WHO classification has superseded the FAB classification and is based on genetic features of the diseases.

Investigations

- Full blood count:
  - Anaemia.
  - Leukopenia/leucocytosis.
  - Thrombocytopenia.
- Blood film – circulating blasts, Auer rods (distinguishes AML from ALL).
- Bone marrow aspirate and trephine biopsy – $\geq$20% blasts.
- Flow cytometry – distinguish AML from ALL.
- Molecular genetic testing.
- Cytogenetic analyses.
- Chest x-ray, computed tomography (CT) chest/abdomen/pelvis – source of infection, mediastinal/abdominal lymphadenopathy.

Differential diagnosis

- Infectious mononucleosis.
- Aplastic anaemia.
- Chronic myeloid leukaemia (CML) blast crisis.

Management
General

- Discuss with Haematologist urgently.
- Blood products
  - Hb aim >70 g/L and >80 g/L if cardiac disease present.
  - Platelets aim >10 if undergoing treatment and not bleeding or septic.
  - Fresh frozen plasma/cryoprecipitate – to correct coagulopathy/disseminated intravascular coagulation (DIC).
- Broad-spectrum antibiotics for febrile neutropenia/sepsis.
- Consider leukapheresis.
- Hydration and tumour lysis prophylaxis (Allopurinol or Rasburicase).

Chemotherapy

- Consider fitness for intensive or non-intensive chemotherapy based on age, co-morbidities and performance status.
- Molecular genetic and cytogenetic results influence prognosis and sometimes treatment.
- Aim of treatment is complete haematological remission, which is defined as no excess blasts (<5%) in the bone marrow and normalisation of the blood count.
- Cure is possible in some intensively treated patients.
  Phases of intensive chemotherapy:
  - Induction
  - Consolidation

  - Maintenance, in some cases
  - Allogeneic stem cell transplant – in fit patients at high risk of relapse
- Targeted therapies.
- Clinical trials.

Acute promyelocytic leukaemia

- Subtype of AML with accumulation of abnormal promyelocytes in the bone marrow.
- Results from the t(15;17) translocation.
- Often multiple Auer rods in acute promyelocytic leukaemia (APML) cells.
- Disseminated intravascular coagulation at presentation puts patient at high risk of life-threatening bleeding and thrombosis (10–20% early mortality).
  Commence emergency treatment as soon as diagnosis is suspected:
- Correct coagulopathy:
  - Platelet transfusions, aiming platelets $>50 \times 10^9$/L.
  - Fresh frozen plasma/cryoprecipitate to normalise PT/APTT and correct low fibrinogen.
- All-trans-retinoic acid (ATRA).
- Risk of differentiation syndrome with ATRA (pulmonary infiltrates, fluid retention and fever). Treatment with Dexamethasone and temporary cessation of ATRA.
  Definitive treatment is chemotherapy with Idarubicin/ATRA or Arsenic trioxide/ATRA.

Myelodysplastic syndromes

Clonal haematopoietic stem cell disorder characterised by ineffective haematopoiesis and manifested by morphological dysplasia, peripheral cytopenias and risk of progression to AML.

Aetiology

- Idiopathic.
- Prior treatment with radiotherapy or chemotherapy, such as alkylating agents or topoisomerase II inhibitors.
- Smoking.
- Genetics – congenital bone marrow failure syndromes, Fanconi syndrome, neurofibromatosis Type 1 and Schwachman–Diamond syndrome.

Clinical features

- Commoner with advancing age.
- May be asymptomatic.
- Anaemic symptoms – fatigue, breathlessness and pallor.
- Infective symptoms – recurrent infections, opportunistic infections and mouth ulcers.
- Thrombocytopenic symptoms – bleeding and bruising and purpuric rash.
- Constitutional symptoms – fatigue and weight loss.
- Hepatosplenomegaly – not usually present.

Classification

- FAB classification, based on morphology.
- WHO classification has superseded the FAB classification and is based on genetic features of the diseases.

Investigations

- Full blood count
  - Anaemia.
  - Leukopenia.
  - Thrombocytopenia/thrombocytosis.
- Blood film
  - Dysplastic features in red cells, white cells and/or platelets.
- Serum EPO level – lower levels predict response to EPO treatment.
- Bone marrow aspirate and trephine – assess cellularity and dysplasia.
- Flow cytometry – identify and quantify blasts.
- Molecular genetic and cytogenetic analyses – to confirm diagnosis and determine prognosis.

Differential diagnosis

- Other causes of cytopenias.
- Reactive bone marrow dysplasia – alcohol excess, HIV, cytotoxic therapy, severe intercurrent illness, drugs.

Management

- Revised International Prognostic Scoring System (IPSS-R) and IPSS-M (molecular) guide prognosis and therapy.
- Supportive care – mainstay of treatment of many patients aiming to maintain quality of life (QoL):
  - Blood products aiming to treat symptoms of anaemia and thrombocytopenia.
  - Antibiotics, antifungals, antivirals where indicated.
  - G-CSF – neutropenia and recurrent infections.
- Non-intensive and intensive chemotherapy.
- Allogenic stem cell transplant – only curable therapy.

Chronic myeloid leukaemia

Leukaemia is associated with uncontrolled proliferation of myeloid cells in the bone marrow and accumulation in the blood. Mature granulocytes and their precursors are seen.

Aetiology

- Idiopathic.
- Ionising radiation is associated with increased risk.
- The hallmark of CML is the presence of the Philadelphia chromosome, t(9;22) translocation. This results in the BCL-ABL1 fusion oncogene, which is a constitutively activated tyrosine kinase that leads to malignant transformation of haematopoietic stem/progenitor cells.

Clinical trajectory, if untreated:

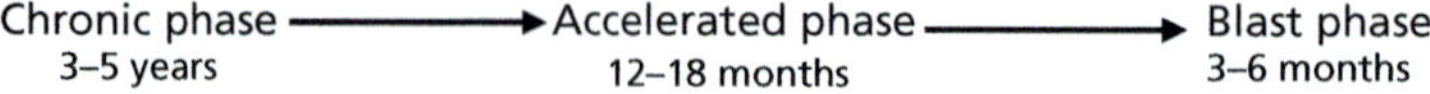

Clinical features

- Asymptomatic, incidental finding on blood test.
- Lethargy, fevers, night sweats and weight loss.

- Symptoms related to splenomegaly – abdominal discomfort/distension, abdominal bloating, early satiety.
- Gout.
- Occasionally leucostatic symptoms – dyspnoea and hypoxia, headache, visual changes and confusion.
- Bruising/bleeding.
- Splenomegaly common.
- Hepatomegaly.
- Lymphadenopathy uncommon.

Investigations

- Full blood count
  - Chronic phase
    - Anaemia.
    - Raised white cell count, often >100 × 10⁹/L.
    - Neutrophilia, basophilia, eosinophilia.
    - Platelets normal or increased.
  - Accelerated phase
    - Basophilia ≥20%.
    - Persistent thrombocytopenia <100 × 10⁹/L not due to therapy; persistent thrombocytosis >1000 × 10⁹/L on therapy.
    - Increased blasts 10–19%.
  - Blast crisis
    - Increased blasts ≥20%.
- Blood film
  - Mature granulocytes (neutrophils, eosinophils and basophils).
  - Myelocytes.
  - Blasts.
- Biochemistry – raised lactate dehydrogenase and urate.
- Bone marrow aspirate and trephine – hypercellular, myeloid hyperplasia
  - Blasts: <10% in chronic phase; ≥10% in accelerated phase; ≥20% in blast crisis.
  Cytogenetics (bone marrow or peripheral blood)
  - t(9;22) by FISH or karyotyping
  - Accelerated phase/blast crisis – clonal evolution with additional cytogenetic abnormalities.
- Molecular analysis with RT-PCR

Management

- Allopurinol – tumour lysis syndrome prophylaxis.
- Hydroxycarbamide – emergency cytoreduction for hyperleukocytosis.
- Tyrosine kinase inhibitor is the definitive treatment
  - Imatinib is usually first line.
  - Other TKIs – Dasatinib, Nilotinib, Bosutinib and Ponatinib.
- Allogenic stem cell transplant is rarely indicated.
- Other agents rarely used – Busulfan and Interferon-alpha.

Disease monitoring

- Molecular monitoring of BCR-ABL1 transcripts with RT-PCR.

Myeloproliferative neoplasms

Group of clonal haematopoietic stem cell disorders characterised by overproduction of mature cells red cells, platelets and/or granulocytes. MPNs are at risk of progression to myelofibrosis or AML. Philadelphia-negative classical MPNs include polycythaemia vera (PV), essential thrombocythemia (ET), and primary myelofibrosis (PMF).

Polycythaemia vera

MPN associated with increased red cell mass.

Aetiology

- *JAK2* mutation – V617F in 95% cases; exon 12 mutation in almost all remaining cases

Clinical features

- Asymptomatic.
- Fatigue, pruritus, headache, dizziness, weakness and paraesthesia.
- Facial plethora and splenomegaly.
- Arterial and venous thromboses.

Investigations

- Full blood count
  - Hb >165 g/L in men; >160 g/L in women.
  - Haematocrit >49% in men; >48% in women.
  - May be associated with thrombocytosis, neutrophilia, eosinophilia and basophilia
- Serum erythropoietin low. Elevated level suggests secondary causes of polycythaemia.
- *JAK2* mutation testing.
- Bone marrow biopsy considered.

Essential thrombocythaemia

MPN associated with elevated platelet count.

Aetiology

- *JAK2* V617F mutation (55%)
- *CALR* mutation (25%)
- *MPL* mutation (5–10%)
- Triple negative (10%)

Clinical features

- Asymptomatic.
- Fatigue, pruritus, headache, dizziness, weakness and paraesthesia.
- Haemorrhagic symptoms – easy bruising and mucosa/GI bleeding.
- Splenomegaly.
- Arterial and venous thromboses.

Investigations

- Full blood count
  - Platelets consistently >450 × 10^9/L.
  - Basophilia.

- Bone marrow biopsy considered.
- Exclude other causes of thrombocytosis, e.g. infection, post-surgery/splenectomy, malignancy, trauma, blood loss, iron deficiency, haemolytic anaemia, severe intercurrent illness and other clonal haematological disorders.

Primary myelofibrosis

MPN characterised by marrow fibrosis, splenomegaly, extramedullary haematopoiesis and a leucoerythroblastic blood film.

Aetiology

- *JAK2* V617F mutation (55%)
- *CALR* mutation (25%)
- *MPL* mutation (5–10%)
- Triple negative (10%)

Clinical features

- Asymptomatic.
- Constitutional symptoms (fevers, night sweats, weight loss and fatigue)
- Symptoms of marrow failure (anaemia, neutropenia and thrombocytopenia) – fatigue, infections and bleeding.
- Symptoms from splenomegaly (abdominal discomfort/distension, abdominal bloating and early satiety)

Investigations

- Full blood count
  - Normochromic normocytic anaemia.
  - Neutrophils and platelets may be elevated, normal or decreased.
  - Eosinophilia and basophilia.
- Raised LDH.
- Raised B12.
- Bone marrow aspirate and trephine – aspirate may be a dry tap. Trephine shows fibrosis and abnormal megakaryocyte morphology.

MPN management

Management for PV and ET:

Treatment is to reduce thrombotic risk.

- Cardiovascular risk factor management:
  - Lifestyle modifications – healthy BMI, stop smoking.
  - Treating reversible factors, e.g. hypertension, hypercholesterolaemia, diabetes mellitus.
- Aspirin.
- Venesections for PV, aiming haematocrit <0.45.
- Cytoreduction – Hydroxycarbamide, Interferon alpha, Anagrelide, Busulfan.
  - For PV, target haematocrit <0.45. For ET, aim platelets $<450 \times 10^9$/L.
- *JAK* inhibitors.

Management for MF:

Prognostic scoring systems (DIPSS Plus and MIPSS70) guide prognosis and treatment.

- Alleviate symptoms of anaemia – red cell transfusion, erythropoietin.
- Cytoreduction – Hydroxycarbamide.

- *JAK* inhibitors in symptomatic patients.
- Allopurinol to treat hyperuricaemia and prevent gout.
- Allogenic stem cell transplant – only curative therapy.

Lymphoma

Group of malignancies resulting from clonal proliferation of lymphoid cells including B-cells, T-cells and NK cells. Subtypes – Hodgkin and non-Hodgkin lymphoma.

Hodgkin lymphoma
Types
- Classical Hodgkin lymphoma (>90%)
  - Nodular sclerosing
  - Lymphocyte-rich
  - Mixed cellularity
  - Lymphocyte-depleted
- Nodular lymphocyte-predominant Hodgkin lymphoma (9%)

Aetiology
- Genetic and environmental predisposition.
- EBV in 40% cases.
- HIV.

Clinical features
- Bimodal age presentation – 20–29 and 60 years.
- Higher prevalence in males.
- B symptoms – fevers ≥38°C, drenching night sweats, unintentional weight loss >10%.
- Pruritus.
- Alcohol-induced lymph node pain.
- Recurrent infections.
- Often presents with painless lymphadenopathy (commonly cervical).
- Spreads from one nodal group to immediate adjacent nodes.
- Haematogenous spread to liver and lungs resulting in:
  - Hepatosplenomegaly.
  - Bulky mediastinum and hilar lymphadenopathy can result in superior vena cava obstruction.
- Extranodal and bone marrow spread – generalised lymphadenopathy.

Investigations
- Full blood count
  - Normocytic anaemia.
  - Leucocytosis, eosinophilia or thrombocytosis may be present.
- Blood film
  - Leucoerythroblastic film if extensive bone marrow involvement, usually accompanied by pancytopenia.
- Deranged LFTs if liver involvement.
- Increased serum urate, LDH and beta2-microglobulin.
- HIV, hepatitis B, C and EBV serology.
- *Helicobacter pylori* screening.

- Serum protein electrophoresis.
- PET-CT or CT neck/thorax/abdomen/pelvis.
- Lymph node biopsy.
- Cytogenetics.
- Molecular genetics.
- Consider bone marrow aspirate and trephine.

Classification
- Ann Arbor staging system – prognosis.

Management
- Treatment takes account of stage, disease bulk, performance status and co-morbidities.
- Cure rates >80%.
- Early stage (I, II) – combined modality with chemotherapy followed by radiotherapy.
- Advanced stage (III, IV) – usually chemotherapy only.
- Common chemotherapy regimen ABVD
  - A – adriamycin (doxorubicin).
  - B – bleomycin.
  - V – vincristine.
  - D – dacarbazine.
- Relapsed/refractory patients treated with salvage chemotherapy, followed by autologous stem cell transplant.
- Balance between effective treatment of the disease against risk of late effects, e.g. therapy-related malignancies, infertility and cardiotoxicity.

Non-Hodgkin lymphoma
>85% are B cell and <15% are T cell.

Some are slowly progressive (low grade) and may not require treatment, whereas others progress rapidly (high grade).

Types
- Low-grade (indolent) lymphomas
  - Follicular lymphoma.
  - Small lymphocytic lymphoma (SLL).
  - Marginal zone lymphoma (MZL).
  - Lymphoplasmacytic lymphoma (LPL)/Waldenström macroglobulinaemia.
- High-grade (aggressive) lymphomas
  - Diffuse large B-cell lymphoma (DLBCL).
  - Mediastinal large B-cell lymphoma.
  - Peripheral T-cell lymphoma.
  - Burkitt lymphoma.
  - HIV-associated lymphoma.
  - Post-transplantation lymphoproliferative disease.

Aetiology
- Genetic mutations – sporadic and hereditary.
- Congenital immunodeficiency – Wiskott–Aldrich syndrome, ataxia telangiectasia.
- Acquired immunodeficiency – immunosuppressed due to drugs or infection, e.g. HIV.
- Infections – EBV, *H. pylori*, HTLV-1.

Clinical features

- Presentation ranges from 'low-grade' indolent to 'high-grade' aggressive.
- Progressive painless lymphadenopathy.
- Extranodal symptoms – oropharyngeal, GI, CNS and skin.
- B symptoms – fevers ≥38 °C, drenching night sweats, unintentional weight loss >10%.
- Hepatosplenomegaly in advanced disease.

Low-grade NHL	High-grade NHL
Widely disseminated at presentation	Localised
Indolent clinical course	Rapid growth
Incurable	>50% curable

Classification

- WHO classification.
- International prognostic index.

Investigations

As for Hodgkin lymphoma
- Blood film
  - Circulating lymphoma cells
- Flow cytometry.
- Consider lumbar puncture for high-grade disease with extranodal disease.

Management

- Treatment takes account of stage, disease bulk, performance status and co-morbidities.
- Indolent B-cell lymphomas
  - Early stage – localised radiotherapy.
  - Advanced stage (most patients)
    - Asymptomatic, no bulk, no organ compromise → Watch and wait.
    - Symptomatic, organ compromise → Rituximab + chemotherapy, e.g. R-CVP or R-CHOP.
    - If good response → Rituximab maintenance.
- Aggressive lymphomas
  - Stage 1A with no bulky disease → R-CHOP (×3 cycles) + involved-field radiotherapy.
  - Other stages → R-CHOP (×6 cycles).
  - Intrathecal chemotherapy may be indicated.
  - Consider adjuvant radiotherapy at site of bulky disease.
- Common chemotherapy regimen R-CHOP
  - R – rituximab. Omit in T-cell lymphomas.
  - C – cyclophosphamide.
  - H – adriamycin (doxorubicin).
  - O – vincristine.
  - P – prednisolone.
- Elderly and less fit patients
  - Consider dose reductions ('R-miniCHOP') or other chemotherapy combinations.

Chronic lymphocytic leukaemia

Cancer of B-lymphocytes, resulting in the accumulation of mature B-cells in peripheral blood, bone marrow, lymph nodes and other organs.

Most common leukaemia in adults.

Aetiology
- Idiopathic.
- Familial in a minority of cases.

Clinical features
- Asymptomatic, incidental finding on blood test.
- Fatigue.
- B symptoms – fevers $\geq 38\,°C$, drenching night sweats, unintentional weight loss >10%.
- Recurrent infections.
- Bruising/bleeding.
- Splenomegaly.
- Hepatomegaly.
- Lymphadenopathy – painless and symmetrical.
- Immune cytopenias
    - Warm antibody autoimmune haemolytic anaemia (AIHA) – jaundice, dark urine and gallstones.
    - Immune thrombocytopenia (immune thrombocytopenic purpura, ITP).

Classification
- Rai and Binet staging use haemoglobin, platelet count and affected lymph nodes to stratify risk.

Investigations
- Full blood count
    - Clonal lymphocytosis $>5 \times 10^9/L$, may present $>400 \times 10^9/L$.
    - Pancytopenia in a more advanced stage.
    - AIHA or ITP may occur at any stage
    - Evidence of haemolysis (AIHA):
        - Increased reticulocytes, LDH and unconjugated bilirubin.
        - Direct Coombs test.
- Blood film
    - Mature lymphocytes.
- Immunoglobulins – hypogammaglobulinaemia.
- Flow cytometry – distinguishes CLL from other causes of lymphocytosis.
- Bone marrow aspirate and trephine – infiltration with mature lymphocytes.
- Lymph node biopsy – consider if diagnosis uncertain or to exclude transformation to high-grade lymphoma if rapidly enlarging nodes.
- *TP53* disruption – prognostic value.
- Imaging as necessary based on symptoms.

Differential diagnosis
- Other chronic lymphoproliferative disorders – morphology and flow cytometry distinguish.

Management
- Asymptomatic patients – monitoring only.
- Indications to treat:
    - Deteriorating blood counts:
        - Anaemia, neutropenia and thrombocytopenia.
        - Lymphocyte doubling time <6 months.
    - Constitutional symptoms (fatigue, fevers, night sweats and weight loss).
    - Progressive lymphadenopathy, splenomegaly and/or hepatomegaly.

- Treatment decisions take account of performance status, age, *TP53* and *IGHV* mutational status.
- Monotherapy or combinations of targeted therapies
  - Bcl-2 inhibitor (venetoclax).
  - Anti-CD20 monoclonal antibody (obinutuzumab).
  - Bruton's tyrosine kinase (BTK) inhibitors, e.g. ibrutinib and acalabrutinib.
- Chemoimmunotherapy in some young fit patients (fludarabine, cyclophosphamide and rituximab).
- Allogenic stem cell transplant is rarely indicated.
- Supportive treatments
  - Blood products.
  - Antibiotics, antifungals and antivirals.
  - G-CSF – to reduce risk of infection with neutropenia.
  - IV Immunoglobulin replacement – low serum immunoglobulins with recurrent infections.
  - Vaccinations (avoid live vaccines).

Myeloma

Definition

Cancer of plasma cells, which accumulate in the bone marrow and usually secrete monoclonal immunoglobulin or immunoglobulin light chains.

Aetiology

- Idiopathic.
- Familial in a minority of cases.
- Radiation.

Clinical features

- Related to classical triad
  - Increased plasma cells in bone marrow.
  - Clonal immunoglobulins or paraproteins.
  - Lytic bone lesions.
- CRAB clinical features
  - Hypercalcaemia.
  - Renal impairment.
  - Anaemia.
  - Lytic bone lesions.
- Symptoms of bone marrow failure – anaemia, thrombocytopenia and leukopenia.
- Spinal cord compression.

Investigations

- Full blood count
  - Normochromic normocytic anaemia.
  - Neutropenia and/or thrombocytopenia.
- Blood film
  - Rouleaux – stacked red blood cells.
- U&Es
  - Renal impairment.
  - Raised calcium.

- Serum beta2-microglobulin.
- Urinalysis – proteinuria.
- Immunoglobulins, serum/urine protein electrophoresis and immunofixation.
  - IgG paraprotein most commonly, followed by IgA. IgM, IgD and IgE paraproteins are uncommon in myeloma. Rarely, no immunoglobulin is secreted.
- Serum-free light-chain assay.
  - Elevated kappa or lambda light chains with skewed kappa/lambda ratio.
- Bone marrow aspirate and trephine – ≥10% clonal plasma cells.
- Flow cytometry.
- Cytogenetics – FISH to identify chromosomal abnormalities to guide prognosis and management.
- Skeletal survey, MRI whole body or PET-CT whole body.
- Consider MRI spine if spinal cord compression is suspected.

Differential diagnosis

- MGUS – associated with a 1% per annum risk of progression to myeloma.
- Other paraproteinaemias – solitary plasmacytoma, POEMS syndrome (polyneuropathy, endocrinopathy, monoclonal gammopathy and skin abnormalities), systemic AL amyloidosis and lymphoproliferative disorders.

Management

- Supportive therapy
  - Pain management.
  - Steroids – spinal cord compression and light chain nephropathy.
  - IV fluids – hypercalcaemia.
  - Bisphosphonates – bone protection and hypercalcaemia.
  - Blood products.
  - Surgery – spinal instability and pathological fractures.
- Combination chemotherapy regimens depending on age, performance status and comorbidities.
  - Monoclonal antibodies (daratumumab and anti-CD38).
  - Chemotherapy (e.g. cyclophosphamide and melphalan).
  - Immunomodulatory drugs, IMiDs (e.g. thalidomide and lenalidomide).
  - Proteasome inhibitors (e.g. bortezomib and carfilzomib).
  - Corticosteroids.
- Radiotherapy – localised pain and spinal cord compression.
- Autologous stem cell transplant extends the duration of remission.

Further reading

Alaggio R, Amador C, Anagnostoopoulos I, *et al.* (2022) The 5th edition of the World Health Organization classification of haematolymphoid tumours: lymphoid neoplasms. *Leukemia* 36, 1720–1748.

Khoury JD, Solary E, Abla O, *et al.* (2022) The 5th edition of the World Health Organization classification of haematolymphoid tumours: myeloid and histiocytic/dendritic neoplasms. *Leukemia* 36, 1703–1719.

CHAPTER 85

Management of anticoagulation

Susan Shapiro

Indications and choice of anticoagulants

The most common indications for therapeutic anticoagulation are atrial fibrillation (AF) and venous thromboembolism (VTE) (see Table 85.1). The main anticoagulatants and their key characteristics are summarised in Box 85.1.

Direct oral anticoagulants (DOACs) are licensed and as efficacious as warfarin for non-valvular AF (i.e. AF not associated with severe mitral stenosis) and VTE. They are associated with approximately 50% reduced risk of intracranial haemorrhage compared to warfarin, do not require monitoring, and have few drug interactions. They are therefore most people's anticoagulant of choice for licensed indications of VTE and AF.

Warfarin is the anticoagulant of choice for metal heart valves, people with recurrent VTE who need a higher therapeutic range, thrombosis (VTE or arterial) associated with triple-positive antiphospholipid syndrome; CrCl <15–30 mL/min.

Table 85.1 Indications for anticoagulation and recommended anticoagulant.

Indication	Low-molecular-weight heparin (LMWH)	Vitamin K antagonists (VKAs)	Direct-acting oral anticoagulants (DOACs)
Primary prevention of VTE post-operatively, in hospital inpatients or post surgery	Yes	No	Yes: for total knee and hip replacements only
Treatment of VTE (acute and long-term-secondary prevention)	Yes	Yes	Yes
Treatment of cancer-associated VTE	Yes (first line for gastrointestinal and genitourinary cancers)	Not recommended (less effective than LMWH)	Yes
Treatment of unstable angina/NSTEMI	Yes	No	No
Atrial fibrillation (AF)	Short-term (bridging) only	Yes	Yes
Prevention of mechanical-heart-valve-associated thromboembolic events and thrombosis	Short-term (bridging) only	Yes	No

VTE, venous thromboembolism.

Box 85.1 Types of anticoagulant and key characteristics.

Heparin	Derived from pig or cow intestines.
	Heparins act indirectly by binding to the endogenous anticoagulant anti-thrombin III (AT), enhancing its inhibition of clotting factors.
	Unfractionated heparin (UFH) is comprised of different-length polysaccharides. It needs to be given intravenously, and monitored using either APTT or antiXa levels.
	It has a short half-life and can be fully reversed with protamine sulphate. It can be used in renal failure.
	LMWH has replaced UFH as the preferred option in most clinical situations. Examples of when UFH would be considered are: patients who might need anticoagulation to be stopped rapidly (those at high risk of bleeding or who may require emergency invasive procedure); patients with acute VTE and CrCl<20mL/min.
	See Table 85.2 for a regimen for administering UFH infusion.
	Low-molecular-weight heparin (LMWH) contains the shorter polysaccharides only.
	LMWH is dosed according to body weight, once or twice daily subcutaneously.
	It has a half-life of approximately 12h.
	It does not require routine monitoring, but antiXa can be used to check levels if required, e.g. renal impairment, overdose.
	Dose adjustments are required if CrCL <20mL/min.
	Commonly used LMWH include dalteparin, enoxaparin and tinzaparin. Each has a specific dosing regimen. See Table 85.3 for dalteparin dosing for VTE by body weight.
	LMWH can only be partially reversed by protamine sulphate.
	Fondaparinux is related, but has pure anti-factor Xa activity.
	It is dosed according to body weight, once daily subcutaneous.
	It has a longer half-life than LMWH (about 17h) and cannot be reversed with protamine. It is most commonly used as an alternative anticoagulation in heparin-induced thrombocytopaenia (HIT) (see Table 85.2).
Warfarin and other vitamin K antagonists (VKAs)	Deplete the level of the reduced form of vitamin K in the liver, which is required for activation of vitamin K-dependent coagulation factors (factors II [prothrombin], VII, IX and X).
	Vitamin K has a slow onset and offset of action. When warfarin is initiated for acute DVT, it must be given with at least 5d LMWH cover initially even if therapeutic INR is achieved before this.
	Everyone requires individualised dosing of warfarin, and monitoring using the INR. For people on long-term warfarin, the majority need INR monitored every 3–4wk.

Warfarin is not usually recommended for people who require a dosette box, and dose adjustments following INR tests are challenging: speak to your local warfarin service or haematologist.

The target INR and range must be stipulated when starting someone on warfarin. The most common target INR is 2.5 (range 2–3). People with recurrent thrombosis may require a higher range, e.g. target INR 3.5 (range 3–4), as well as people with metallic heart valves.

Drug interactions with warfarin are common and can be serious. When starting or stopping a treatment in a patient taking warfarin, check the list in the *British National Formulary* for an interaction.

An example initiation of a patient on warfarin (dosing and blood tests) is shown in Table 85.4.

Warfarin can be reversed with vitamin K (oral or intravenous) and prothrombin complex concentrate (PCC) which contains factors II/VII/IX/X.

Direct Oral Anticoagulants (DOACs)

There are currently four DOACS: dabigatran is a direct inhibitor of factor IIa, and apixaban/rivaroxaban/edoxaban are direct inhibitors of factor Xa.

They are taken orally at fixed dose, once or twice a day.

Similar to LMWH, they have a half-life of approximately 12 h, and are largely renally cleared; and so should not be used when CrCl <15–30 mL/min.

They do not require routine monitoring. They have a variable effect on PT/APTT and the coagulation screen may be normal despite therapeutic levels of DOAC.

DOAC levels might be helpful in certain circumstances, e.g. renal impairment, overdose, emergency surgery. Specific DOAC tests have to be requested, e.g. apixaban levels; many, but not all, hospitals will be able to do these tests.

They have few drug interactions but key contraindications include: rifampicin, azole antifungals, HIV protease inhibitors and the antiepileptics carbamazepine and phenytoin.

Standard dosing regimens are shown in Table 85.5.

In case of bleeding: dabigatran has a direct reversal agent (idaricizumab), and andexanet alfa is licensed for reversal of apixaban and rivaroxaban. Tranexamic acid and PCC can be used to counteract the effects of edoxaban, or the other DOACs if specific reversal agents are not available.

Low-molecular-weight heparin (LMWH) is generally used short-term as it is subcutaneous and long-term use is associated with osteoporosis. It has minimal drug interactions but is renally excreted, and dosing should be reduced if CrCl <20 mL/min. It remains the anticoagulant of choice for cancer-VTE associated with gastrointestinal and genitourinary cancers as it has reduced bleeding risk compared to DOACs for these cancers in clinical trials.

Patient counselling of risks/benefits of anticoagulation and choice of anticoagulant is crucial.

Table 85.2 Example of protocol for unfractionated heparin by infusion for adults weighing up to 120 kg. Local hospital guidelines should be followed in practice.

Loading dose
5000 units IV over 5 min
Infusion
Give as a continuous infusion via a syringe pump using 1000 units/mL concentration.
Start the infusion at 1400 units/h (1.4 mL/h of the 1000 units per mL solution).
Monitoring
Check the activated partial thromboplastin time (APTT) at 4 h.
Ensure that the request form clearly states the patient is receiving heparin.

Table 85.3 Example of LWMH dosing: DALTEPARIN for the treatment of deep vein thrombosis/pulmonary embolism (DVT/PE) in adults (month 1 dosing).

Weight (kg)	Dose for DVT/PE treatment Subcutaneous administration (units)
Less than 46 kg	7500 once daily
46–56	10,000 once daily
57–68	12,500 once daily
69–82	15,000 once daily
83–98	18,000 once daily
More than 98 kg	Consult local guidelines: some local guidelines advise higher doses of dalteparin as weight increases

Table 85.4 Starting warfarin. Example fast loading regiment for acute VTE. Use local guidelines in practice.

Day	International Normalized Ratio (INR)	Dose of warfarin (mg) to be given that evening
1	1.3 or above	Establish cause of coagulation disorder. Do not start warfarin before discussion with a haematologist.
	<1.3	5
2		5
3	10	10
	1.5–2	5
	2.1–2.5	3
	2.6–3	1
	>3	0
4	<1.6	10
	1.6–1.7	7
	1.8–1.9	6
	2–2.3	5
	2.4–2.7	4
	2.8–3	3
	3.1–3.5	2
	3.6–4	1
	>4	0

Table 85.5 Dosing of direct oral anticoagulants by indication.

	Dabigatran	Rivaroxaban	Apixaban
Acute VTE	150 mg BD following five days of LMWH	Day 1–21 : 15 mg BD; Day 22 : 20 mg OD*	Days 1–7 : 10 mg BD; Day 7 : 5 mg BD
Prevention of recurrent VTE	150 mg BD	10 mg OD, or 20 mg OD* for high-risk patients	2.5 mg BD
	110 mg BD**		
Thromboprophylaxis	220 mg OD	10 mg OD	2.5 mg BD
	150 mg OD**		
Atrial fibrillation	150 mg BD	20 mg OD*	5 mg BD
	110 mg BD**		2.5 mg BD†

* 20 mg OD rivaroxaban should be taken with food, to aid absorption.

** A dose of 150 mg OD for thromboprophylaxis or 110 mg BD for AF/recurrent VTE should be considered in patients >75 yr or patients with eGFR <50 mL/min.

† The reduced doses of apixaban and dabigatran in atrial fibrillation are recommended for patients with two of the following: age >60 yr, weight <60 kg, serum creatinine >133 µmol/L.

Adjust the dose as follows:

APTT (target 1.5–2.5 × control)	Action
>5	Stop for 1 h then reduce infusion rate by 1.0 mL/h.
4.1–5	Reduce infusion rate by 0.5 mL/h.
3.1–4	Reduce infusion rate by 0.3 mL/h.
2.6–3	Reduce infusion rate by 0.1 mL/h.
1.5–2.5	No change.
1.2–1.4	Increase infusion rate by 0.1 mL/h.
1.0–1.2	Increase infusion rate by 0.2 mL/h.

After each change in infusion rate, recheck APTT in 4–6 h, and every 24 h if stable.

Check the platelet count at least on alternate days. Heparin-induced thrombocytopenia (HIT), which may be complicated by thrombosis, is most likely to occur 4–10 days after starting heparin. Stop heparin immediately and take advice from a haematologist if there is a significant fall in platelet count. See Table 82.1 and Appendix 82.1 (Chapter 82) for further information on the diagnosis of HIT.

Atrial fibrillation

The CHA$_2$DS$_2$VASc score (Table 85.6) estimates annual risk of stroke or systemic thromboembolism in non-valvular AF (Table 85.7). All patients with AF, whether paroxysmal, persistent or permanent are at increased risk of thromboembolism. Anticoagulation should be considered with a score of ≥2 for women ≥1 for men. With anticoagulants, the reduction in the risk of thrombosis must always be balanced against the increased risk of bleeding by being on an anticoagulant. The HASBLED score (Table 85.8) estimates the annual risk of major bleeding for patients on warfarin for AF (Table 85.9); and the ORBIT score is a new score which is similar to the HASBLED but does not take into account the choice of anticoagulant (Tables 85.10 and 85.11). NICE recommend the ORBIT score over other bleeding scores as evidence shows it has better accuracy in

Table 85.6 CHA_2DS_2VASc score (estimates the annual risk of stroke or systemic thromboembolism in non-valvular AF).

	Variable	Score
C	**Congestive heart failure** or left ventricular systolic dysfunction	1 for yes
H	**Hypertension**	1 for yes
	Blood pressure consistently above 140/90 mmHg (or treated hypertension on medication)	
A_2	**Age > 75 yr**	2 for yes
D	**Diabetes mellitus**	1 for yes
S_2	Prior **stroke or TIA or systemic thromboembolism**	2 for yes
V	**Vascular disease** (peripheral arterial disease, coronary artery disease and aortic atheroma)	1 for yes
A	**Age 65–74 yr**	1 for yes
Sc	**Sex category**	1 for female
	Total score	0–9
	(as age < 65 scores 0, age 65–74 scores 1 and age ≥ 75 scores 2)	

Table 85.7 Cumulative CHA_2DS_2VASc score and risk of stroke or systemic thromboembolism.

Cumulative CHA_2DS_2 VASc score	Annual risk of stroke or systemic thromboembolism (%)
0	0.3
1	1.3
2	2.2
3	3.2
4	4
5	6.7
6–8	9.8
9	15.2

Table 85.8 The HAS-BLED score (estimates the annual risk of major bleeding for patients on warfarin for atrial fibrillation).

	Variable	Score
H	**Hypertension**	1 for yes, 0 for no
	Systolic BP > 160 mmHg	
A	**Abnormal renal or liver function**	1 for yes, 0 for no
	Renal disease:	1 for yes, 0 for no
	Dialysis, transplant or serum creatinine >200 μmol/L	
	Liver disease:	
	Cirrhosis, serum bilirubin >2× normal or AST/ALT/alkaline phosphatase >3× normal	
S	**Stroke history**	1 for yes, 0 for no
B	**Bleeding risk**	1 for yes, 0 for no
	Prior major bleeding or predisposition to bleeding	
L	**Labile INR**	1 for yes, 0 for no
	Time in therapeutic range <60%	
E	**Elderly**	1 for yes, 0 for no
	Age > 65	
D	**Drug/alcohol history**	1 for yes, 0 for no
	Medication usage predisposing to bleeding (antiplatelet agents, NSAIDs)	1 for yes, 0 for no
	Alcohol consumption ≥8 units/wk	
	Total score	0–9

Table 85.9 Cumulative HAS-BLED score and risk of major bleeding.

HAS-BLED score (1–9)	Annual risk of major bleeding (%)
0	0.9
1	3.4
2	4.1
3	5.8
4	8.9
5–9	9.1

Table 85.10 The ORBIT score (estimates the annual risk of major bleeding for people with AF on anticoagulation).

Variable	Score
Haemoglobin <13 g/dL or haematocrit <40%	Yes +2
	No 0
Age > 74 yr	Yes +1
	No 0
Bleeding history:	Yes +2
Any history of gastrointestinal bleeding, intracranial bleeding or haemorrhagic stroke	No 0
Glomerular filtration rate (GFR) <60 mL/min/1.73 m^2	Yes +2
	No 0
Treatment with antiplatelet agents	Yes +1
	No 0

Table 85.11 Cumulative ORBIT score and risk of major bleeding.

ORBIT score	Bleeds per 100 patient-years
Low (0–2)	2.4
Medium (3)	4.7
High (≥4)	8.1

predicting absolute bleeding risk than other bleeding risk scores. However, patients at the highest risk of bleeding are often those who have the highest risk of stroke; it is therefore advised that these bleeding scores should be used as a tool to identify and control reversible bleeding risks in order to help reduce the bleeding risk.

Duration of anticoagulation following VTE and predicting risk of recurrence

Three months of anticoagulation is required to treat acute VTE (deep vein thrombosis or pulmonary embolism). In general, VTE **provoked** by a reversible risk factor (see Chapter 31) has a low probability of recurrence and anticoagulation can be safely stopped after this point.

Long-term anticoagulation (beyond the initial three months treatment) should be considered for secondary prevention, that is to prevent recurrent VTE, in people with **unprovoked** VTE, or a significant ongoing VTE risk factor (e.g. disseminated malignancy) following acute proximal deep venous thrombosis (DVT) and pulmonary embolism (PE). Conversely, if the VTE was **unprovoked** or provoked secondary to an irreversible risk factor, for example incurable disseminated malignancy, indefinite anticoagulation should be considered.

Management of bleeding in a patient taking an anticoagulant or antiplatelet drug

General measures are summarized in Table 85.12, and specific measures in Tables 85.13–85.15.

Table 85.12 Management of bleeding in a patient taking an anticoagulant or antiplatelet drug.

General measures
Stop the anticoagulant drug
Document the timing and amount of the last drug dose and presence of pre-existing renal or hepatic impairment
Estimate the half-life and length of functional defect induced by the drug
Assess the source of bleeding
Request full blood count, prothrombin time, APTT, thrombin time, fibrinogen; renal function
If available, request a specific laboratory test to measure the antithrombotic effect of the drug, e.g. INR, antiXa, apixaban level
Correct haemodynamic compromise with intravenous fluids and red cell transfusion
Apply mechanical pressure, if possible
Use endoscopic, radiological or surgical measures to achieve haemostasis

Source: Adapted from British Society for Haematology. Reproduced with permission of John Wiley & Sons.

Table 85.13 Specific measures according to the anticoagulant/antiplatelet agent.

Anticoagulant/antiplatelet	Specific measures
Heparins **Unfractionated heparin by continuous IV infusion** (half-life 1–2 h)	Stop the infusion. For rapid reversal in major bleeding, give IV protamine sulphate. 1 mg protamine neutralizes 80–100 units of heparin. If the infusion has been stopped for 30 min or longer, give protamine 25 mg IV by slow injection over 10 min. If the infusion has only just been stopped, give protamine 50 mg IV by slow injection over 10 min.
LMWH (half-life 12 h)	Stop the LMWH. Check FBC, coagulation screen and fibrinogen. Check anti-Xa level. If last dose of LMWH heparin was <8 h, give protamine. 1 mg per 100 anti-Xa units of LMWH IV, by slow injection over 10 min (maximum 50 mg). Consider 1 g tranexamic acid IV.
Warfarin and other VKAs	For rapid reversal in major bleeding or in head injury*, give four-factor prothrombin complex (contains factors II, VII, IX and X), e.g. Beriplex® or Octaplex®: give Beriplex or Octaplex 50 units/kg (to a maximum single dose of Beriplex 5000 units or Octaplex 3000 units). Fresh frozen plasma produces suboptimal anticoagulation reversal and should only be used if prothrombin complex is not available.

(continued)

Table 85.13 (*Continued*)

Anticoagulant/antiplatelet	Specific measures
	Give vitamin K 5–10 mg IV by slow injection.
	For non-major bleeding give 1–3 mg intravenous vitamin K (correction of the INR is seen within 6–8 h; this has a faster time to effect than oral administration).
DOACS (half-life about 12 h)	
Dabigatran	Stop dabigatran and ascertain time of last dose.
	Consider use of PRAXBIND (idaracizumab): 5 mg bolus by IV injection.
Rivaroxaban/apixaban	Stop drug and ascertain time of last dose.
	Consider andexanet alfa for licensed indications, e.g. life-threatening gastrointestinal bleeding.
	For situations when andexanet alfa is not licensed, consider 1 g tranexamic acid and PCC.
	Consider discussing with haematologist.
Edoxaban	Stop edoxaban and ascertain time of last dose.
	Consider 1 g tranexamic acid and PCC.
	Consider discussing with haematologist.
Antiplatelet agents, e.g. aspirin, clopidogrel, ticagrelor	Consider transfusion of two pools of platelets.

NB Protamine is contraindicated if the patient has a fish allergy. Protamine can cause hypotension, bradycardia and anaphylaxis.

* In head injury sufficient to cause facial or scalp laceration, bruising or haematoma, arrange for urgent CT head. If there is a suspicion of intracerebral bleed, reverse warfarin before the results of the CT head and INR are known. Even in patients with a normal CT head, a supra-therapeutic INR should be corrected with oral or IV vitamin K because of the risk of delayed bleeding. Adapted from: British Society for Haematology.

Table 85.14 Management of over-anticoagulation in a patient taking warfarin or another vitamin K antagonist who is *not* bleeding.

INR	Action
<5	Reduce maintenance dose
5–8	Omit 1–2 doses and reduce maintenance dose
>8	Give 1–5 mg oral vitamin K

Source: Adapted from: British Society for Haematology.

Table 85.15 Management of oral anticoagulation for elective surgery and invasive procedures.

Warfarin	For patients on warfarin, some minor procedures such as joint injections can be carried out without interrupting warfarin therapy; however, for major procedures, warfarin needs to be stopped and the INR normalised.
	Warfarin would standardly be stopped 5 d prior to surgery, with the INR measured the day before surgery; allowing correction with vitamin K if it is >1.5.
	Warfarin can usually be resumed at the normal maintenance dose on the evening of surgery.
	Patients at high thrombotic risk (e.g. mechanical heart valves and acute VTE within last 3 mo) require bridging therapy with LMWH when the INR is subtherapeutic (pre/post procedure).

Table 85.15 (*Continued*)

DOACS	**Apixaban/rivaroxaban/edoxaban** should be stopped 24 h before a low-risk bleeding procedure, and 48 h prior to a high-risk bleeding procedure (for people with CrCl >30 mL/min). If CrCl is <30 mL/min, then this duration needs to be increased. **Dabigatran** should be stopped 24 h before a low-risk bleeding procedure and 48 h prior to a high-risk bleeding procedure in people with CrCl >80 mL/min. For those with CrCl<80 mL/min, then this duration needs to be extended (dabigatran is more reliant on renal clearance than the other DOACs). Following a low bleeding risk procedure, a DOAC can be recommenced once haemostasis is secure, usually at 48 h. Following major surgery, or procedure with high bleeding risk, a DOAC should not be reintroduced until at least 48 h post procedure. Prophylactic LMWH should be considered in the interim (providing haemostasis is secure). Due to the short half-lives of DOACs, bridging with therapeutic LMWH is not required.

Management of oral anticoagulation for elective surgery and invasive procedures

The perioperative/periprocedural management of patients who are receiving anticoagulation depends on the underlying thrombotic risk and the risk of bleeding associated with the surgery/procedure.

Apart from in an emergency, for example insertion of a central line in a critically unwell patient, it is safer to allow anticoagulants to be metabolized/excreted rather than attempting to reverse them before a planned invasive procedure (e.g. lumbar puncture, chest drain and ascitic drain), as reversal agents are potentially pro-thrombotic and may expose the patient unnecessarily to plasma products. Safe timing of a procedure requires knowledge of when the last dose of anticoagulant was taken, the half-life of the drug, the excretion pathway, and any factors in the patient that may alter this, for example deranged renal function.

Renal Medicine

CHAPTER 86

Acute kidney injury

ELEANOR SMITH AND MICHELLE GOONASEKERA

Acute kidney injury (AKI) is defined as an absolute rise in serum creatinine of ≥27 mmol/L or oliguria (<0.5 mL/kg/h) for >6 h and is staged as in Box 86.1. AKI is present in 10–20% of hospital admissions and is an independent risk factor for morbidity and mortality. Hypovolaemia and sepsis account for the majority of AKI seen in acute medicine, with the remainder due to urinary tract obstruction and rarer systemic or intrinsic renal diseases.

Management is based on the following principles:

- Focused history, (including drug history); features suggestive of specific causes of AKI are found in Table 86.1. Drug causes of AKI are found in Table 86.2.
- Examination with particular reference to haemodynamic and fluid balance assessment.
- Structural imaging of the renal tract (ultrasound or non-contrast CT in the first instance to exclude obstruction).
- Urinalysis – increasingly dipstick analysis and urine protein quantification (albumin : creatinine or protein : creatinine ratio) replaces microscopy for casts.

Box 86.1 Definition and staging of acute kidney injury.

AKI is defined by:

- A rise in serum creatinine by ≥27 μmol/L, in 48 h or less
- A >50% rise in serum creatinine from baseline, in seven days, or
- A urine output of <0.5 mL/kg/h for >6 h.

AKI is staged by the magnitude of the rise in serum creatinine or decrease in urine output:

Stage of AKI	Serum creatinine	Urine output
1	Rise in serum creatinine ≥27 μmol/L in 48 h, or rise 1.5–1.9 times from baseline	<0.5 mL/kg/h for 6–12 h
2	Rise in serum creatinine 2.0–2.9 times from baseline	<0.5 mL/kg/h for ≥12 h
3	Rise in serum creatinine three times from baseline, or increase in serum creatinine to ≥354 μmol/L, or initiation of renal replacement therapy irrespective of serum creatinine	<0.3 mL/kg/h for ≥24 h or anuria for ≥12 h

AKI, acute kidney injury.

Acute Medicine: A Practical Guide to the Management of Medical Emergencies, Sixth Edition.
Edited by Mridula Rajwani, Leila Vaziri, and Ivie Gbinigie.
© 2026 John Wiley & Sons Ltd. Published 2026 by John Wiley & Sons Ltd.

Table 86.1 Causes of acute kidney injury: clinical features, typical findings on examination of the urine and confirmatory tests.

Cause of AKI	Clinical features suggesting diagnosis	Typical urinalysis	Confirmatory tests
Hypovolaemia/ hypotension	Systolic BP <100 mmHg or a decrease in baseline BP of >40 mmHg or postural hypotension; low JVP.	Normal urinalysis	Resolution of AKI on correction of hypovolaemia/ hypotension.
Sepsis	Fever or reduced body temperature (<36 °C); clinical focus of infection.	May be normal, or show pyuria if UTI.	Microbiological confirmation of infection.
Nephrotoxic drugs and toxins	Exposure to known nephrotoxic drug or toxin (Table 86.2).	May be normal, some drugs, e.g. immune checkpoint inhibitors can cause proteinuria and glomerulonephritis (GN).	Resolution of AKI on withdrawal of drug or toxin (see below tubulointerstitial nephritis).
Hepatorenal syndrome	Chronic or acute liver disease with liver failure and portal hypertension, *in the absence of volume depletion*. Note that sepsis and hypovolaemia are also prevalent in this group and distinct from hepatorenal syndrome.	Typically normal	Resolution of AKI with improvement in liver function.
Diseases involving large renal vessels			
Renal artery thrombosis/ embolism/dissection	Flank pain	Mild proteinuria, haematuria, or can be bland.	CT or MR angiography
Renal vein thrombosis	Background of nephrotic syndrome	Nephrotic range proteinuria >300 mg/ mmol and macro- or microscopic haematuria.	CT venogram or duplex US where available
Diseases of small vessels and glomeruli			
Glomerulonephritis/ vasculitis	See Chapter 90. Evidence of multi-system disease.	Proteinuria, usually 50–300 mg/mmol, microscopic or macroscopic haematuria.	Condition-specific blood tests, renal biopsy
HUS/TTP	In particular thrombocytopenia, red cell fragments on blood film.	May be normal or low-grade proteinuria 50–300 mg/mmol, microscopic haematuria.	Evidence of microangiopathic haemolytic anaemia (MAHA) on blood film, renal biopsy, targeted complement tests for atypical HUS.
Severe hypertension with acute hypertensive nephrosclerosis	Severe hypertension, with retinal haemorrhages and exudates, may have evidence of MAHA on blood film.	Microscopic haematuria or moderate proteinuria	Renal biopsy
Scleroderma renal crisis (SRC)	Skin signs of scleroderma Moderate to severe hypertension, often with retinal haemorrhages and exudates. Association with high steroid dose >20 mg prednisolone/day.	Normal or mild proteinuria	Renal biopsy confirmatory, but often high risk, and diagnosed clinically.

Table 86.1 (*Continued*)

Cause of AKI	Clinical features suggesting diagnosis	Typical urinalysis	Confirmatory tests
Diseases of the tubulointerstitium			
Tubulointerstitial nephritis	Recent drug exposure. Fever, rash and arthralgia. Eosinophilia.	Usually bland	Renal biopsy
Cast nephropathy	Transient or mild hypotension followed by oligoanuria. Hypercalcaemia, bone pain or atypical fractures, anaemia, monoclonal paraprotein.	Heavy proteinuria or monoclonal proteinuria (NB can appear 'bland' as dipstick is specific for albumin).	Renal biopsy, serum electrophoresis and free light chain quantification.
Rhabdomyolysis	Raised serum creatine kinase, history of crush injury, long lie or compartment syndrome. Disproportionate acidosis, hyperkalaemia and hypocalcaemia.	Dipstick haematuria (cross-reactivity of myoglobin).	Usually clinical, renal biopsy confirmatory if needed.
Acute bilateral/single kidney pyelonephritis	Fever, flank pain, renal tenderness.	Pyuria, bacteriuria.	Urine microscopy and culture
Urological			
Urinary tract obstruction	Abdominal or flank pain	May be normal	Ultrasonography or non-contrast CT

Table 86.2 Drugs and toxins in acute kidney injury.

Nephrotoxic drugs/exposures	Exogenous toxins	Endogenous toxins
Radiocontrast agents	*Amanita phalloides*	Free haemoglobin (intravascular haemolysis)
Aminoglycosides	Ethylene glycol	Free myoglobin (rhabdomyolysis)
Amphotericin	Paracetamol poisoning	Free light chains (myeloma)
NSAIDs	Salicylate poisoning	
β-lactam antibiotics		
Sulphonamides		
Aciclovir		
Methotrexate		
Cisplatin		
Calcineurin inhibitors (ciclosporin and tacrolimus)		
ACE-inhibitors		
Angiotensin-receptor blockers		
Immune checkpoint inhibitors		
Proton pump inhibitors		

Table 86.3 Approach to clinical assessment of the patient with AKI.

Element	Comment
What is the volume status?	History of volume depletion (diarrhoea or vomiting, haemorrhage, recent surgery or trauma, sepsis and diuretic medications). Tachycardia, hypotension or postural hypotension. JVP raised or not seen, mucus membranes, presence of third or fourth heart sounds, lung bases for crepitations, ascites and peripheral oedema.
Has there been anuria, oliguria or polyuria?	Anuria is seen in severe hypotension or complete urinary tract obstruction. It is more rarely due to bilateral renal artery occlusion (e.g. with aortic dissection), renal cortical necrosis, acute cast nephropathy or necrotizing glomerular disease. Established acute tubular injury gives rise to anuria following a prolonged period of hypotension in critical illness. Assume that anuria is due to bilateral urinary obstruction until proven otherwise. Polyuria, for example in hyperglycaemia or hypercalcaemia, may be a cause of volume depletion leading to AKI.
Is there evidence of sepsis or infection?	Fever, localising signs, neutrophilia or lymphopenia, positive blood or urine cultures. NB infective endocarditis is a cause of GN.
Drug history	Note specific drug causes of AKI as per Table 86.2, also drugs that are renally excreted, and diuretics that can exacerbate hypovolaemia. Note the variable phenotype of drug-induced AKI that can include acute GN.
Are there lower urinary tract symptoms suggestive of obstruction? Are there features suggestive of systemic disease?	Poor stream, hesitancy, incomplete voiding and urgency are most associated with bladder outflow obstruction. Obstruction higher up the urinary tract should be excluded by imaging. In particular: Vasculitis: low-grade fever, malaise, weight loss, joint pains or myalgia, purpuric rash, ENT symptoms, haemoptysis and frank haematuria Myeloma: weight loss, bone pain, anaemia and hypercalcaemia Rhabdomyolysis: history of crush or electrical injury, compartment syndrome, prolonged immobility or seizures, extreme exercise and genetic syndromes with predisposition HUS/TTP: history of diarrhoea (may be absent), evidence of MAHA (thrombocytopenia, bilirubinaemia, raised LDH with reduced haptoglobins and red cell fragments on blood film) +/– neurological symptoms.
Is there hypertension?	Hypertension can be a cause or consequence of AKI: accelerated-phase hypertension, aortic dissection, pre-eclampsia and SRC are causes. Hypertension may be seen as a consequence where acute GN leads to severe AKI (the so-called 'nephritic syndrome').
Is there heart failure?	Acute heart failure with hypotension leading to hypoperfusion of the kidney. Medications in chronic heart failure include nephrotoxins (ACEis/ARBs) and diuretics which exacerbate hypovolaemic states leading to AKI.
Is there liver failure?	Important to differentiate hepatorenal syndrome, due to splanchnic vasodilatation and reduction in renal blood flow, from hypovolaemia or sepsis which are also common in acute or chronic renal failure and have different management. Human albumin solution (e.g. 100 mL 20% solution given twice daily) in treatment of sepsis for patients with chronic liver disease is protective against AKI. Role for terlipressin in treatment of hepatorenal syndrome. In acute liver disease associated with AKI consider paracetamol overdose and leptospirosis.
Is there vascular disease?	Recent endovascular intervention associated with cholesterol embolus causing AKI. Critical renal artery stenosis can precipitate AKI in hypovolaemia or with new ACEi/ARB.

Priorities

1 Identify and respond to sepsis and hypovolaemia with appropriate antibiotic therapy and prompt fluid resuscitation:

- Volume resuscitation should be accompanied by regular assessment of fluid balance, especially where confounding conditions such as heart failure coexist.
- Point-of-care ultrasound (POCUS) assessment of left and right ventricular filling and collapsibility of the inferior vena cava (IVC) with respiration have increasingly replaced invasive measurement of central venous pressure.
- Urinary catheterisation is not essential for fluid balance measurement but should be considered where a patient is confused, or incontinent, or where there are concerns about bladder outflow obstruction.
- If a patient is adequately volume resuscitated and remains hypotensive (mean arterial pressure <65 mmHg), discussion with intensive care unit (ICU) regarding whether vasopressor therapy is indicated, if appropriate.
- Management of sepsis is discussed in detail in Chapter 5.

2 Structural imaging of the renal tract to exclude obstruction:

- Where bladder outflow obstruction cannot be confidently excluded by a bedside bladder scan, or to confirm suspected anuria, urinary catheterisation can be performed. Routine catheterisation of the AKI patient is no longer recommended if fluid balance can be monitored without this.
- Ultrasound of the renal tract is the ideal imaging modality; where this cannot be offered quickly, a non-contrast CT is a good alternative. This should be obtained within 24 h. Where there is a single kidney, transplant kidney, or suspected pyonephrosis, imaging should be obtained urgently.
- If identified, urinary tract obstruction should be discussed with a urologist.

3 Management of complications of AKI:

- The criteria for renal replacement therapy in AKI are found in Box 86.2.
- Hyperkalaemia is defined as K > 6.5 mmol/L.
  - **i.** Where electrocardiogram (ECG) changes are present, initial management is with calcium gluconate or calcium chloride, 10 mL 10% solution given intravenously. This can be repeated if necessary, until ECG changes resolve or until serum-adjusted calcium reaches 3 mmol/L.
  - **ii.** Where there is metabolic acidosis (serum bicarbonate <22 mmol/L) and no fluid overload, intravenous sodium bicarbonate 1.26% 500 mL can be given over 1–2 h.
  - **iii.** Insulin (up to 10 units fast-acting) and dextrose 50% 50 mL or 20% 75 mL is given over 30 min where K > 6.5. Nebulised salbutamol 5 mg also has a small effect and can be used as a temporising measure.

Box 86.2 Criteria for initiation of renal replacement therapy (RRT) in AKI.

Hyperkalaemia >6.5 mmol/L despite medical treatment.

Pulmonary oedema not responsive to diuretics, or with oligoanuria.

Severe or profound metabolic acidosis pH <7.1 despite medical treatment.

Uraemic complications: pericarditis and encephalopathy.

NB Absolute urea levels *alone* in AKI are not an indication for RRT, and urea levels >40–50 mmol/L are needed before uraemia should be suspected as the cause of obtundation or pericarditis. Urea *itself* is not toxic even at levels 10× the upper limit of normal, but its levels mirror those of other toxic small molecules that accumulate in renal failure and which are not measured routinely.

Specific drug overdoses or poisons that are cleared rapidly on dialysis, e.g. lithium and ethylene glycol

    iv. Sodium zirconium cyclosilicate 10g up to three times daily is effective in treating persistent but non-life-threatening hyperkalaemia, with onset of action as quick as 1h. Although also effective in life-threatening hyperkalaemia, sodium zirconium cyclosilicate monotherapy should not replace the interventions above.

    v. Where hyperkalaemia persists despite vigorous medical treatment of potassium and underlying causes, or in the presence of oligoanuria, renal replacement therapy may be indicated and early discussion with ICU or local renal unit is advised.

- Pulmonary oedema is treated with oxygen to target saturations >94%:
  - **i.** High-flow nasal oxygen or continuous positive airway pressure can be used to provide positive end-expiratory pressure and supplement oxygenation.
  - **ii.** Sit the patient upright.
  - **iii.** Furosemide at minimum 80mg IV should be given if diuretic naïve. If established on diuretics, double the usual oral dose should be given intravenously.
  - **iv.** A nitrate infusion can be used if systolic BP >110mmHg.
  - **v.** Assessment for underlying cardiac disease with ECG and echocardiogram or POCUS.
  - **vi.** Where there is pulmonary oedema in the presence of oligoanuria, urgent discussion with ICU or renal unit regarding renal replacement therapy is required.

7 Further management of AKI:

- Review of medications with a view to cessation of nephrotoxins, and diuretics where hypovolaemia is present, and review of dosing and schedule of renally excreted drugs (the renal drug database provides comprehensive drug information in renal impairment; specialist pharmacy advice should be sought where needed).
- Where AKI persists despite resolution of hypovolaemia, treatment of sepsis and cessation of nephrotoxic drugs, renal advice should be sought.
- Complete list of recommended investigations in AKI can be found in Box 86.3.

Box 86.3 Investigations in acute kidney injury.

All patients
Serum urea, creatinine, sodium, potassium, calcium, phosphate and bicarbonate
Full blood count
Blood gases: venous usually sufficient, for lactate, pH, point of care bicarbonate and haemoglobin estimation
Blood glucose
Coagulation screen
C-reactive protein
Blood and urine cultures, if there is a suspicion of infection
Urine dipstick test for blood, protein and glucose
Urine protein:creatinine ratio if any protein evident on dipstick (>50mg/mmol may suggest glomerular disease, NB this can be longstanding, e.g. in diabetes)
ECG
Chest x-ray
Imaging of the renal tract to exclude obstruction: usually ultrasound, but non-contrast CT is an alternative

Further investigation: depending on results and progress
Creatine kinase if risk factors or suspicion of rhabdomyolysis
Myeloma screen (serum immunoglobulins, electrophoresis and serum free light chain measurement)
Antinuclear antigen (ANA) if suspicion of SLE, then endonuclear antigens if ANA is positive
Complement (C3, C4) plus rheumatoid factor: hypocomplementaemia is present in SLE, cryoglobuli-naemia, membranoproliferative GN, HUS, post-infective GN and others
Antineutrophil cytoplasmic antibody (ANCA): NB a positive ANCA should be accompanied by measure-ment of myeloperoxidase (MPO) and proteinase-3 (PR3) – if both are negative, the positive ANCA may be spurious and unrelated to the AKI
Anti-glomerular basement membrane (GBM) antibody: if strong suspicion of anti-GBM disease this should be arranged urgently, so that prompt plasma exchange can begin
Hepatitis B, C and HIV serology: both as a potential factor in AKI, and for infection control purposes if dialysis is needed
Group and antibody screen: if there is active bleeding, or if plasma exchange may be required

Further reading

Johnson RJ, Floege J, Tonelli M (Eds.). (2023) *Comprehensive Clinical Nephrology*, 7th edition. Section XIV Acute kidney injury.
Turner NN. (2015). In: *Oxford Textbook of Clinical Nephrology*, Lameire N, Goldsmith DJ, Winearls CG, *et al.* (Eds), 4th edition. Section 11 The patient with acute kidney injury (and critical care nephrology).

CHAPTER 87

Chronic kidney disease, including end-stage kidney disease

KHIZR NAWAB AND MATTHEW BROOK

Definition

- Chronic kidney disease (CKD) refers to the presence of varying degrees of renal dysfunction, categorised by abnormal estimated glomerular filtration rate (eGFR) and albuminuria, for three months or longer.
- CKD is classified based on the underlying cause and staged based on calculated eGFR (G1 through G5, with higher stages reflecting lower eGFR) and degree of albuminuria (A1 through A3, with higher stages reflecting greater degrees of albuminuria); see Figure 87.1.
- End-stage kidney disease refers to CKD stage V in addition to patients receiving renal replacement therapy.
- Renal replacement therapies include haemodialysis (which can be delivered in-centre or at home), peritoneal dialysis or transplant.

Evaluation of cause of CKD

- The most common causes of CKD worldwide include diabetes, hypertension, glomerulonephritis and polycystic kidney disease.
- Once chronicity has been established (see Table 87.1), establishing a cause for CKD involves a multi-faceted approach (see Table 87.2) including a detailed medical history and examination with a particular focus on the following:
  - Medications: Focus on newly started agents, particularly those known for their nephrotoxicity and any over-the-counter herbal remedies and allergies which may not be volunteered directly. Analgesics such as non-steroidal agents are commonly used *ad hoc* by patients.
  - **Symptoms and signs of systemic diseases** should be elicited systematically as renal dysfunction can be a prominent feature of conditions such as systemic lupus erythematosus, connective tissue disorders and vasculitis. This includes asking patients about weight loss, anorexia, night sweats, a reduction in appetite, general lassitude with no obvious alternative cause, upper respiratory symptoms, haemoptysis, general myalgia, arthralgia, rashes, ulcers, hair loss.
  - **Symptoms and signs of urinary tract abnormalities**, particularly in men, can provide clues towards potential obstructive uropathies. Nocturia, starting and stopping of the flow of urine, hesitancy and poor stream are all suggestive of potential bladder outflow obstruction and warrant prompt imaging and further discussion with urological surgeons. A large palpable mass arising from the suprapubic region, with dullness to percussion may suggest a grossly enlarged bladder with chronic urinary retention, warranting urgent

KDIGO: prognosis of CKD by GFR and albuminuria categories			Persistent albuminuria categories Description and range		
			A1	**A2**	**A3**
			Normal to mildly increased	Moderately increased	Severely increased
			<30 mg/g <3 mg/mmol	30-300 mg/g 3-30 mg/mmol	300 mg/g >30 mg/mmol
GFR categories (mL/min/1.73 m^2) Description and range	**G1**	Normal or high	≥90		
	G2	Mildly decreased	60–89		
	G3a	Mildly to moderately decreased	45–59		
	G3b	Moderately to severely decreased	30–44		
	G4	Severely decreased	15–29		
	G5	Kidney failure	<15		

Green: low risk (If no other markers of kidney disease, no CKD); Yellow: moderately Increased risk; Orange: high risk; Red: very high risk. GFR, glomerular filtration rate.

Figure 87.1 Adapted from KDIGO 2024 clinical practice guideline for the evaluation and management of chronic kidney disease.

Table 87.1 Adapted from executive summary of the KDIGO 2024 clinical practice guideline for the evaluation and management of chronic kidney disease: known knowns and known unknowns.

   i. **Proof of chronicity (duration of a minimum of three months) can be established by:**
  ii. **Review of past estimated or measured GFR**
 iii. **Review of past measurements of albuminuria, proteinuria or urinary microscopic examinations**
  iv. **Imaging findings such as reduced kidney size and reduced cortical thickness**
   v. **Histopathological interstitial fibrosis and tubular atrophy based on a previous renal biopsy sample**
  vi. **Repeat measurements within and beyond the three-month point**

catheterisation and further urology investigations. Flank pain associated with macroscopic haematuria may be suggestive of ureteric calculi. It is important to note that patients will often report passing normal volumes of urine despite evidence of urinary retention or upper tract obstruction causing hydronephrosis.

- ***Abnormalities of urine*** such as gross haematuria, particularly in relation to recent upper respiratory infections, and frothy urine, which can be due high levels of proteinuria, are suggestive of glomerular disorders.
- ***Eliciting any history of diabetes*** is important due to the sheer ubiquity of this condition. Remember that advanced CKD, unfortunately, can sometimes be the first presentation of diabetes mellitus. For established diabetics, it is important to establish the age at diagnosis, type 1 versus type 2 diabetes, glycaemic control over the years and microvascular (retinopathy, neuropathy) and macrovascular complications of diabetes. Diabetic nephropathy typically causes a chronically progressive, proteinuric CKD, in association with other microvascular complications, particularly retinopathy. It is important to use this opportunity to comprehensively establish the impact diabetes has on their health as a whole and to involve the diabetologists if needed.

Table 87.2 Adapted from KDIGO 2024 clinical practice guideline for the evaluation and management of chronic kidney disease.

Establishing a cause of CKD	
Physical examination	Look for signs of systemic disease or weight loss. Volume assessment, percussing for palpable bladder, blood pressure (including postural measurements), listening for a pericardial rub or renal bruit.
Medication history	Newly started medications and correlations with renal function; focus on penicillin-based antibiotics (risk of TIN), proton pump inhibitors (risk of TIN), non-steroidal agents (risk of ATN, TIN, membranous nephropathy), medications acting on the renin–angiotensin–aldosterone axis (can cause haemodynamic changes within the kidney, causing decreased filtration (often acceptably so and then associated with renal protection)).
Identifying urinary tract abnormalities	Lower urinary symptoms (frequency, dysuria), macroscopic haematuria, obstructive symptoms (hesitancy, poor stream, terminal dribbling), strangury. Also, focus on changes in quantity of urine passed and nocturia.
Eliciting signs and symptoms of systemic diseases	Seek out symptoms and signs of connective tissue disorders, lupus, vasculitis, especially in at-risk patients. Remember non-specific symptoms of weight loss, lethargy, night sweats are often a dominant feature of presentation.
Eliciting signs and symptoms of common diseases causing renal dysfunction	Diabetes: age at onset, type, anti-diabetic drugs and their history, glycaemic control, macro- and microvascular complications (especially retinopathy). Hypertension: age at onset, degree of control, number of agents needed for control, evidence of end-organ damage (encephalopathy, cardiomyopathy), evidence of complications (retinopathy, strokes), investigation of secondary causes.
Detailed family history	Pedigree to map out mode of inheritance, genetic testing in family members, age at onset, degree to which family members are affected by condition, extra-renal manifestations (e.g. sensorineural deafness with Alport's, intracranial aneurysms with autosomal dominant polycystic kidney diseases).
Detailed social history	Other than helping to build rapport with patient, will inform the management options offered to the patient in terms of renal replacement therapy. Useful to identify environmental triggers to certain conditions (e.g. smoking for anti-GBM disease)
Bedside investigations	Urinalysis: active urinary sediment guides one towards glomerular inflammation, proteinuria crucial for diagnosis of nephrotic syndrome. Bladder scan: useful to identify retention.
Formal laboratory investigations	Identifying anaemia, renal bone disease, secondary hyperparathyroidism (all signs of relative chronicity); non-invasive acute renal screen (ANA, ANCA, anti-GBM, serum electrophoresis, light chain ratio, immunoglobulin and complement levels), urinary proteinuria quantification and electrophoresis.
Imaging	US or CT KUB – to identify size, number of kidneys, corticomedullary differentiation, hydronephrosis. CT or MR angiogram to assess renal vessels if indicated.
Kidney biopsy	Gold standard for diagnosis of various intrinsic renal conditions.

- ***Eliciting a history of hypertension*** is also similarly important. Secondary hypertension is more likely than primary hypertension to be associated with renal impairment, and there is typically evidence of other end-organ damage (cardiomyopathy and retinopathy). Persistent hypertension, refractory to multiple agents, in an ambulatory setting is far more likely to be associated with renal impairment. It is important to note, however, that with advanced CKD and attendant fluid overload, hypertension is exceedingly common and there must be a convincing antecedent history of severe hypertension if renal failure is to be blamed on it. Certain nephritic syndromes also present with hypertension as part of the clinical syndrome.

- ***Eliciting a detailed family history*** is critically important in diagnosing familial conditions such as autosomal dominant polycystic kidney disease. If there is a 'positive' family history, a pedigree of affected family members will be useful in identifying the mode of inheritance and can guide further imaging and genetic analysis.

- The judicious use of various bedside and laboratory tests and evaluation techniques can yield clues as to the cause of CKD:
  - ***Imaging,*** obtained promptly, is essential to rule out bladder outflow obstruction or upper urinary tract obstruction, both of which can present with CKD. The presence, size, symmetry, and morphology of kidneys can be appreciated via an ultrasound or cross-sectional imaging techniques such as computed tomography or magnetic resonance imaging. Ultrasonography is safe and imminently useful but requires a skilled operator, and its utility may be limited by the patient's body habitus. An unenhanced computed tomography scan of the kidneys, ureter and bladder can act as a substitute. Where indicated, renal arteries and veins can be specifically imaged via CT or MR angiograms as ultrasound is not typically diagnostic.
  - ***Urinalysis*** is a cheap, widely available test which can be obtained at the point of care. The presence of blood and protein on urinalysis can bring into play various intrinsic renal diseases, thus alerting the assessing clinician of the need to involve nephrology services early.
  - ***Quantification of proteinuria*** is advisable if there is proteinuria on urinalysis. Urine albumin:creatinine ratio measurements are used widely. A 24 hour collection is rarely necessary. In certain cases, non-albumin proteinuria (light-chain cast nephropathy, tubular proteinuria) can account for the majority of proteinuria and for this reason, sending urine for both albumin:creatinine ratio and protein:creatinine ratio is advisable.
  - ***Serological tests*** are particularly helpful in diagnosing various causes of CKD due to systemic and intrinsic renal diseases and the history, examination and urinalysis should be used to determine which tests need to be sent. In patients with microscopic haematuria and/or macroscopic proteinuria with CKD consideration should be given in liaison with renal services to sending a renal acute screen including: antinuclear antibodies (ANA), anti-neutrophil cytoplasmic antibodies (ANCA), anti-glomerular basement membrane (GBM) antibodies, serum free light chains, serum and urine protein electrophoresis, immunoglobulin and complement (C3 and C4) levels alongside more routine biochemistry. Active infection, if suspected, should be sought with blood cultures and further investigations targeting the potential source (e.g. echocardiogram for potential infective endocarditis). Anti-streptolysin O titre is useful in diagnosing post-infection glomerulonephritis.

Managing complications of CKD

- It is important to note at the outset that most CKD is asymptomatic until at an advanced stage and discovered incidentally in primary or secondary care.
- Patients with CKD are more susceptible to acute kidney injury (AKI), and the investigation and management of AKI remains largely the same in spite of the presence of underlying renal dysfunction. Such ***acute-on-chronic kidney injury (AoCKI)*** as well as advanced chronic kidney disease (stage IV and V) can be associated with some specific management concerns, outlined below:
  - ***Hypovolaemia*** leading to hypotension due to numerous reasons can lead to AoCKI and judicious fluid resuscitation with a temporary halting of diuretics and medications with haemodynamic effects on the kidney is indicated. If crystalloid boluses are used for fluid resuscitation, repeated fluid balance assessments and urine output monitoring should be used to guide fluid replacement with small boluses being used where there is uncertainty.

- ***Fluid overload*** can occur in AoCKI if the patient becomes oliguric/anuric. The value of an accurate fluid balance assessment, repeated at regular intervals to guide fluid management, cannot be underestimated. This involves assessment of thirst, assessing mucous membranes, skin turgor, assessing the jugular venous pressure remaining mindful of potential right heart failure or valvular disease which can confound this assessment, peripheral oedema (which tends to be pedal in ambulant patients and sacral in bed-bound patients) and auscultation and imaging of the lung fields to identify pulmonary oedema. Regular patient weights and monitoring of urine output are indispensable for guiding diuresis in such cases. Managing acute pulmonary oedema is described elsewhere (Chapter 14). Patients with existing CKD may already be on high doses of diuretics to manage their fluid balance. If an acute insult renders them anuric, renal replacement therapy will be needed urgently; early involvement of nephrology services would be prudent. Where patients retain some urine output and sufficient blood pressure, a trial of higher-than-usual dose of loop diuretic might be helpful as a temporising measure (higher doses are required in AKI and CKD to meet a diuretic threshold). Heart disease often co-exists with renal disease and concomitant assessment of the heart with an electrocardiogram and echocardiogram is recommended.
- ***Hyperkalaemia*** can be life threatening and typically occurs due to reduced renal potassium excretion by the failing kidney but also due to the acidosis which tends to dominate. Emergent management of hyperkalaemia as outlined in Chapter 86 is recommended with a particular focus on cessation of agents promoting hyperkalaemia, typically those affecting the renin–angiotensin–aldosterone axis. Where acidosis exists, intravenous bicarbonate can encourage transcellular movement of potassium into cells and high doses of loop diuretics can aid a kaliuresis. Ultimately, renal replacement therapy will need to be considered.
- ***Uraemic complications*** include uraemic encephalopathy, pericarditis or gastritis. The symptoms of uraemia are non-specific and attribution of confusion to uraemia can result in diagnostic over-shadowing and missing other more convincing contributory factors such as delirium, intracranial pathology, sepsis, other metabolic and electrolyte abnormalities. Evidence of mental slowness will be obvious in the course of history-taking and often, a collateral is useful in shedding light on hitherto unappreciated cognitive decline. Tests of cognitive function and attention are useful in quantifying cognitive decline. Pericarditis and uraemic pericardial effusions can be diagnosed with an electrocardiogram and an echocardiogram, respectively. A pericardial rub in the context of uraemia warrants urgent renal advice. Ultimately, the presence of suspected complications of advanced uraemia necessitates renal replacement therapy. Patients with CKD are more prone to gastrointestinal bleeding and prompt recognition of this in the context of a disproportionate urea rise is key.

Contrast nephropathy

- The use of iodinated contrast media is thought to cause, in certain vulnerable individuals, a transient, non-oliguric reversible AKI.
- The proposed underlying mechanisms include vasoconstriction causing medullary hypoxia, direct tubular toxicity and altered levels of various vasoactive mediators.
- The risk of AKI should certainly be assessed and mitigated before offering iodinated contrast media to adults, but this **must not delay emergency or essential contrast imaging**.
  - Increased risk is associated with:
    - eGFR less than $40\,mL/min/1.73\,m^2$
    - Diabetic with eGFR less than $40\,mL/min/1.73\,m^2$
    - Heart failure
    - Renal transplant

- Age 75 and over
- Hypovolaemia
- Increased volume of contrast agent
- Intra-arterial administration of contrast medium with first-pass renal exposure
- Historically, the literature on contrast media nephrotoxicity has been limited due to a lack of adequate and robust control groups and a failure to adequately account for significant predisposing risk factors when making comparisons between patients with CKD who were administered contrast or spared contrast.
- A relatively recent meta-analysis analysed propensity score-matched pairs obtained from 21 cohort studies finding no increased risk for AKI, dialysis or mortality after contrast-enhanced CT among patients with eGFR >45 mL/min/1.73 m². The use of multivariable logistic regression identified an association between eGFR <30 mL/min/1.73 m² and AKI, but even here the absolute increase in risk in patients exposed to contrast compared to those who were not was low (19% versus 15%).
- There is no convincing evidence for the use of N-acetylcysteine to prevent or mitigate contrast-associated AKI.
- Volume expansion, via the intravenous or oral route, is sometimes recommended and this is not unreasonable, but the volume and rate of crystalloid infusion must be guided by the patient's fluid balance and not given without thought.

Anaemia in patients with CKD/ESKD

- Anaemia is invariably associated with advanced CKD and ESKD and is typically a result of attenuated erythropoietin reserve in the diseased kidneys alongside a functional iron deficiency.
- The degree of anaemia correlates with the stages of CKD such that most patients with CKD G4 and higher tend be on some form of erythropoiesis-stimulating therapy (ESA). Iron replacement can be via the oral route in less advanced CKD with the intravenous route often required for higher stages of CKD and for ESKD.
- The adjustment of ESA and iron doses is usually the preserve of outpatient nephrology with a target haemoglobin of 100–120 g/L.
- When patients with CKD/ESKD present acutely unwell in a general medicine setting, they can be anaemic (or more anaemic than usual) for a number of reasons including bleeding from a hitherto unknown source, sepsis, haemolysis, abnormalities of bone marrow, etc. As such, a comprehensive medical history, examination and appropriate supplementary investigations (elemental iron, transferrin saturation, ferritin, LDH, haptoglobin, reticulocyte count, blood film, B12, folate, etc.) are often required to tease out the contributory factors for a new and/or worsening anaemia in an otherwise stable patient with CKD/ESKD.
- Once such reversible causes have been considered and ruled out, iron and ESA doses can then be adjusted in conjunction with the patient's overseeing nephrologist.
- For patients with an ongoing acute driver for anaemia, such as active bleeding necessitating urgent surgery or a haemolytic process, there may be no choice but to transfuse blood as this is the only means of rapidly correcting haemoglobin (ESA therapy adjustments take a few weeks to have an effect).
- For patients with CKD/ESKD who are candidates for a transplant in the future, the immune-sensitising effect of a red cell transfusion must be considered, and it would always be wise to involve the patient's nephrologist in such discussions unless in an emergency situation.

Comprehensive conservative care in patients with CKD

- The increasing prevalence of CKD in elderly, frail and heavily co-morbid patient populations has necessitated a focus on so-called comprehensive conservative care.
- Comprehensive conservative care is an encompassing term which includes delaying progression of CKD, minimising complications of CKD and engaging in detailed communications with patients and their families

on goals of treatment, advanced care planning, including the provision of psychological support, as required. Crucially, it does not involve the provision of renal replacement therapy.
- There are two main scenarios where renal replacement therapy may not be considered:
  - Stable: This refers to the elderly patient presenting to nephrology clinic or a medical setting with CKD diagnosed either in primary care or discovered incidentally, with a significant burden of medical co-morbidities (such as heart failure or ischaemic heart disease), significant frailty and/or cognitive and functional impairment or the presence of pre-existing conditions which curtails life expectancy (e.g. disseminated malignancy). Alternatively, it could also refer to the patient for whom the physical, psychological, and time-related burdens of renal replacement therapy are simply incompatible with the maintenance of their quality of life.
  - Critically ill: This is where a critical illness has rendered a patient acutely in need of renal replacement therapy. In some cases, due to chronic disease burden and/or frailty, the impact of potentially long-term dialysis on quality of life is felt to be unacceptable. The prospect of renal recovery is often uncertain. Patients may not be physiologically able, in acute illness, to tolerate the haemodynamic challenges of renal replacement therapy meaning it is not considered to be an option. In many cases, the patient may not wish for invasive access procedures or dialysis to be performed. In other situations they may be willing to tolerate renal replacement therapy if recovery is a short term meaningful prospect but not otherwise and a time limited period of dialysis is occasionally used with ongoing review.
- Kidney Disease Improving Global Outcomes (KDIGO) suggest comprehensive conservative care should be introduced as a viable treatment option for patients who are unlikely to benefit from dialysis.
- In one of the larger studies in this area to date in stable CKD, Chandna et al studied 844 patients over an 18 year period (82% treated by RRT and 18% conservatively) and found that median survival (gauged from onset of stage V CKD) was 21.2 months in the conservative care group versus 67.1 months in the RRT group. **However, this survival advantage was reduced to 4 months for those over 75 years, once age, comorbidity and diabetes were corrected for**.
- In a general medicine setting, the elderly, frail and/or co-morbid patient presenting with CKD (either incidentally discovered or in association with an acute illness), presents arguably an even greater challenge in terms of discussing prognosis and the utility of RRT in terms of its impact on survival and quality of life.
  - The early involvement of a nephrologist to aid the caretaking team in undertaking these delicate, emotionally charged discussions in an acute situation is essential unless the patients does not wish to consider RRT or the clinical judgment that RRT is inappropriate is clear.
  - Once a decision to pursue comprehensive conservative care has been agreed by all parties, there will need to be an open dialogue between the nephrology or treating team, local palliative care, including hospice-level care if needed, the patient, their family and primary care to enact a robust plan for the management of symptoms. This should be undertaken wherever possible in the patients location of choice.

Further reading

Chandna SM, Da Silva-Gane M, Marshall C, *et al*. (2011) Survival of elderly patients with stage 5 CKD: comparison of conservative management and renal replacement therapy. *Nephrol Dial Transplant* 26(5), 1608–1614.

Davison SN, Levin A, Moss AH, *et al*. (2015) Executive summary of the KDIGO controversies conference on supportive care in chronic kidney disease: developing a roadmap to improving quality care. *Kidney Int* 88(3), 447–459.

Levin A, Ahmed SB, Carrero JJ, *et al.* (2024) Executive summary of the KDIGO 2024 Clinical Practice Guideline for the Evaluation and Management of Chronic Kidney Disease: known knowns and known unknowns. *Kidney Int* 105(4), 684–701.

Mullasari A, Victor SM. (2014) Update on contrast induced nephropathy. *EJ ESC Counc Cardiol Pract* 13, 4.

Murtagh FE, Burns A, Moranne O, *et al.* (2016) Supportive care: comprehensive conservative care in end-stage kidney disease. *Clin J Am Soc Nephrol* 11(10), 1909–1914.

National Institute for Health and Care Excellent (2013) 2023 exceptional surveillance of acute kidney injury: prevention, detection and management (NICE guideline NG148). https://www.nice.org.uk/guidance/NG148/documents/162

Obed M, Gabriel MM, Dumann E, *et al.* (2022) Risk of acute kidney injury after contrast-enhanced computerized tomography: a systematic review and meta-analysis of 21 propensity score–matched cohort studies. *Eur Radiol* 32(12), 8432–8442.

Stevens PE, Ahmed SB, Carrero JJ, *et al.* (2024) KDIGO 2024 clinical practice guideline for the evaluation and management of chronic kidney disease. *Kidney Int* 105(4), S117–S314.

CHAPTER 88

Renal tubular disorders

Michael Turner and Katherine R. Bull

Priorities

The renal tubule processes glomerular filtrate and regulates homeostasis of fluid, electrolytes and pH. Apart from acute tubular injury (ATI), renal tubular disorders are rare, but can present to the general medical take and should be considered as part of the differential in people with unexplained electrolyte, acid base or complex renal stone disorders.

Tubular disorders may be inherited or acquired, and cause electrolyte imbalances that need supplementation and dietary/lifestyle changes. Presentations depend on the underlying defect.

Suspected inherited or acquired tubular disorders should usually be discussed with or referred to Nephrology for further investigation and on-going management. Where a genetic cause is suspected, discuss with Nephrology or Clinical Genetics service. In the United Kingdom, panel testing for renal tubulopathy and tubular acidosis genes is available (see links at end of this section).

Acute tubular injury (ATI)

Pathophysiology: The commonest tubular disorder and most commonly caused by ischaemia due to pre-renal acute kidney injury (AKI, Chapter 86), it is self-limiting unless cortical or tubular necrosis occurs. The former can result in chronic kidney disease (CKD) or renal replacement therapy (RRT) dependence and the latter in acquired Fanconi's syndrome (see below).

Presentation: Persistent renal impairment after precipitating illness has resolved. Urine will typically not contain blood and protein (but catheterised samples can mislead). May take days-weeks to resolve.

Key investigations: Urine dipstick, renal US to exclude obstruction, screen for other causes of AKI (Chapter 25). Fractional excretion of sodium (FENa) >1% is suggestive of tubular rather than pre-renal injury but not reliable. When injury persists, renal biopsy may exclude other pathology.

Management: Removing precipitating cause, ensuring euvolaemia and treating infection, and supportive care, including renal replacement therapy (RRT). Suspected ATI that does not respond to initial and supportive measures should be discussed with nephrology.

Disorders by segment

Specific tubular disorders are now considered by tubular segment (Figure 88.1).

Acute Medicine: A Practical Guide to the Management of Medical Emergencies, Sixth Edition.
Edited by Mridula Rajwani, Leila Vaziri, and Ivie Gbinigie.
© 2026 John Wiley & Sons Ltd. Published 2026 by John Wiley & Sons Ltd.

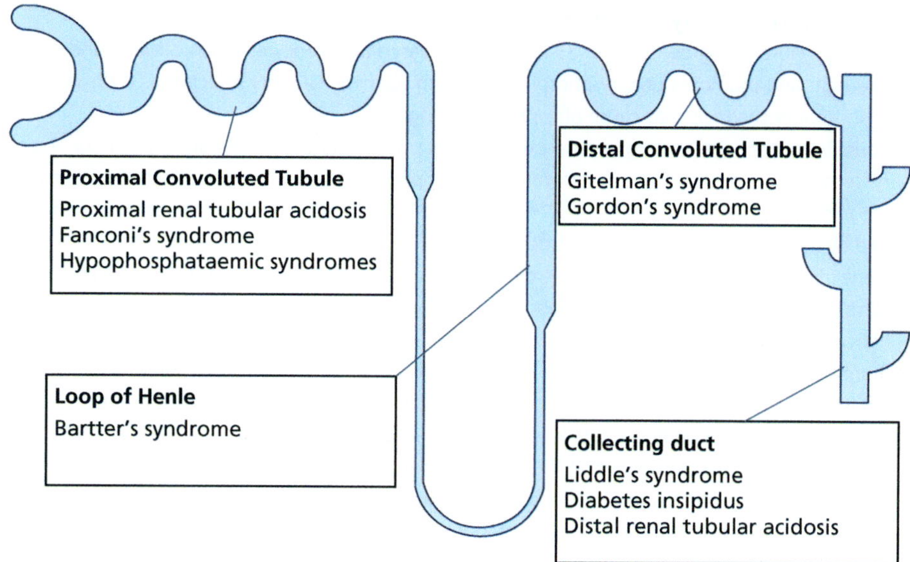

Figure 88.1 Segments of the kidney tubule and selected conditions affecting them. Source: Adapted from Walsh and Unwin, Clin Med (Lond) 2012/Royal College of Physicians.

The proximal convoluted tubule

The proximal convoluted tubule is responsible for most reabsorption of essential metabolites. Due to high rates of aerobic metabolism, the proximal tubule is sensitive to insults such as hypoperfusion, mitochondrial disorders or heavy metals.

Fanconi's syndrome

Pathophysiology: Fanconi's syndrome describes impaired proximal reabsorption of sodium, potassium, phosphate, amino acids, glucose and bicarbonate. This causes metabolic acidosis, hypokalaemia and hypophosphataemia. Genetic causes underly most paediatric cases. Acquired causes dominate in adults, including ATI, lead and cadmium poisoning, myeloma, amyloidosis, Sjögren's syndrome and medications such as tenofovir and aminoglycoside antibiotics.

Presentation: In childhood, delayed growth and rickets, plus features related to underlying cause, e.g. neurological impairment in Wilson's disease. Adults may present with symptoms of osteomalacia or muscle weakness, or with incidental urine and blood abnormalities.

Investigations: Paired urine and serum pH, phosphate, potassium, sodium and glucose levels may reveal hypokalaemia, hypophosphataemia and hyperchloraemic metabolic acidosis. Glycosuria and generalised aminoaciduria are expected. Screen for monoclonal gammopathy. Isolated glycosuria in the absence of diabetes mellitus can be due to pregnancy, or mutations in the SGLT2 channel. Differential may include Vitamin D or calcium deficiencies, see also hypophosphatemia syndromes and renal tubular acidosis (RTA), below.

Management: Treat underlying cause if acquired. Potassium citrate treats both hypokalaemia and acidosis. Phosphate and vitamin D supplementation are also required (alfacalcidol since hydroxylation may be impaired). Intercurrent illnesses may severely dehydrate people with Fanconi's syndrome, low threshold for IV fluids.

Proximal renal tubular acidosis

See RTA below.

Hypophosphataemia syndromes

Pathophysiology: Fibroblast growth factor 23 (FGF23) is released by osteocytes when calcitriol and phosphate levels are high and promotes urinary phosphate wasting. Genetic variants affecting FGF23, vitamin D or tubular phosphate channels may cause phosphate wasting.

Acquired tubular phosphate-wasting can be caused by vitamin D deficiency (dietary, lack of sun exposure), primary, secondary or tertiary hyperparathyroidism. Hypophosphataemia is a side effect of intravenous iron infusion, particularly Ferric carboxymaltose, due to FGF23 stabilisation. FGF23-mimicking proteins can be produced by tumours causing oncogenic osteomalacia.

The non-renal differential for hypophosphataemia includes gastrointestinal (malnutrition, reduced absorption, alcoholism), and increased intracellular phosphate sequestration (refeeding syndrome, haematological malignancy and diabetic ketoacidosis).

Presentation: Hypophosphataemia and rickets in childhood. Weakness, confusion, muscle and bone pain in acquired forms. Nephrocalcinosis or stones due to hypercalciuria when vitamin D is elevated.

Investigations: Serum and urine phosphate levels. ionised calcium levels, alkaline phosphatase (ALP), parathyroid hormone (PTH), measurement of 25(OH) vitamin D and where available consider 1,25(OH) vitamin D and FGF23 dependent on initial results. Consider imaging for malignancy in acquired forms.

Management: Phosphate and calcitriol supplementation. Treatment of underlying cause.

The loop of Henle

The loop on Henle establishes the corticomedullary counter current which allows urinary concentration.

Bartter's syndrome

Pathophysiology: Results from loss of sodium and chloride reabsorption due to autosomal recessive mutations in *SLC12A1*, encoding NKCC2 (type 1), *KCNJ1* (type 2), *CLCLNKB* (type 3), *CLCNKA* and *CLCNKB* (type 4b) or *BSND* (type 4a).

Presentation: Bartter's syndrome type 1, 2 and 4 present antenatally with polyhydramnios and lethargy. Type 3 may present in adolescence or early adulthood with hypokalaemia, metabolic alkalosis, hypomagnesaemia and hypercalciuria. Patients prefer salty snacks. Blood pressure is low-normal. Hypercalciuria can lead to nephrocalcinosis or stones.

Investigations: Paired urine and serum pH, potassium, sodium, chloride and calcium will show hypokalaemic metabolic alkalosis, with high fractional urinary excretion of potassium, calcium and chloride. Urinary tract US shows nephrocalcinosis in type 1, 2 and sometimes 3.

Management: By a nephrologist or experienced clinical biochemist. Encourage a salty diet, slow-release potassium chloride. If blood pressure permits, potassium-sparing diuretics may be useful, but caution is needed because of the risk of hypovolaemia. NSAIDs have been used (to suppress prostaglandin) but may increase the risk of CKD. Often it is not feasible to achieve potassium levels in the normal range. Intercurrent illnesses can result in serious dehydration so low threshold for IV rehydration. Anaesthesia needs careful planning. Pregnancy, particularly if hyperemesis occurs, can present additional risks.

Distal convoluted tubule

Reabsorbs sodium and chloride, as well as magnesium and calcium via transcellular mechanisms.

Gitelman's syndrome

Pathophysiology: loss of function mutations in the thiazide receptor (Na^+/Cl^- channel NCC) in the distal convoluted tubule.

Presentation: Mild hypotension, hypokalaemia, hypomagnesaemia, metabolic alkalosis and hypocalciuria (unlike hypercalciuria in Bartter's syndrome). Symptoms are variable, but may include lethargy, tetany, paraesthesia, and polydipsia. Often diagnosed in adolescence or adulthood. Take a detailed and sensitive history exploring eating disorders, laxative and diuretic abuse. Proton pump inhibitors can cause hypomagnesaemia.

Investigations: Serum potassium and magnesium are low, and serum bicarbonate high, with low urine calcium:creatinine ratio. Urine chloride may distinguish from gastrointestinal (GI) potassium loss (urinary chloride is inappropriately high in Gitelman's syndrome). If blood pressure is high consider hyperaldosteronism and check cortisol, aldosterone and renin. Exclude hyperthyroidism which can cause low potassium.

Management: Encourage a salty diet. The need for electrolyte supplements varies, but slow-release oral potassium and magnesium supplements are typically required. Aim for K>3mmol/L and Mg>0.6mmol/L. Potassium will be difficult to correct unless hypomagnesaemia treated. Magnesium supplements can cause GI symptoms, Mg lactate may be better tolerated than Mg glycerophosphate. Intercurrent illnesses can result in serious dehydration so low threshold for IV rehydration.

Gordon's syndrome (pseudohypoaldosteronism type II)

Pathophysiology: The mirror image of Gitelman's syndrome, caused by activation of the thiazide receptor.

Presentation: Na^+ and Cl^- retention with hypertension, metabolic acidosis, hypercalciuria may present as kidney stones. Differential includes autosomal recessive 11β-hydroxysteroid dehydrogenase deficiency (apparent mineralocorticoid excess), which itself can be mimicked by excessive liquorice intake.

Investigation: Consider and investigate for other causes of hypertension. Genetic testing for *WNK4* and *HSD11B2* gene mutations. CT KUB if renal colic present.

Management: Responds well to thiazide diuretics.

The collecting duct

The collecting duct comprises principal cells which reabsorb water and sodium and secrete potassium, and intercalated cells which secrete bicarbonate or H^+.

Nephrogenic diabetes insipidus

Pathophysiology: Antidiuretic hormone (ADH) is released in response to hypertonic serum and binds V2 receptors in the collecting ducts. This increases water reabsorption, maintaining serum osmolality and concentrating urine. Failure of the kidney to respond to ADH is nephrogenic diabetes insipidus (DI). Failure of posterior pituitary ADH secretion is central DI. Both cause polyuria and polydipsia.

Nephrogenic DI is most commonly acquired, due to lithium toxicity or hypercalcaemia. Rarely, nephrogenic DI is inherited due to variants in *AVPR2* (X-linked) and *AQP2*.

Presentation: Polyuria and polydipsia, with polyuria persisting and marked dehydration when access to water is restricted (e.g. by illness and/or hospital admission). Other causes of polyuria (e.g. diuretic use, diabetes mellitus, post-obstructive diuresis and psychogenic polydipsia) should be excluded.

Investigation: Urine osmolality will be low (<300mOsm). Serum osmolality is high (>300mOsm) when access to water is insufficient. A water deprivation test can demonstrate this. A desmopressin challenge will differentiate central from nephrogenic DI.

Management: Treat precipitating conditions. Plentiful access to fluids, ensure adequate supplementary fluid is given when illness prevents patients from drinking freely (e.g. peri-operatively). Thiazide diuretics help limit hypernatraemia.

Liddle's syndrome

Pathophysiology: Genetic variants prevent vesicular sequestration of ENaC, resulting in unregulated sodium reabsorption and hypertension. Corresponding effluxes of potassium and protons into the tubular lumen drive hypokalaemia and metabolic alkalosis.

Presentation: Resistant hypertension, metabolic alkalosis and hypokalaemia.

Investigation: Serum pH and potassium level. Blood pressure. Measure renin aldosterone ratio. Trial of amiloride. Genetic testing should include *SCNN1A*, *SCNN1B* and *SCNN1G*, coding for the ENaC subunits.

Management: Treatment with amiloride achieves good outcomes.

Distal renal tubular acidosis

See below.

Renal tubular acidoses

Endogenous production, combined with animal protein-containing diets, results in net gain of acid, requiring renal excretion of hydrogen ions. Additionally, the kidneys must reabsorb the large amount of filtered bicarbonate. RTA disorders are caused by failures of acid-base handling at varying points in the tubule.

General points about the investigation of suspected RTA

Normal anion gap (Na^+ − (Cl^- + $HCO3^-$)) metabolic acidosis with elevated urine pH may suggest RTA, but exclude urinary tract infection or severe volume depletion. Trans-tubular potassium gradient, fractional excretion of potassium, or urine potassium to creatinine ratio, *when measured in the context of hypokalaemia, off supplementation,* can help distinguish inappropriate renal potassium wasting from non-renal causes. Take a careful history including diuretic or laxative use and eating disorders, which can present with hypokalaemia and either acidosis or alkalosis.

Type 1 (distal)

Pathophysiology: Distal RTA (dRTA) results from failure of H^+ secretion in the distal tubule. It can be due to autosomal dominant pathogenic variants in the anion exchanger 1, which may be accompanied by spherocytosis. Autosomal recessive dRTA is due to genes encoding the H^+ATPase (which pumps H^+ into the tubular lumen), sometimes associated with sensorineural deafness. dRTA is more commonly acquired, e.g. in autoimmune disease, particularly Sjögren's syndrome or systemic lupus erythematosus – or secondary to chronic obstructive uropathy, drugs (e.g. cyclosporin A, amphotericin B, and lithium- see also diabetes insipidus), sickle cell anaemia and renal transplant.

Presentation: Failure to thrive, rickets, fatigue and weakness. Kidney stones and nephrocalcinosis may occur. Features of the underlying cause.

Investigations: Blood tests show hypokalaemic metabolic acidosis. Blood film may show spherocytes with *SLC4A1* variants. Anti-nuclear antibodies and autoimmune screen. Renal US for nephrocalcinosis and stones. Partial RTA, where acidaemia is only apparent with challenge, can be detected with a furosemide fludrocortisone urine acidification test.

Management: Potassium citrate supplementation treats acidosis and hypokalaemia. Sodium bicarbonate supplementation may also be needed. Correction of acidosis may lead to normalisation of potassium. Risk of osteoporosis if inadequately treated in adults. Management of any underlying autoimmune disorder.

Type 2 (proximal)

Pathophysiology: Proximal RTA (pRTA) rarely occurs due to isolated bicarbonate reabsorption defects which may be due to genetic variation in the Na^+/HCO_3^- co-transporter gene (*SLC4A4*) or medications (topiramate or carbonic anhydrase inhibitors). They most commonly occur as part of Fanconi syndrome (see above).

Failure of bicarbonate reabsorption in the proximal tubule can be partially compensated for in the TALH and collecting duct, so acidaemia is often less marked than in dRTA.

Presentation: Failure to thrive, rickets, fatigue and weakness. Kidney stones and nephrocalcinosis may occur.

Investigations: Blood tests show hypokalaemic metabolic acidosis. Investigate for features of a more generalised proximal defect (see Fanconi's syndrome above).

Management: High doses of alkali are often needed as supplemented filtered bicarbonate load will exceed proximal reabsorptive capacity. Potassium citrate treats both acidosis and hypokalaemia.

Type 3 (mixed)

Type 3 RTA can be considered as combined proximal and distal RTA due to mutations in carbonic anhydrase 2 and is exceedingly rare. It combines features of type 1 and type 2 and has a profound acidaemia.

Type 4 (aldosterone deficiency/hyperkalaemic RTA)

Pathophysiology: Hypoaldosteronism results in less sodium reabsorption in the collecting duct and consequently less H+ excretion and potassium loss in the urine. Causes include adrenal insufficiency or hyporeninaemic hypoaldosteronism due to kidney damage (frequently caused by diabetic nephropathy, NSAIDs or calcineurin inhibitors).

Presentation: Patients may experience weakness, lethargy and hypotension. Hyperpigmentation suggests adrenal insufficiency (including autoimmune Addison's disease) with elevated adrenocorticotrophic hormone and melanocyte-stimulating hormone.

Investigations: Blood tests show hyperkalaemic metabolic acidosis. Urine sodium remains high on a sodium-restricted diet. Renin and aldosterone levels distinguish primary from secondary hypoaldosteronism. Review drug history for potassium-sparing diuretics, ACE inhibitors or Angiotensin II receptor blockers.

Management: Fludrocortisone treats the mineralocorticoid deficiency and hyperkalaemia. However, in CKD fludrocortisone may exacerbate fluid retention and hypertension. Low potassium diet and loop or thiazide diuretics may be used in addition or as an alternative in this context. If required, glucocorticoids can be given for more generalised adrenal insufficiency.

Common presentations of tubular disease

Presentation	Renal causes	Non-renal causes	Key first-line tests
Hyperkalaemia	Reduced glomerular filtration (AKI and/or CKD), type 4 renal tubular acidosis.	Cell lysis (tumour lysis syndrome and rhabdomyolysis), increased potassium intake, iatrogenic, Artefactual (sample haemolysis).	U and Es, bone profile, blood gas for pH, LDH, CK.
Hypokalaemia	Bartter's, Fanconi's, Gitelman's and Liddle's syndromes, renal tubular acidosis (types 1-3), loop diuretic overuse.	Malnutrition, GI losses, excess insulin, beta-agonist use.	U and Es, blood gas analysis, serum glucose, C-peptide, urine chloride. Fractional excretion of potassium, measured *off supplements* when serum K low.
Acidosis	AKI, CKD, Gordon's syndrome, renal tubular acidosis.	Hypoventilation, diarrhoeal illnesses, laxative over-use, hyperlactataemia (tissue hypoxia and metformin), diabetic ketoacidosis, Poisoning.	Blood gas analysis (arterial if raised pCO_2 suspected), U and Es, bone profile, ketones, Urinary pH and chloride, Anion gap.
Alkalosis	Bartter's, Gitelman's and Liddle's syndromes	Vomiting, hyperventilation, hypovolaemia (contraction alkalosis)	Blood gas analysis (arterial if decreased pCO_2 suspected)
Polyuria	Nephrogenic diabetes insipidus, diuretic over-use, post-obstructive diuresis, osmotic diuresis (e.g. hypercalcaemia)	Psychogenic polydipsia, central and gestational diabetes insipidus, diabetes mellitus.	U and Es, bone profile, glucose (+/− ketones)

Further reading

Downie ML, Garcia SC, Kleta R, Bockenhauer D. (2021) Inherited tubulopathies of the kidney: insights from genetics. *Clin J Am Soc Nephrol* 16(4), 620–630.
European Rare Kidney Disease Reference Network Guidelines and Pathways: Tubulopathies https://www.erknet.org/guidelines-pathways/tubulopathies.
Gallagher H, Soar J, Tomson C. (2016) New guideline for perioperative management of people with inherited salt-wasting alkaloses. *Br J Anaesth* 116(6), 746–749.
Walsh SB, Unwin RJ. (2012) Renal tubular disorders. *Clin Med J* 12, 476.

Genetic Testing

Eligibility Criteria: https://www.england.nhs.uk/publication/national-genomic-test-directories/.
Renal tubular panel: https://nhsgms-panelapp.genomicsengland.co.uk/panels/292/v4.0.

CHAPTER 89

Nephrotic syndrome

EDWARD DROSCHER AND MATTHEW BROOK

Nephrotic syndrome is one of the major presentations of intrinsic kidney disease and describes the presence of:

- Nephrotic-range proteinuria (for adults: >3.5g total protein per day or urine protein:creatinine ratio >300mg/mmol which approximates a urine albumin:creatinine ratio >230mg/mmol)
- Hypoalbuminaemia (serum albumin<35g/L)
- Oedema

Nephrotic syndrome is the consequence of disruption of components of the glomerular filtration barrier, typically podocyte cells, resulting in loss of basement membrane integrity. A loss of basement membrane integrity is permissive to protein leaking into the glomerular filtrate and eventually the urine.

Nephrotic syndrome is not a diagnosis but represents the common clinical presentation of numerous possible disease processes. The underlying cause must be identified to allow specific treatment where appropriate.

Some diagnoses can be made through serological testing or by identifying a clearly associated trigger. However, in many cases a kidney biopsy is required to facilitate a diagnosis and initiate appropriate treatment.

Nephrotic syndrome may present as part of a nephritic picture with variable evidence of progressive renal dysfunction, haematuria and/or hypertension. Urgent nephrology advice is generally indicated in this scenario.

History

Presentation is typically due to oedema (patients may complain of tight-fitting clothes/jewellery/shoes or rapid weight gain). Oedema can affect the upper limbs, trunk and face (especially periorbital oedema) and is not necessarily gravity dependent. Patients may have incidentally noted 'frothy' or 'foamy' urine.

History taking should focus on establishing the symptom burden and identifying clues about possible etiologies resulting in the nephrotic syndrome (Table 89.1). This is especially important as some infections, drugs, and systemic diseases are known triggers (Table 89.3).

Acute Medicine: A Practical Guide to the Management of Medical Emergencies, Sixth Edition.
Edited by Mridula Rajwani, Leila Vaziri, and Ivie Gbinigie.
© 2026 John Wiley & Sons Ltd. Published 2026 by John Wiley & Sons Ltd.

Table 89.1 Focused history for patients presenting with the nephrotic syndrome.

History	Relevance
Description of symptom onset, did the symptoms start suddenly or slowly?	• Rapid onset of symptoms suggest minimal change disease or primary focal segmental glomerulosclerosis (FSGS) • Gradual onset is more typical of membranous nephropathy or secondary causes
Degree of weight gain and impact of oedema on daily activities	• Helps to assess symptom burden and guides the need for conservative measures and targeted treatments • Asymmetry in leg swelling should prompt consideration of deep vein thrombosis (thrombotic risk is increased in many cases of nephrotic syndrome)
Any history of breathlessness	• Patients may develop pulmonary oedema, pleural or pericardial effusions • Unexplained or sudden onset breathlessness associated with the nephrotic syndrome requires exclusion of pulmonary embolism
Is there a previous personal history of nephrotic syndrome?	• Relapse is common in many causes of the nephrotic syndrome particularly as treatment is weaned or stopped. Relapse may occur years later, especially important if nephrotic during childhood (~ one third will relapse in adulthood after a quiescent period)
Systems enquiry (red flags) for symptoms of malignancy	• Almost any malignancies can be associated with a secondary nephrotic syndrome • Multiple myeloma, sometimes initially presents as AL-amyloidosis, and is a specific cause to look out for
Are there any features of a systemic disease (known diabetes, rash, ulcers, weight loss, night sweats, fevers, hearing or visual changes, Raynaud phenomenon, joint pains, chest pains, extrarenal organ dysfunction)	• Presence of these features raises suspicion of secondary causes that warrant further investigation (e.g. diabetes, chronic infection, lupus, IgG4-related disease) • Chronic inflammatory/infectious conditions may present with AA amyloidosis
Any recent infections? Infection history should also include risk factors for viral hepatitis infection, HIV and syphilis as well as a travel history.	• Patients with the nephrotic syndrome are at higher risk for secondary infections. Screening questions including skin breakdown or ulceration should be asked about • Infection can often trigger an underlying disease process associated with the nephrotic syndrome, such as C3 glomerulopathy • Specific infections have strong associations with nephrotic syndrome (HIV and collapsing glomerulopathy, HCV and cryoglobulinaemic vasculitis) • Travel acquired conditions such as malaria or schistosomiasis may be associated with nephrotic syndrome
A detailed drug history (prescribed, over the counter, supplements, misuse)	• E.g. non-steroidal anti-inflammatory drugs (NSAIDs), lithium or bisphosphonates are recognised triggers • Supplements such as alpha lipoic acid have been associated with nephrotic syndrome as have some traditional remedies • Drugs of misuse may have an association (anabolic steroids and FSGS, heroin and FSGS)
Is there a family history of kidney disease, kidney failure, dialysis or transplantation	Genetic testing can sometimes identify causes of nephrotic syndromes including minimal change disease or FSGS

Investigations

- Quantitation of urine protein concentration:
  - Reagent test strips are calibrated such that 3+ typically correlates to a urine protein concentration of >3 g (Those with an existing diagnosis may have already tested their urine with a reagent test strip at home). Some proteins (especially cationic proteins) are not detected by reagent test strips: know the false negatives of your reagent strips.
  - The presence or absence of blood on dipstick testing should be noted.
  - Send a spot urine sample for formal quantification with both urine protein:creatinine ratio and urine albumin:creatinine ratio. Twenty-four-hour urine collections are not required.
- Measure weight. Weight change is a crude, but clinically useful measure of water gains/losses and is used to assess diuresis adequacy.
- Measure blood pressure. Blood pressure control is a key management goal both to reduce proteinuria and for safety should a kidney biopsy be required.
- Send blood for routine and specific blood tests (Table 89.2).
- Chest imaging for evidence of pulmonary oedema, pleural or pericardial effusions.
- Imaging or investigations targeted towards the clinical history and possible secondary causes may be required, e.g. looking for evidence of malignancy where this is suspected.
- Ultrasound of the kidneys for structural abnormalities such as kidney asymmetry (single kidney as a cause adapative FSGS, for example) and to assess kidney anatomy prior to consideration of kidney biopsy.
- If there is a clinical suggestion of a thrombotic event (most commonly pulmonary embolism, deep vein thrombosis, renal vein thrombosis or Budd–Chiari), then urgent diagnostic imaging is indicated. This may include contrast imaging, which should generally be performed without delay to avoid life- or organ-threatening consequences.

Table 89.2 Routine and specific laboratory tests to send in a patient presenting with the nephrotic syndrome.

Test	Rational
Full blood count	• May play a role in diagnosing an underlying haematological malignancy • Anaemia may be common in systemic disease • Anaemia may need correcting prior to kidney biopsy
Clotting	• Important as a prerequisite test before a kidney biopsy • Abnormalities may reflect loss of clotting factors that can be clinically relevant and require correcting
U&E	• To assess kidney filtration function and electrolytes • Recognition of acute kidney injury (AKI) as part of the presentation requires independent consideration for cause and expedited nephrology review • May impact diuretic choice for managing oedema (for example, using amiloride if hypokalaemic)
Liver function tests (LFTs)	• Primarily to assess serum albumin level to make the diagnosis of the nephrotic syndrome and guide need for anticoagulation • Abnormal LFTs may focus investigations on underlying causes with a liver association such as IgG4-RD or malignancy • Abnormalities in the right clinical context might raise suspicion of the Budd–Chiari syndrome as a thrombotic complication of the nephrotic syndrome or viral hepatitis as an underlying aetiology
Lipid profile	• Significant dyslipidaemia is typical in nephrotic syndrome and may require targeted therapy if duration of nephrotic state is likely to be prolonged

(continued)

Table 89.2 (*Continued*)

Test	Rational
C-reactive protein (CRP)	• May point to an infective complication or a cause of the nephrotic syndrome, or associate with a systemic condition as the underlying cause • Not usually elevated in a primary nephrotic syndrome in absence of infective complication
Total immunoglobulin G/M/A levels	• Immunoglobulin wasting due to proteinuria can result in a generalised *hypo*-gammaglobulinaemia • Isolated elevation in one immunoglobulin class occasionally suggests an underlying haematological malignancy (e.g. multiple myeloma-associated presentations)
Serum protein electrophoresis	• To detect the presence of a monoclonal protein
Serum-free light chains	• Free kappa:lambda light chain ratio is important for detecting a monoclonal gammopathy of renal significance (MGRS) • In AL-amyloid, small amounts of an amyloid-forming light chain, too small to be detected by electrophoresis, can be pathogenic and are only detected if serum-free light chains are quantified
Urine electrophoresis	• Detection of a Bence–Jones protein strongly suggests an MGRS
Antinuclear antibody (ANA) and, if positive, extractable nuclear antigens (ENA) and double-stranded DNA (dsDNA)	• To detect an underlying autoimmune disease • Caution with over-interpretation of low-level titre of ANA in the absence of other immunological abnormalities
Complement C3 and C4	• Low levels can be associated with a number of nephrotic-associated conditions including C3 glomerulopathy (low C3) and SLE (low C3 and C4 during active disease)
Rheumatoid factor	• Rheumatoid factors might be found in nephrotic syndrome-associated conditions such as cryoglobulinaemia, Sjögren syndrome or mixed connective tissue disease
Viral/infectious serology	• HIV, HBV and HCV testing should be sent as routine in nephrotic syndrome • Syphilis, cytomegalovirus (CMV), Epstein-Barr virus (EBV), parvovirus B19 and other viral causes might be considered in the right clinical circumstances
Anti-PLA2R antibody and if available, anti-THSD7A antibody	• Specifically looking for membranous nephropathy • anti-PLA2R autoantibodies are found in primary membranous nephropathy and strong positivity may be considered diagnostic without the need for kidney biopsy

Table 89.3 Common causes of the nephrotic syndrome.

Nephrotic syndrome associated with systemic conditions	
Diabetes mellitus	Diabetic kidney disease is often associated with nephrotic-range proteinuria and oedema. Albumin does not always fall sufficiently to classify patients with the nephrotic syndrome. Onset of proteinuria is gradual, often over many years, tracked through annual diabetic checks. A new sudden increase in proteinuria to nephrotic levels should prompt consideration of an alternative cause.
Systemic lupus erythematosus	Systemic lupus erythematosus is associated with multiple classes of kidney disease (lupus nephritis), often presenting with a nephritic picture. 5–10% of all lupus nephritis cases are pure class V, which has microscopy features of membranous nephropathy and a nephrotic presentation. 10–30% of patients will eventually progress to end-stage kidney disease. All patients with such a presentation should be seen by nephrology.

Table 89.3 (*Continued*)

Haematological disease	Plasma cell dyscrasias can present with nephrotic-range proteinuria. In these scenarios the protein:creatinine ratio is often markedly elevated due to detectable light chains in the urine, which are freely filtered, whilst the albumin:creatinine ratio is disproportionately low (as the filtration barrier is intact). Multiple myeloma-associated AL-amyloidosis can disrupt the filtration barrier and present as the nephrotic syndrome. Other haematological diagnoses such as lymphoma or leukaemias can rarely present with the nephrotic syndrome with varying histological patterns.
	Histopathological patterns and associations
Membranous nephropathy	Membranous nephropathy (MN) is the most common cause of the nephrotic syndrome in non-diabetic adults. MN has peak incidence in the sixth and seventh decades of life and occurs more frequently in males (two-thirds) than females (one-third). Primary disease occurs in about 70% of cases and is often associated with anti-phospholipase A2 receptor (PLA2R) antibodies, which can be diagnostic and prevent need for biopsy. Secondary MN is associated with another trigger or disease process (e.g. malignancy, NSAIDs, IgG4-RD and syphilis). Membranous nephropathy has a higher thrombotic risk than other causes of the nephrotic syndrome.
Focal segmental glomerulosclerosis (FSGS)	FSGS is the second most common cause of the nephrotic syndrome in adults and can be classified most simply as primary or secondary. Primary FSGS typically has an abrupt onset. Diagnosis is on kidney biopsy. Response to corticosteroids is often poor, with only about half of those treated achieving complete remission. Outcomes are determined by remission of proteinuria, and progression to ESKD occurs in up to 50% presenting with heavy proteinuria or kidney impairment. Secondary FSGS may be seen in people who are obese, those who are born with (e.g. dysplastic kidneys) or acquire (e.g. nephrectomy, reflux nephropathy and sickle cell disease) a reduced nephron mass. Collapsing GN is a rapidly progressing variant of FSGS and the characteristic finding in HIV-associated nephropathy and other viral or infectious triggers. The drugs pamidronate, anthracyclines and interferon as well as anabolic steroids and heroin are also associated. FSGS may have a genetic cause or a genetic predisposition, including APOL1 polymorphisms seen typically in those of West African descent.
Minimal change disease (MCD)	At light microscopy, the glomeruli look normal (there is minimal change). Accounts for up to 20% of nephrotic syndrome cases in adults. An association with atopy is frequently recognized. In primary disease, the response to high doses of corticosteroids for a prolonged course is frequently excellent with up to 90% of patients attaining a complete response. However, relapse often occurs (reported in about two-thirds) and may require transition to second- or third-line treatment options for frequently relapsing or steroid-resistant cases. MCD may also be secondary to drugs (NSAIDs, rifampicin, lithium, interferon alpha and beta), solid organ and haematological malignancy, autoimmunity (sarcoidosis, Grave's disease and myasthenia gravis) or infections (syphilis, HIV and hepatitis B/C).

Management

Referral to nephrology is indicated for all patients found to have nephrotic syndrome to assess the urgency for kidney biopsy and guide periprocedural anticoagulation, to determine any indication for immunosuppression, and to guide the need for specialist tests (autoimmune screening or genetic testing).

Management is divided into conservative measures to control oedema, minimise proteinuria and mitigate complications of the nephrotic syndrome followed by targeting of the underlying condition when the cause has been identified. Specific treatments of an underlying cause are the remit of a nephrologist or relevant specialist and will not be covered here. Conservative measures can be instigated from the outset by any assessing physician. Management of the nephrotic syndrome is generally outpatient-based.

Treatment of an underlying cause may result in remission of the nephrotic syndrome at differing rates. Conservative measures that have been established will require modification with the changing clinical picture as the nephrotic syndrome resolves (e.g. diuretic reduction).

Conservative measures

Oedema

Managing oedema is typically the first concern in nephrotic syndrome. Patients may have gained significant amounts of weight (often >10 kg) through fluid retention and may have tightly fitting clothes and shoes, often limiting mobility.

Oedema is often generalised (anasarca) and not necessarily gravity dependent. Patients might present symptomatic with pleural effusion, pericardial effusion or ascites. Skin breakdown results in pain and potential for superadded soft tissue infection. Significant genital oedema can be particularly uncomfortable and concerning for patients.

The oedema in the nephrotic syndrome is often resistant to diuretics. In part, this may be related to the third spacing of fluid into the extravascular tissues with blood volume only mildly if at all increased. This may predispose to intravascular depletion and acute kidney impairment with diuretic use. Patients requiring high-dose diuretics for fluid management in these scenarios may inevitably develop a need for kidney replacement therapy (dialysis), which in the acute presentation may be temporary whilst treatment of the underlying cause is initiated.

Strategy

- **Serial weights** are a crude way to monitor fluid gain/loss and are used to guide diuretic regimen and dosing, aiming for 0.5–1 kg weight loss per day until euvolaemia. Patients may often titrate diuretics themselves, aiming for an agreed individual target weight.
- **Loop diuretics** are first line. High doses are often required to achieve adequate diuresis for a number of reasons. First, the volume of distribution is increased because of fluid retention leading to reduced drug delivery to the kidney. Second, loop diuretics are highly protein bound therefore significant urinary losses are seen with nephrotic-range proteinuria. Third, increased metabolic clearance occurs because of greater unbound diuretic in hypoalbuminaemia (loop diuretics are highly albumin-bound).
- Starting doses are guided by severity of oedema-related symptoms, kidney function (impaired estimated glomerular filtration rate (eGFR) may warrant higher starting doses unless there is a concern for intravascular depletion as a cause of AKI), electrolyte disturbance and tolerability.
- In patients without severe oedema, then high-dose oral loop diuretics may be sufficient to achieve diuresis and facilitate outpatient management. Severe oedema causing compromise may require admission or ambulatory intravenous loop diuretics (which assures good bioavailability; oral loop-diuretics suffer from highly variable oral bioavailability).
- Loop diuretics work by increasing sodium and water loss from the kidneys. **Fluid restriction** (typically 1 L/24 h) and **salt restriction** are needed to facilitate a net reduction of total body water and lessen oedema.
- Patients often become tolerant/resistant to loop diuretics. Increasing the dose (often doubled initially) can be effective. Switching from oral to intravenous diuresis is a commonly used strategy but would usually require escalation of the dose as well.
- **Sequential tubular blockade** (of sodium and water retention) alongside a loop diuretic through the concomitant administration of a thiazide or thiazide-like diuretic and/or potassium-sparing diuretics can overcome resistance in some cases.
- Loop and thiazide diuretics frequently cause hypokalaemia, which can be mitigated by the addition of potassium-sparing diuretics.
- Overdiuresis is a potential cause of AKI in this patient population, although this is sometimes a necessary complication of managing the disabling symptoms of oedema where present.

- Where oedema is minimal or well controlled in the steady state, then patients should be counselled on the possible need for temporary diuretic suspension in certain circumstances (diarrhoea, vomiting, febrile illness and extreme heat).

Antiproteinuric therapy

In most cases, significant reduction in proteinuria will require treatment targeted at the underlying cause however conservative measures can help and are particularly useful where there is a more chronic presentation. The severity of proteinuria is recognised as one of the best predictors for risk of kidney disease progression and reduction in proteinuria is a trackable marker of remission. Many causes of the nephrotic syndrome lead to progressive chronic kidney disease and end-stage kidney disease. Strategies to minimise urinary protein loss are considered protective from both a renal and cardiovascular perspective.

Strategy

- **Angiotensin converting enzyme inhibitors (ACEi) or angiotensin II receptor blockers (ARB)** are considered 'renoprotective' medications as they result in significant proteinuria reduction.
- Introduction of an ACEi/ARB is expected to cause an increase in serum creatinine (up to 30%) and this should not be a reason to discontinue these medications.
- If eGFR is rapidly changing in the acute phase of a nephrotic syndrome presentation, then the introduction of an ACEi/ARB, with the expected change in serum creatinine, can make it challenging to monitor disease trajectory and might be a reason to delay initiation.
- ACEi/ARB can cause acute kidney impairment in intravascularly depleted patients and initiation may be best delayed in those with an abrupt onset of nephrotic syndrome with florid oedema whilst diagnosis and targeted treatment is being established.
- Where chronicity is a feature of presentation or the clinical course, then prompt recognition of this and introduction of an ACEi/ARB should occur and the **dose maximally titrated** as tolerated.
- After initiation and dose changes blood testing between one and two weeks is recommended to check potassium and for changes in kidney function.
- Discontinuation due to hyperkalaemia may associate with worse long-term outcomes. Stable non-life-threatening hyperkalaemia (typically less than 6.0 mmol/L assuming asymptomatic and no ECG changes) can be tolerated.
- **SGLT2 inhibitors** have been shown to significantly slow progression of renal disease in proteinuric chronic kidney disease (CKD) and confer cardiovascular risk benefits.
- SGLT2i may cause a reduction in eGFR on initiation, similar to an ACEi/ARB, and the approach to starting these medications in nephrotic syndrome should be similar (as described earlier).
- Early repeat blood tests after initiation of an SGLT2i are not considered necessary.
- **Blood pressure control** is consistently shown to result in proteinuria reduction. The latest guidelines recommend that the blood pressure target should be 120 mmHg systolic where tolerated. An ACEi/ARB is the preferred agent.
- High sodium intake can worsen hypertension, worsen interstitial oedema, negate the pharmacological effect of both diuretics and ACEi/ARB, and is independently associated with proteinuria. **Dietary salt restriction** is recommended.

Complications

The potential complications of nephrotic syndrome can be life-threatening and need to be recognized at an early stage to mitigate risk. These commonly include hypercoagulability and risk of thrombotic events, risk of infection and acute kidney injury.

The risk of **thrombotic events** is higher in nephrotic syndrome than in the general population and may be the presenting feature. Any individual presenting with thrombus and low albumin should have a measurement of urinary protein for completion.

The best predictors for thrombotic events are the histological diagnosis (membranous nephropathy is associated with the highest risk of thrombosis), the degree of proteinuria and a serum albumin <25 g/L.

Thrombosis can affect any and multiple vascular beds simultaneously and occur in both arterial and venous systems. Thrombosis has been described as pulmonary embolism, DVT, renal artery/vein thrombosis, Budd–Chiari syndrome, cerebral vein thrombosis, acute limb ischaemia, cardiac ischaemia and others.

Strategy

- Be suspicious of thrombotic events with a low threshold for investigations including contrast scans where indicated to ensure a diagnosis.
- An identified thrombotic event should be treated in the usual manner, urgently with full anticoagulation unless otherwise contraindicated.
- If confirmed thromboembolic events are identified in the context of the nephrotic syndrome, then full-dose anticoagulation is required for a minimum of three months but more likely for as long as the patient remains nephrotic.
- Blanket guidelines for prophylactic anticoagulation as primary prevention are controversial. Any underlying conditions and individual risk factors for thrombosis and bleeding need to be considered.
- Prophylactic treatment-dose anticoagulation should be considered in those with other risk factors for thrombosis (obesity, smoking, thrombophilia, immobilisation, recent orthopaedic or abdominal surgery, previous venous thrombolembolism (VTE)), in those with serum albumin <25 g/L, and in those with 10 g/day proteinuria as well as in those with a histological diagnosis of membranous nephropathy.
- Low molecular weight heparin and warfarin are established anticoagulants for this indication. There is interest in direct-acting oral anticoagulants as an alternative but practice may vary according to local protocols.

AKI is sometimes seen in the index presentation of the nephrotic syndrome and in future relapses. It has a greater association with minimal change disease, in the setting of which it has been reported in 25–40% of patients. AKI warrants more urgent nephrology involvement and assessment of all the usual causes alongside nephrotic-specific considerations.

Strategy

- Rapidly progressive glomerulonephritis can occur in association with nephrosis. Typically, there will be additional urinary abnormalities such as haematuria, severe hypertension +/− high serum CRP depending on cause. Such presentations require urgent discussion with nephrology, expedited immunology samples and usually inpatient management.
- Consider the possibility of renal vein thrombosis (loin pain, haematuria, kidney enlargement on imaging), renal artery thrombosis or thrombosis involving the inferior vena cava in discussion with nephrology.
- Significant fluid shifts between intravascular and extravascular compartments are often a feature of nephrotic syndrome and predispose to AKI. This might be due to intravascular depletion from fluid moving into the extravascular space during presentation or relapse but also over diuresis when nephrotic syndrome is going into remission. Frequent re-assessment of fluid state is required.
- AKI might reflect glomerular damage from the underlying disease process, e.g. SLE or collapsing GN. Treatment in these cases is aimed at the underlying cause and directed by nephrology.
- The nephrotic syndrome might be triggered by infection or medications (e.g. NSAIDs) that can also result in impairment of kidney function. Treatment of any trigger or withdrawal of medications associated with nephrotic syndrome is appropriate.
- The usual management of AKI remains relevant in the nephrotic syndrome (see Chapter 86).

Infection is a common complication of the nephrotic syndrome. In some cases, infectious triggers represent the underlying cause. Loss of immunoglobulins, complement components and other immune mediators in the urine are contributory to general infection risk. Treatment of an underlying cause often requires significant doses of immunosuppression further enhancing this risk. Oedema leading to skin breakdown can result in cellulitis as part of the presenting complaint.

Strategy

- Vigilance for infection is key. A good history, as detailed above, and appropriate serology might identify an underlying infectious trigger to be addressed.
- Assess for any evidence of infection with prompt treatment where concerns arise.
- Patients should be encouraged to engage with vaccination programs where offered.

Significant laboratory abnormalities such as hyperlipidiaemia (in nearly all cases) and abnormal thyroid hormone testing (loss of thyroid hormones and thyroxine-binding globulin) is common. Accelerated atherosclerosis is a concern in those patients presenting with a chronic history or where the clinical course is prolonged.

Strategy

- Patients should be advised to increase **exercise, lose weight** (where relevant), and **stop smoking** as these interventions have beneficial effects on blood pressure and overall cardiovascular health.
- Initiation of statin therapy unless rapid resolution is anticipated.

Summary

- Diagnosing the nephrotic syndrome represents the start of a search for the underlying cause.
- Prompt referral to nephrology is appropriate in all cases.
- Conservative measures such as loop diuretics, fluid and salt restriction and daily weights are appropriate for nearly all.
- Complications such as severe oedema, thrombosis, infection and AKI need to be recognised with prompt treatment alongside addressing the underlying cause of nephrotic syndrome.
- Rapid deterioration in renal function warrants urgent discussion with nephrology and likely inpatient management.
- Longer-term strategies include initiation of an ACE-I, SGLT2i and lipid-lowering medication as well as blood pressure control to prevent or delay kidney disease progression and reduce cardiovascular risk.

Further reading

Assessment of nephrotic syndrome - Differential diagnosis of symptoms | BMJ Best Practice

Executive summary of the KDIGO. (2021) Guideline for the Management of Glomerular Diseases. *Kidney Int* 2021(100), 753 779.

Minimal Change Disease. (2017). *Clin J Am Soc Nephrol* 12(2), 332–345.

Nephrotic Syndrome for the Internist. (2023). *Medi Clin North America* 107(4), 727–737.

The Immune System and Idiopathic Nephrotic Syndrome. (2022 Dec). *Clin J Am Soc Nephrol.* 17(12), 1823–1834.

CHAPTER 90

Glomerular diseases

JOSEPH GAIED AND JEREMY LEVY

Introduction

Consider glomerular disease (Box 90.1) in all patients with unexplained urine abnormalities (blood and/or protein), and acute kidney injury (AKI) with or without systemic features, especially without a cause for volume depletion or hypotension.

Box 90.1 Causes and Pathology of glomerular diseases.

Pathology
- Glomerular diseases present in two main prototypical ways: with nephrotic syndrome (see Chapter 89) or with haematuria, proteinuria and acute kidney injury of varying degrees.
- The glomerular filtration barrier is responsible for creating an ultrafiltrate (and ultimately urine) of water and low-molecular-weight solutes, while retaining most high-molecular-weight proteins and blood cells within the vasculature.
- Highly specialized glomerular endothelial and epithelial cells build a size- and charge-dependent barrier to serum proteins.
- The glomerular microvasculature is particularly vulnerable to immune-mediated injury because the filtration process involves delicate anatomical structures that are exposed to substantial shear stress and perfusion pressure.
- In the nephrotic syndrome (see Chapter 89), leakage of plasma proteins without inflammation is the primary pathogenic mechanism.
- In glomerulonephritis (GN), inflammation within the glomerulus leads not only to the passage of plasma proteins but also of inflammatory cells (leukocytes) and RBCs into the renal tubule.
- These classifications are not completely exclusive, as some conditions may present with both patterns, and some disorders (e.g. lupus nephritis) may progress from one pattern to the other.

Classification
Glomerulonephritis should be classified by the underlying cause where possible rather than by the histological pattern:
- Immune-complex glomerulonephritis (including infection-related glomerulonephritis, IgA nephropathy, lupus nephritis and cryoglobulinaemic GN).

- Pauci-immune GN: anti-neutrophil cytoplasmic antibody (ANCA)-associated glomerulonephritis
- Anti-glomerular basement membrane antibody glomerulonephritis
- C3 glomerulopathy
- Monoclonal immunoglobulin-associated glomerulonephritis.
  Precise classification usually requires a kidney biopsy.

Priorities

- Prompt recognition of a possible acute glomerulonephritis (Box 90.2 and Table 90.1) and referral to nephrologist is key, since if left untreated, acute GN can lead to irreversible kidney failure or chronic kidney disease.
- If there is AKI with urine abnormalities (blood or protein), send urgent work-up (see below).
- If AKI with no urine abnormalities (bland urine), think acute tubular necrosis (ATN) or acute interstitial nephritis (AIN) as a cause of AKI, and hence possible drugs as a cause or hypotension and hypovolaemia. The urine dipstick is critical.
- If AKI + suspected GN + oligo-anuria, refer urgently for advice from a nephrologist

Box 90.2 Presentation of glomerular disease.

Glomerular diseases can present in various ways.
- Asymptomatic urinary abnormalities: proteinuria, now usually measured as a urine protein:creatinine ratio (uPCR: rather than 24-hour collections), usually 30–300 mg/mmol, haematuria (>2 red blood cells/high power field), often found on dipstick and non-visible.
- Visible haematuria: usually painless, typically coincides with intercurrent infections.
- Nephrotic syndrome: triad of heavy proteinuria uPCR >300 mg/mmol, hypoalbuminemia <30 g/L and oedema.
- Nephritic syndrome (GN): Usually abrupt onset, self-limiting with oliguria, haematuria, proteinuria (usually uPCR <300 mg/mmol), oedema, hypertension.
- Rapidly progressive glomerulonephritis (RPGN): renal failure occurring over days to weeks, proteinuria (usually uPCR <300 mg/mmol), haematuria, may have other features of systemic disease such as vasculitis (e.g. pulmonary haemorrhage and skin rash).
- Chronic GN: Hypertension, renal impairment, proteinuria (often uPCR >3 mg/mmol) and small kidneys on imaging. This can be the final outcome of any chronic glomerular disease.

Table 90.1 Assessment of the patient with suspected glomerulonephritis.

History and Examination

- Usually no symptoms
- Specific questioning may reveal oedema, foamy urine, incidental urinary abnormalities or hypertension noted during previous routine testing (e.g. pre-employment).
- Patient may report leg swelling (shoes no longer fit), morning eye puffiness.
- Any systemic diseases associated with glomerular involvement? (e.g. diabetes, hypertension, amyloid, lupus and vasculitis).
- Glomerular disease may be limited primarily to the kidney or may be associated with systemic conditions such as infections, autoimmune disorders, malignancy, and drug reactions. Thus, in patients with suspected glomerular disease, the history and examination, should include evaluation for a systemic disorder.

(continued)

Table 90.1 (*Continued*)

History and Examination

Constitutional symptoms	• Fever, chills, weight loss, fatigue and night sweats, may be found in infection-associated GN or vasculitis.
Gross haematuria	• May sometimes accompany GN and be associated with upper respiratory infection. • The time elapsed between the respiratory infection and the appearance of haematuria may sometimes be helpful: Gross haematuria occurring concurrently with the onset of infection ('synpharyngitic') is typical of IgA nephropathy but may occasionally accompany C3 glomerulopathy and Alport syndrome. • If a latent period of 7–10 days occurs between the onset of infection and haematuria, post-streptococcal glomerulonephritis (especially in children) is more likely.
Oedema	• Surprisingly oedema can be massive before patients seek medical help with fluid gains up to 20 kg or more not unusual, in nephrotic states. • Examine calves for deep vein thrombosis (DVT). Many glomerular diseases are prothrombotic.
Blood pressure	• Always critical to measure blood pressure. • Check lying and standing BP: postural hypotension may indicate reduced intravascular volume. • Acute onset of hypertension (HTN) in a previously normotensive patient, or acute worsening of a preexisting controlled HTN raises the suspicion of glomerular disease, particularly if other manifestations (e.g. haematuria and oedema). Hypertension is virtually universal as chronic GN progresses towards kidney failure and is a key modifiable factor in preserving kidney function in the long term.
ENT/respiratory	• Epistaxis, sinus congestion/discharge • Shortness of breath, haemoptysis • May occur in infection-associated GN or vasculitis/RPGN
Eyes	• Puffiness of eyelids (in oedematous states), retinitis, uveitis (in systemic vasculitis).
Skin and joints	• Look for skin rash carefully. If rash is visible, press to assess if blanchable (vasculitis rash is non-blanching). • Any evidence of arthritis
Drugs	• Always ask about drugs: e.g. NSAIDs, Hydralazine, Penicillamine, Interferon, Pamidronate, mercury (in skin lightening creams) etc can all cause glomerular pathology. • Obtain timelines for medications (particularly for patients in hospital), most commonly prescribed antibiotics or NSAIDs, in relation to developing AKI or urine abnormalities.
Family history	• of renal diseases may indicate genetic disorders, e.g. Alport syndrome, familiar forms of FSGS, complement-mediated GN, and thrombotic microangiopathies. • Any possibility of underlying genetic disorders, particularly in young patients, e.g. hearing loss in Alport syndrome.

Investigations

• Urine dipstick: a critical test but often missed. Blood and protein in urine frequently indicates glomerular disease, also very helpful in distinguishing from other causes of AKI, e.g. acute tubular necrosis or interstitial nephritis.

• Urine protein quantification by protein:creatinine measurement is critical.

• A dipstick-positive catheter sample is difficult to interpret. Look for a urine dip result before the catheter was inserted, a negative result may help to reassure you about the absence of glomerular disease.

• Most isolated haematuria (not associated with proteinuria) is not due to renal disease and urological investigations are the first line for all those aged >40 years.

• Urine abnormalities should be evaluated carefully in the settings of urinary infections, most are not indicative of GN. Repeat after resolution of infection.

Renal ultrasound (US)

- Small size kidneys (<9 cm on US scan) and or severe cortical thinning suggest advanced chronic kidney disease hence likely irreversible and may preclude renal biopsy. Large kidneys (>14 cm) are sometimes seen in amyloidosis, HIV nephropathy and early diabetic nephropathy.

Kidney biopsy

The gold standard for the diagnosis of a glomerulonephritis with a hallmark glomerular inflammation that translates into various histopathological patterns depending on the location and severity of the glomerular injury. This should only ever be done by a renal team since the result needs careful interpretation.

Blood tests

All patients

- Urea and electrolytes, always obtain previous serum creatinine values to assess trend and acuity.
- Acute GN may present with AKI, especially in patients with crescentic GN, which is often due to ANCA or anti GBM antibody-associated glomerulonephritis. Repeat U&Es daily in an acute presentation.
- CRP, venous bicarbonate and serum lactate, important if any hint of sepsis/hypotension
- FBC: any anaemia or thrombocytopenia? (may indicate thrombotic microangiopathy (TMA)). If present, send urgent blood film, LDH and reticulocyte count.
- Liver Function Tests (LFT), Parathyroid hormone (PTH), bone profile: serum albumin is typically low in nephrotic syndrome.
- Lipid profile
- Clotting profile: may aid in planning for kidney biopsy, and also distinguishing causes of TMA.

In selected patients

- Serum protein electrophoresis, serum free light chains and urine Bence Jones Protein (BJP): if any suspicion of monoclonal gammopathy or myeloma and always in older patients over 50 years of age or anaemia worse than expected or hypercalcemia.
- Serum complement levels (C3 and C4): can be low in SLE, infection-associated GN and cryoglobulinaemia.
- Autoantibodies: ANCA (in vasculitis), anti-dsDNA, ANA (in lupus), anti-phospholipase A2 receptor (PLA2R) in membranous GN, anti-glomerular basement (GBM) antibodies. Contact laboratory to run these tests urgently if high clinical suspicion since urgent treatment is needed.
- Blood culture, ASOT, hepatitis B and C and HIV serology.
- If the patient seems to likely have AKI from ATN, with no blood or protein in urine, then all the above tests may not be needed. They are all critical when glomerular disease is suspected.

Common causes of glomerulonephritis

These might present with AKI, RPGN, asymptomatic urine abnormalities, proteinuria, hypertension or even 'CKD'.

IgA nephropathy

Commonest primary GN in high-income countries. About 20–50% progress to kidney failure over 30 years. May present with asymptomatic non-visible haematuria, episodic visible haematuria which may be 'synpharyngitic', CKD or new onset hypertension, and very rarely as RPGN. Hypertension is common. Proteinuria (uPCR) usually <100 mg/mmol. Renal biopsy shows: IgA deposition in mesangium and is diagnostic and prognostic. Treatment includes blood pressure control (with ACE-i/ARB) and SGLT2 inhibitors. Increasing evidence for use of gut-delivered steroids and anti-complement therapies in those at high risk of progression.

Henoch–Schönlein purpura (HSP)

More commonly known as IgA Vasculitis, considered as a systemic variant of IgA nephropathy with IgA deposition in skin, joints, gut as well as kidneys. Presents with purpuric rash typically on legs, abdominal pains, flitting polyarthritis and nephritis. Diagnosis is clinical, confirmed by IgA and C3 deposition in skin or renal biopsy. Treatment is supportive, but steroids may be used for gut involvement; kidney disease managed as IgA Nephropathy.

Post-streptococcal GN (PSGN)

Primarily occurs in resource-limited countries, now rare in developed countries, most commonly in children and older adults (>60 years). Occurs after a throat (~two weeks) or skin (~three to six weeks) infection. Streptococcal antigen deposits in the glomerulus lead to immune complex formation and inflammation. Most commonly presents with oedema, visible haematuria and hypertension, evidence of streptococcal infection (e.g. raised ASOT, anti-DNAse B antibodies and low complement C3). Renal biopsy is diagnostic: Differential diagnosis include C3 glomerulonephritis and IgA nephropathy. Treatment: no specific therapy, management is supportive, with focus on diuretic to address volume overload and hypertension. Dialysis may be required. Prognosis is favourable with most patients recovering within a few weeks.

Infection-associated GN

This term encompasses the entities of post-streptococcal GN, IgA dominant (staphylococcus-associated) GN, endocarditis-associated GN and other infections driving GN. Various infectious agents including some viruses may be the cause. Clinical and pathologic manifestations vary depending on underlying pathogen, duration and intensity of infection. Pathology is largely driven by complement deposition followed by subsequent inflammatory/immune response. Renal biopsy is characteristic but cannot define underlying infective cause. Usually self-limiting but must exclude underlying complement abnormalities.

Rapidly progressive GN (RPGN)

Aggressive GN, rapidly progressing to kidney failure over days/weeks. Acute onset of haematuria with variable degrees of proteinuria, oliguria, AKI and sometimes hypertension. Renal biopsy characterised by extensive 'crescent' formation. Causes include Pauci-immune RPGN (in association with small vessel/ANCA vasculitis), anti-GBM antibody disease and Immune complex RPGN (lupus nephritis and IgA nephropathy). Deterioration can be very rapid. Diagnosis by appropriate serological testing and urgent renal biopsy.

Management: Seek very urgent nephrology input to allow rapid start of treatment, which includes immunosuppression with corticosteroids and cyclophosphamide or Rituximab. Other treatments depend on aetiology, e.g. plasma exchange for anti-GBM antibody disease, mycophenolate for lupus nephritis.

Anti-glomerular basement membrane (anti-GBM) disease

Caused by antibodies arising to type IV collagen in glomerular and alveolar basement membranes. Presents usually with fulminant RPGN with or without pulmonary haemorrhage (causing haemoptysis), often visible haematuria and painful swollen kidneys, oligo-anuria, dialysis dependence and biopsy features predict poor prognosis. Diagnosis by detecting GBM antibodies in circulation and kidney biopsy. Treatment: corticosteroids and cyclophosphamide (to stop antibody production) and urgent plasma exchange (to remove circulating antibody).

ANCA-associated vasculitis (AAV)

Comprise three main disorders, microscopic polyangiitis (MPA), granulomatosis with polyangiitis (GPA) and eosinophilic granulomatosis with polyangiitis (EGPA). All are small vessel vasculitides, defined by the presence of inflammatory leucocytes in blood vessel walls leading to loss of blood vessel integrity and downstream tissue ischemia. AAV causes a necrotising GN without the deposition of immune complexes. Suspect AAV in patients who present with systemic (constitutional) features in combination with evidence of single or multiorgan involvement. Isolated kidney involvement is common. ANCA testing is not fully diagnostic on its own, but the presence of ANCA directed to proteinase 3 (PR3) or myeloperoxidase (MPO) can be >95% specific.

Management

Making an urgent diagnosis is critical, since all management will follow, and often have rapid deterioration. Specific treatments usually include immunosuppression often with corticosteroids and cyclophosphamide or rituximab or newer agents. All patients need control of blood pressure, frequent monitoring, avoiding additional nephrotoxic insults where possible.

In a patient with suspected glomerulonephritis ask yourself

- Have you sent all the appropriate tests to make a rapid diagnosis?
- How ill is the patient, and does the patient need emergency haemodialysis or haemofiltration? This may be the case in RPGN. The major indications are hyperkalaemia, pulmonary oedema, profound acidosis and severe uraemia.
- Are there features of 'pulmonary renal' syndrome? With haemoptysis (from pulmonary haemorrhage) or features suggestive of pulmonary involvement with vasculitis on imaging which may cause severe hypoxia and is an urgent indication for immunosuppression and possibly dialysis or haemofiltration.
- What is the urine output? Complete anuria is highly suggestive of total urinary tract obstruction but may also occur in patient with RPGN, especially anti-GBM disease.
- Ensure the patient has daily blood tests (including at weekends) as the clinical condition can change rapidly and needs at least daily if not twice daily formal clinical review of observations, urine output, oxygenation, volume status and blood pressure. Check the drug chart at least daily and avoid nephrotoxins where possible.

When to contact a nephrologist?

- If you suspect RPGN, ANCA vasculitis, anti-GBM antibody disease or acute lupus nephritis.
- If renal biopsy may be indicated, usually for unexplained urinary abnormalities, unexplained progressive AKI or other systemic features suggestive of autoimmune disease.
- If dialysis is anticipated, regardless of suspected underlying aetiology.

Further reading

Johnson RJ. (2023) *Comprehensive Clinical Nephrology*, 7th edition. Elsevier.
Turner N. (2015) *Oxford Textbook of Clinical Nephrology*, 4th edition. OUP Oxford.

Rheumatology

CHAPTER 91

Acute arthritis

KEHINDE SUNMBOYE

Arthralgia in the strictest sense refers to joint pain without swelling, while arthritis signifies joint pain with swelling. In acute mono-arthritis, exclusion of septic arthritis is the immediate priority. Acute oligo- or polyarthritis has a broad differential diagnosis (Table 91.1), and if it has persisted >six weeks, is unlikely to resolve spontaneously and needs urgent referral to a rheumatologist. Assessment of the patient with acute arthritis is summarized in Figure 91.1. Focussed assessment of an acute arthritis is important and this is highlighted in Table 91.2. The relevant investigations that should follow the clinical assessment carried out are detailed in Table 91.3. The management of an acute arthritis ensures that the patient has the required intervention as soon as possible and the steps to take depending on the underlying diagnosis is highlighted in Table 91.4.

Table 91.1 Causes of acute arthritis.

Cause	Monoarthritis	Usually oligoarthritis (2–4 joints)	Usually polyarthritis (5 or more joints)
Common	Septic arthritis	Ankylosing spondylitis	Rheumatoid arthritis Systemic lupus erythematosus
	Gout, Pseudogout Trauma*	Inflammatory bowel disease	
			Viral diseases (e.g. rubella, hepatitis B and C, infectious mononucleosis)
	Haemarthrosis secondary to anticoagulation	Reactive arthritis following gut or genitourinary infection	
	Flare of osteoarthritis (overuse or minor trauma)	Psoriatic arthritis	
		Endocarditis (acute synovitis or tenosynovitis)	
Uncommon or rare	Osteonecrosis	Sarcoidosis	Post-streptococcal infection
	Pigmented villonodular synovitis	Whipple disease	
			Leukaemia
			Vasculitis
	Tuberculosis		Syphilis
	Haemophilia		Adult Still's disease
	Palindromic		Familial
	Rheumatism		Mediterranean fever

* Causing internal derangement, haemarthrosis or fracture, or acute synovitis from penetrating injury.

Acute Medicine: A Practical Guide to the Management of Medical Emergencies, Sixth Edition.
Edited by Mridula Rajwani, Leila Vaziri, and Ivie Gbinigie.
© 2026 John Wiley & Sons Ltd. Published 2026 by John Wiley & Sons Ltd.

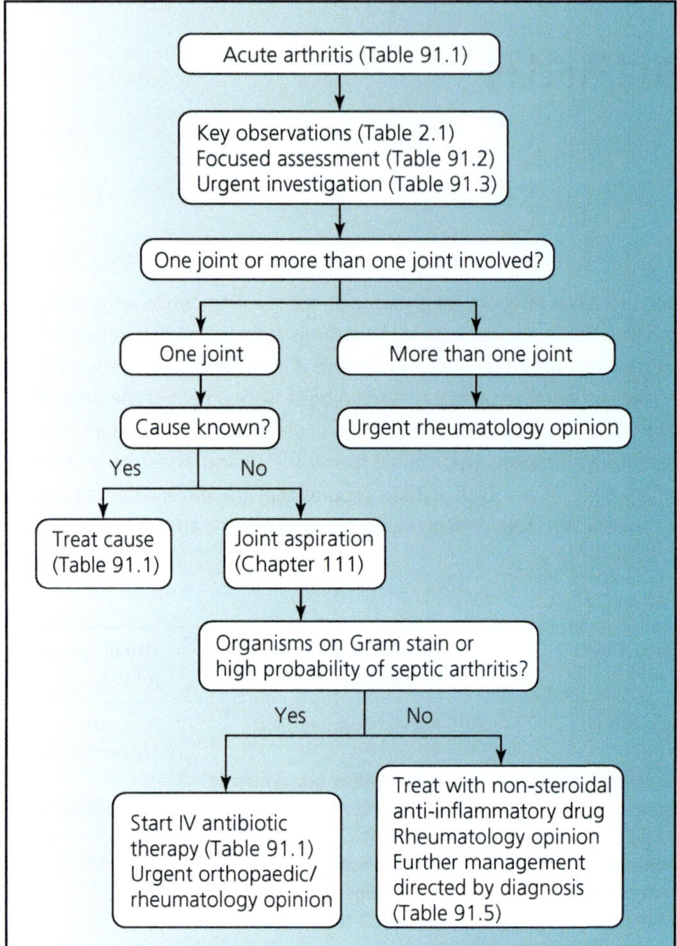

Figure 91.1 Assessment of the patient with acute arthritis.

Table 91.2 Focused assessment of acute arthritis.

History
- Duration and time course of arthritis and other symptoms (e.g. fever, rash, diarrhoea, urethritis and uveitis).
- Known arthritis or prosthetic joint?
- Previous similar attacks of arthritis?
- History of trauma?
- Possible septic arthritis? Septic arthritis usually follows a bacteraemia (e.g. from IV drug use) in a patient at risk because of rheumatoid arthritis, the presence of a prosthetic joint or immunocompromised individuals.
- Risk of gonococcal arthritis?
- Other illness?
- Current medication

Examination
- Key observations plus systematic examination.
- Pattern of joint involvement: monoarthritis, oligoarthritis (two to four joints) or polyarthritis (five joints or more) (see Table 91.1).
- Arthritis or periarticular inflammation (bursitis, tendinitis or cellulitis)? Painful limitation of movement of the joint suggests arthritis.
- Extra-articular signs (e.g. fever, rash, mouth ulcers, anterior uveitis and urethritis).

Table 91.3 Urgent investigation in acute arthritis.

- Joint aspiration (Chapter 111)
- Blood culture (×2) (especially if septic arthritis is suspected)
- Blood glucose
- Creatinine and electrolytes
- Liver function tests
- Full blood count
- Erythrocyte sedimentation rate and C-reactive protein
- Viral serology if indicated
- X-ray joint for baseline and to exclude osteomyelitis
- Urine stick test, microscopy and culture
- Swab of urethra, cervix and anorectum if gonococcal infection is possible

Table 91.4 Management of acute arthritis.

Cause of acute arthritis	Management
Septic arthritis	Antibiotic therapy
See Chapter 79	Joint drainage
	Seek advice from orthopaedic surgeon/rheumatologist
Gout	High-dose NSAID (consider PPI cover)
See Chapter 92	Colchicine if NSAID contraindicated Oral corticosteroid (prednisolone 40 mg daily for 1–2 days, then tapered over 7–10 days) if NSAID/colchicine contraindicated or not tolerated
	Consider intra-articular corticosteroid in place or oral corticosteroid if only one joint affected
Pseudogout	Joint drainage
See Chapter 92	Intra-articular corticosteroid
	NSAID (consider PPI cover)
	Colchicine if NSAID contraindicated
Flare of rheumatoid arthritis	Seek advice from rheumatologist
Flare of osteoarthritis	NSAID (consider PPI cover), intra-articular corticosteroid

NSAID, non-steroidal anti-inflammatory drug; PPI, proton pump inhibitor.

Further reading

Carlin E, Flew S. (2016) Sexually acquired reactive arthritis. *Clin Med* 16, 193–196. http://www.clinmed.rcpjournal.org/content/16/2/193.full.pdf+html.

Helfgott SM. (2015) Overview of monoarthritis in adults. UpToDate. https://www.uptodate.com/contents/overview-of-monoarthritis-in-adults?source=search_result&search=acute%20arthritis&selectedTitle=2~150.

Senthelal S, Li J, Ardeshirzadeh S, Thomas MA. (2024) Arthritis. In: StatPearls. [Online], Singh JA (Ed). Treasure Island (FL): StatPearls Publishing. Available from: http://www.ncbi.nlm.nih.gov/books/NBK518992/. [Accessed: 8 May 2024].

Smolen JS, Aletaha D, McInnes IB. (2016) Rheumatoid arthritis. *Lancet* 388, 2023–2038.

CHAPTER 92

Crystal arthropathies

KEHINDE SUNMBOYE

Gout and pseudogout are the two most common crystal arthropathies. Gout is caused by deposition of monosodium urate monohydrate crystals, and pseudogout by calcium pyrophosphate crystals. Their epidemiology is summarized in Table 92.1.

Table 92.1 Epidemiology of gout and pseudogout.

	Gout	Pseudogout (calcium pyrophosphate dihydrate deposition (CPPD) disease)
Age	Predominantly 30–60 years, risk increases with advancing age	>60 years, risk increases in the elderly
Sex	Male predominance, post-menopausal women, very rare in premenopausal women	Male: female ratio 1 : 1
Risk factors	Conditions that promote hyperuricaemia, due to overproduction or under-excretion of urate Overproduction of urate Genetic diseases: • Hypoxanthine-guanine phosphoribosyltransferase deficiency (Lesch–Nyhan syndrome) • Superactivity of phosphoribosyl pyrophosphate synthetase (PRPS) High cell turnover: • Cell lysis from chemotherapy for malignancies • Lympho- and myelo-proliferative diseases Under-excretion of urate: • Chronic alcohol abuse (beer and hard liquor) • Renal insufficiency (also below) • Dehydration	Conditions that promote altered concentrations of calcium, inorganic pyrophosphate (PPi) and the solubility products of these ions Genetic diseases: • Mutations in the ANKH gene, leading to altered PPi metabolism (familial CPPD deposition disease) Metabolic conditions causing CPPD deposition: • Hyperparathyroidism • Haemochromatosis • Hypomagnesaemia • Hypophosphataemia • Familial hypocalciuric hypercalcaemia (The five Hs of CPPD disease)
Related comorbid conditions	Hypertension Diabetes mellitus Renal insufficiency Hypertriglyceridaemia Hypercholesterolaemia Obesity Anaemia	Hyperparathyroidism Haemochromatosis Hypomagnesaemia (Chapter 52) Hypophosphataemia (Chapter 52) Familial hypocalciuric hypercalcaemia
Dietary Factors	Foods rich in purines such as red meat and seafood	No clear dietary causes

Acute Medicine: A Practical Guide to the Management of Medical Emergencies, Sixth Edition.
Edited by Mridula Rajwani, Leila Vaziri, and Ivie Gbinigie.

Priorities

- Septic arthritis (Chapter 79) must be excluded in any patient presenting with an acute monoarthritis.
- The clinical assessment of a patient with suspected gout or pseudogout is given in Table 92.2 and investigation is needed urgently in Table 92.3. Management is summarized in Figure 92.1.

Table 92.2 Focused assessment in suspected acute gout or pseudogout.

Element	Comment
Time course and duration of joint and other symptoms	In gout, attacks begin abruptly, usually overnight, and typically reach maximum intensity within 12 h.
	In pseudogout, attacks may resemble those of acute gout or follow a sub-acute course over several days.
Pattern of joint involvement	In gout, the first MTP joint (podagra) is the initial joint involved in 50% of cases and is eventually involved in >90% of cases. Monoarticular involvement occurs commonly, although polyarticular acute flares do occur.
	In pseudogout, large joint involvement such as the knee, wrist, elbow or ankle.
Context and comorbidities	See Table 92.1.
History of trauma	Trauma may cause agitation, with subsequent deposition of urate and CPPD crystals in patients with tophi and chondrocalcinosis, respectively.
Examination of involved joint(s) other signs	Swelling, warmth, redness (sometimes resembling cellulitis) and tenderness. In gout, tophi may be present in the helix of the ear, fingers, toes, prepatellar bursa and olecranon bursa.
Fever	May be present in polyarticular presentations of gout or pseudogout (septic arthritis must be excluded).

Table 92.3 Urgent investigation for suspected acute gout or pseudogout.

X-ray of involved joints
Aspiration of involved joint (samples for crystal analysis, microscopy and culture)
Blood culture (×2) if febrile
Creatinine and electrolytes
Urate level (may be normal in acute gout; gout and pseudogout may coexist)
Full blood count
If pseudogout confirmed:
Bone profile: calcium and phosphate, alkaline phosphatase
Magnesium
Ferritin, serum iron and total iron binding capacity (to assess for haemochromatosis)
Thyroid-stimulating hormone (hypothyroidism and pseudogout often coexist)
Parathyroid hormone levels (if hypercalcaemia)

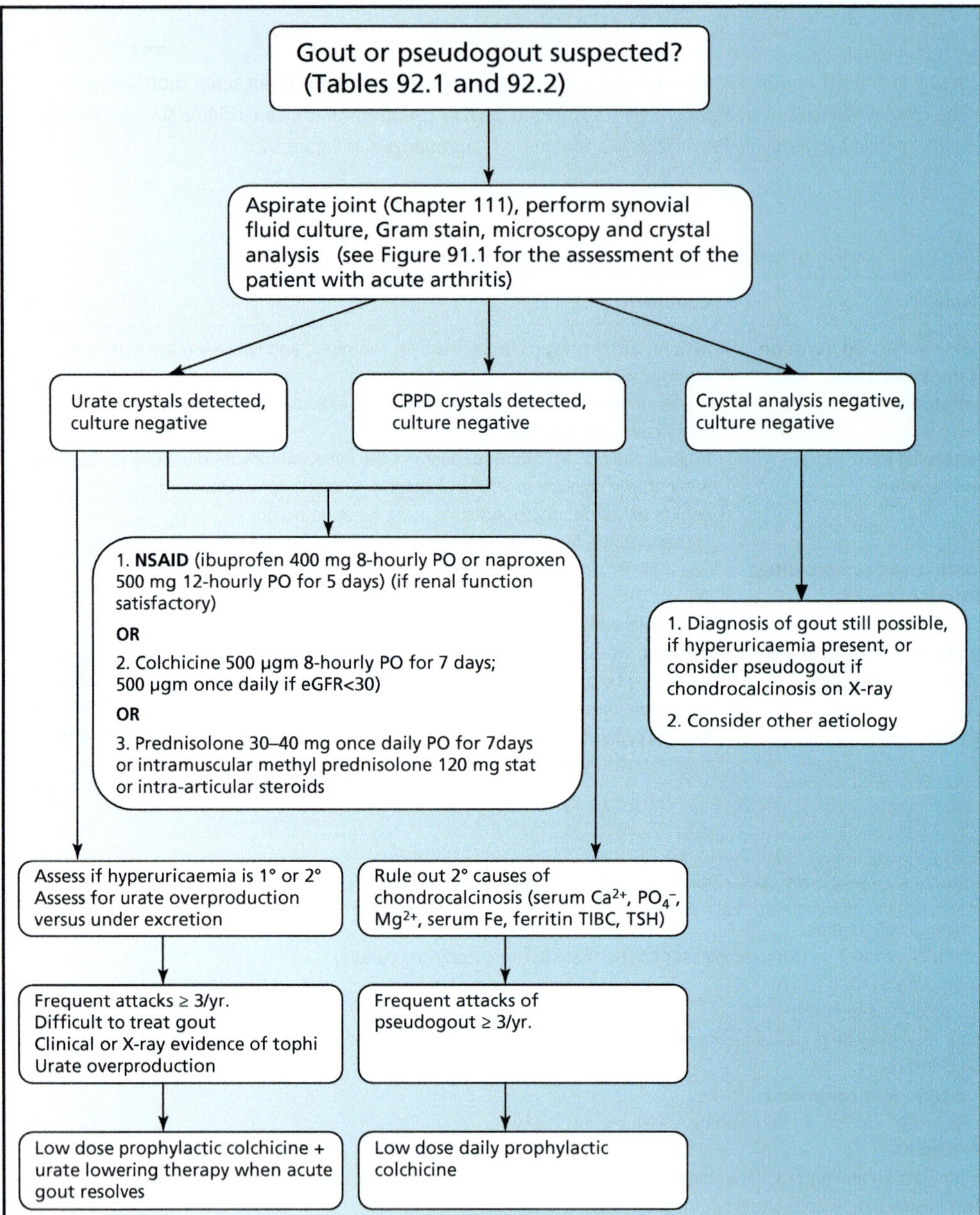

Figure 92.1 Treatment algorithm for acute gout and pseudogout.

Further reading

Cowley S, McCarthy G. (2023) Diagnosis and treatment of calcium pyrophosphate deposition (CPPD) disease: a review. *Open Access Rheumatol* 15, 33–41. DOI: 10.2147/OARRR.S389664. PMID: 36987530; PMCID: PMC10040153.

Dalbeth N, Merriman TR, Stamp LK. (2016). *Gout Lancet* 388, 2039–2052.

NICE guidelines (2022) Recommendations | Gout: diagnosis and management|Guidance|NICE. Available from https://www.nice.org.uk/guidance/ng219/chapter/Recommendations. [Accessed: 8 May 2024].

Rosenthal AK, Ryan LM. (2016) Calcium pyrophosphate deposition disease. *N Engl J Med* 374, 2575–2584.

CHAPTER 93

Rheumatoid arthritis

CHARLOTTE DAVID AND JOEL DAVID

Introduction

Rheumatoid arthritis (RA) is an auto-immune inflammatory disease of the joints, typically presenting with pain, stiffness and swelling of symmetrical small and large joints and can progress to joint destruction and extra-articular manifestations (EAMs, see Table 93.1), if insufficiently treated.

RA affects women three times more commonly than men, with the highest incidence in the fifth and sixth decades.

Priorities

- Early and effective management can prevent deformity, development of EAMs and reduce mortality.
- Diagnostic investigations include elevated CRP, rheumatoid factor (RF) and anti-cyclic citrullinated peptide (anti-CCP) and imaging of the joints, usually by ultrasound.
- Treatment includes initiation of a conventional disease-modifying anti-rheumatic drug (cDMARD) with optional bridging of glucocorticoids dependent on the level of inflammation.
- Biological therapies are used if low disease activity or remission is not achieved with optimisation of cDMARDs.
- The multi-disciplinary team (MDT) plays a key role in the holistic management of patients with RA.

Table 93.1 EAMs by system.

System	EAM
Skin	Nodules, Raynaud's phenomenon, petechiae, purpura, ulcers and gangrene.
Pulmonary	Bronchiolitis obliterans, organizing pneumonia, interstitial lung disease (UIP more than NSIP) and pleural disease.
Cardiac	Valvular disease, myocarditis, arrhythmias, vasculitis and pericarditis.
Neurological	Mono/polyneuritis multiplex.
Eyes	Sicca syndrome, episcleritis and scleritis.
Haematological	Felty's syndrome (RA, neutropenia and splenomegaly) and anaemia of chronic disease.
Renal	Glomerulonephritis, interstitial nephritis and amyloid deposition.

Acute Medicine: A Practical Guide to the Management of Medical Emergencies, Sixth Edition.
Edited by Mridula Rajwani, Leila Vaziri, and Ivie Gbinigie.

Pathology

The cause of RA, like other auto-immune conditions, is unknown. It is thought that genetic and environmental factors play a role in causation and development. The pathology is characterized by activation of endothelial cells resulting in neovascularization within the synovial membrane. The resultant hypertrophy causes bony erosion and cartilage destruction within the joint. Cytokines such as tumour necrosis factor (TNF), interleukin-1 (IL-1) and IL-6 are key in this inflammatory process).

The disease can be classified into seropositive and seronegative disease, based on the presence of the rheumatoid factor and anti-citrullinated C-peptide antibody. (ACPA). More than half of patients with RA are seropositive. RF is produced by B cells present in the inflamed synovium. RF activates complement and leukocyte infiltration within the synovium. It may be present in patients with other auto-immune diseases and therefore has a limited specificity in the diagnosis of RA.

Anti-CCP has a specificity of 98% and can be used as a prognostic indicator of erosive disease.

Natural history

The natural history of the disease is relapsing and remitting, and if left untreated, may lead to progressive joint destruction, deformity, and premature mortality secondary to EAMs, and also accelerated atheromatosis which correlates with untreated inflammation. Methotrexate has played a seminal role in reducing this premature mortality, with a 70% reduction when compared to other disease-modifying drugs.

History and examination

The typical presentation of RA is with polyarticular symmetrical joint disease, mainly in the hands and feet.

Key features in the history
- One in four patients has an acute or subacute onset.
- Presents with small joint pain, often multiple at a time.
- Morning joint stiffness, lasting >30 min, improves with movement.
- Swelling of joints.
- Limitations to activities of daily living (ADLs).
- Joint-specific symptoms such as carpal tunnel syndrome in wrist disease.
- Systemic symptoms are present in up to a third of patients and include fevers, malaise, weight loss and fatigue.

Key examination findings
- 'Soft' swelling of joints secondary to joint effusions. The joint may also be described as 'boggy' secondary to synovial thickening.
- Tenderness on palpation or passive movement of the joint.
- Distribution is symmetrical involving small joints* or large joints**.
- Reduced grip strength (a useful biomarker).
- Palmar erythema.
- Thickening of the flexor tendons in the palm.
- Rheumatoid nodulosis, including along the palmar tendon sheaths which may result in trigger finger, and subcutaneously near bony prominences.

- Deformities (prevalent in advanced disease):
  - Boutonniere (flexion of the PIP with hyperextension of the DIP) and Swan Neck (PIP hyperextension with DIP flexion) deformities – resulting from damage and subluxation of PIPs and tendons.
  - Z thumb (flexion of the MCP with hyperextension of the interphalangeal joint).
  - Ulnar deviation or drift of the MCPs.

Small joints: metacarpophalangeal (MCPs), metatarsophalangeal (MTPs), proximal interphalangeal (PIPs) and wrist joints.

**Large joints: ankle, knee, elbow and shoulder joints.*

Investigations

Investigation	For diagnosis	Following diagnosis
Blood tests	• RF +/– anti-CCP • Full blood count (FBC): anaemia of chronic disease, thrombocytosis, mild leucocytosis. • Erythrocyte sedimentation rate (ESR) and C-reactive protein (CRP) are elevated in inflammation.	• ESR and CRP are elevated during an acute phase of the disease and can therefore be used as biomarkers of active disease. • Anti-CCP can be used as a prognostic indicator of disease severity.
Imaging	• X-ray* hands/feet if persistent synovitis. • If X-ray changes are not yet present, Magnetic Resonance Imaging (MRI) may be helpful in identifying hypertrophic synovial tissue. • Ultrasound scan (USS) may also be used to identify joint inflammation.	• X-ray hands/feet to assess for bony erosions. • MRI and USS can be used as biomarkers of disease activity through measurement of the volume of inflamed tissue.
Questionnaires	• Health Assessment Questionnaire (HAQ) is used to assess the patient's functional status in relation to disease.	• HAQ. • Disease Activity Score (DAS28)**.

Synovial fluid analysis may help to identify when a rheumatoid joint is complicated by infection.
* Pathognomonic x-ray findings of the hands/feet are soft tissue swelling, periarticular osteopenia and osteoporosis, narrowing of the joint spaces, cysts and bony erosions.
** DAS28 is a quantitative index to measure disease activity in rheumatoid arthritis and response to treatment. It's comprised of information on the number of swollen tender joints, the acute phase response and the patient's self-assessment of disease activity.

Differential diagnoses

Differential diagnosis	
Connective Tissue Disorders (CTDs) – for example systemic lupus erythematosus (SLE)	• Usually not associated with deformity or erosive disease. • More likely to present with additional signs and symptoms such as rashes, mouth ulcers and Raynaud's phenomenon (although 10% of patients with RA will have Raynaud's).
Fibromyalgia	• 'Trigger points' at non-articular sites with absence of joint swelling/reduced range of motion, and normal blood tests.
Viral arthritis	• Usually polyarthritis. • < six-week course. • Diagnosis aided by history and serological testing.
Septic arthritis	• Single hot, red, swollen joint. • Often systemically unwell. • Requires aspiration to isolate organism.

Differential diagnosis

Osteoarthritis	• Joint distribution is different – in hands, the distal interphalangeal joints (DIPs) are more affected than the PIPs. • Associated with Heberden's and Bouchard's nodes. • Swelling feels bony. • Stiffness lasting <30 min, often toward the end of the day and worse on movement. • X-ray features: joint-space narrowing, loss of cartilage and osteophyte formation.
Crystalline arthritis	• Look for gout risk factors and tophi. • Serum urate level is elevated. • Synovial fluid analysis shows presence of crystals.
Polymyalgia rheumatica (PMR)	• More associated with shoulder/pelvic girdle pain/stiffness. • Joint involvement is milder, associated with synovitis of the shoulders, hips and occasionally the wrists. • It has a significant response to steroids.
Psoriatic arthritis	• Joint involvement is usually asymmetric. • May have DIP involvement. • 90% of patients have associated psoriasis or a family history of psoriasis.
Reactive arthritis	• Recent viral/bacterial infection. • Causes symmetrical inflammation of the joints in the hands/feet.
Sarcoidosis	• Usually associated with respiratory disease – chest X-ray advisable if sarcoid is suspected. • Elevated serum angiotensin-converting enzyme (ACE)
Seronegative spondylarthritis	• If there is a history of inflammatory bowel disease, psoriasis or back pain and a family history this differential should be suspected.
Palindromic rheumatism	• Episodes of intense joint inflammation that affects one or several joints sequentially, with asymptomatic periods in between. • May progress to RA particularly in the presence of anti-CCP.

Management

The management of RA is guided by a treat-to-target strategy. The strategy aim is remission. The response to treatment is assessed using the biomarkers – namely acute phase markers and scoring systems, such as DAS28.

Conventional disease-modifying anti-rheumatic drugs

First line treatment of RA is cDMARD monotherapy. Treatment is started within the first three months of persistent symptoms. cDMARDs include oral or subcutaneous methotrexate (first line, with supplemental folic acid), leflunomide, sulfasalazine or hydroxychloroquine (as an alternative or in addition to the aforementioned drugs, in mild disease). The doses are up-titrated as tolerated and can be given in combination if the target has not been achieved.

A short-term course of steroids (either orally or three IM depomedrone at monthly intervals) may be used to bridge treatment with the cDMARD to reduce the symptoms of inflammation. If the disease is less active, the steroid bridging may be omitted.

Steroids can, although not ideally, be used long-term, and only when all other treatment options have been offered and the patient is properly counselled on the complications and side effects of treatment. They may also be offered when there are EAMs present.

Biological therapies

There are different classes of biological DMARDs (bDMARDs) available to use for RA if remission is not achieved. These include TNF-alpha inhibitors, CD80/CD86 inhibitor, IL-6 inhibitors, CD-20 reducing agents and anti-IL1 antibody (although this is no longer licensed in the United Kingdom). Anti-TNF is often used as first line. Biological therapies may be used concurrently with cDMARDs or as a monotherapy if cDMARDs are not tolerated. It is advisable to change class of biological therapy if treatment is not tolerated or ineffective.

Biological therapies are expensive and may sometimes be associated with a slightly higher risk of infection when steroids are used concomitantly, therefore guidelines exist for their commencement. Infections such as latent tuberculosis and reactivation of hepatitis B are of main concern, and therefore patients are required to have blood tests (Hepatitis B and C, interferon-gamma release assay and HIV serology) and a chest X-ray prior to commencing therapy. Administration of live vaccines is also contraindicated in patients taking biological therapies.

Target	Examples	Pharmacology	Notes
TNF-alpha	Infliximab, adalimumab, etanercept, golimumab, certolizumab	Blockade of the pro-inflammatory cascade involved in formation of the pannus.	1st line
CD80/CD86	Abatacept	Inhibits T-cell activation through binding to CD80/86 on the antigen-presenting cells.	Useful in TNF-inhibitor refractory disease.
IL-6	Tocilizumab, sarilumab	IL-6 is a key cytokine involved in the pathogenesis of RA.	Greater efficacy than TNF-inhibitors when used as monotherapy. Also useful as a monotherapy if cDMARDs are poorly tolerated.
CD20	Rituximab	CD20 is found in B lymphocytes, which produce auto-antibodies. Binding to CD20 causes B cell depletion.	Useful in sero-positive patients who do not tolerate anti-TNF therapy.

Surgical interventions

Referral to surgical specialties should be considered if there has been significant joint damage and inadequate response to conservative management of pain, joint function, deformity or persistent synovitis.

Complications of RA such as carpal tunnel syndrome, cervical myelopathy or tendon rupture also require referral.

Remission

After six months of complete remission, therapies may be tapered. The bDMARD is the first to taper, with continuation of the cDMARD. If remission is maintained, the cDMARD may be tapered after six months.

The management of therapies therefore requires regular review – initially at six months following remission and from then on, annually.

Multi-disciplinary team

RA has a significant impact on patient lives through pain, disease activity and EAMS, fatigue, functional impact, libido, appetite and mood. There is an important role for the MDT.

Physiotherapy is used to improve muscle strength, general fitness and management of functional impairments. Occupational therapists can assist with management of associated functional limitations. Podiatrists may be of assistance if there is presence of foot problems and can advise on footwear. Psychological interventions should also be offered to patients with RA. Collaboration with other medical specialties such as ophthalmology, respiratory and gastroenterology is often necessary. Rapid access to services should be available to patients, such as nurse specialist hotlines. Self-help through recognized charities, such as Versus Arthritis and Arthritis Research, are also very important.

Further reading

Aletaha D, Smolen JS. (2018) Diagnosis and management of rheumatoid arthritis: a review. *Jama* 320(13), 1360–1372.

Findeisen KE, Sewell J, Ostor AJ. (2021) Biological therapies for rheumatoid arthritis: an overview for the clinician. *Biologics* 15, 343–352.

NICE CKS. Rheumatoid arthritis: what else might it be?Available at: https://cks.nice.org.uk/topics/rheumatoid-arthritis/diagnosis/differential-diagnosis/. [Accessed: 20/12/2023].

Prete M, Racanelli V, Digiglio L, *et al.* (2011) Extra-articular manifestations of rheumatoid arthritis: an update. *Autoimmun. Rev.* 11(2), 123–131.

CHAPTER 94

Acute vasculitis

GAGANDEEP SUKHIJA AND ARTI MAHTO

"The only certainty is that nothing is certain."
– *Pliny the Elder*

Introduction

Vasculitis, characterized by inflammation of blood vessels and leading to organ damage, presents a significant challenge in acute medicine due to its diverse clinical manifestations and potential for serious complications. Early recognition and prompt management are crucial to prevent end-organ damage and improve outcomes. This chapter provides a comprehensive overview of acute vasculitis, covering its basic concepts, classification, symptoms, examination findings, diagnosis and management strategies.

Pathophysiology

The specific pathophysiology varies depending on the type and severity of vasculitis, influencing the clinical manifestations and outcomes of the disease.

The pathogenesis involves immune-mediated processes where immune cells activate and release pro-inflammatory cytokines, leading to the formation of immune complexes that deposit in blood vessel walls, initiating inflammation. This results in endothelial cell dysfunction, infiltration of inflammatory cells like neutrophils and lymphocytes, and subsequent tissue damage. Additionally, the release of harmful enzymes and reactive oxygen species exacerbates vascular injury. Genetic predisposition and environmental factors such as infections or medications can contribute to its development.

Classification of vasculitis

The classification of vasculitis is essential for understanding its diverse clinical presentations and guiding management. Vasculitis can be classified based on the size of the affected vessels: small, medium and large vessels (Table 94.1 and Figure 94.1). They are also classified based on aetiology into primary (occurring in isolation) and secondary vasculitis (associated with other conditions, e.g. systemic lupus erythematous, rheumatoid arthritis or infections etc.). Some vasculitides do not fit these classifications and could be systemic like Behcet's syndrome or limited to one organ (primary CNS vasculitis).

Acute Medicine: A Practical Guide to the Management of Medical Emergencies, Sixth Edition.
Edited by Mridula Rajwani, Leila Vaziri, and Ivie Gbinigie.
© 2026 John Wiley & Sons Ltd. Published 2026 by John Wiley & Sons Ltd.

Table 94.1 Classification of vasculitis.

Classification	Description
Small vessel vasculitis	Diseases affecting small vessels; includes ANCA-associated granulomatosis with polyangiitis (GPA), microscopic polyangiitis (MPA) and eosinophilic granulomatosis with polyangiitis (EGPA) or anti-glomerular basement membrane antibody vasculitis
Medium vessel vasculitis	Diseases affecting medium-sized vessels; includes polyarteritis nodosa and Kawasaki disease
Large vessel vasculitis	Diseases affecting large vessels, predominantly the aorta and its branches; prominent examples are giant cell arteritis (GCAs) and Takayasu arteritis

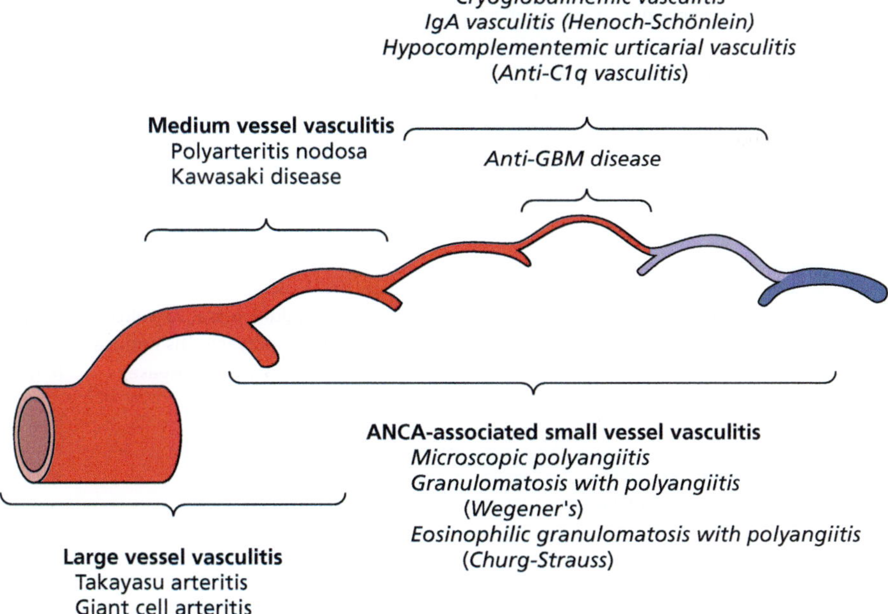

Figure 94.1 Classification of vasculitis.

Symptoms and organ involvement

Systemic vasculitis can present with a wide range of clinical manifestations (Table 94.2). The pattern of involvement can vary between each type of vasculitis but there is considerable overlap in these conditions (Table 94.3).

Diagnosis

Diagnosis of acute vasculitis relies on a combination of clinical evaluation, laboratory investigations, imaging studies and histopathological examination.

Table 94.2 Typical presentations of acute vasculitis.

Symptom	Description
General symptoms	Fatigue, malaise, unintentional loss of body weight
Headache	Often severe, persistent and localized, especially in temporal arteritis (GCAs)
Fever	May be present, particularly in systemic vasculitis
Skin manifestations	Varied, including purpura, ulcers, nodules, and livedo reticularis
Joint involvement	Arthritis (joint inflammation), arthralgia (joint pain), commonly affecting small or large joints
Neurological symptoms	Neuropathy (mononeuritis multiplex, polyneuropathy), cranial nerve palsies (facial nerve palsy, abducens nerve palsy), stroke, transient ischaemic attacks, cognitive impairment, encephalopathy and seizures
Pulmonary involvement	Cough, dyspnoea, haemoptysis, pleuritic chest pain, lung nodules, interstitial lung disease and cavitating lung lesions
Cardiac manifestations	Chest pain, dyspnoea, arrhythmias, myocarditis, pericarditis and heart failure
Gastrointestinal symptoms	Abdominal pain, gastrointestinal bleeding, diarrhoea and mesenteric ischemia
Renal involvement	Haematuria, proteinuria, renal insufficiency and rapidly progressive glomerulonephritis
Ophthalmological symptoms	Visual disturbances (e.g., blurring, diplopia), amaurosis fugax, anterior ischemic optic neuropathy, uveitis and scleritis
ENT symptoms	Epistaxis, sinusitis, hearing loss, otalgia and nasal septal perforation
Testicular pain	Pain or tenderness in the testes, may indicate vasculitis involving the testicular arteries

Table 94.3 Symptoms and system involvement in various vasculitis.

System	Examination findings	Small vessel vasculitis (e.g. GPA and MPA)	Medium vessel vasculitis (e.g., polyarteritis nodosa and Kawasaki disease)	Large vessel vasculitis (e.g. GCA)
Skin	Purpura, ulcers, livedo reticularis	++	++	+
Joints	Arthritis, arthralgia	++	+++	+
Neurological	Mononeuritis multiplex, peripheral neuropathy	++	++	+
Cardiac	Chest pain, dyspnoea, arrhythmias	+	++	++
Pulmonary	Cough, dyspnoea, haemoptysis	++	+	+
Renal	Haematuria, proteinuria, renal insufficiency	++	++	+
Ophthalmological	Visual disturbances, anterior ischemic optic neuropathy	++	+	+++
ENT	Epistaxis, sinusitis, hearing loss	++	+	+
Gastrointestinal	Abdominal pain, gastrointestinal bleeding	++	++	+
Head	Headache, jaw claudication	+	+	+++
General	Fatigue, malaise, weight loss	++	++	++

Note: The prominence of symptoms may vary within each type of vasculitis and depends on factors such as disease severity and individual patient characteristics.

Consider vasculitis in a patient presenting with constitutional upset, systemic symptoms or headache (after the age of 50), with or without evidence of organ dysfunction after ruling out common causes (Table 94.4). Diagnosis of specific vasculitis is based on pattern of organ involvement, laboratory features, imaging and histopathological findings on biopsy.

Clinical history and physical examination are crucial for identifying specific symptoms and signs suggestive of vasculitis (Table 94.5) and ruling out differentials (Table 94.4).

Table 94.4 Differential diagnosis of systemic vasculitis.

Cause/ subtype	Clinical features	Laboratory features	Imaging	Histopathological findings
Infectious vasculitis	Sepsis with multiorgan failure	Elevated inflammatory markers (ESR and CRP)	CT/MRI showing vascular abnormalities	Micro abscesses, thrombi, fibrinoid necrosis
	Infective endocarditis	Positive blood cultures	PET scan for active inflammation	
	Tuberculosis	Raised ESR	CT showing cavitating lesions	Caseating granuloma
	Falciparum malaria Mycoplasma and legionella infection Syphilis, Lyme disease, leptospirosis Fungal infection (coccidioidomycosis and histoplasmosis)			
Neoplastic diseases	Metastatic cancer	Specific tumour markers (e.g. PSA and CA-125)	Imaging (CT, MRI and PET)	Variable (may show tumour emboli, infiltration)
	Cancer with paraneoplastic syndrome Acute leukaemia Lymphoma			
Vascular diseases	Multifocal embolism from the heart (e.g. infective endocarditis, atrial myxoma and intracardiac thrombus)	Echocardiography (for cardiac emboli)		Emboli, dissection, thrombosis
	Aortic dissection involving multiple branch arteries	CT angiography (for aortic dissection)		
Other disorders	Disseminated intravascular coagulation (DIC)	Coagulation studies (e.g. D-dimer and fibrinogen)		
	Thrombotic thrombocytopenic purpura (TTP)	ADAMTS13 activity (for TTP)		
	Drug toxicity (prescribed and recreational)	Drug levels (if suspected)		
	Pre-eclampsia			
	Systemic lupus erythematosus	ANA, DsDNA, Complement C3 and C4		
	Antiphospholipid syndrome (recurrent venous or arterial thromboses, foetal loss, mild thrombocytopenia, anticardiolipin antibodies and lupus anticoagulant antibodies)	Lupus anti-coagulant and anti-cardiolipin		

Table 94.5 Focused assessment of the patient with possible systemic vasculitis.

History
- Gather comprehensive medical history, focusing on previous episodes and therapies administered. Evaluate for potential flare-ups, intercurrent infections or comorbidities.
- Inquire about illicit drug use.
- Consider past symptoms to identify patterns indicative of systemic involvement (e.g. weight loss, fever, rash, with a history of chronic nasal discharge, hearing loss or neuropathy).
- Recognize characteristic features such as upper and lower airway involvement in granulomatosis with polyangiitis (GPA) and predominant lung and renal involvement in microscopic polyangiitis (MPA), with rare upper airway symptoms.

Examination
- Conduct a thorough physical examination, including weight assessment for diagnosis aid and treatment dosing.
- Evaluate eyes for signs of inflammation or haemorrhage, consider slit lamp examination for suspected uveitis.
- Assess for sensorineural hearing loss.
- Inspect oral and genital mucosa for ulceration.
- Examine skin for lesions indicative of vasculitis, including infarcts, purpura or gangrene.
- Palpate lymph nodes for enlargement.
- Assess pulses in all limbs and compare blood pressure in both arms (and legs if indicated for large vessel vasculitis suspicion).
- Check for artery tenderness and listen for bruits.
- Auscultate chest and heart for signs of inflammation, effusion or murmurs.
- Palpate abdomen for organomegaly and evaluate the aorta.
- Assess for neuropathy or central nervous system involvement through cranial nerve examination, reflexes, power, sensation and orientation.

Laboratory investigations typically include assessment of inflammatory markers such as erythrocyte sedimentation rate (ESR) and C-reactive protein (CRP), renal function, full blood count (FBC), blood cultures (to rule out infection), urine dip, culture and urine protein creatinine ratio, Electrocardiogram (ECG), chest X-ray as well as autoantibody testing (e.g. ANCA, PR3, MPO and anti-GBM), myeloma screen and other autoantibody testing in case of overlapping symptoms and signs.

Imaging such as angiography, ultrasound, Computed Tomography (CT), magnetic resonance imaging (MRI), and positron emission tomography (PET-CT) scan aid in visualizing vessel inflammation and identifying affected areas.

Nerve conduction studies, echocardiography and pulmonary function tests may be required based on presenting symptoms.

Management of acute vasculitis

The focus of management is to recognise suspected new onset vasculitis and contacting a specialist for advice while at the same time ruling out other differential diagnoses (Table 94.4).

Early intervention with high-dose steroids should be considered in patients with GCA. Early specialist input is required for all patients, especially those with organ or life-threatening presentations. Patients require close observation and repeated examinations as clinical symptoms can evolve rapidly. Patients with non-organ threatening presentation can be managed on an ambulatory basis.

Management of acute vasculitis aims to control inflammation early, prevent long-term end-organ damage and improve patient outcomes.

Look for evidence of organ or life-threatening disease that may warrant contacting the ITU/HDU team early on for supportive care.

Corticosteroids are the cornerstone of therapy, with high-dose initial therapy followed by a tapering regimen based on clinical response.

Other immunosuppressive agents such as cyclophosphamide, rituximab, methotrexate or azathioprine are often used as steroid-sparing agents usually by the specialist particularly in severe cases or those with relapsing disease. Avacopan (complement 5a receptor antagonist) is a new steroid-sparing agent being used to treat ANCA vasculitis (GPA and MPA).

Biologic agents including tocilizumab (GCA) and may be considered in refractory cases.

Supportive care and adjunctive therapies are essential to address specific complications and optimize patient well-being.

Giant cell arteritis (GCAs): diagnosis and management

The commonest vasculitis in adults is giant-cell arteritis (GCAs), usually presenting with new-onset headache in older people (patients over 50 years of age).

Associated symptoms include constitutional upset, malaise, weight loss, jaw claudication and scalp tenderness.

It carries a significant risk (20–30%) of visual loss from ischaemic optic neuropathy and so needs urgent assessment and treatment.

Diagnosis is based on pretest probability, TA US and biopsy demonstrating characteristic inflammatory infiltrates (Figure 94.2).

Management involves high-dose corticosteroids to prevent vision loss and long-term therapy with careful monitoring for steroid-related complications. Adjunctive therapies such as methotrexate and tocilizumab may be considered in refractory cases.

Prognosis and complications

The prognosis of acute vasculitis varies depending on the specific subtype, extent of organ involvement and response to therapy. Common complications include organ damage (e.g. renal failure and pulmonary haemorrhage), infection (related to immunosuppressive therapy) and long-term sequelae of corticosteroid use (e.g. osteoporosis and diabetes). Long-term follow-up is essential to monitor disease activity, assess treatment response, and manage complications effectively.

Conclusion

Acute vasculitis poses significant challenges in acute medicine, requiring a multidisciplinary approach for optimal management.

Early recognition, prompt diagnosis and tailored treatment strategies are essential to improve outcomes and prevent complications.

Giant Cell Arteritis (GCA)

Consider GCA if >50 years with the following features:
- Acute new headache/facial pain
- Scalp tenderness
- Jaw/tongue claudication
- Visual symptoms (amaurosis fugax, diplopia, visual loss)
- PMR symptoms
- Fevers, weight loss
- Temporal artery abnormality: non
- Raised ESR/CRP

Immediate referral

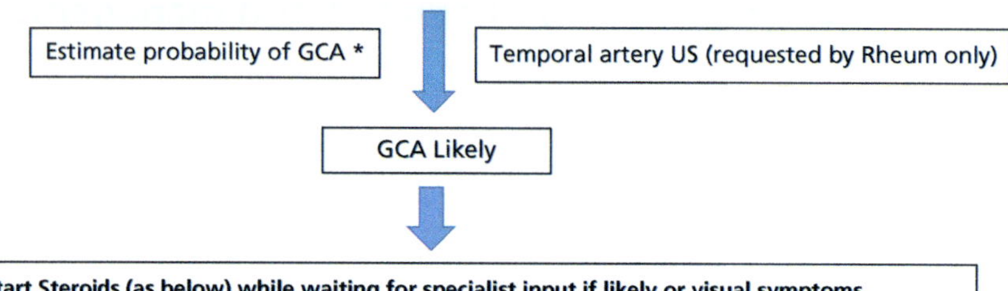

- Check full blood count, C reactive protein, ESR, renal and liver function and blood glucose.
- Consider checking Myeloma screen, ANCA ab in patients with other symptoms.
- Seek Urgent advice from Rheumatologist or refer to your local GCA pathway.

Estimate probability of GCA *

Temporal artery US (requested by Rheum only)

GCA Likely

- Start Steroids (as below) while waiting for specialist input if likely or visual symptoms.

Suspected/confirmed GCA management:

Commence Steroid treatment and PPI cover

- Prednisolone 60 mg OD – if jaw claudication, but no visual symptoms
- Prednisolone 40 mg OD – if no jaw claudication or visual symptoms
- Pulsed IV methylprednisolone 500 mg-1g OD for 3 days – acute/intermittent visual loss.

*estimate probability based on Sounthend GCA Probability score

Figure 94.2 Diagnosis and management of GCA.

Further reading

Jennette JC, Falk RJ, Bacon PA, et al. (2013) revised international Chapel Hill consensus conference nomenclature of vasculitides. *Arthritis & Rheumatology* 65(1), 1–11. DOI: 10.1002/art.37715.

Merkel P. Overview of and approach to the vasculitides in adults. In: UpToDate, Connor RF (Ed), Wolters Kluwer. (Accessed on January 4, 2024). Available from Overview of and approach to the vasculitides in adults - UpToDate

Vasculitis UK website: www.vasculitis.org.uk.

Zarka F, Veillette C, Makhzoum JP. (2020) A review of primary vasculitis mimickers based on the Chapel Hill consensus classification. *Int J Rheumatol* 2020, 8392542.

CHAPTER 95

Multisystem rheumatic disorders

SUNG-HEE KIM AND JOEL DAVID

Many autoimmune rheumatic diseases are multi-system. However, it is important to remember that the commonest presentations of multi-system disorders are due to infection and malignancy. Only 2–3% of presentations with unintentional weight loss have underlying autoimmune disease. A quarter of these presentations are due to a malignancy and a third have a gastrointestinal cause. Therefore, it is imperative to exclude other major differentials such as infection and malignancy when considering the underlying diagnosis of multisystem rheumatic disorders.

When to suspect rheumatic disease

- Prolonged fever in the absence of infection or malignancy
- Rash associated with joint pains
- Persistently elevated inflammatory markers (Erythrocyte Sedimentary Rate /C-Reactive Protein)
- Presence of auto-antibodies

Diagnostic approach

- Detailed history and meticulous examination seeking out involvement of all organ systems. Symptoms and signs for different organ systems are detailed in Table 95.1 and Figure 95.1. Characteristics of specific multisystem rheumatic diseases are shown in Table 95.2.
- It is also important to consider the patient's demographics (age, gender and ethnicity). For example, Behcet's disease is more common in people from Turkey and Silk Route countries, connective tissue diseases are more prevalent within Afro-Caribbean population. Para-neoplastic syndromes would be more relevant in older patients.
- Drug history is important as some diseases can be triggered by certain drugs. For example, SLE can be triggered by drugs such as carbimazole, allopurinol, hydralazine, penicillamine and phenytoin. Cocaine use can mimic symptoms of granulomatous polyangiitis or relapsing polychondritis.

Investigations

In most systemic autoimmune disorders, there would be raised inflammatory markers (CRP and ESR). However, CRP can also be mild-moderately raised in the context of high BMI (especially truncal obesity) and with smoking. ESR may be affected by concentration of immunoglobulins, fibrinogen, age, food intake and has a diurnal

---

Acute Medicine: A Practical Guide to the Management of Medical Emergencies, Sixth Edition.
Edited by Mridula Rajwani, Leila Vaziri, and Ivie Gbinigie.

Table 95.1 Systems approach in taking thorough history and examination for a patient with possible multisystem autoimmune rheumatic disease.

Systems	Symptoms	Signs	Investigations
General	Fever Loss of appetite Weight loss Fatigue/malaise Night sweats	Pyrexia Cachexia Sarcopenia Lethargy	FBC, ESR, CRP Renal profile LFT, CPK, LDH ANA, ANCA C3/C4, Immunoglobulins
Skin and Mucous membranes	Rash – type and distribution Hair loss Mouth ulcers	Erythema nodosum, photosensitivity Raynaud's, digital ulcers, infarcts, gangrene, skin ulceration	Skin biopsy including immunofluorescence, CT angiogram, US arteriogram
Cardiovascular	Chest pain Palpitations Shortness of breath Peripheral oedema	Cardiomegaly Murmurs Pericardial rub Arrhythmia Reduced pulses bruits	ECG, Echo, Arteriogram
Respiratory	Cough, shortness of breath, haemoptysis, wheeze	Lung crepitations Low saturation Cyanosis	CXR HRCT Lung function tests CTPA ANCA
Gastrointestinal	Abdominal pain Nausea, vomiting Diarrhoea Bloody stools	Ascites, abdominal distension, organomegaly	Abdominal XR US abdomen CT abdomen Endoscopy
Renal	Oedema Frothy urine Reduced urine output Blood in urine	Periorbital, facial, ankle oedema Hypertension Ascites Sacral oedema	ANA, ENA Anti-ds DNA ab Anti-GBM ab Renal function 24-h urine protein Urinary ACR Renal biopsy
Musculoskeletal	Arthralgia, EMS, muscle tenderness Difficulty getting up from floor	Joint swelling, tenderness, reduced ROM Muscle weakness	X-ray Ultrasound MRI/CT Muscle enzymes MRI Muscle biopsy EMG
Central nervous system	Headache, giddiness, seizures, stroke, cognitive decline, reduced GCS Psychiatric features Pins and needles Weakness of limbs Facial asymmetry	Reduced GCS, focal neurological signs Peripheral neuropathy Mononeuritis multiplex Cranial nerve palsies	CT/MRI head/spine Nerve conduction tests Temporal artery ultrasound
Ophthalmological	Red eye, painful eye, visual loss	Episcleritis, uveitis, scleritis	Slit lamp examination
Ear nose and throat	Nosebleeds, nose crusting, nasal collapse, past ear infections, deafness	Nose crusting, saddles nose, chondritis	CT nasal sinuses Nasal endoscopy/ laryngoscopy
Haematological	Pallor, purpuric rash, bruises	Pallor, jaundice, purpura, petechiae, bleeding gums, hepatosplenomegaly, lymphadenopathy, venous or arterial thrombosis	FBC, DAT, bone marrow aspirate, clotting Gene testing
Genitourinary	Ulcers, testicular pain	Genital ulcers	Testicular US

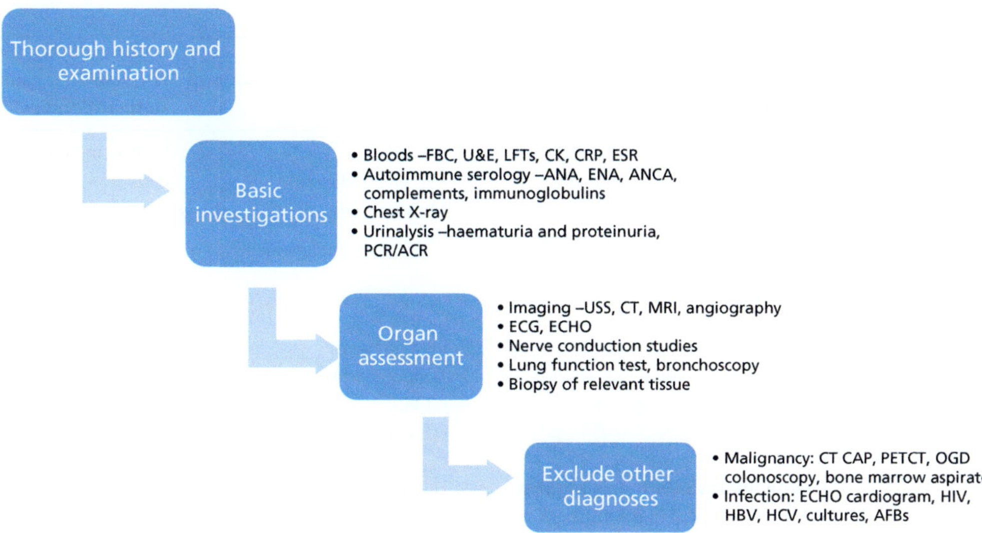

Figure 95.1 Approach to investigating a patient with possible multisystem autoimmune rheumatic disease. Source: Adapted from How to investigate multisystem disease by Watts RA. Best Pract Res Clin Rheumatol. 2014 Dec.

Table 95.2 Characteristics of specific multisystem rheumatic diseases.

Connective tissue disease			
	Clinical features	**Investigations**	**Auto-antibodies**
Rheumatoid arthritis	Synovitis Interstitial lung disease Pleural effusion Scleritis, keratitis Felty's syndrome – splenomegaly and neutropenia	US hands	Rheumatoid factor Anti-CCP antibodies
Systemic lupus erythematosus	Non-erosive arthralgia Malar, discoid rash, mouth ulcers Non-scarring alopecia Serositis, pericarditis Libman Sack's endocarditis Glomerulonephritis CNS lupus: headache, cognitive disorders, seizures Previous pregnancy losses	Leukopenia, thrombocytopenia, pancytopenia Low complements ECHO	ANA dsDNA ENA, e.g. Sm, RNP, Ro, La anti-phospholipid antibody
Sjögren's syndrome	Severe fatigue Severe eye and mouth dryness Neuro or pulmonary disease Associated with lymphoma	Hypergammaglobulinaemia	ANA anti-Ro, anti-La
Systemic sclerosis	Raynaud's, skin fibrosis, sclerodactyly, calcinosis, telangiectasia, digital ulcers Interstitial lung disease and pulmonary hypertension Oesophageal dysfunction, GORD Renal crisis (in diffuse systemic sclerosis)	BP ECHO HRCT Urine dip	ANA Anti Scl-70 (diffuse) Anti-centromere (limited) PMScl

(continued)

Table 95.2 (*Continued*)

Connective tissue disease			
	Clinical features	**Investigations**	**Auto-antibodies**
Inflammatory myositis	Significant muscle weakness and pain Rash (dermatomyositis – gottron's papules, heliotropic rash) ILD (associated with anti-synthetase syndrome) dysphagia	Raised CK MRI affected muscle Muscle biopsy HRCT	Positive myositis blot E.g. Jo1, PL7, PL12, Ku, MDA,
Systemic vasculitides			
	Clinical features	Investigations	ANCA
Large vessel vasculitis	GCA- headache, visual loss, jaw/tongue claudication, PMR symptoms Absent pulses, Bruits	Temporal artery ultrasound CT PET MR Aorta	ANCA-negative
ANCA- associated vasculitis (small vessel vasculitis)	**Granulomatosis with polyangiitis** • ENT involvement (nasal crusting, nosebleeds, sinusitis, hearing loss) • Destruction of upper airways • Granulomatous inflammation • Haemoptysis, granulomas in lungs, pulmonary nodules • Glomerulonephritis	HRCT, CT sinus, Audiogram, Renal biopsy	80–90% c-ANCA (PR3)
	Eosinophilic Granulomatosis with polyangiitis • Adult onset asthma • Nasal polyps and rhinitis • Eosinophilic gastroenteritis • Tender skin nodules • Mononeuritis multiplex • Glomerulonephritis	Eosinophilia HRCT	40% pANCA (MPO)
	Microscopic polyangiitis • No granulomatous inflammation • Alveolar haemorrhage • Glomerulonephritis • Mononeuritis multiplex	Renal biopsy	75% pNACA (MPO)
Polyarteritis nodosa	Medium vessel vasculitis Renal hypertension Abdominal pain/bleeding, myocarditis, scleritis, painful rash, testicular involvement	HBV serology Colio-mesenteric angiography Renal angiography	ANCA negative
Behcet's disease	Oro-genital ulcers Arthritis Recurrent venous and arterial thrombosis Erythema nodosum Uveitis	CT venogram	ANCA negative HLA-B51

variation. However, it is useful in context – for example, high ESR with low CRP suggests there is hypergammaglobulinaemia which is present in Sjögren's syndrome or SLE.

Paraneoplastic syndrome

Paraneoplastic syndromes associated with malignancies can present with multisystem features as well as general malaise. Around 8–20% with cancer develop paraneoplastic syndromes. The types of cancer most commonly associated with paraneoplastic syndromes are breast, GI, lymphoma, small cell lung, ovarian, pancreatic, prostate, renal and testicular cancers. It can be challenging to differentiate this presentation from autoimmune rheumatic diseases. Paraneoplastic syndromes often affect the following systems:

System	Symptoms	Conditions
Nervous system • Central and peripheral	Dizziness, diplopia, dysphasia, memory loss, seizures, myopathy, reduced reflexes, sensation, neuropathies	Encephalitis, Lambert-Eaton myasthenic syndrome, myasthenia gravis, myelopathy, neuropathy
Endocrine	Fatigue, hypertension, nausea and vomiting, weight gain	Cushing's syndrome Hypercalcaemia SIADH
Rheumatological	Joint pains, stiffness	Hypertrophic osteoarthropathy, Dermatomyositis, eosinophilic fasciitis
Dermatological	Itching, flushing, thickened skin	Sweet's syndrome, leukocytoclastic vasculitis, dermatomyositis, acanthosis nigricans

Role of the PET-CT scan in investigation

Positron emission tomography (PET) uses mildly radioactive tracer (fluorine 18 fluorodeoxyglucose – FDG) which accumulates in metabolically active tissues. It is useful in evaluation of inflammation, infection and malignancy. It is especially useful in the context of general malaise, constitutional symptoms or raised inflammatory markers with no clear cause. It can be used for diagnosis of large vessel vasculitis or aortitis.

Although PET-CT scans are highly sensitive for detecting inflammation, the uptake itself is not very specific. It can detect incidental lesions that have no relevance to the pathology in question. Furthermore, concurrent use of steroids can impair its sensitivity. It is generally recommended to reduce or completely stop steroids to increase the sensitivity of this investigation (prednisolone <10 mg OD).

Further management

Management of autoimmune rheumatic diseases often involves immune suppression and it is important to ensure infection is sufficiently excluded.

Due to the multisystem nature of these conditions, a multi-disciplinary approach is central to management of patients with autoimmune rheumatic diseases. Early involvement of relevant specialties and the rheumatology team will lead to improved outcome for these patients. Choice of immune suppression will depend on the patient's frailty, co-morbidities, severity of disease and type of autoimmune rheumatic disease: the rheumatology team will lead on this aspect of treatment. It is important not to rush into treatment with steroids as this may hinder diagnosis and delay definitive treatment.

Further reading

Goldblatt F, O'Neill SG. (2013) Clinical aspects of autoimmune rheumatic diseases. *The Lancet 382*(9894), 797–808. DOI: 10.1016/s0140-6736(13)61499-3.
Watts RA. (2014) How to investigate multisystem disease. *Best Pract Res Clin Rheumatol.* 28(6), 831–843. DOI: 10.1016/j.berh.2015.04.011. Epub 2015 May 18. PMID: 26096088.

Oncology and Palliative Care

CHAPTER 96

Complications of cancer

IRENE MATHIAS, ANIL BABAR, AND LAURA SPIERS

Patients with cancer often present acutely, with
- Complications or progression of cancer (Table 96.1)
- New symptoms, with a range of diagnostic possibilities (Tables 96.2–96.5)
- Complications of chemotherapy (Table 96.6), checkpoint inhibitor immunotherapy (Tables 96.7–96.12) or radiotherapy (Table 96.13)

Seek urgent help from the oncology team if the patient is critically ill or you suspect:
- Neutropenic sepsis (Chapter 74)
- Spinal cord compression (Chapter 66)
- Superior vena caval obstruction (Table 96.5)

Where possible, before contacting your oncology team, establish
- The primary origin and staging of the tumour including known spread
- The type and timing of any systemic therapy or radiotherapy
- The presence of comorbidities
- Functional status

Common symptoms and management

Table 96.1 Complications or progression of cancer.

Complication	Reference
Superior vena caval obstruction (SVCO)	Table 96.5
Upper airway obstruction	Chapter 105
Acute kidney injury	Chapter 86
Bowel obstruction	Chapter 32
Delirium	Chapter 69
Paraneoplastic neurological syndromes	
Pleural effusion	Chapter 28
Cardiac tamponade	Chapter 6
Ascites	Chapter 36
Hyponatraemia	Chapter 52
Hypercalcaemia	Chapter 52
Raised intracranial pressure	Chapter 64
Spinal cord compression	Chapter 66
Deep vein thrombosis	Chapter 82
Pulmonary embolism	Chapter 82

Acute Medicine: A Practical Guide to the Management of Medical Emergencies, Sixth Edition.
Edited by Mridula Rajwani, Leila Vaziri, and Ivie Gbinigie.
© 2026 John Wiley & Sons Ltd. Published 2026 by John Wiley & Sons Ltd.

Table 96.2 Causes of breathlessness in the patient with cancer.

Cause	Onset and progression	Additional clinical features	Investigation	Management
Pulmonary embolism (Chapter 31)	Acute onset Variable progression	Dyspnoea Pleuritic chest pain Tachycardia	CT Pulmonary angiogram	Anticoagulation (Chapter 85)
Progression of disease	Gradual onset Gradual progression		Chest X-ray CT	Cancer-specific, e.g. radiotherapy, chemotherapy
Heart failure	Gradual onset Gradual progression Consider in patients on trastuzumab or doxorubicin	See Chapter 14	BNP Echocardiogram	See Chapter 14
Pneumonitis due to chemotherapy, e.g. paclitaxel, immunotherapy, e.g. nivolumab or radiation	Acute onset Days-weeks after chemotherapy 2–24 months after immunotherapy 2–12 months after radiotherapy Rapid progression	Cough Fever Chest pain	Chest X-ray CT Bronchoscopy	Corticosteroids
Bronchial obstruction (Chapter 105)	Gradual onset. Slow progression over days to weeks. Can lead to lung collapse, lung consolidation, or pleural effusion	Reduced chest movements Dullness to percussion Reduced breath sounds on affected side.	Chest X-ray Bronchoscopy Ultrasound Aspiration with cytology	Aspiration Drainage Stenting Pleurodesis Laser therapy
Upper airway obstruction (Chapter 105)	Gradual onset Relentless progression Can rapidly progress to cause complete occlusion of airway	Stridor Wheeze	Flow-volume loop Flexible laryngoscopy CT	Radiotherapy Corticosteroids Endobronchial debulking for intraluminal lesions Stenting for extrinsic compression
Acute superior vena caval obstruction from e.g. Lung cancer, lymphoma	Rapid onset Rapid progression	Facial swelling Cyanosis or plethora Distended neck and chest veins Cough	CXR CT	Stent if severe Dependant on cancer: Corticosteroids Radiotherapy Chemotherapy
Cardiac tamponade (Chapter 6)	Rapid onset Rapid progression: clinical emergency	Beck's Triad: Hypotension Jugular venous distension Muffled heart sounds	Chest X-ray Urgent echocardiogram	Pericardiocentesis Pericardial window
Lymphangitis carcinomatosis	Gradual onset Gradual progression		High-resolution CT	Corticosteroids Chemotherapy

BNP, brain natriuretic peptide; CT, computed tomography.

Table 96.3 Causes of vomiting in the patient with cancer.

Cause	Additional clinical features	Investigation	Management	
			First line	**Second line**
Meningeal irritation/ stretch from, e.g. Intracranial tumours Meningeal infiltration Skull metastases	Headache Neurological symptoms	CT head MRI head Lumbar puncture	Dexamethasone Radiotherapy	Cyclizine Levomepromazine
Chemotherapy			Dexamethasone Ondansetron Metoclopramide	Levomepromazine
Gastric stasis from, e.g. Opioids Anticholinergic drugs Mechanical pressure, e.g. ascites, hepatomegaly, tumour Paraneoplastic autonomic gastroparesis			Metoclopramide Haloperidol	Levomepromazine
Hypercalcaemia from, e.g. Dehydration, Parathyroid hormone related protein, Bone metastasis	Constipation Polydipsia, polyuria Muscle weakness Fatigue, confusion Bone pain Palpitations	Parathyroid hormone levels	Treat underlying cause IV fluid +/− IV bisphosphonates Haloperidol	Cyclizine
Malignant bowel obstruction Mechanical: Intrinsic or extrinsic by tumour Functional: malignant involvement of blood supply, bowel muscles, or paraneoplastic neuropathy	Constipation Abdominal distension Absent bowel sounds	Abdominal X-ray CT abdomen-pelvis	Haloperidol Cyclizine Dexamethasone Complete bowel obstruction may need surgery	Reduce gastric secretions with ranitidine or octreotide Treat underlying cause
Abdominal and pelvic tumour from, e.g. Mesenteric metastases Liver metastases Retroperitoneal cancer Ureteric obstruction	Local symptoms, e.g. liver failure, PV bleeding, haematuria	CT abdomen pelvis	Cyclizine Stent to relieve obstruction Treat underlying cause	Levomepromazine
Tumour lysis syndrome	See Table 96.6			

Source: Adapted from https://www.england.nhs.uk/mids-east/wp-content/uploads/sites/7/2018/04/antiemetic-policy-2016.pdf.

Table 96.4 Causes of diarrhoea in the patient with cancer.

Cause	Onset	Investigation	Management
Infection, e.g. C difficile	Acute onset over days	Stool culture C difficile toxin and antigen PCR	Local guidelines, e.g. oral vancomycin Hold causative antibiotics and chemotherapy
Chemotherapy related colitis, e.g. Capecitabine	Acute onset usually two to three weeks after starting	Abdominal X-ray CT abdomen-pelvis Flexible sigmoidoscopy	Hold chemotherapy Octreotide for Capecitabine-related colitis
Immunotherapy-related colitis, e.g. pembrolizumab	Acute onset usually eight weeks after treatment starts	Flexible sigmoidoscopy if >grade 1 Abdominal X-ray if >grade 2 CT abdomen and pelvis if persistent pain, peritonism or fever	IV rehydration Loperamide Hold immunotherapy if >grade 1 Corticosteroids If severe, infliximab under gastroenterology guidance
Tyrosine kinase inhibitors, e.g. imatinib	Acute onset usually in two to three days after treatment starts	Exclude other pathologies	Loperamide Specialist input for dose reduction or withholding drug
Radiation colitis	Gradual onset six months to five years after radiation	See Table 96.13	

Table 96.5 Causes of cancer-related pain.

Cause	Pain characteristics	Investigations	Management
Mucositis and oral ulceration from chemotherapy and radiation	Painful mucosal inflammation with ulcers	Examination	Benzydamine mouthwash Dispersible paracetamol and aspirin
Pleural irritation, e.g. tumour infiltration or PE	Sharp well-localised pain Worse on inspiration	CT chest CT pulmonary angiogram for PE	Paracetamol NSAIDs
Visceral pain from malignant or non-malignant causes	Poorly localised pain which may refer to other sites May be tender to palpation over affected organs	CT abdomen-pelvis	Paracetamol NSAIDs Dexamethasone, e.g. for liver capsular pain Anti-muscarinic, e.g. hyoscine butylbromide for smooth muscle spasm
Tumour in bone, stretching periosteum	Constant, dull, poorly localized pain Worse on weight bearing	X-ray of affected bone MRI of affected bone	Paracetamol NSAIDs Bisphosphonates, e.g. zoledronic acid Radiotherapy Surgical options
Pathological fracture	Severe sharp pain Worse on any passive movement.	X-ray of affected bone	
Neuropathic pain from chemotherapy, spinal radiation, nerve compression	Paraesthesia (e.g. burning, cold, numb, stabbing) in the distribution of a peripheral nerve or nerve root. Hypersensitivity or allodynia (pain on light touch) Can by continuous, e.g. tumour compression, or intermittent, e.g. skeletal instability	MRI spine Electromyography	Anti-epileptics, e.g. pregabalin or gabapentin Atypical antidepressants, e.g. amitriptyline, mirtazapine or duloxetine

Table 96.5 (*Continued*)

Cause	Pain characteristics	Investigations	Management
Central nervous system	Spinal pain first Then motor and sensory signs Sphincter disturbance causing incontinence is late sign	Metastatic spinal cord compression is an oncological emergency MRI spine within 4 h	Dexamethasone 8 mg BD once suspected Radiotherapy
Tumour flare after starting hormonal therapy for prostate cancer	Pressure-like pain around rectum		Reassurance and monitoring Anti-androgens, e.g. Enzalutamide can reduce flare from hormone therapy Analgesic ladder

Table 96.6 Complications of chemotherapy.

Complication	Common drugs	Symptoms	Management
Blood: **Bone marrow suppression** **(anaemia, thrombocytopenia, neutropenia)**	Any	Anaemia • Breathlessness • Fatigue • Pallor Thrombocytopenia • Bruising/bleeding	Check MCV; iron studies, B12/folate, TSH Remember anaemia can also be from tumour bleed, dietary changes (loss of appetite with SACT), gastric irritation . . . Replace as per local guidelines. Septic screen Disseminated Intravascular Coagulation (DIC). Remember low platelets can also be from other drugs (e.g. anticoagulants) or marrow infiltration
Blood: **Neutropenic sepsis** (Infection with neutrophil count $<1 \times 10^9$/L)	Any	Consider in any patient who has received chemotherapy in the previous four weeks and is feeling unwell/with signs of infection	Antibiotic therapy within 1 h of presentation, if temperature is >38 or <36 °C – you do not need to wait for a neutrophil count. The use of point-of-care testing is recommended for timely results, treat if neutrophil count is $<1 \times 10^9$/L. See Chapter 74
Blood: **Tumour lysis syndrome** Metabolic derangements because of tumour breakdown: hyperuricaemia, hyperkalaemia, hyperphosphataemia, uraemia hypocalcaemia,	Especially in Haematological Malignancies, and Gastro-Intestinal Tumours (GIST) with high disease burden	Usually occurs 12–72 h after start of treatment. • lethargy • nausea • vomiting • fluid overload • muscle cramps • cardiac arrythmias, • tetany • seizures • syncope • sudden death.	Prophylaxis: rasburicase or xanthine oxidase inhibitors Rehydration to reduce acute kidney injury. Treatment: Renal replacement therapy may be necessary if uncontrolled hyperkalaemia, hyperphosphataemia or severe acute kidney injury occurs

(*continued*)

Table 96.6 (*Continued*)

Complication	Common drugs	Symptoms	Management
			Hyperphosphataemia: phosphate >2.1 mmol/L. Oral phosphate binding resins may be required. See Chapter 52
			Hyperkalaemia: Calcium gluconate and insulin/glucose infusion. See Chapter 52.
			Hypocalcaemia: calcium gluconate 50–100 mg/kg cautiously if symptomatic, need to avoid precipitation of calcium phosphate. See Chapter 52.
Cardiac toxicity: Heart failure	Anthracyclines e.g., doxorubicin HER-2 receptor inhibitors e.g. trastuzumab (Herceptin)	• Breathlessness • Fluid overload	Baseline ECHO, surveillance as per local guidance Cardiology input
Cardiac toxicity: Acute coronary syndrome	Fluorouracil (5FU), capecitabine, vincristine	• Cardiac chest pain • nausea	Baseline ECG Troponin ACS protocol
Cardiac toxicity: Arrhythmia	Cisplatin Alkylating agents e.g. cyclophosphamide CDK4/6 inhibitors e.g. ribociclib	• may be asymptomatic • palpitations • breathlessness • chest pain • cardiac failure	Baseline ECG Replacement of electrolytes (magnesium, potassium) Cardiology input
Cardiac toxicity: Hypertension	Monoclonal antibodies, e.g. VEGF inhibitors (bevacizumab), Tyrosine kinase inhibitors e.g. sunitinib	• Haematological: haemorrhage, • Cardiovascular: hypertension, cardiac failure • Renal: proteinuria • Cerebrovascular: posterior reversible encephalopathy syndrome	Seek urgent advice from a consultant with experience in the management of anti-angiogenic therapy
Dermatology: Rash	Allergic/hypersensitivity reactions e.g. platinum agents (cisplatin, carboplatin), photosensitivity e.g. doxorubicin Maculopapular/acneiform rashes e.g. targeted agents e.g. EGFR inhibitors (cetuximab), TKIs (Lenvatinib, imatinib), BRAF inhibitors (dabrafenib)	See Chapter 98 for assessment of rash.	

Table 96.6 (*Continued*)

Complication	Common drugs	Symptoms	Management
Dermatology: Palmar-Plantar Erythema (Hand-foot Syndrome)	5FU, capecitabine	Progressive redness of hands and feet which may progress to pain, cracking or blistering of skin and eventually desquamation with concomitant progressive functional impairment.	Emollient and topical NSAIDs Give antibiotics if secondary infection occurs. Pyridoxine 50–100 mg 8-hourly PO may be helpful.
Endocrine; Diabetes Mellitus	PI3K inhibitors e.g. alpelisib Can also be secondary to steroid (given with chemotherapy)	Secondary to corticosteroid therapy	See Chapter 44
Endocrine; Altered Thyroid Function	Radioactive iodine TKI e.g. sunitinib		See Chapters 49
Gastric: Diarrhoea	All Colitis more common with 5FU and capecitabine (check for DYPD deficiency now standard)		See Table 96.7 and Chapter 34.
Hepatic: Altered Liver Function Tests	All	See Chapter 42	Brain MRI (to exclude e.g. brain metastases, intracerebral haemorrhage or infarction) and demonstrate hyperintense lesions involving the parieto-occipital regions
Neurological: Posterior Leucoencephalopathy Syndrome	Gemcitabine, Cisplatin, Bevacizumab, TKI e.g. sunitinib.	Visual symptoms, increasing confusion, generalized headaches, seizures and hypertension	Treat hypertension, and seizures Monitor fluid balance. Neurology specialist input Symptomatic improvement usually occurs over several days
Respiratory: Pneumonitis	Antibiotics: bleomycin, mitomycin C Alkylating agents: carmustine, busulfan Antimetabolites: methotrexate, fludarabine Taxanes: paclitaxel, docetaxel Targeted agents: trastuzumab	Increased breathlessness, dry cough	Oxygen support, High-resolution CT, Respiratory input

General diarrhoea management

- Check baseline bloods: Full blood count, urea and electrolytes, magnesium, phosphate, liver function tests, C reactive protein and thyroid function tests.
- Take stool cultures and test for C difficile. Do not start loperamide until stool cultures are back negative.
- A stool chart should be strictly filled out.

Table 96.7 Colitis guidelines.

Grades	Actions	Follow-up
Grade 1 Increase of <4 stools per day Mild increase in ostomy output compared to baseline Clinically well with normal vital signs	**Investigations** • Baseline bloods: FBC, CRP, U&E, LFTs, full TFTs, cortisol • Faecal calprotectin • Stool culture including C. *difficile* **Management** • Continue ICI therapy • Low fibre diet, spasmolytic	**If remains stable/resolves** • Early review within one to two weeks • Monitor closely and advise patient to report worsening symptoms immediately • Ensure patient is completing stool diary **If worsens/persists >15 days or deranged U+Es:** • Treat as G2 or 3/4
Grade 2 4–6 stools per day over baseline/moderate increase in ostomy output compared to baseline Mild abdominal pain	**Investigations** • As per G1 • Stool chart, faecal elastase • Whole blood PCR CMV • Consider viral pathogen screen e.g. Norovirus • Flexible sigmoidoscopy **Management** • Hold I-O therapy • Start oral prednisolone 1 mg/kg/day (maximum 60 mg OD) • PPI cover	**Review in one week.** **If improves to G1** • Taper oral steroids over eight weeks • Resume I-O therapy **If worsens or persists more than five to seven days with steroids** • Treat as G3/4
Grade 3–4 7 or more stools per day over baseline/severe increase in ostomy output Severe or continuous abdominal pain Fever 37.5 °C Tachycardia over 90 bpm Dehydration Consider: Rising CRP or CRP over 30 if previously normal Falling Hb or Hb less than 105 g/L if previously normal Falling albumin or low albumin if previously normal	**Investigations** • As per G2 • AXR • CTAP if persistent pain, peritonitic or febrile **Management** • Discontinue I-O therapy • Admit patient • 1 mg/kg/day IV Methylprednisolone OD (+ PPI) • IV fluid replacement • Daily U&Es with fluid balance chart • Continue accurate stool chart • Refer to gastroenterology	**If symptoms resolving** • Continue IV for at least three to five days then switch to PO prednisolone 1 mg/kg OD (maximum 60 mg OD) and taper as per standard regimen **If symptoms persist more than three to five days or recur after improvement** • Refer to gastroenterology for ongoing guidance • Add infliximab (5 mg/kg if no contraindication) **If persists more than three to five days or worsens after infliximab** • Consider switching to other biologics/treatments guided by gastroenterology • Refer to surgeons for consideration of colectomy

- Admit for IV rehydration if there are adverse features: fever, neutropenia, blood or mucus in stool, dehydration, vomiting, or poorly controlled diabetes.
- Manage as neutropenic sepsis if there is bloody diarrhoea, neutropenia and right lower quadrant tenderness.

In general, follow the World Health Organisation analgesia ladder. The management column shows specific additional treatments that may be beneficial for different causes of pain.

Table 96.8 Nephritis guidelines.

Grades	Actions	Follow-up
Grade 1 Creatinine greater than baseline and ULN but less than or equal to 1.5× baseline (Lowest value in last three months is baseline)	**Investigations** • Review hydration status and medications • Urine dip – for PCR if proteinuria • Urine cultures if UTI symptoms • If obstruction suspected, then renal US to exclude obstruction **Management** • Continue I-O therapy	**If remains stable/resolves** • Continue I-O therapy but *monitor creatinine weekly* **If worsens** • Treat as G2 or 3/4
Grade 2 Creatinine 1.5–3× ULN	**Investigations** • Urinalysis • Renal USS • Glomerulonephritis screen **Management** • Hold I-O therapy • Repeat Creatinine in 48–72 h – if not improving then for discussion with renal for biopsy • Start prednisolone 1 mg/kg with gastric protection	**If improves to G1:** • Taper oral steroids over six to eight weeks • Consider resuming I-O therapy if creatinine returns to baseline and steroid treatment complete. **If elevation persists more than five days or worsens after initial improvement:** • Treat as G3/4
Grade 3–4 Creatinine more than 3× ULN or more than 3× baseline	**Investigations** • As per G2 • Refer to renal team for consideration of biopsy **Management** • Discontinue I-O therapy • Admit patient • 1–2 mg/kg IV Methylprednisolone OD or pulse dose with 250–500 mg IV Methylprednisolone for three days (+ gastric protection) • Daily weight and fluid balance • Daily U+Es	**If improves to G1:** • Switch to oral prednisolone 1 mg/kg OD (max 60 mg OD) • Taper oral steroids over at least two months. • Weekly renal function as OP after discharge • PCP prophylaxis and bone protection for all patients on high-dose steroids (>20 mg PO prednisolone for >four weeks) **If worsens:** • Consider MMF 250–500 mg BD +/− 10 mg prednisolone directed by renal team.

Table 96.9 Guidelines for management of IO Induced liver toxicities.

Grades	Actions	Follow-up
Grade 1 ALT/AST > ULN but ≤ 3× ULN and/or Bilirubin < 1.5× ULN	• Weekly LFT monitoring • Consider alternative causes	• Continue I-O therapy with close monitoring of LFTs If worsens, treat as G2
Grade 2 ALT/AST > 3× ULN but ≤5× ULN and/or Bilirubin > 1.5× ULN but ≤ 3× ULN	• Twice weekly LFTs and INR • Review other medications • Review alcohol history • Liver screen including viral hepatitis (hepatitis A, B, C and E), EBV, CMV, HIV, liver autoantibodies, iron studies • Liver USS +/− portal vein doppler • Consider hepatology advice Consider other causes e.g. metastases, biliary obstruction, pre-existing liver disease	• **Delay I-O therapy.** • Avoid hepatotoxic drugs • If no improvement in LFTs when rechecked, commence **oral prednisolone (1 mg/kg, max 60 mg OD)** with PPI cover • Can taper steroids as per regime below after one week if LFTs ≤ Grade 1 limits • **Consider resuming I-O therapy** if LFTs return to baseline and stable on prednisolone ≤ 10 mg OD • Consider bone protection with AdCalD3 +/− bisphosphonates

(continued)

Table 96.9 (*Continued*)

Grades	Actions	Follow-up
		If no improvement or flare on steroid wean: • Refer to hepatology • Increase prednisolone dose by 10 mg (max 60 mg OD) then slowly taper
Grade 3 ALT/AST > 5× ULN and/or Bilirubin > 3× ULN OR symptomatic liver dysfunction	• Admit to hospital • Daily LFTs and INR • **Urgent hepatology referral** (including out of hours) • Other investigations and recommendations as above • Consider IV vitamin K 10 mg for three days if raised INR • Monitor BMs • Consider liver biopsy if steroid refractory	• **Discontinue I-O therapy.** • **Commence 1 mg/kg/day IV methylprednisolone sodium succinate** (consider 2 mg/kg/day if ALT/AST > 400) • Once LFTs improved to ≤ G2 limits, switch to oral prednisolone (1 mg/kg, max 60 mg) and wean as per Oncology advice. **If no improvement after three to five days or rebounds:** • Continued discussion with hepatology Consider adding 1 g BD PO mycophenolate mofetil (under guidance of hepatology only) once infection excluded
Grade 4 ALT/AST > 20× ULN and/or Bilirubin > 10× ULN OR decompensated liver disease e.g. ascites, coagulopathy, hepatic encephalopathy	Recommendations as per Grade 3	• **Discontinue I-O therapy.** • **Commence 2 mg/kg/day IV methylprednisolone sodium succinate** Recommendations otherwise as above

Table 96.10 Guidelines for management of IO related skin toxicities:

Grade	Action	Follow-up
Grade 1 Localised maculopapular rash (<10% BSA)	**Investigations** • Examination – exclude other causes i.e. viral illness, infection, other drug reaction **Management** • Continue IO therapy • Photograph rash and record BSA • Symptomatic management i.e. emollient with paraffin (Cetraben), consider antihistamines if itching • Consider mild topical steroid (Eumovate)	**If remains stable/resolves:** No further follow up required **If worsens/persists:** Treat as Grade 2
Grade 2 Rash affecting 10–30% BSA	**Investigations** • As per G1 • FBC, U&Es, LFTs, Cortisol, TFTs, Glucose **Management** • Photograph rash and record BSA • Symptomatic management • Consider moderate (Betnovate) to high (Dermovate) potency topical steroids	**If improves:** • If improving on topical steroids, continue for two weeks. Repeat treatment if flare. **If worsens or persists:** • If persists for over five days or worsens then then treat as grade 3

Table 96.10 (*Continued*)

Grade	Action	Follow-up
Grade 3 Rash >30% BSA or Red flags: mucosal involvement, blistering, bullous, SCAR, skin shedding, fever, hypothermia, pustules	**Investigations** • As per G2 • Bacterial and viral wound swabs **Management** • Consider admission. • Photograph rash and record BSA • Hold I-O therapy. • Urgent Dermatology referral +/− biopsy • Symptomatic management • Initial high potency topical steroids • Abx and antivirals not indicated unless proven infection. • Antihistamines for itching.	**If symptoms worsen or persist:** • If refractory to topical steroids or **extensive rash**, then start oral prednisolone at 30 mg/day and can increase up to 1 mg/kg/day (max 60 mg per 24 h) **If symptoms resolving:** • If improving and on oral steroids to wean over >four weeks. • Can re-start I-O therapy when grade 1 and prednisolone <10 mg/day (check with primary team)
Grade 4 Rash >50% BSA with severe symptoms, life threatening, requiring immediate intervention.	**Investigations** • As per G3 **Management** • Admission • Photograph rash and record BSA • Consider permanently discontinuing I-O therapy. • Urgent Dermatology referral +/− biopsy • Symptomatic management • IV methylprednisolone 1–2 mg/k/day • IV fluid hydration and fluid balance	**If symptoms resolving:** • If improving convert to oral prednisolone 1 mg/kg/day and wean slowly under guidance of dermatology **If symptoms worsen or persist:** • If refractory to IV steroids, then continue management under guidance of dermatology.

Table 96.11 Guidelines for management of IO related pneumonitis.

Grade	Action	Follow-up
Grade 1 Clinically Asymptomatic and radiographic changes <25% of lung parenchyma or changes confined to one lobe	**Investigations** • FBC, U&E, LFT, Ca, TFT, ESR, CRP • CT Chest with Contrast • Clinical assessment (incl. oxygen sats) • Consider screening for viral, opportunistic or specific bacterial infections* **Management** Consider holding I-O Consider non-urgent communication to Respiratory interstitial lung disease team Inform Primary Oncology Team	**If remains stable/resolves:** • Single check-in and safety-netting **If worsens/persists:** • If becomes symptomatic treat as grade 2 • If sarcoid node type reaction, consider early EBUS to ensure not progressive malignancy

(*continued*)

Table 96.11 (*Continued*)

Grade	Action	Follow-up
Grade 2 New onset or worsening of symptoms i.e. dyspnea, cough, fever, chest pain, new oxygen requirement	**Investigations** • As per G1 • Additional bloods: beta-d-glucan, BNP • Additional infection screening: Sputum MCS + AFB • Consider CTPA to exclude PE • Consider bronchoscopy with BAL to rule out infection **Management** • Hold I-O therapy • Consider admission • Consult Respiratory (urgent referral if sats <94% on RA at rest) • Consult Infectious Diseases team • Inform primary oncology team • Start Prednisolone 1 mg/kg/day (max 60 mg/day) + PPI • Start antibiotics as per local protocol if suspicion of infection • Optimise underlying respiratory disease i.e. COPD	**If improves:** • Repeat CXR, baseline bloods and lung function tests incl TLCO weekly • Once symptoms return to baseline wean steroids over four to six weeks, titrating to symptoms **If worsens or persists:** • If no improvement in 48 h treat as grade 3 • Discuss use of second-line agents (Tacrolimus, or MMF or Infliximab) early in cases of patients with multiple toxicities- Guided by respiratory team. • If recurrent G2 pneumonitis discontinue I-O therapy
Grade 3–4 Severe new symptoms, including: new or worsening hypoxia, life-threatening difficulty in breathing, ARDS	**Investigations** • As per G2 • Additional bloods: ILD bloods (ANA and ANCA) **Management** • Admission • Urgent Respiratory Consult • Discontinue I-O therapy • Discuss escalation, ceiling of care and ventilation • Start IV methylprednisolone 1–2 mg/kg/day (250 mg max for 3 doses only and step down to oral) • Cover with empirical antibiotics +/− PCP treatment depending on clinical risk • Optimise underlying respiratory disease i.e. COPD • Inform primary Oncology team	**If symptoms resolving:** Step down to oral prednisolone 60 mg once daily, then wean by 10 mg every seven days until at 10 mg. At this point consider clinically re-assessment and re-imagine at 8–12 weeks before considering cessation of steroid treatment. **If symptoms worsen or persist:** • Depending on clinical performance; CXR every one to three days • If not improving after 48 h: re-discuss with urgently with respiratory and acute oncology, re-review all results, with advice of respiratory team can add alternative immunosuppressants

Table 96.12 Guidelines for management of IO related endocrine toxicities.

Adrenal	Action	Follow-up
9 a.m. Cortisol: <100 nmol/L Cortisol insufficiency likely	**Investigations:** • Urgent ACTH, U and E, glucose, PRL, fT4, TSH, LH/FSH and testosterone or oestradiol (T or E2) **Emergency (severe symptoms):** • 100 mg hydrocortisone iv/im (after blood drawn but do not wait for results) • Followed by 50 mg hydrocortisone every 6 h and fluid resuscitation as required • Contact endocrinology on-call for advice.	Once stable, Start hydrocortisone 20 mg/10 mg/10 mg and reduce to 10 mg/5 mg/5 mg after three days Steroid advice, steroid card and emergency pack. If ACTH low; pituitary ACTH deficiency or exogenous glucocorticoid • ACTH ≥2 ULN primary adrenal insufficiency
9 a.m. Cortisol: >100 nmol/L and ≤350 nmol/L	Possible acute pituitary failure; review symptoms. If unwell, assess pituitary profile and start hydrocortisone replacement as above.	If asymptomatic; repeat 9 a.m. cortisol in one week and warn patient of symptoms of concern. • Contact endocrinology on-call for advice

Thyroid dysfunction	Action	Follow-up
Hypothyroidism: TSH > 10 mU/L and free T4 <12 pmol/L	**Investigations** • Send full endocrine panel (see Adrenal section), specifically ensure cortisol is normal • Check thyroid peroxidase antibodies **Management** • Continue I-O therapy • Levothyroxine ~50 mcg OD (0.5–1.5 mcg/kg)	• Recheck TFTs and cortisol with each treatment cycle • Increase levothyroxine in 25 mcg increments every six weeks if required • Aim for T4 15–20 pmol/L and TSH on lower end of normal range if on levothyroxine replacement (usual replacement dose 125 mcg OD) • Consider referral to endocrine team if unable to stabilize thyroid function
Hyperthyroidism: TSH <0.4 mU/L and free T4 >22 pmol/L	**Investigations** • Complete endocrine panel • If TSH low but T4 normal/low need to exclude pituitary dysfunction (see hypophysitis section) **Management** • Treatment only indicated if symptomatic • Trial propranolol 40–80 mg OD • Carbimazole rarely indicated unless associated with anti-TSH antibodies (consult endocrinology) • If painful thyroiditis discuss with endocrine regarding steroids (prednisolone PO 0.5 mg/kg)	**If patient asymptomatic:** • Recheck TFTs and cortisol within three weeks and then three weekly thereafter (*majority of cases will turn hypothyroid*) **If symptomatic:** • Recheck TFTs within two weeks and two weekly thereafter

(*continued*)

Table 96.12 (*Continued*)

Grades of pituitary toxicity	Action	Follow-up
Vague symptoms Of tiredness/reduced appetite with no headache etc or asymptomatic and low cortisol PD-1/PD1-L inhibitors alone, or CTLA4 +/− PD-1 inhibitors or withdrawal from LT exogenous glucocorticoid Typically later in ICI treatment	**Investigations:** Ideally 9 a.m. cortisol and ACTH, U and E, glucose, PRL and fT4 and TSH MRI Pituitary Urgent	See Management of Possible Adrenal Insufficiency (9 a.m. cortisol <350 nmol/L)
Acute Hypophysitis Severe mass effect symptoms (Severe headache, nausea and vomiting, visual symptoms, visual field defects, mass on MRI pituitary) CTLA4 +/− PD-1 inhibitors (often within 12 w of commencing ICI)	**Investigations:** Urgent cortisol, ACTH, U and E, glucose, PRL, fT4, TSH, LH/FSH and testosterone or oestradiol (T or E2) MRI Pituitary Urgent **Emergency Rx:** 100 mg hydrocortisone iv/im (after blood drawn but do not wait for results) Followed by 50 mg hydrocortisone every 6 h and fluid resuscitation as required	• Contact endocrinology on-call for advice Consider IV methylprednisolone 1 mcg/kg if optic chiasm compression • Oral prednisolone e.g. 20 mg/day if severe headache with no resolution Subsequent pituitary assessment: Reassess LH/FSH and T/E2 (if pre-menopausal) when recovered from acute phase • If persistent deficiency; consider sex hormone replacement if not in context of acute illness (via Endocrinology)
Acute Hypophysitis Moderate symptoms- Headache but no other severe symptoms, no visual disturbances CTLA4 +/− PD-1 inhibitors (often within 12 w of commencing ICI)	**Investigations:** Same as above MRI Pituitary Urgent **Emergency Rx:** Same as above Once stable, oral hydrocortisone replacement (double dosing for three days then standard replacement).	Steroid advice, steroid card and emergency pack. Contact endocrinology on-call for advice Subsequent pituitary assessment: As above
Acute ACTH deficiency causing adrenal crises, acute cortisol deficiency CTLA4 +/− PD-1 inhibitors or PD-1/ PD1-L inhibitors alone or withdrawal from LT exogenous glucocorticoid Typically later in ICI treatment	**Investigations:** • Urgent cortisol, ACTH, U and E, glucose, PRL, fT4, TSH, LH/FSH and testosterone or oestradiol (T or E2) • MRI Pituitary **Emergency:** • 100 mg hydrocortisone iv/im (after blood drawn but do not wait for results) • Followed by 50 mg hydrocortisone every 6 h and fluid resuscitation as required.	• Contact endocrinology on-call for advice Consider IV methylprednisolone 1 mcg/kg if optic chiasm compression. • Oral prednisolone e.g. 20 mg/day if severe headache with no resolution Subsequent pituitary assessment: Reassess LH/FSH and T/E2 (if pre-menopausal) when recovered from acute phase • If persistent deficiency; consider sex hormone replacement if not in context of acute illness (via Endocrinology)

Table 96.13 Complications of radiotherapy.

Complication	Timing	Symptoms	Management
Head and neck: Xerostomia (salivary glands make less saliva)	During/early after treatment	Dry/sore mouth or throat Hoarse voice	Artificial saliva Oral fluids
Head and neck: Mucositis	Early after treatment	Oral ulcers Difficulty swallowing pain	Oral hygiene Analgesia If unable to manage oral intake, then a percutaneous endoscopic gastrostomy (PEG) or nasogastric tube (NGT) may be needed for nutrition
Respiratory: Pneumonitis	Early: radiation pneumonitis Late: radiation-related pulmonary fibrosis	Breathlessness with or without a dry cough	Chest X-ray may be normal or show some interstitial shadowing. CT chest: ground glass shadowing within the area of the radiotherapy Corticosteroids and oxygen support may be needed. Symptoms should improve, but if fibrosis occurs then long-term oxygen may be required.
Dermatology	Early (10–14 days after the start of radiotherapy)	Skin discomfort Erythema Ulceration Secondary infection can occur, causing cellulitis	Moisturisers Analgesia Treatment of secondary infection (bacterial or fungal)
Pelvic	Early:	Diarrhoea and gastrointestinal mucositis Bladder (dysuria, frequency	Adequate hydration Anti-diarrhoeal agents (ensure no superadded infection e.g. *C difficile*; see Chapter 34). Bladder: oral fluids are important although patients may try to avoid this to reduce the urinary frequency
	Late effects:	Sexual dysfunction Impaired fertility Dysfunction of bowel (urgency and frequency of defaecation) and bladder (rarely incontinence) Psychological distress	Referral to relevant specialist teams (may be co-ordinated via Late Effects Radiotherapy team)
Central nervous system toxicity	Can be related to toxicity of treatment (usually early) or due to disease progression, with variable timings	Nausea/vomiting Somnolence Encephalopathy (rare)	Corticosteroids (e.g. dexamethasone 4 mg for nausea, or 8–16 mg daily PO with gastroprotection for encephalopathy)

Systemic Anti-Cancer Therapy (SACT)

SACT includes chemotherapy, immunotherapy and targeted biological agents.

It can be given in the neoadjuvant (before surgery), adjuvant (after surgery) and metastatic setting, and can be administered in combination with localised therapies, e.g. radiotherapy.

Chemotherapy

The aim of chemotherapy is to arrest the cell cycle of dividing cells and/or cause cell death. Cancer cells are active and, hence take up proportionally more drug than non-cancerous cells – side effects occur from uptake into healthy cells.

Chemotherapy may be intravenous or orally administered.

Immunotherapy toxicities

Immuno-oncology (I-O) agents are being increasingly used in the treatment of cancers including melanoma, lung cancer, RCC, CRC and bladder cancer. These agents are associated with immune-related adverse events that can differ in nature, severity and duration from adverse events caused by other classes of anti-cancer therapy. Early recognition of symptoms and treatment of potential immune-related adverse events is critical to ensuring appropriate management and, in some cases, may require the use of immunosuppressants.

Immunotherapy toxicities include

1 Colitis
2 Nephritis
3 Hepatitis- liver toxicity
4 Pneumonitis
5 Skin toxicities (rash, inflammation)
6 Endocrine side effects (hypothyroidism or hyperthyroidism, hypoadrenalism, hypophysis's)

Less common

Myocarditis, neurological side effects (autoimmune neuropathy, Guillain-Barré syndrome (GBS), myasthenia gravis), uveitis, iritis, cytokine release syndrome.

Radiotherapy

Radiotherapy is the use of localised radiation (usually X-rays) to induced DNA damage in the cancer cells. It can be given as External Beam Radiotherapy (EBRT), or internally.

The radiation treatment may be given as a single dose (usually with palliative intent to help with pain or bleeding) or divided into a number of smaller doses (fractions) to allow healthy cells to recover between treatments and enable larger overall dose delivery (with curative intent, or to reduce recurrence risk).

Radiotherapy can be combined with chemotherapy (chemo-radiotherapy) or can be given in combination with surgery (neoadjuvant or adjuvant settings).

EBRT is usually shaped to fit the cancer outline (to spare healthy tissue) and may be intensity modulated (IMRT) to deliver different amounts of radiation to different parts of the tumour.

Stereotactic radiotherapy (SABR) delivers radiotherapy from different directions, all focused to deliver the full dose to the target. This is very precise and suited to treating small cancers.

Further reading

Acute Oncology Guidelines: Acute Oncology Society version 4 (2023). Accessed by hyperlink Acute Oncology Guidelines: UK Acute Oncology Society.

Marshall E, Young A, Clark PI, Selby S (Eds.). (2014) *Problem Solving in Acute Oncology*. Oxford: Published in association with the Association of Cancer Physicians. Clinical Publishing.

CHAPTER 97

Palliative and end-of-life care

MARY MILLER

The number of patients dying in acute care settings will rise as the population grows and ages. In the United Kingdom, 10% of inpatients in hospital today will die and one in four will die in the following 12 months. Patients will present to the acute take with multiple chronic conditions, and both cognitive and physical frailty.

Acute physicians should be aware of local guidelines and palliative care support services. A definition of palliative care may be found in Box 97.1. Information regarding the patient's wishes and preferences for medical care as death approaches and care at the end of life should be ascertained as soon as possible, particularly when the patient has had multiple admissions in the preceding three months. These wishes and preferences may be formally recorded as an advance care plan (including ReSPECT: recommended summary plan for emergency care and treatment) or a legally binding ADRT (advance decision to refuse treatment). Where written guidance is not available, discussion with the patient is important where they have the capacity to make decisions regarding their treatment. Alternatively, information may be gathered from those who know the patient to inform a best interest decision. Both the law and professional ethical guidance regarding advance care planning vary by country. Physicians need to be aware of guidance that is relevant to their practice.

Do not attempt cardiopulmonary resuscitation (DNACPR) is a decision made by the medical and healthcare team leading the patient's care. It is important to gather information about DNACPR on presentation to acute care. As aforementioned, it is important to practice within local legal and ethical frameworks.

Pain management

- Diagnose the cause/s and address reversible causes (e.g. antibiotics for cellulitis and fixation of a fracture).
- Prescribe 'by mouth (oral), by the clock (regularly) and by the ladder' (WHO ladder) (Figure 97.1). Note: Step 2 is often omitted.
- Give regular 4-hourly doses of immediate-release morphine 2.5–5 mg PO (lower if the patient is elderly, frail or has liver disease or renal impairment). Prescribe PRNs (at same dose) every 4–6 h for breakthrough pain.
- Once a stable daily dose is established, convert the opioid to a twice daily modified release preparation, e.g. 20 mg/24 h to 10 mg MR BD.
- Review daily requirements after 24–48 h and adjust the regular and breakthrough doses as needed.
- Adjuvants (Table 97.1) may be added at any step of the ladder.
- When prescribing opioids, co-prescribe an antiemetic PRN and regular laxatives.
- Pain may be 'total pain', a combination of psychological, social, spiritual as well as physical pain. Consider the person and try to address all causes of pain.
- Consider non-pharmacological management of pain alongside analgesics, e.g. heat/cool pads, TENS.
- If the oral route is not possible or reliable, drugs may be given by subcutaneous infusion (SC) via a syringe driver.

Acute Medicine: A Practical Guide to the Management of Medical Emergencies, Sixth Edition.
Edited by Mridula Rajwani, Leila Vaziri, and Ivie Gbinigie.
© 2026 John Wiley & Sons Ltd. Published 2026 by John Wiley & Sons Ltd.

Box 97.1 Palliative care

'Palliative care is an approach that improves the quality of life of patients and their families facing the problems associated with life-threatening illness, through the prevention and relief of suffering by means of early identification and impeccable assessment and treatment of pain and other problems, physical, psychosocial and spiritual.'

Source: Adapted from World Health Organization (2013)

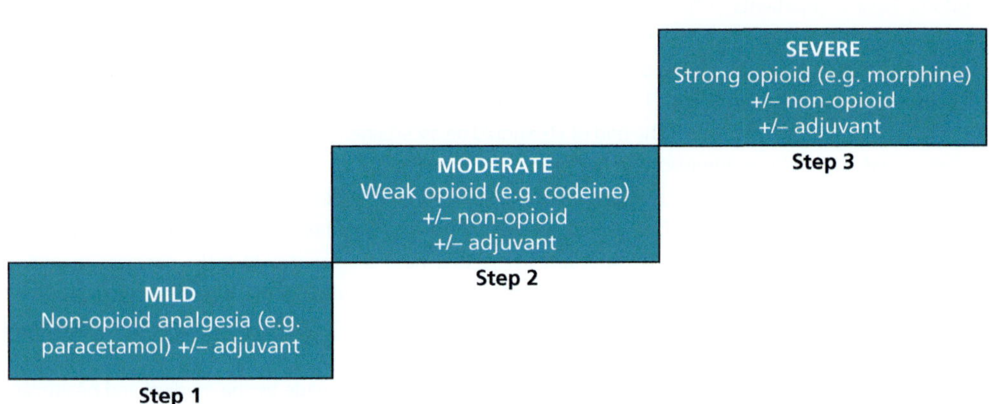

Figure 97.1 WHO analgesic ladder.

Table 97.1 Adjuvant analgesics.

Class of drugs	Indication	Example	Adverse effects/comments
Non-steroidal anti-inflammatory drugs (NSAIDs)	Inflammation Bone metastases Soft tissue infiltration	Individual drug choice based on patient's risk factors and adverse effect profile of drug	Peptic ulceration, bleeding and perforation
		Use PPI cover	Renal impairment Fluid retention Caution in elderly
Steroids	Inflammation Soft tissue infiltration	Dexamethasone (4–8 mg daily, give in morning to reduce insomnia)	Fluid retention GI irritation and bleeding
	Bone metastases	Titrate down to the lowest dose that controls pain	Cushingoid appearance
	Nerve compression		Diabetes
	Liver capsule pain Raised intracranial pressure	Short course with PPI cover	Candidiasis Osteoporosis
Anti-muscarinics	Smooth muscle colic	Hyoscine butylbromide	Dry mouth, constipation, urinary retention, blurred vision, flushing, tachycardia

Table 97.1 (*Continued*)

Class of drugs	Indication	Example	Adverse effects/comments
Bisphosphonates	Painful bone metastases	Various regimens (usually IV infusion)	Hypocalcaemia Flu-like symptoms Osteonecrosis of the jaw (need dental review before commencing)
Neuropathic agents **Gabapentin**	Neuropathic pain (Anticonvulsant)	300 mg PO dose at night and titrate by 300 mg/24 h every two to three days (Slower titration in elderly/frail: 100 mg at night and titrate by 100 mg/24 h every two to three days)	Mild sedation Tremor Confusion Reduce dose in renal impairment
Pregabalin	Neuropathic pain (Anticonvulsant)	75 mg 12-hourly PO and titrate at intervals of three to seven days (in debilitated patients start with 25–50 mg BD).	Dizziness, drowsiness (usually improve) Confusion, tremor, dry mouth Reduce dose in renal impairment
Amitriptyline	Neuropathic pain (antidepressant)	10 mg PO at night and titrate to 25 mg after three to seven days if tolerated	Sedation, dizziness, confusion, dry mouth, constipation, urinary retention Caution in heart failure

Breathlessness

- Diagnose the cause/s and address reversible causes (Table 97.2).
- Consider non-pharmacological measures before pharmacological therapy (Table 97.3).

Nausea and vomiting

- Diagnose the cause/s and tailor treatment to the cause.
- Ensure appropriate route of administration. Use parenteral route if drug is not being absorbed enterally: intravenous or subcutaneous.
- Use stepwise approach to management: start with the most appropriate narrow-spectrum antiemetic and either switch to an alternative or add in a second if symptomatic control is not achieved (Table 97.4).
- Consider non-pharmacological measures (e.g. reassurance, positioning and placement of a nasogastric tube).

Table 97.2 Specific causes of breathlessness and their management.

Cause	Management
Hypoxia	Oxygen (see Chapter 30)
Infection	Antibiotics (see Chapter 25)
Pulmonary embolism	Anticoagulation (see Chapter 31)
Bronchospasm	Beta-2 agonist by nebuliser (see Chapters 22 and 23)
Pleural effusion	Drainage of effusion (see Chapters 28 and 110)
Heart failure	Diuretic, ACE-inhibitor (see Chapter 14)
Anaemia	Blood transfusion
Pericardial effusion	Pericardiocentesis

Table 97.3 Management of breathlessness.

Non-pharmacological measures
Sit the patient up (increases vital capacity and reduces abdominal splinting)
Arrange cool airflow over the patient's face with a fan or by opening a window
Maintain a calm empathic approach and presence
Reassurance
Physiotherapy
Breathing/relaxation exercises
Activity pacing
Complementary therapies
Pharmacological therapy

Oxygen **Beta-2 agonists** **Opioids**	May be helpful if patient is hypoxic (i.e. arterial SaO_2 <92%) Give salbutamol by inhaler or nebuliser if there is bronchospasm. Start with oral morphine 1 mg as required, if tolerated and beneficial then consider using this regularly every 4 h and as required. After two days: calculate the total dose given over 24 h and use this to recalculate the 4-hourly dose (the new 4-hourly and 'as required' dose is one-sixth of the new total daily dose). Once a stable dose has been reached, this can be converted to once- or twice-daily modified-release morphine. If the patient is already on regular (analgesic) morphine: increase the dose of regular morphine by 30–50% every two to three days until symptoms are controlled, or use >30 mg/24 h
Anxiolytics	If anxiety-related breathlessness, consider the use of long-term anxiolytic (e.g. mirtazapine). For panic-related breathlessness in patients approaching the end of life then consider the use of low-dose lorazepam (0.5–1 mg up to 12-hourly).

Table 97.4 Antiemetic therapy.

Drug	Receptors	Indications	
Cyclizine	H_1 Muscarinic – Anticholinergic	Raised intracranial pressure Motion sickness Inoperable bowel obstruction Inoperable bowel obstruction	
Metoclopramide – central and peripheral action	D_2 $5HT_4$	Gastric stasis Gastric irritation	
Domperidone – peripheral action only	D_2 and D_3	Inoperable bowel obstruction if no colic	
Haloperidol	D_2	Opioid induced Metabolic causes, e.g. hypercalcaemia Inoperable bowel obstruction Inoperable bowel obstruction	

Table 97.4 (*Continued*)

Drug	Receptors	Indications
Ondansetron	$5HT_3$	Chemotherapy Radiotherapy Bowel obstruction
Hyoscine butylbromide	Muscarinic – Anticholinergic	Inoperable bowel obstruction with colic
Levomepromazine	D_2 H_1 Muscarinic – anticholinergic	Broad-spectrum antiemetic Often used third line

Delirium

- Common causes and their management are summarised in Table 97.5. Refer also to Chapter 69.
- Terminal agitation is seen in dying patients and is distinct from delirium.
- Contact the specialist palliative care team for advice if the patient is not settling with the suggested management.

Table 97.5 Common causes of delirium in palliative care and their management.

Diagnose the cause and address reversible issues

Pain	Adverse effect of drugs (e.g. opioid toxicity)
Infection	Brain or meningeal metastases
Urinary retention	Electrolyte disorder (e.g. hyponatraemia and hypercalcaemia)
Constipation	Paraneoplastic effect
Hypoglycaemia	

Non-pharmacological measures to manage delirium

Explain delirium to patient and their family	Support hearing and vision
Reduce over-stimulation: quiet side room	
Maintain a day/night rhythm	

Pharmacological therapy to manage hyperactive delirium

Aim is limiting danger to the patient and others
Haloperidol 1–1.5 mg (0.5–1 mg elderly) once daily
Benzodiazepine: e.g. lorazepam 0.5–1 mg sublingually prn or midazolam 2.5 mg SC

End-of-life care

Recognise the patient is dying
Signs that are commonly seen in the last few days of life include
- Rapid deterioration in condition (often day by day) despite active treatment
- Increasing weakness – bed-bound, requiring help with personal care
- Barely able to take liquids and unable to take medicines by mouth
- Impaired concentration, muddled thinking and difficulty sustaining conversation
- Increasing drowsiness

Consider potentially reversible disorders contributing to the patient's deterioration

These include infection, acute kidney injury, hypercalcaemia, opioid toxicity and oversedation. Decide if treatment is appropriate at this point in the patient's illness and consider whether specialist opinion should be sought.

Communicate with the patient and their family

You should speak to the patient and those close to the patient, involving a translator if needed. Assess the patient's insight into their condition. If the patient does not have capacity, you should consult with those close to the patient and the multidisciplinary team and make decisions in the best interests of the patient.

Make a plan of care

Elements that should be included in an individualised plan of care are summarised in Table 97.6.
- Expect that the patient will lose their oral route as they die and plan ahead. Deprescribe all medications for secondary prevention and all non-essential medication. Ensure a parenteral route for essential medication e.g. opioids via a continuous subcutaneous infusion delivered using a syringe driver.
- As per NICE guidance, prescribe anticipatory subcutaneous symptom control medications.

Table 97.6 Elements that should be included in an individualised plan of care for a patient nearing the end of life.

Review the patient's preferred place of death: has it changed, is it appropriate or possible to transfer the patient in time?
Review and update resuscitation status, treatment escalation plan, ADRT, LPA/IMCA.
Consider deactivation of ICD if present.
Review current medications and deprescribe non-essential drugs.
Develop a plan for management of diabetes: seek advice from diabetes service (see Further reading).
Plan ahead to administer essential medication parenterally
Prescribe as required medications for anticipatory symptom control according to local guidelines (Table 97.7).
Consider if artificial nutrition and hydration should be continued. Discuss with patient and family
Encourage oral intake if not harmful to patient.
Discontinue inappropriate interventions (e.g. observations and turning regimens). Focus is on comfort observations
Regular care of the patient's mouth and pressure areas.
Assess and meet the spiritual and psychological needs of the patient and those close to the patient.
Find out how those close to the patient wish to be informed of the patient's death, wishes about care as the patient dies and care of the patient's body after death.

Table 97.7 Common symptoms in dying patients for which anticipatory as-required prescribing is appropriate.

Symptom	Drug	Dose for subcutaneous prn administration Comment administration*
Pain	Morphine**	2.5 mg 4-hourly
Restlessness or agitation	Midazolam	2.5 mg 4-hourly
Breathlessness	Morphine**	1–2 mg 4-hourly
Nausea and vomiting	Haloperidol	0.5 mg 8-hourly
Retained bronchopulmonary secretions	Hyoscine butylbromide	20 mg 4-hourly

* Usual starting dose in opioid-naive patient with normal renal function; lower doses may be required for elderly or frail patients. For patients with liver or renal impairment (eGFR <50), consult local guidelines or contact palliative care team for advice.
** Opioid drug conversions are given in Table 97.8.

Table 97.8 Opioid drug conversions.

SC morphine is twice as strong as PO morphine
PO oxycodone is 1.5–2 times as strong as PO morphine
SC oxycodone is 1.5–2 times as strong as PO oxycodone
PO morphine to SC morphine ÷ 2 for example 10 mg PO morphine = 5 mg SC morphine
PO morphine to PO oxycodone ÷ 2 for example 10 mg PO morphine = 5 mg PO oxycodone
PO oxycodone to SC oxycodone ÷ 2 for example 10 mg PO oxycodone = 5 mg SC oxycodone

- Review PRN requirement every 24 h. Assess whether PRN is used in anticipation (turn or would dressing). If PRN is used to manage an episode of unprovoked pain and three or more doses are required, consider the need for a continuous subcutaneous infusion (CSCI), if not already in place. If CSCI is in place increase background analgesia by 25–50%.
- If the patient has reliable IV access and difficult-to-control symptoms (e.g. pulmonary oedema), then the continued use of IV administration (e.g. for diuretics) may be appropriate.

Keep good notes

Details of the plan of care and summaries of conversations with the patient and family members should be documented in the medical record.

Review the patient

The patient should be seen at least daily, reviewing care plans.

Consider if specialist palliative care advice is needed – escalating symptoms, patient or family distressing not settling with explanation and to provide a second opinion when the patient has plateaued and is not dying as expected.

After death

The body of the deceased person should be cared for in accordance with their spiritual and cultural beliefs. Bereavement support should be offered to close family members.

Further reading

Blinderman CD, Billings JA. (2015) Comfort care for patients dying in the hospital. *N Engl J Med* 373, 2549–2561.

Clark D, Armstrong M, Allan A, *et al.* (2014) Imminence of death among hospital inpatients: prevalent cohort study. *Palliat Med* 28(6), 474–479. DOI: 10.1177/0269216314526443. PMID: 24637342; PMCID: PMC4845030.

Diabetes UK (2013) End-of-life diabetes care. Available online at: http://www.diabetes.org.uk/upload/Position%20statements/End-of-life-care-Clinical-recs111113.pdf.

General Medical Council (2010) Treatment and care towards the end of life: good practice in decision making.

National Institute for Health and Care Excellence. Care of dying adults in the last days of life (2015) NICE guideline (NG31). https://www.nice.org.uk/guidance/ng31?unlid=976936892016102725548.

Dermatology

CHAPTER 98

Acute rash

NEMESHA DESAI AND RUTH LAMB

'Rash' is a non-specific term for any abnormal skin finding:
- Acute rash develops over <four weeks and is described by morphology and distribution (Box 98.1 and Figure 98.1). Acute rashes account for 3% of emergency department presentations. Causes are given in Table 98.1.
- Sub-acute rash develops over four to six weeks, chronic rash is present for >six weeks. Sometimes patients report itchiness. It is important to clarify if a rash preceded the itch or whether the eruption seen results from scratching a generalized itch with another cause.

Priorities

1 Assessment is summarised in Table 98.2 and urgent investigation in Table 98.3.
- Acute erythroderma, a dermatological emergency, is defined as >90% inflammation of the skin surface. Assess the cardiovascular system. See Chapter 99 for management.
- Examination of the skin includes mucosal membranes (oral/genital), the nails and scalp and must be performed in good lighting. Start with the hands; then the extensor surfaces of the elbows, moving on

Box 98.1 Definition of skin abnormalities

Skin abnormality	Definition
Macule	Flat skin lesion <10 mm diameter
Patch	Flat skin lesion >10 mm diameter
Papule	A raised/palpable lesion <10 mm diameter
Plaque	A raised/palpable lesion >20 mm diameter
Nodule	A larger, firm papule >10 mm diameter
Vesicle	A papule containing clear serous fluid <5 mm diameter
Bulla	A larger vesicle >5 mm diameter
Pustule	A papule containing purulent fluid
Wheal	An oedematous, erythematous elevation in the skin, often round in shape
Purpura	Non-blanching red-purple discolouration of the skin. May be palpable or non-palpable.

Acute Medicine: A Practical Guide to the Management of Medical Emergencies, Sixth Edition.
Edited by Mridula Rajwani, Leila Vaziri, and Ivie Gbinigie.
© 2026 John Wiley & Sons Ltd. Published 2026 by John Wiley & Sons Ltd.

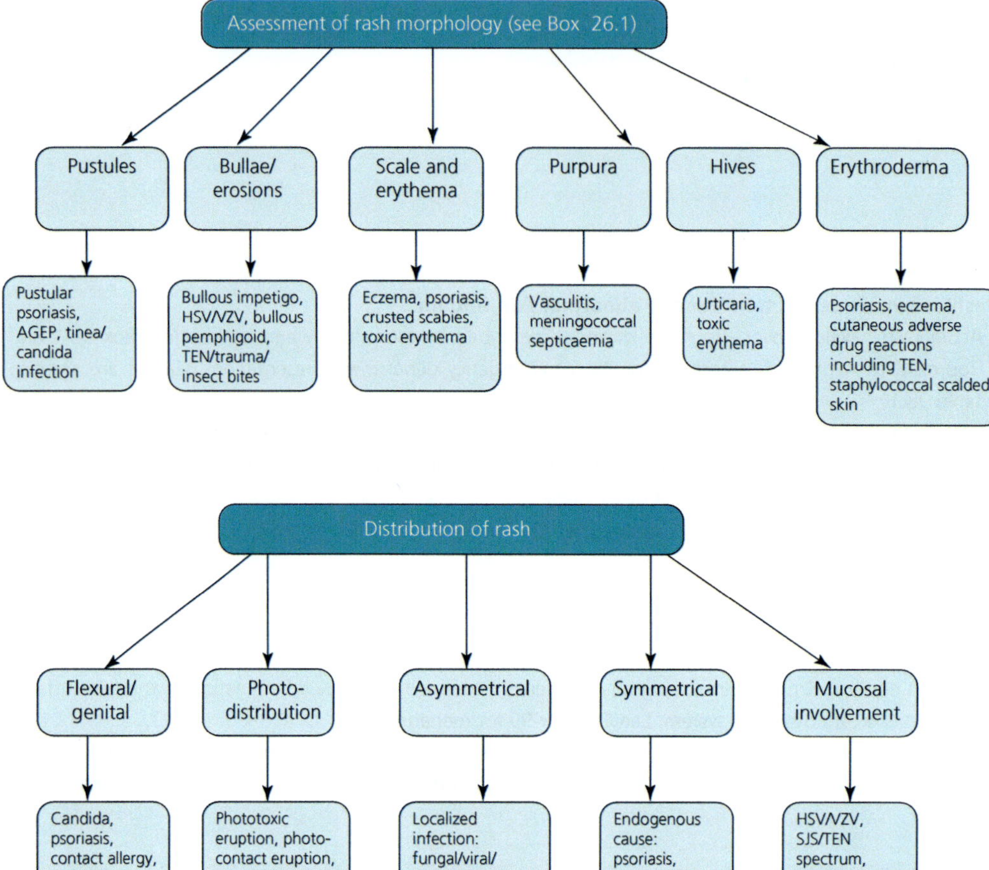

Figure 98.1 Assessment of an acute rash by morphology and distribution.

to the scalp, face, mucosal surfaces (eyes/mouth) followed by general and closer inspection of the trunk, limbs, other joints and genital skin if relevant. Assessment of morphology and distribution will inform the differential diagnosis (Figures 98.1 and 98.2).

- Additional examination depending on clinical suspicion includes examination for lymphadenopathy (seen in infection, inflammatory and malignant causes of rash), and other systems as appropriate, for example toxic erythema with pneumonia, splenomegaly with Epstein Barr Virus (EBV) infection.

2 Address haemodynamic compromise: fluid and electrolyte imbalance (see Chapter 2).

3 Pain control: erythematous, eroded skin is painful and patients may require opioid analgesia.

4 Assess for and treat suspected infection (primary or superadded), according to local antibiotic policies, **send bacterial and viral swabs.**

5 Stop any implicated drugs.

6 Seek dermatology advice if the diagnosis or management is uncertain. Involvement of mucosal surfaces may require review by ENT/Ophthalmology to advise on supportive care (HSV/VZV/SJS).

Table 98.1 Common eruptions seen acutely in the emergency department and in inpatients.

Aetiology	Localized	Widespread
Infectious		
• **Any**	Cutaneous vasculitis	Toxic erythema
• **Viral**	Varicella zoster virus (VZV) Eczema herpeticum	Eczema herpeticum virus (HSV) VZV Epstein Barr viral infection (+/– penicillin) Measles HIV seroconversion Erythema multiforme
• **Bacterial**	Impetigo Erysipelas Cellulitis Necrotizing fasciitis	Meningococcaemia Staphylococcal scalded skin Staphylococcal/Streptococcal toxic shock syndrome
• **Rickettsial**		Spotted fevers/typhus group
• **Treponemal**		Secondary syphilis
• **Other**	Tinea infection	Crusted scabies
Cutaneous adverse drug reactions	Cutaneous vasculitis Toxic erythema	Stevens–Johnson syndrome (SJS), toxic epidermal necrolysis (TEN) Drug hypersensitivity syndrome (also known as drug reaction with eosinophilia and systemic symptoms [DRESS] and drug-induced hypersensitivity syndrome [DIHS]) Acute generalized exanthematous pustulosis (AGEP) Phototoxic drug eruption
Inflammatory and autoimmune	Pompholyx Pyoderma gangrenosum	Infected exacerbation of atopic eczema Psoriasis (including pustular variants) Pityriasis rubra pilaris Bullous pemphigoid Cutaneous lupus
Allergic		Contact dermatitis Urticaria +/ angioedema (see Chapter 100, Urticaria and angioedema)
Malignancy		Cutaneous T cell lymphoma and Sezary syndrome

Criteria for escalation of care

- Cutaneous adverse drug reactions lie on a spectrum and may progress over days from mild erythema to toxic epidermal necrolysis. Close monitoring is required. See Chapter 99 for further guidance.
- Patients with eczema herpeticum are at risk of aseptic/viral meningitis: assess frequently. If inflammation is widespread and/or infection affects periorbital skin then the patient is likely to require IV aciclovir and ophthalmology input.
- Any erythrodermic patient is at risk of haemodynamic decompensation and should be monitored in a high-dependency unit.

Further management

Specific treatment is guided by the diagnosis. Often when a rash is seen in the early stages it can be difficult to diagnose with certainty. If the patient is systemically well, one approach is 'watch and wait'. In this situation, however, it is prudent to attempt to exclude exogenous causes (infection/drug) first and then treat symptomatically.

Table 98.2 Focused assessment of the patient with acute rash.

	Key points to cover in history	Differential diagnosis
History of presenting complaint	Itch	Atopic eczema, scabies, contact dermatitis, urticaria
	Pain	Cutaneous adverse drug reaction, TEN, VZV, eczema herpeticum, unstable psoriasis
	Mucosal involvement? For example gritty eyes, mouth/genital ulceration?	SJS/TEN spectrum, HSV/VZV, Autoimmune bullous disorders
	Site of onset: flexural,	Atopic eczema, flexural psoriasis
	extensor, dermatomal	Psoriasis, VZV
	Associated systemic symptoms: Unwell in addition to rash? And/or pyrexia?	Infection/inflammatory/cutaneous adverse drug reaction
	Joint symptoms	Inflammatory/autoimmune skin conditions, for example psoriasis, Behçet's disease, adult onset Still's disease
	History of inflammatory skin condition	Inflammatory conditions: atopic eczema, psoriasis
Past medical history	Atopy (asthma/hayfever)	Atopic eczema
Family history	Inflammatory skin conditions	Atopic eczema, psoriasis
Medications	New medicines in the last three to six months: in particular antibiotics/ antiepileptics Dosage increase in existing drugs	Cutaneous adverse drug reactions
Social history	Foreign travel Occupational history Social circumstances	Tropical infections, phototoxic/sensitive eruptions Contact/irritant dermatitis Nursing home/institution: scabies At-risk individuals: HIV seroconversion, secondary syphilis

Table 98.3 Urgent investigation in acute rash.

Swabs (bacterial and viral (VZV/HSV)) from eroded, crusted areas, blisters and pustules (use a sterile needle to burst vesicle/pustule)
Skin scrapings if fungal infection suspected
Blood culture if febrile
Full blood count (neutrophilia: infection/inflammation, eosinophilia: Drug hypersensitivity syndrome, allergic/atopic disease)
C-reactive protein
Blood glucose
Sodium, potassium, urea and creatinine
Liver function tests (deranged in cutaneous adverse drug reactions, erythroderma from any cause)
Urinalysis if vasculitic eruption suspected
Consider skin biopsy: consult a dermatologist

General principles of management include

- Use of emollients to restore skin barrier function.
- Avoidance of soap/fragranced products that can further impair the skin barrier; use of soap substitutes.
- Avoid topical steroids and occlusion in patients with infected (bacterial/viral) skin. Consider early NG feeding to maintain protein losses, if patient has mucosal erosions preventing normal oral intake.

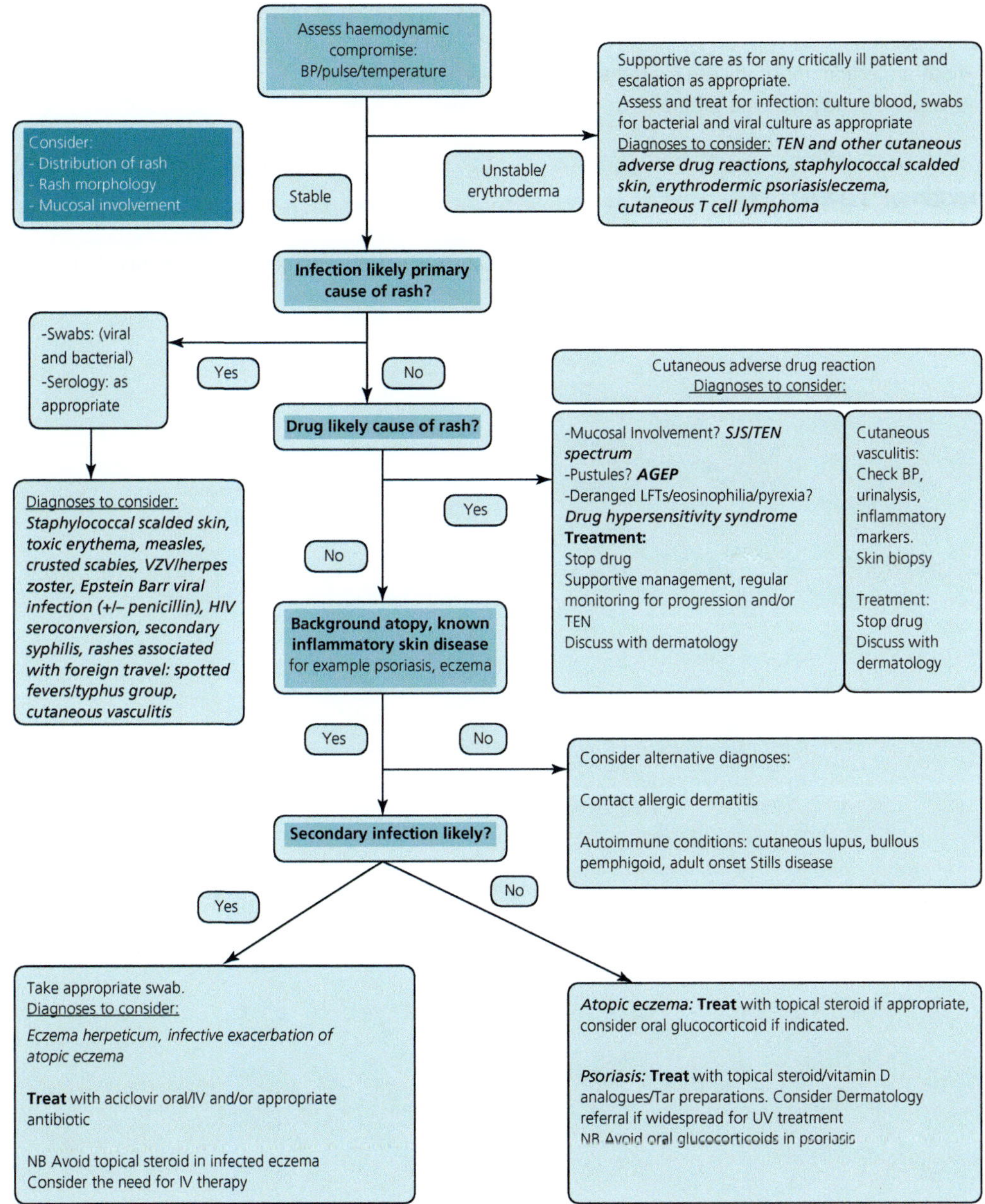

Figure 98.2 Approach to diagnosis and initial management of the patient with acute rash. AGEP, acute generalized exanthematous pustulosis; HIV, human immunodeficiency virus; SJS, Stevens–Johnson syndrome; TEN, toxic epidermal necrolysis; UV, ultraviolet; VZV, varicella-zoster virus.

- Consider catheter insertion if patient compromised or has involvement of mucosal surfaces making passing urine painful.
- Photo-protection: for conditions exacerbated by ultraviolet light.
- Reassurance and psychological support.

Further reading

Baibergenova A, Shear NH. (2011) Skin conditions that bring patients to emergency departments. *Arch Dermatol* 147, 118–120.

CHAPTER 99

Erythroderma and toxic epidermal necrolysis

NEMESHA DESAI AND SALLY AZIZ

Erythroderma

Erythroderma describes redness and exfoliation of the skin, affecting more than 90% of the body surface area. It is a dermatological emergency as patients are at risk of associated haemodynamic and metabolic complications.

Aetiology

- The aetiology of erythroderma is broad and included in Table 99.1. The most common causes include underlying inflammatory skin disease (e.g. eczema or psoriasis), drug reactions, haematological malignancies (e.g. subcutaneous T cell lymphoma or Hodgkin's lymphoma) and idiopathic.

Table 99.1 Causes of erythroderma.

Inflammatory skin disease	Atopic eczema
	Psoriasis
	Pityriasis rubra pilaris
Drug reactions	Stevens–Johnson syndrome/toxic epidermal necrolysis
See Table 99.6 for common culprit	Drug rash with eosinophilia and systemic symptoms (DRESS)
drugs	Acute generalised exanthematous pustulosis (AGEP)
Neoplastic	Primary skin malignancies, e.g. cutaneous T-cell lymphoma, cutaneous B-cell lymphoma
	Haematological or solid organ malignancy, e.g. Hodgkin's lymphoma
Infective	Scabies
	HIV
	Staphylococcal scaled skin syndrome
Others	Idiopathic
	Autoimmune blistering conditions
	Connective tissue disease
	Graft versus host disease

Clinical assessment

- The patient with erythroderma requires urgent assessment. History taking should enquire about the timing and symptoms of the rash, underlying diseases and a drug timeline. Examination involves general assessment of the patient with specific inspection of the skin, nails, scalp and mucosal surfaces. A general approach to history and examination is described in Table 99.2.
- Investigations required will vary from patient to patient, depending on the possible differential diagnoses and are listed in Table 99.3.
- Key clinical features during your assessment may guide you towards the underlying cause of erythroderma. These are shown in Table 99.4.

Table 99.2 Focused assessment of the patient with erythroderma.

History

Take a full medical and drug history, focusing on a personal and family history of underlying skin disease, atopy and new medications in the preceding eight weeks, to include topical agents, complementary and over-the-counter therapies.

Establish the timing of onset of the rash; drug reactions tend to evolve rapidly, whereas inflammatory skin disease may be more insidious.

Assess for cutaneous symptoms; skin pain may be experienced with drug rashes and unstable psoriasis, itch with atopic dermatitis.

Systemic symptoms should be sought including fever and prodromal flu-like illness.

Examination

Physiological observations and general examination.

Examine the palms and nails.

Inspect scalp, oral mucosa, natal cleft and genitalia in addition to the body skin. Observe carefully for pustules or vesicles.

Multiple sterile micropustules are seen in erythrodermic psoriasis and drug reactions.

Examine for Nikolsky sign (see TEN skin failure).

Palpate for lymph nodes; widespread lymphadenopathy can occur in erythroderma as a non-specific reaction to the inflammatory process ('dermatopathic' lymphadenopathy) and/ or secondary to the underlying aetiology (e.g. cutaneous T- cell lymphoma).

In chronic erythroderma, ectropion, hair loss and thickening of the skin on the palms and soles are seen.

Table 99.3 Urgent investigation in erythroderma.

Full blood count and coagulation

Sodium, potassium, urea and creatinine: to monitor for derangement secondary to fluid loss

Liver function tests: drug reactions are often associated with hepatic derangement

C reactive protein, erythrocyte sedimentation rate

Bone profile

Immunoglobulins

Blood culture if febrile, mycoplasma serology

Skin swab to screen for secondary infections: bacterial and viral

ECG

Chest X-ray to assess for high-output cardiac failure

Skin biopsy should be performed if there is a negative history of established skin disease

Table 99.4 Common causes of erythroderma.

Cause	Key points on history	Clinical features seen in particular disease	Important specific tests
Psoriasis	Personal or family history of psoriasis, withdrawal of recent oral steroids	Scalp scale, nail changes (pitting, onycholysis), pustules. Joint involvement	
Eczema	Personal or family history of atopy	Lichenification of skin Periorbital disease	Serum immunoglobulin E (IgE), eosinophilia
Drug-related	New medications in the past eight weeks	Morbilliform rash Flexural erythema Pustules	Monitor eosinophils and liver function for DRESS*
Cutaneous T cell lymphoma (CTCL)		Generalized erythema	Circulating atypical T cells
Pityriasis rubra pilaris (PRP)		'Islands' of clear skin	

* DRESS, drug reaction with eosinophilia and systemic symptoms: a severe idiosyncratic drug reaction with a broad range of clinical features (which may include raised ALT) appearing two to eight weeks after starting the causative drug.

Management

- Erythroderma can extend rapidly and hence requires urgent intervention, as patients who appear well may decompensate abruptly due to the extent of skin barrier impairment. All cases should be discussed with the on-call dermatologist.

Patients are at risk of
- Dehydration and electrolyte abnormalities due to increased transepidermal water loss through inflamed skin
- High-output cardiac failure due to increased blood flow through the skin
- Hypothermia due to excessive heat loss through increased skin perfusion
- Hypoalbuminemia due to exfoliation of the skin and associated protein loss
- Infection due to compromise of mechanical skin barrier function

Priorities

Management is summarized in Figure 99.1.

General supportive measures
- Patients should be cared for in a monitored bed with close nursing input
- Discontinue any possible culprit drug causes and unnecessary medications
- Monitor and correct fluid balance and electrolytes
- Monitor body temperature. A Bair–Hugger blanket or equivalent can be applied to prevent heat loss and maintain core temperature
- Initiate nutritional support early
- Treat secondary sepsis
- Copious bland emollient should be applied to whole body, 50 : 50 white soft paraffin/liquid paraffin is recommended
- Topical steroids may be indicated and the choice of potency depends on the underlying diagnosis. A potent topical steroid may be used in suspected drug reactions or eczema. A mild/moderate potency topical steroid may be used in psoriasis. Potent topical steroids are avoided in psoriasis due to the risk of developing generalised pustular psoriasis.

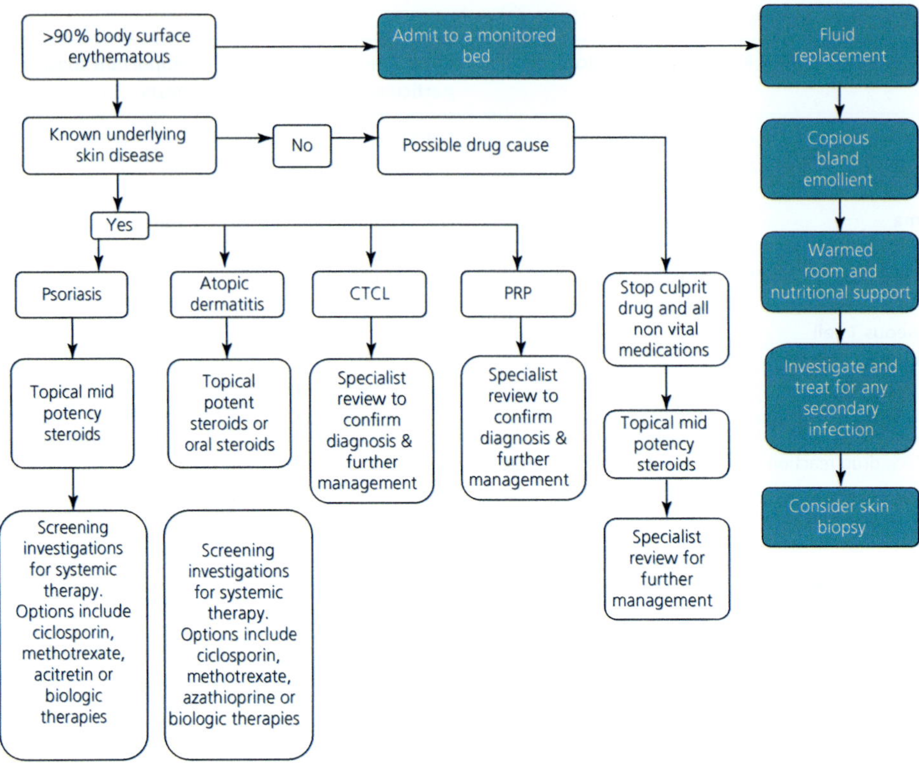

Figure 99.1 Management of erythroderma. CTCL, cutaneous T-cell lymphoma; DRESS, drug reaction with eosinophilia and systemic symptoms; PRP, pityriasis rubra pilaris.

Disease-specific measures

- Systemic therapies can be used to treat patients where the underlying cause of erythroderma is known. These treatments are usually patient dependant, initiated by specialists and drug-specific screening and monitoring investigations are required.
- Treatments for erythrodermic atopic eczema include oral corticosteroids, antibiotics and systemic immunosuppression with ciclosporin, methotrexate or biologic therapies.
- Treatments for severe psoriasis include ciclosporin, methotrexate, acitretin or biologic therapies.
- Cutaneous T-cell lymphoma (CTCL) requires specialist review for specific treatment.
- Pityriasis Rubra Pilaris (PRP) requires intensive topical steroids; second-line therapies include acitretin.
- For a large proportion of erythrodermic patients, an aetiology is not found; for such patients, continual emollients and topical steroids should be considered, alongside supportive therapy to prevent and monitor for complications.

Toxic epidermal necrolysis

- Toxic epidermal necrolysis (TEN) is the most severe form of skin failure. It is rare, affecting 1–2 persons per million population per year and associated with significant morbidity and mortality. It is a severe mucocutaneous reaction, usually drug-induced, characterized by fever, full-thickness skin necrosis affecting more than 30% of the body surface area, erosion or ulceration of at least two mucous membrane sites (ocular, oral or anogenital) and variable systemic organ involvement.

Table 99.5 Features of toxic epidermal necrolysis (TEN), Stevens–Johnson syndrome (SJS) and erythema multiforme major.

	TEN	SJS	Erythema multiforme major
Percentage of body skin affected	>30%	10%	n/a
Initial skin lesions	Painful dusky erythematous cutaneous and mucosal skin	Erythema in mucous membranes	Dusky erythema
Skin signs	Mucosal involvement Full thickness epidermal necrosis resulting in friable bullae Nikolsky positive	Mucosal involvement Erosions and bullae	Targetoid skin lesions Mucosal involvement
Mortality	>30%	<10%	Rare

Table 99.6 Medications which are likely causative agents in toxic epidermal necrolysis/Stevens-Johnson syndrome.

Allopurinol
Aromatic anticonvulsants, e.g. carbamazepine, phenytoin, sodium valproate, phenobarbitone, lamotrigine
Antibiotics, e.g. amoxicillin, cotrimoxazole, penicillin, trimethoprim
HAART drugs, e.g. nevirapine
Analgesics, e.g. paracetamol, NSAIDs
Others: sulphasalazine, omeprazole, diuretics

- TEN lies on a spectrum with Stevens–Johnson syndrome (SJS) and erythema multiforme major (see Table 99.5). The aetiology is often drug-related (Table 99.6), rarely infections such as *Mycoplasma* and herpes simplex virus are implicated.
- At-risk individuals include the elderly (relating to polypharmacy), patients with systemic lupus erythematosus (SLE), HIV/AIDS and recipients of bone marrow transplants.
- The leading cause of death is secondary sepsis. Morbidity relating to chronic pain, Stricturing of mucosal sites (e.g. urethral stenosis and vaginal synechiae causing chronic dyspareunia; ocular symblepharon, corneal scarring and sicca symptoms), oesophageal strictures and bronchiolitis obliterans can persist long after the acute cutaneous reaction has resolved.

Priorities

- Clinical assessment is given in Table 99.7 and investigation is needed urgently in Table 99.8. The SCORTEN criteria predict mortality (Table 99.9).
- The main stay of management is supportive, focusing on high-level nursing care. The aims are prevention of further skin injury, prevention of infection and maintenance of haemostasis and thermoregulation.
- Stop the suspected drug immediately. All drugs started within 7–21 days of the first manifestation of the skin eruption should be discontinued. Consider any drug started within the previous eight weeks as a candidate.
- Early referral to a multidisciplinary, high dependency/intensive care unit for 1 : 1 specialist nursing with aseptic technique and close monitoring of vital parameters and respiratory function.
- Nurse in a side room, warmed to 30–32 °C to reduce percutaneous heat loss, on a pressure relieving mattress with non-adherent bed lining such as Exu-dry* or Lyofoam* lined with copious bland emollient such as 50 : 50 white soft paraffin.
- Cleanse the skin gently using warmed sterile water, saline or an antiseptic wash, e.g. chlorhexidine (1/5000).
- Cover skin with copious bland emollient such as 50 : 50 white soft paraffin and liquid paraffin.

Table 99.7 Focused assessment in toxic-epidermal necrolysis.

History

A careful history of comorbidities and detailed drug history of the last eight weeks is imperative, including prescribed, over-the-counter and complementary therapies. Specific symptoms to support a diagnosis of incipient TEN include skin pain, involvement of the mucous membranes presenting as ocular pain, grittiness, photophobia, sore throat, odynophagia, dysuria and systemic malaise, specifically flu-like symptoms and fever. Muco-cutaneous symptoms in established disease include a spectrum of extensive blistering, erosions and haemorrhagic mucositis.

Examination

Careful skin and mucous membrane examination is required to assess the extent of involved sites. The skin may be friable and denude easily on examination; hence assistance will be required to minimize direct handling of the skin during examination. Assessment of the percentage body surface area involved should be made, to include erythema (which may take the appearance of subtle slate grey pigmentation in darker skin types or where full thickness skin necrosis is already established), erosions and bullae. Nikolsky sign is positive in TEN: gentle lateral pressure applied to the skin results in separation of the epidermis from the dermis. The ocular, oral, genital and urethral mucous membranes should be examined for involvement. Systemic examination should focus on respiratory and gastrointestinal systems, which may exhibit early involvement, although any organ can be involved.

Table 99.8 Urgent investigation in toxic epidermal necrolysis.

Full blood count and coagulation
C-reactive protein
Urea, creatinine and electrolytes
Liver function, bone profile, glucose, magnesium, lactate
Immunoglobulins
Mycoplasma serology
Blood culture
Skin and mucosal swabs to screen for secondary infections: viral and bacterial
Skin biopsy
ECG
Chest X-ray to assess for high-output cardiac failure

Table 99.9 SCORTEN scoring system for toxic epidermal necrolysis.

SCORTEN criteria	Points	Total SCORTEN score	Predicted mortality
Age >40 years	1	0–1	1–3%
Heart rate >120/min	1	2	12%
Comorbid malignancy	1	3	35%
Epidermal detachment >10% body surface	1	4	58%
area on day 1		5+	>90%
Serum urea >10 mol/L	1		
Bicarbonate level <20 mmol/L	1		
Serum glucose >14 mmol/L	1		

- Blisters should be decompressed, by piercing with a sterile needle. The epidermal roof of the blister may be left in situ to act as a biological dressing.
- Denuded dermis should be covered with a primary non-adherent dressing, e.g. Mepitel, followed by a secondary foam to help collect exudate, e.g. Mepilex.
- Careful fluid balance. IV fluid and electrolyte replacement may be needed. Where possible, site peripheral venous cannulas through intact skin and change every 48 h to reduce the risk of infection.

- Daily assessment of eye, oral and genital involvement is necessary.
- Referral to ophthalmology for daily ocular hygiene, lubricating eye drops and preservative-free topical antibiotics/steroids. Severe causes may require amniotic membrane transplantation to help prevent ocular sequalae.
- Urinary catheters are effective in keeping the urethra patent, but meticulous aseptic technique must be observed on insertion.
- Regular oral toilette with sterile water and soft applicator sponge to remove crusts and exudates.
- Supplement nutrition orally or with careful siting of a nasogastric tube.
- Ensure adequate analgesia, especially during dressing change.

Further management

- There are few large clinical trials on the therapeutic management of TEN/SJS, thus treatment remains supportive. Treatments that have been employed on a case-by-case basis include intravenous immunoglobulin (IVIG), systemic corticosteroid and ciclosporin. However, in the absence of high-quality evidence supporting any single agent, therapy remains supportive, with vigilant prevention of secondary infection.
- The patient and all doctors involved in the patient's case, including the GP, should be provided with written information regarding the episode and details regarding the culprit drug which they must avoid. Patients should be encouraged to wear MedicAlert bracelet or amulet with this information.

Further reading

Creamer D, Walsh SA, Dziewulski P, *et al*. (2016) UK guidelines for the management of Stevens-Johnson syndrome/toxic epidermal necrolysis in adults 2016. *Br J Dermatol* 174, 1194–1227. http://www.bad.org.uk/shared/get-file.ashx?id=3968&itemtype=document.

Scwartz R. (2013) Toxic epidermal necrolysis Part II. Prognosis, sequelae, diagnosis, differential diagnosis, prevention, and treatment. *J Am Acad Dermatol* 69(2), 182.

Tso S, Satchwell F, Moiz H, *et al*. (2021) Erythroderma (exfoliative dermatitis). Part 1: underlying causes, clinical presentation and pathogenesis. *Clin Exp Dermatol* 46(6), 1001–1010.

CHAPTER 100

Urticaria and angioedema

ALEXANDRA CROOM

Urticaria (nettle rash, hives) arises from mast cell degranulation in the skin. Angioedema (tissue swelling) may be due to mast cell degranulation in deeper tissues (with or without accompanying urticaria). Alternatively, it may be independent of mast cells and be mediated by bradykinins. The majority of urticaria is not allergic.

The clinical features of urticaria and angioedema are described in Box 100.1 and angioedema emergency management in Box 100.2.

- Angioedema can cause life-threatening upper airway obstruction and airway management should be a priority (Chapter 105).
- Urticarial vasculitis may resemble urticaria in appearance but has distinct clinical features and may be part of a systemic process.
- Bradykinin-mediated isolated angioedema will not respond to emergency treatment with antihistamines, corticosteroids or adrenaline.

Box 100.1 Clinical features of urticaria, angioedema and urticarial vasculitis

Urticaria	**Weals**
	• Itchy, raised, central pallor with surrounding erythema
	• Variable size – pinprick to dinner plate
	• Single or multiple
	• Local or generalized
	• Individually may last a few minutes to around 24 h
	• Rash may move around the body (flitting)
	• On resolution skin returns to normal (unless damaged by excoriation)
Angioedema	**Swelling**
	• Discrete swelling(s) – overlying skin may be normal in appearance or erythematous
	• May occur anywhere but favours distensible skin (eyelids, lips and genitalia); may involve mucosal surfaces (including oropharynx and gut)
	• Painful (due to tissue distension) rather than itchy
	• Resolution may take up to three days (longer if bradykinin mediated)
Urticarial vasculitis	**Weals**
	• Tender rather than itchy
	• Individual weals may persist for days
	• Leaves bruising or discolouration on resolution
	• Vasculitis may be confined to skin or be part of a systemic process

Box 100.2 Angioedema emergency management

Angioedema can cause life-threatening upper airway obstruction; early recognition and airway management should be a priority (Chapter 105)

If airway obstruction is present or imminent alert anaesthetist; consider intervention early as advanced laryngeal oedema will distort anatomy and make intubation difficult.

If features of anaphylaxis are present
Give adrenaline 500 μg IM into anterolateral thigh using a 23G needle (blue – length 25 mm); in morbidly obese use 21 G needle (green – length 38 mm) or administer to calf. Repeat after 5 min; if no improvement consider low-dose adrenaline infusion (see Chapter 4).

If features of anaphylaxis are absent
Give hydrocortisone 200 mg IV and cetirizine 20 mg orally or chlorphenamine 10 mg IV

Consider nebulized adrenaline (5 mL of 1 : 1000 solution)

Continue to observe for progression or biphasic reactions

If related to angiotensin-converting-enzyme inhibitor (ACEi)
Consider treatment with icatibant 30 mg SC – discuss with on-call immunologist

If hereditary angioedema (HAE) or acquired angioedema (AAE) known
Diagnosed patients should already have written self-management plan for C1 inhibitor concentrate IV and/or icatibant SC (maximum 3 doses in 24 h)

Discuss with on-call immunologist

Urticaria

When looking for a cause it is helpful to divide urticaria by duration of symptoms
- Acute: symptoms of less than six weeks' duration
- Chronic: symptoms more or less daily for six weeks or more

The underlying causes of each group are different (Table 100.1). No cause is identified (idiopathic) in 50% of acute urticaria and 98% of chronic urticaria; chronic urticaria is rarely allergic, i.e. mediated by allergen specific IgE (but is often mistakenly perceived as being so).

Urticaria management

Identify a cause
Urticaria is a symptom rather than a diagnosis. Although most urticaria is idiopathic, an underlying cause may become apparent on clinical assessment (Table 100.2, Figure 100.1). Some patterns of symptoms are typical, for example the urticaria in an IgE-mediated reaction will be accompanied by other allergic symptoms and is of rapid onset after allergen exposure (typically within 60 minutes), peaks in severity within 2-4 hours and resolves within 1-2 days. Urticaria and/or angioedema that evolves over hours or days is not allergic.

The investigations required for urticaria depend on its type and the suspected underlying cause.

In acute urticaria, investigations are normally unnecessary other than for the identification of allergens in suspected IgE-mediated reactions, e.g. skin prick testing and/or spIgE assays. Testing should be deferred until specialist review.

Table 100.1 Causes of urticaria.

Acute urticaria

IgE mediated	For example, food allergy, drugs, latex
Drugs	For example, NSAIDs, codeine, vaccines
Infection	
Idiopathic	
Chronic urticaria	
Spontaneous (idiopathic)	
Inducible (physical) urticaria	For example, dermographism, cold, exercise, solar, pressure, delayed, vibration, aquagenic
Chronic infection	For example, *H. pylori*, cholecystitis, parasitic infestation, hepatitis B and C, dental caries and gingivitis
Autoimmune	Antibody directed at FcεR1α or IgE on mast cells
	Thyroid autoimmunity (patient usually euthyroid)
Stress	
Iron deficiency	With or without anaemia - transferrin saturation <20%
Miscellaneous	Urticaria pigmentosa, CAPS (cryopyrin-associated autoinflammatory syndrome)
	Dietary pseudoallergens, e.g. dietary salicylates

Table 100.2 Focused assessment in urticaria (occurring with or without angioedema).

Duration and frequency of symptoms
Provoking factors
Relationship to food
Use of medications – prescribed, over the counter and naturopathic – regular or intermittent
Recent infective illness and/or vaccinations
Use of recreational drugs in particular cannabis
Comorbidities
Foreign travel
Occupation
Relationship to menses
Stress

In chronic urticaria testing should be determined by the history and clinical findings, but as a minimum an FBC and ESR/CRP (as a screen for underlying inflammation as a driver) should be performed. Most chronic urticaria is 'spontaneous', i.e. without a known cause or trigger.

Laboratory testing is not normally required for inducible urticaria, with the exception of cold urticaria, which is associated with thyroid autoimmunity and, rarely, with the presence of cryoglobulins or cold agglutinins.

Pre-existing chronic spontaneous urticaria may be exacerbated by stress, use of NSAIDs, and iron deficiency without anaemia.

Where there is an underlying condition 'driving' the urticaria, effective treatment of that will be required before there is clinical improvement.

Treatment

Urticaria in the context of anaphylaxis should be treated as per the anaphylaxis algorithm (see Chapter 4, figure 4.1).

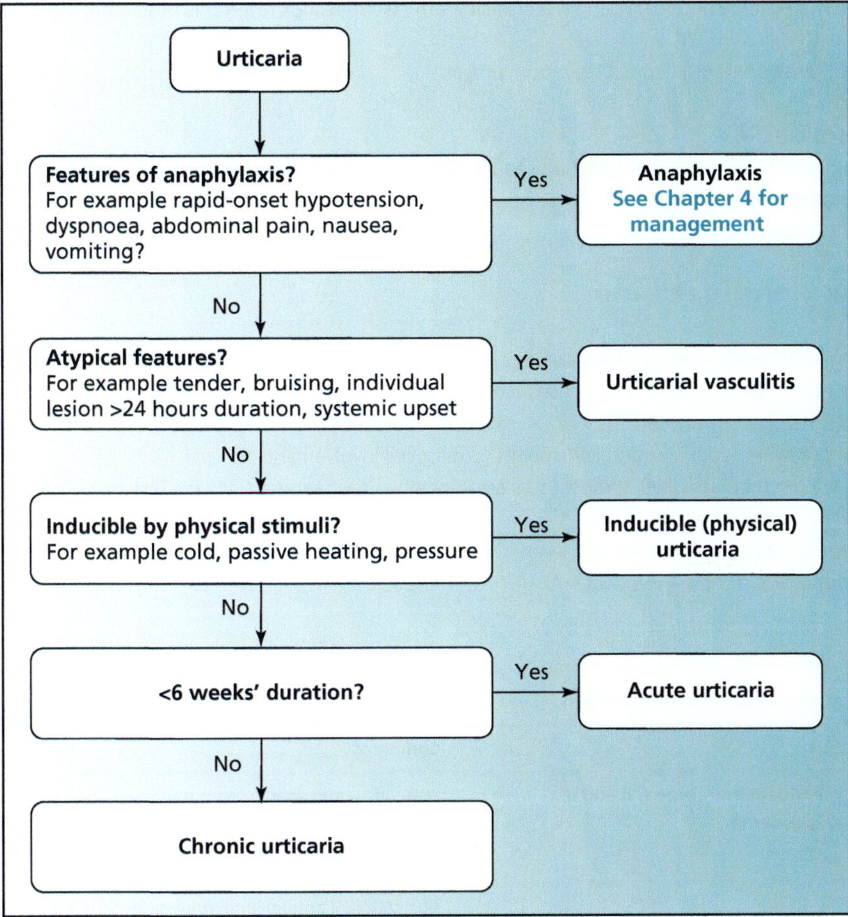

Figure 100.1 Assessment of urticaria.

Antihistamines

Second-generation antihistamines, for example cetirizine, loratidine and fexofenadine are mostly well tolerated. The onset of action of oral antihistamines is around 20–25 min. Chlorphenamine (and other first-generation antihistamines) should, where possible, be avoided as it can cause sedation, and confusion and falls in the elderly.

Higher than licensed doses (e.g. cetirizine up to 40 mg daily, fexofenadine up to 540 mg daily) are recommended for chronic urticaria not responding to conventional doses. Sedation is more likely as doses are increased.

Loratidine is the antihistamine of first choice for pregnant women. Cetirizine is the second choice.

Corticosteroids

Corticosteroids may be used, particularly if angioedema dominates the clinical picture or urticaria does not immediately come under control with antihistamines. Short courses should be used (prednisolone 30–40 mg daily for five to seven days). Avoid protracted courses (> two weeks) as tachyphylaxis will result in diminishing efficacy and increasing adverse side effects. Specialist referral is required if steroid requirements persist.

There is no role for topical corticosteroids in urticaria.

Tranexamic acid

Tranexamic acid 1–1.5 g TDS can be helpful as an add-on for prophylaxis when chronic urticaria is accompanied by angioedema.

Isolated angioedema

Angioedema occurring without coexistent urticaria may be due to mast cell degranulation but can also occur independent of mast cells and as a consequence be poorly responsive to antihistamines, corticosteroids or adrenaline. Distinction between the two is important, particularly when there is the potential for airways threatening swelling. Coexistent urticaria points to mast cell involvement.

Causes are given in Table 100.3; most cases are idiopathic. Key features from the history are summarized in Table 100.4.

If urticaria is absent, the complement levels, C1-inhibitor level and functional assay should be checked. Seek immunology advice if the C4 is low or HAE or AAE is suspected.

Table 100.3 Causes of isolated angioedema.

Cause	Comment
Hereditary angioedema – type I, II and III	20% arise from spontaneous mutation- absent family history
Acquired angioedema	Associated with lymphoproliferative and autoimmune conditions
Drugs	Angiotensin-converting-enzyme inhibitors
	Non-steroidal anti-inflammatory drugs
	Oral contraceptives
	Statins
Idiopathic	

Table 100.4 Focused assessment in angioedema

Presence/absence of urticaria (this episode or recently)
Speed of onset and duration
Sites affected by swelling
Symptoms (voice change, stridor with laryngeal swelling; vomiting and abdominal pain with gut involvement)
Precipitating factors (drugs, trauma, menses, infection and stress)
Number of previous episodes
Age of onset
Family history
Response to treatment, e.g. antihistamines
Use of medications – prescribed, over the counter or naturopathic – regular or intermittent
General health and comorbidities

Hereditary angioedema (HAE)

This is due to low or dysfunctional C1-inhibitor.
Clinical features suggestive of this group of conditions include

- Repeated episodes of angioedema developing from childhood/adolescence
- Triggered by trauma, stress, oral contraceptive pill, menses and infection
- Non-painful, non-itchy swelling developing over a few hours and lasting three to five days
- Life-threatening laryngeal obstruction (30% mortality rate)
- Abdominal symptoms – vomiting, abdominal pain, hypotension, ascites; may be confused with acute abdomen

Acute episodes are treated with plasma-derived or recombinant human C1-inhibitor concentrate or icatibant (a bradykinin B2 receptor antagonist), according to the patient's individualised management plan; supportive management of the airway may be necessary. FFP should only be used if none of these are available and patients should be counselled about risk of transmission of blood-borne disease. Androgens, tranexamic acid and kallikrein inhibitors are used long term for prophylaxis but have no acute role.

Acquired angioedema (AAE)

This occurs in the context of autoimmune or lymphoproliferative disease. C1 inhibitor production is normal but functional activity is lost either due to increased consumption of C1 inhibitor (type 1) or due to an autoantibody directed at C1 inhibitor (type 2). In contrast to HAE, there is no family history and the onset is from middle age in 90% cases. AAE may improve as the underlying condition is treated. Acute episodes with life-threatening airway obstruction are rare but should be treated as per HAE.

Angiotensin-converting-enzyme inhibitor (ACEi) – associated angioedema

ACEi drugs may be a primary cause of angioedema or make coexisting angioedema worse. In the primary type, localised swelling lasting up to 72 hours is characteristically confined to the head and neck; those of West African descent, women and smokers are at increased risk. The onset of episodes of swelling can be from months to years after initiation of treatment; episodes can recur for up to 3 months after discontinuation of therapy. A switch to an angiotensin receptor-blocking agent is normally well-tolerated. Treatment is usually supportive. Swelling is not mast cell-mediated and antihistamines, corticosteroids and adrenaline are ineffective. Airways obstruction may be life-threatening and require anaesthetic or ENT management; if present icatibant may be used (off-license) and specialist immunology input should be sought early.

Further reading

Maurer M *et al*. (2022) The international WAO/EAACI guideline for the management of hereditary angioedema – the 2021 revision and update. *Allergy* 77(7), 1961–1990.
Zuberbier T, Abdul Latiff AH, Abuzakouk M, *et al*. (2022) The international EAACI/GA²LEN/EuroGuiDerm/ APAAACI guideline for the definition, classification, diagnosis, and management of urticaria. *Allergy* 77(3), 734–766.

Same Day Emergency Care

CHAPTER 101

Same-day emergency care

VINCENT CONNOLLY

Acute (Internal) Medicine

The specialty of acute medicine was developed to streamline the assessment and care of patients with acute illness or exacerbations of long-term conditions. Patients accepted on an acute medical unit are assessed on arrival by a senior doctor and assigned to one of four streams of care:

- Same-day emergency care, for same-day treatment and discharge without using a hospital bed
- Short-stay (<72 h) inpatient care
- Organ-specific disease requiring inpatient care from a specialist team
- Frail older patients, for whom comprehensive geriatric assessment (Chapter 68) is needed.

An acute physician requires the clinical skills to manage patients with a broad range of clinical problems, and in each of the care streams described above. This chapter focuses on same-day emergency care (Box 101.1). Same-day emergency care evolved from ambulatory emergency care and they are, for all practical purposes, synonymous.

Same-day emergency care (SDEC)

This is usually run by specialists in acute medicine, but can also be part of emergency medicine, surgery or paediatrics. Delivery requires rapid assessment by a senior physician, usually a consultant.

Referrals are accepted from (Figure 101.1)

- The emergency department
- General practitioners and community nurses

Box 101.1 Same-day emergency care (SDEC)

> An effective SDEC service can improve patient care and system efficiency.
> The essentials for a highly functioning service are:
> - Senior clinician presence throughout the opening hours
> - Clear patient-selection criteria
> - Agreed pathways for high-volume clinical presentations
> - Access to a multi-disciplinary team to support care plans for older people
> - Appropriate infrastructure to meet the demand, particularly staffing

Acute Medicine: A Practical Guide to the Management of Medical Emergencies, Sixth Edition.
Edited by Mridula Rajwani, Leila Vaziri, and Ivie Gbinigie.
© 2026 John Wiley & Sons Ltd. Published 2026 by John Wiley & Sons Ltd.

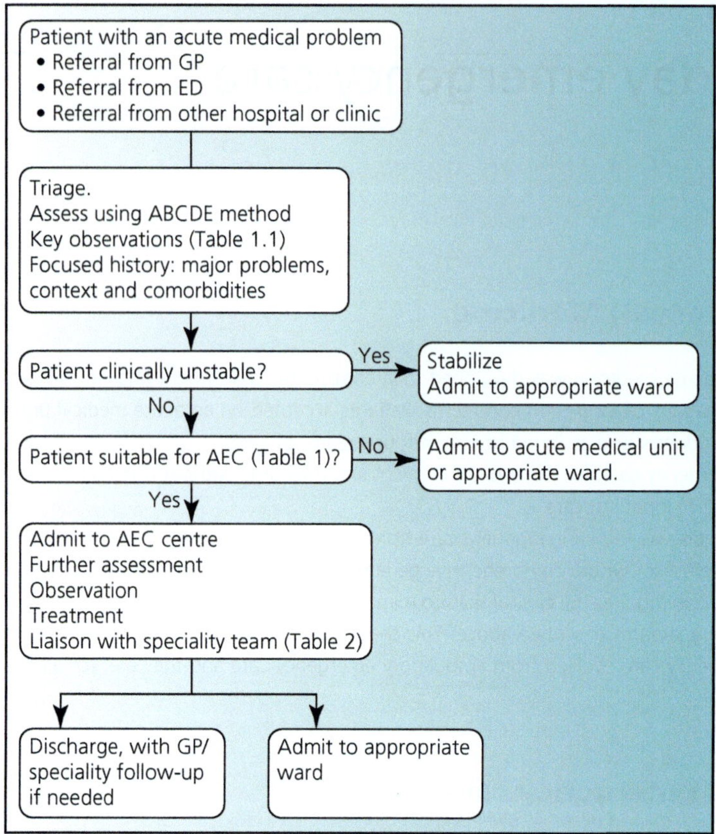

Figure 101.1 Same-day emergency care (SDEC) in acute medicine.

- Inpatient wards as part of a step-down approach to discharge
- Other hospitals and clinics

Many SDEC units will receive patients directly from the ambulance service usually preceded by a telephone referral to a senior clinician.

- If suitable for SDEC, the patient and relatives or carers must be informed that the plan is for same-day care then discharge, since the initial expectation after referral is often that an inpatient admission will be needed.
- The initial assessment must establish that the patient is safe in the SDEC setting.

Is the clinical condition suitable for SDEC?

Is the patient actually well enough for early outpatient review? Alternatively, is the patient sick enough to require inpatient admission? National Early Warning Score (NEWS) can help, but must be interpreted individually in the clinical context and working diagnosis. For example, a patient on long-term domiciliary oxygen may have a high NEWS but be clinically stable and suitable for AEC; a young person with low oxygen saturation levels may not trigger concern, even with a sub-massive PE. A clinical conversation between the referring and accepting clinicians is important in establishing that an individual patient can be safely managed in SDEC.

Table 101.1 The Amb score.

Factor	Score
	1 if applicable, 0 if not applicable
Female sex	
Age <80 years	
Has access to personal/public transport	
IV treatment not anticipated	
Not acutely confused	
National Early Warning Score = 0	
Not discharged from hospital within previous 30 days	
Total Amb score	0–7
	A score of 5 or more suggests the patient is suitable for AEC

The Amb score (Table 101.1) is also useful. A composite score of 5 or more suggests that the patient is suitable for AEC. The Amb score can be a particularly useful tool when less experienced staff are responsible for streaming, to help build confidence in the process.

Can the AEC unit deliver the required care?

Is there access to required back-up services: diagnostics; support by a community heart failure team; and ability to give parenteral antibiotics seven days a week?

Are staffing levels adequate in the face of current patient load and concerns like sickness and annual leave?

Can the SDEC unit cope with the patient's personal needs?

These include feeding, toileting and behaviour. It is possible, indeed it should be encouraged, to manage frail older people with confusion or delirium in the AEC unit if the appropriate staff and facilities are available.

Patient presentations to SDEC

The clinical scenarios suitable for management in the SDEC unit are in four main categories.

Diagnostic exclusion

Examples include
- Chest pain with no acute ECG changes and low coronary risk. The patients can await troponin assays on SDEC.
- Sudden onset severe headache in the absence of other neurological symptoms or signs. Exclusion of subarachnoid haemorrhage or other potentially serious diagnoses, with a computed tomography (CT) of the brain and possibly a lumbar puncture, can be delivered in SDEC.

- Suspected pulmonary embolism if haemodynamically stable. A CT pulmonary angiogram (CTPA) (see Chapter 31) according to clinical scores can be performed.
- Non-specific abdominal pain can be assessed and investigated in SDEC with appropriate onward referral if required.

Management of specific conditions

Patients may present with an easily recognizable diagnosis, for example DVT, cellulitis, atrial fibrillation, for which the patient requires a clinical management plan. There is often a need for confirmatory diagnostic tests, which should be readily available, or in the case of cellulitis, an outpatient parenteral intravenous antibiotic service. The patient may need to return to the SDEC service for ongoing management or referral to another service for follow-up.

Management after risk-stratification

This group of clinical scenarios uses validated risk stratification tools to identify suitable patients for SDEC. Examples include the Glasgow–Blatchford score for acute upper gastrointestinal bleeding, the Hestia score for suspected pulmonary embolism and the CURB-65 score for pneumonia. These scoring systems stratify patients as to their suitability for an SDEC management pathway. This supports clinical decision-making but is not a substitute for it. The stratification tools should be readily available for use, with the result recorded in the healthcare records.

Procedures

Some important clinical procedures can be performed, for example lumbar puncture, drainage of pleural effusions, knee aspiration and abdominal paracentesis. These may not be true emergencies, but are needed quickly for therapeutic or diagnostic purposes. Referrals in the evening can be seen the next day for the procedure, with follow-up investigations and referral as individually appropriate.

The procedures should always be carried out or directly supervised by a competent senior clinician. Another benefit of this model is that it is a training opportunity for junior medical staff.

The frail older patient

Frail older people are often admitted to hospital beds, although the clinical presentation with significant functional decline does not suggest serious illness. The involvement of a multi-disciplinary team within SDEC or closely aligned to SDEC can support the patient's needs. For example, an elderly patient who has fallen and fractured the inferior pubic ramus requires analgesia, walking and toileting aids at home and regular home visits until their functional status has returned to normal. This can all be initiated in an SDEC service without hospital admission.

Many SDEC services do not care for confusion or delirium, but some tailor their resources to support management at home.

Alignment with other services

Virtual ward and hospital-at-home services have developed rapidly since the COVID-19 pandemic. These services and SDEC have a similar ethos which is to provide effective safe care close to home. There is significant overlap in respect of
- Patient groups, e.g. frail elderly, chronic respiratory disease
- Clinical skills
- Supporting services

While each of these three services has important individual features, it is important that they operate in a coordinated way, e.g. sharing protocols and guidelines and that the staff have skills to enable them to work across boundaries rather than move the patient between services.

SDEC infrastructure and processes

Location

Many of the lessons concerning the development of SDEC mirror those learned in the development of day surgery.

The unit consists of offices and trolleys and placing it close to the emergency department or acute medicine unit increases referrals. The importance of a specified unit is that it helps the team work toward a culture of supporting patient care at home.

Staffing

Adequate staffing capacity to match the demand for services. Typically, a consultant should be available for 12 h/day with support from junior medical staff. There will be a mix of nurse practitioners, staff nurses and healthcare assistants. Some units combine medical and surgical SDEC by sharing the facilities and nursing staff.

Diagnostic support

Diagnostic support for the SDEC service is needed, for example designated slots for Doppler ultrasound for DVT, CTPAs for suspected pulmonary embolism or an agreement to provide imaging within specified time scales, such as CT head scans within 1 h of request. Others offer a designated number of slots for radiological tests. The time scales for diagnostics need to reflect the overall timescales for the effective operation of the AEC unit; this should include the reporting of any imaging. Many units have individuals trained in the use of ultrasound. Increasingly near patient testing is being used to reduce delays in blood test results.

Pathways and checklists

Local pathways for common clinical scenarios reduce the variability of care and increase speed and efficiency. Exclusion criteria should be minimized.

A safety checklist incorporated into the healthcare records helps to ensure that vital checks are carried out, for example:
- NEWS check
- Pain management
- Cannula check
- Radiology results
- Medication advice

Follow-up arrangements should be agreed.

Table 101.2 Clinical teams in the same-day emergency care network.

- Chronic obstructive pulmonary disease outreach team
- Rapid access chest pain clinic
- Transient ischaemic attack/stroke clinic
- Pleural diseases clinic
- Pain management team
- Falls clinic
- Multi-disciplinary functional assessment team
- Rapid response team
- Diabetes nurse specialist
- Palliative care team
- Heart failure team
- Hospital at home
- Virtual ward

Patient information

Patients should be provided with a simple information booklet explaining the SDEC service, the working diagnosis, treatment plan and follow-up arrangements. The booklet should include what to do in the event of symptom recurrence or treatment complications, with a contact telephone number for in hours and out of hours. This provides a safety net for the patient and feedback for the team.

Networking

The back-up network of services (Table 101.2) should be made aware of the SDEC service, in particular where it is and how it operates. The option of being able to make direct patient referrals especially out of hours and at weekends can significantly improve the quality of patient care. These services contribute to educating the patient about their chronic conditions.

Audit

Audit data should be collected to monitor the AEC unit's safety and effectiveness:
- Outcome metrics:
  - Mortality rate in acute medicine
    - Proportion of patients returning directly to their own home
- Process metrics:
  - Percentage of patients assessed within 15 min of arrival
  - Percentage of patients that have a medical assessment within 60 min
- Balancing metric:
  - Percentage of patients with unexpected re-attending or re-admission within seven days

Further reading

Connolly V, Thompson D. (2014) *Acute Care Toolkit 10: Ambulatory Emergency Care*. London: RCP. https://www.rcplondon.ac.uk/guidelines-policy/acute-care-toolkit-10-ambulatory-emergency-care.

Dean S, Barratt J. (2023) What is the existing evidence base for adult medical same day emergency care in UK NHS hospitals? A scoping review protocol. *BMJ Open* 13(10), e071890. doi: 10.1136/bmjopen-2023-071890.

CHAPTER 102

Hospital at home

ALEX BUNN AND DANIEL LASSERSON

Key points

- **Acute Hospital at Home (H@H) services substitute the need for admission (admission avoidance) or enable earlier discharge from hospital (early supported discharge) by delivering hospital-level processes of care in the home or care home.**
- **Point-of-care (POC) testing (including blood and ultrasound) supports acute medical decision-making within the home.**
- **Intravenous treatments such as antibiotics, fluids, and diuretics, as well as oxygen can be delivered in the home, using regimens that are adapted to the home environment.**
- **Multidisciplinary team working is essential to deliver comprehensive geriatric assessment, as most patients are older and live with frailty.**

Introduction

H@H services offer an alternative care model for patients who traditionally would require acute assessment and treatment of their problems through conveyance and/or admission to a hospital setting. H@H usually constitutes two workflows; avoiding a hospital admission from the offset (named 'admission avoidance') or supporting early discharge from hospital by providing ongoing care in the community. This approach is particularly well-suited for older patients living with frailty who can receive interventions corresponding to their ceiling of treatment, whilst minimising the potential risk of complications faced within inpatient environments such as delirium, nosocomial infection and deconditioning.

A growing body of evidence supports its safety and clinical effectiveness, with clinical trials demonstrating comparable mortality rates to standard hospital care, along with a lower incidence of delirium. Moreover, there is a wider system value, with a reduced likelihood of requiring a transition to residential care in the six months following an acute medical illness. This innovative approach proves to be cost-effective and can offer a more economical alternative compared to in-patient care.

Nonetheless, the decision regarding the location of care for an acute medical illness should be made through an informed choice by patients, their families and caregivers, considering both the benefits and risks associated with hospital-based and home-based care.

Acute Medicine: A Practical Guide to the Management of Medical Emergencies, Sixth Edition.
Edited by Mridula Rajwani, Leila Vaziri, and Ivie Gbinigie.
© 2026 John Wiley & Sons Ltd. Published 2026 by John Wiley & Sons Ltd.

Common acute medical conditions and presenting syndromes treated by H@H

H@H care addresses various acute symptoms and syndromes often associated with underlying frailty, such as:

- Breathlessness
- Delirium
- Diarrhoea and/or vomiting
- Falls
- Functional decline
- New incontinence
- Palliative care support
- Pyrexia

H@H is adept at diagnosing and treating a range of underlying conditions supported by POC testing in the home, including:

- Acute kidney injury
- Atrial fibrillation with a fast ventricular response
- Bacteraemia with an unclear focus (requires collaboration with infectious diseases specialists)
- Cellulitis
- COVID-19 pneumonitis, and other respiratory viral illnesses
- Dehydration
- Electrolyte disturbance
- Heart failure decompensation
- Pneumonia
- Urinary tract infection

H@H services

There are currently no universal benchmarking standards of what H@H services should deliver locally, although supportive policy frameworks without mandating particular processes of care have been developed at the national level. H@H services work closely with existing acute care services, whilst also bridging the interface between hospital and community care as seen in Figure 102.1.

The two main workstreams of H@H services are admission avoidance and supporting early discharge from hospital. Importantly, H@H is distinct from out-patient parenteral therapy (OPAT) or virtual wards (which are purely for remote monitoring without in-person delivery of hospital-level care in the home).

Admission avoidance

Admission avoidance aims to replace hospital admission, and H@H teams should receive direct referrals of acutely unwell patients from clinical staff who have assessed the potential for H@H care including GPs, paramedics, and allied healthcare professionals.

Considerations for H@H assessment, as an alternative to hospital conveyance, should encompass:

- An acute illness syndrome mapping to common conditions treated by the H@H team.
- An advanced care plan stipulating H@H as opposed to hospital-based care.
- Patient-informed decision, ideally supported by family members and/or caregivers.
- Home environment suitable for healthcare delivery, ensuring the absence of any potential safety risks to healthcare staff attending to the patient alone.

Admission avoidance referrals to H@H should provide essential details about presenting symptoms, any available past medical history, vital signs, current medications, and ongoing social care support. Furthermore,

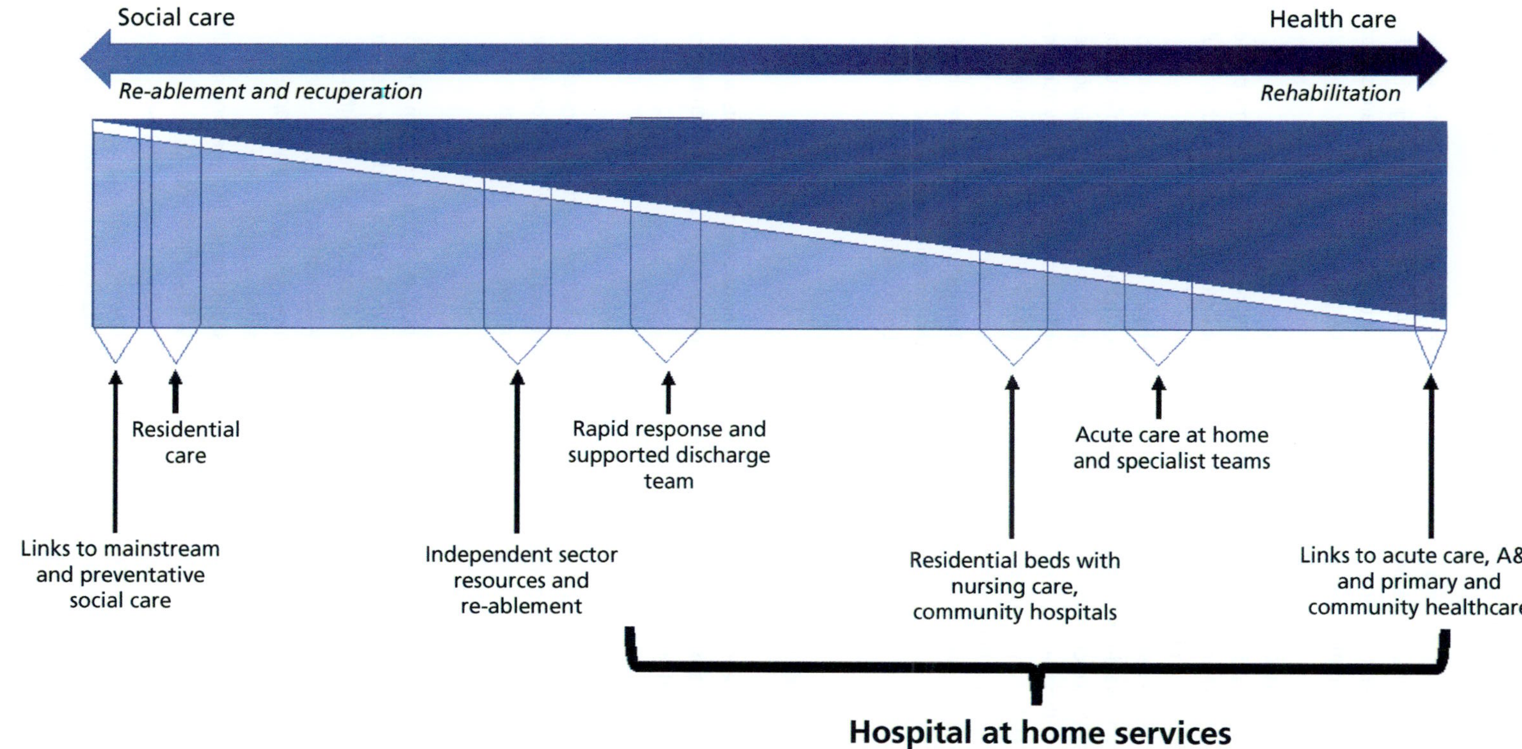

Figure 102.1 The continuum of intermediate care. Source: Adapted from Brophy 2008.

previous advanced care plan decisions and resuscitation status, as this information aids the H@H team in planning the initial visit and determining the need for additional medication or equipment alongside their standard stock.

Syndromes or conditions carrying a high risk of deterioration, especially when an advanced care plan specifies critical care admission, are deemed inappropriate for H@H care. If there is a high risk of deterioration, but the patient prefers, and can receive their ceiling of treatment care at home, H@H care is appropriate when necessary, conversations outline the risks and benefits involved.

Early discharge support

H@H services supporting discharge from hospital generally aim to provide short-term post-discharge care within the patient's own home/residential setting. This care is at a more intensive level than would normally be provided by primary care professionals.

H@H services should receive referrals after an initial hospital-based assessment and treatment, typically from on-call medical teams, ward-based medical teams, or emergency department teams. Early supported discharge H@H requires less reliance on point-of-care (POC) testing, as patients would have undergone extensive diagnostic assessment within their initial hospital assessment. The higher diagnostic certainty at referral enables the referring team to outline an initial medical management plan for the H@H team to execute.

Referrals for early supported discharge H@H should encompass essential information for safe ongoing management in a community setting for an acute medical illness. This includes diagnosis, results of key investigations, a medical management plan, social support, any outstanding investigations and a clarification on whether the medical responsibility is retained by the referring consultant or transitioning to the H@H team's oversight.

Processes of care

H@H patients should receive the same prioritised access to key investigations as patients who are admitted to hospital. This should be a balance between POC tests and if necessary, single-day attendance at hospital for more advanced investigations.

Phlebotomy
- POC tests in the home including blood gases, lactate, glucose, ketones, electrolytes, renal function and CRP.
- Samples taken at home and sent back to the laboratory: Full blood count, liver function, blood cultures, and additional tests as required, e.g. haematinics, thyroid function and paired osmolalities.

Intravenous treatments
- Intravenous fluid can be given for rehydration, usually 1 L boluses of 0.9% sodium chloride or balanced crystalloid over 60 minutes if patients are not hypernatraemic or at risk of circulatory overload.
- For hypernatraemic patients, slow infusions of 'free water' solutions are required: either 5% glucose intravenously, or subcutaneous infusions of 4% glucose/0.18% sodium chloride.
- Intravenous antibiotics guided by the local antimicrobial formulary, pragmatically adapted to the availability of visiting nurses in the H@H team, e.g. use of once or twice daily dosing.
- For antimicrobial stewardship, narrow-spectrum antibiotics should be the first line, and if multiple dosing is required, the use of 24-h infusions should be considered, e.g. flucloxacillin 8 g/24 h.
- Patients with fluid overload requiring high-dose furosemide (e.g. 300 mg) should have infusions delivered using monitored infusion pump devices to ensure accurate infusion rates.
- Most H@H patients can be managed with peripheral cannulae, ensuring the standard daily monitoring for skin reactions is completed, and replaced when necessary. For prolonged intravenous treatment, midlines are preferred.

Imaging

- Point-of-care ultrasound (POCUS) has a major role within H@H care through rapid identification of underlying causes for acute illness syndromes and/or confirming clinical suspicion from physical examination.
- Conditions commonly identified using POCUS include: pleural effusion, pneumonia, COVID-19 pneumonitis, pericardial effusion, reduced left ventricular function, hydronephrosis, urinary retention, ascites, small bowel obstruction and deep vein thromboses.
- Sharing of POCUS images with specialty teams can support the H@H team in management decisions.
- Transfer to hospital may be needed for plain X-ray (e.g. hip fracture post fall), CT scanning (e.g. CT pulmonary angiogram if PE suspected and CT chest abdomen pelvis for suspected metastatic malignancy) or MRI (e.g. suspected cauda equina syndrome). Most patients transferred for such investigations can subsequently continue to receive care at home under the H@H team, with changes in management determined by imaging results.

Respiratory support

- Short-duration oxygen therapy can be given through H@H. If long-term therapy is subsequently needed, a referral should be made to the community respiratory team.
- Portable oxygen concentrators allow flow rates of 4–5L/min and can be used with venturi masks for controlled FiO_2 of 24% or 28%.
- Safety assessments must be made about the use of oxygen in the home (e.g. smoking).
- Nebulised salbutamol and/or ipratropium bromide can be given to support discharge for patients with exacerbations of airway disease.

Specialist investigations

- Other investigations, e.g. gastrointestinal endoscopy should be performed within the same timeframes as if the patient is in hospital. This can be facilitated through same-day emergency care (SDEC) units with H@H teams providing ongoing care afterwards if needed.

Broadening the scope for H@H

Utilising the processes aforementioned, H@H services are increasingly delivering novel patient care pathways, such as:

- Electrolyte replacement for patients with eating disorders, who traditionally are referred to the medical take for intravenous treatment
- Supporting acute oncology in the management of check-point inhibitor complications
- Intravenous fluids and anti-emetics for patients with hyperemesis gravidarum
- Acute paediatrics, for example assessing and managing conditions such as bronchiolitis or gastroenteritis.

Multidisciplinary working in H@H

- When working at the interface between acute and community settings, it is important to develop a H@H workforce that encompasses staff from acute and community backgrounds, in order to benefit from their multidisciplinary skill sets.
- This workforce comprises nurses, doctors, physiotherapists, occupational therapists and clinical pharmacists. Furthermore, this versatile workforce enables the completion of comprehensive geriatric assessments for older adults with frailty who are managed at home.
- Similarly, this person-centred, multi-disciplinary holistic approach is advantageous in assessing patient's functional, medical, social and environmental needs.
- Specialist teams such as heart failure and infectious diseases can support H@H in managing particular patients as appropriate.

H@H communication

- The primary care team should be notified that their patient is currently being managed at home by the H@H team. This notification should occur at the time of referral, for either admission avoidance or early supported discharge.
- Primary care teams may have queries about patients being managed by H@H, therefore, the H@H team should be accessible daily about patients they are currently managing.
- Similar to hospital care, extensive medical documentation is unlikely to be easily accessible by primary care. Therefore, it is imperative that at the point of discharge back to primary care, the H@H team should provide a comprehensive summary of care provided during a clinical episode. This includes; details of assessment and diagnosis, progress during treatment, results of key investigations, changes to existing treatments and medications, plans for necessary further monitoring as well as advanced care planning discussions or changes.

Further reading

Chen H, Ignatowicz A, Skrybant M, Lasserson D. (2024) An integrated understanding of the impact of hospital at home: a mixed-methods study to articulate and test a programme theory. *BMC Health Serv Res* 24(1), 163. DOI: 10.1186/s12913-024-10619-7. PMID: 38308304; PMCID: PMC10835828.

Knight T, Harris C, Mas MÀ, *et al.* (2021) The provision of hospital at home care: results of a national survey of UK hospitals. *Int J Clin Pract* 75(12), e14814. DOI: 10.1111/ijcp.14814.

Levine DM, Ouchi K, Blanchfield B, *et al.* (2020) Hospital-level care at home for acutely ill adults: a randomized controlled trial. *Ann Intern Med* 172(2), 77–85. DOI: 10.7326/M19-0600. Epub 2019 Dec 17. PMID: 31842232.

National Guideline Centre (UK). (2018) Emergency and acute medical care in over 16s: service delivery and organisation. London: National Institute for Health and Care Excellence (NICE). (NICE Guideline, No. 94) Chapter 12, Alternatives to hospital care. Available from: https://www.ncbi.nlm.nih.gov/books/NBK564910/.

National Institute for Health and Care Excellence (2018) Emergency and acute medical care in over 16s: service delivery and organisation. NICE Guideline (NG94)

NICE guideline 82.

Shepperd S, Ellis G, Schiff R, *et al.* (2021) Is comprehensive geriatric assessment admission avoidance hospital at home an alternative to hospital admission for older persons? *Ann Intern Med* 174(11), 1633–1634. DOI: 10.7326/L21-0615. PMID: 34781721.

Singh S, Gray A, Shepperd S, *et al.* (2022) Is comprehensive geriatric assessment hospital at home a cost-effective alternative to hospital admission for older people? *Age Ageing* 51(1), afab220. DOI: 10.1093/ageing/afab220.

CHAPTER 103

Pregnancy-related medical conditions

HANNAH IRVINE AND LUCY MACKILLOP

Pregnant women may present with problems related to pre-existing medical conditions, problems related to pregnancy or unrelated disorders. Achieving good maternal and fetal outcomes requires close collaboration between the medical and obstetric services.

Breathlessness

Breathlessness in the absence of underlying pathology occurs in up to 70% of pregnant women. This can be related to physiological adaptations of pregnancy including reduced residual functional capacity related to diaphragmatic splinting. Pathological causes that should be considered include primary respiratory causes and other non-respiratory causes which include metabolic dysfunction and cardiorespiratory issues (Table 103.1).

Priorities

- End of the bed assessment: if there is cyanosis, distress or a reduced conscious level, get help urgently.
  - Senior anaesthetist input at an early stage is required as intubation of a pregnant woman is particularly difficult.
  - An intensivist, obstetrician and neonatologist (if pregnancy >22 weeks or unsure of gestation) should be contacted.
  - Give high-flow oxygen.
  - Nurse the patient in the left lateral position to avoid vena caval compression by the gravid uterus.
- For women not in extremis, a detailed history should be taken including the onset of symptoms and their relationship to the pregnancy; past medical and obstetric history.
- Use pregnancy-specific normal ranges for investigations so they are interpreted correctly (Table 103.2).
- Do not withhold critical investigations (such as CTPA) or treatment for fear of the effects on the fetus.
- Chest x-ray confers negligible radiation to the fetus at any gestation.

Chest pain/shock

The pregnant patient with shock presents unique medical and management challenges. The differential diagnosis needs to include obstetric complications not often presenting to acute medical services, for example amniotic fluid embolus (Table 103.3). Furthermore, resuscitation of the pregnant woman carries particular challenges, including optimum position of the gravid uterus and potentially difficult airway management.

Table 103.1 Differential diagnosis of breathlessness in pregnancy.

Diagnosis	Key features	Management
Physiological breathlessness of pregnancy	Gradual onset in second/third trimester. Present at rest/talking and paradoxically improves with activity.	Exclude pathology and reassure.
Anaemia	Physiological haemodilution means anaemia is defined as Hb < 105 g/L.	Exclude serious pathology. Check iron status and correct as appropriate. Oral iron given as first line.
Cardiorespiratory causes:		
Asthma	As in non-pregnant, but pregnancy may exacerbate the condition. Reflux can also exacerbate or mimic asthma symptoms.	Manage acute exacerbation as with non-pregnant patient (Chapter 22). Ensure compliance with prescribed medications/effective inhaler technique.
Pneumonia/ Pneumonitis	As in non-pregnant; however, some organisms are associated with particularly severe disease, for example H1N1, VZV, SARS-CoV.	As for non-pregnant. Lower threshold for admission. Use antimicrobial guidelines in pregnancy. If VZV pneumonitis suspected – IV acyclovir. If delivery is within 10 days – neonate needs varicella-zoster immunoglobulin (ZIG)
Pneumothorax	Associated with the valsalva of second stage of labour.	Chest radiography.
Pulmonary embolus	~fivefold increase risk in pregnancy. ~25-fold increase risk immediately postnatal. Sudden onset chest pain (CP), unexplained tachycardia and breathlessness. Signs of right heart strain. Classical clinical features of DVT are much less common in pregnancy therefore need high index of suspicion.	CXR, ECG, ABG. Make the diagnosis with available imaging (Q scan or CTPA); both of which have high negative predictive values and low foetal fetal radiation exposure. Anticoagulate with low molecular weight heparin (LMWH). Consider IV heparin or thrombolysis if cardiovascular instability. Involve obstetricians with timing of delivery. Consider Echo.
Pulmonary oedema	Rare. Associated with tocolytic use, pre-eclampsia or peripartum cardiomyopathy. Shortness of breath with widespread respiratory crackles, peripheral oedema and orthopnoea.	If clinical suspicion, urgent ECG/CXR/Echo. Treat with diuretics/oxygen. Liaise with obstetricians regarding timing and management around delivery.
Peripartum cardiomyopathy	Most common in first month after delivery in older, multiparous black women. Progressive, exertional dyspnoea, orthopnoea, peripheral oedema, fatigue	Involve cardiology early – manage as per pulmonary oedema. BNP/Echo. Avoid late gadolinium MRI in pregnancy unless potential benefits to mother outweigh potential risks to fetus (i.e. pregnant cancer patients). Multidisciplinary team (MDT) decision.
Pulmonary hypertension	Rare but is associated with 25% mortality in pregnancy; needs to be excluded.	Refer to specialist pulmonary hypertension centre.
Heart valve disease	MS can present for the first time in pregnancy (usually in second trimester) with breathlessness/palpitations, tachyarrhythmia, pulmonary oedema or stroke.	ECG, CXR, Echo, BNP Treat if decompensated HF Anticoagulate if in AF, β-blockers once failure treated. Liaise with obstetricians for management plan for delivery.
Other causes		
Amniotic fluid embolus	See chest pain/shock.	Emergency Mx See chest pain/shock.
Metabolic	Starvation ketoacidosis can occur in the third trimester in association with a short duration of vomiting or reduced oral intake.	ABG/Ketones. Treatment is with intravenous glucose/electrolyte replacement. Treat cause of vomiting. Re-establish oral intake.

Table 103.2 Interpreting investigations in pregnancy.

Investigations	Normal values	
	Pregnant	Non-pregnant
Haemoglobin g/dL	105–140	120–150
White cell count ×10⁹/L	6–16	4–11
Platelets ×10⁹/L	150–400*	150–400
Haematocrit	0.3–0.4	0.36–0.47
MCV fL	80–100	80–100
Sodium mmol/L	130–140	135–145
Potassium mmol/L	3.3–4.1	3.5–5.0
Urea mmol/L	2.4–4.1	2.5–7.5
Creatinine µmol/L	44–73	65–101
Bicarbonate mmol/L	18–22	22–28
C-reactive protein (CRP) g/L	0–7	0–7
ESR	Unreliable – high	0–10
D-dimer mg/L	Unreliable – high**	<0.5
pH	7.35–7.45	7.40–7.48
$PaCO_2$ kPa/mmHg	3.6–4.3/27–32	4.7–6.0/35–45
PaO_2 kPa/mmHg	12.6–14.0/94–105	10.6–14.0/80–105
Base excess	+2–2	+2–2
Peak expiratory flow (PEF)	No change	
Forced expiratory volume in 1 second (FEV1)	No change	

* A 10% fall in platelet count maybe expected during pregnancy.

** Difference especially marked in late pregnancy.

Priorities

- Institute advanced life support (Chapter 1).
- Call a senior anaesthetist, intensivist, obstetrician and neonatologist.
- Nurse in left lateral position to avoid vena caval compression by the gravid uterus.
- Give high-flow oxygen and gain intravenous access with large-bore cannulae.
- If output is lost, return patient to the supine position to initiate chest compressions and laterally displace the gravid uterus.
- Peri-mortem caesarean section should be considered within 5 min of loss of output to aid maternal resuscitation.

Headache/seizures (see Chapters 53 and 57)

Headaches in pregnancy and post-partum are a common symptom and although generally benign, can herald a more serious underlying pathology in some cases. (Table 103.4).

Seizures are uncommon in pregnancy, but when they occur, are potentially life-threatening to both mother and fetus (Table 103.5).

Table 103.3 Differential diagnosis of chest pain/shock in pregnancy.

Diagnosis	Key features	Management
Pulmonary embolism	See breathlessness	
Myocardial infarction • **ACS from atherosclerosis** • **Coronary artery dissection**	As in non-pregnant (atypical presentations more common in women).	ECG, troponin (not altered by pregnancy). Medical management (as in non-pregnant), that is primary PCI, except avoid IIb/IIIa inhibitors and statins.
Stroke CVT/SAH/ICH/ infarction	As in non-pregnant	Appropriate imaging depends on availability and most likely cause of symptoms, but MRI is usually preferred after the first first trimester Aspirin and other antiplatelet agents can be given in pregnancy as can UFH and LMWH.
Aortic dissection	Associated with pregnancy particularly in women with Marfan syndrome, Ehlers–Danlos type IV or coarctation of the aorta.	CXR, CT In some cases, a combined caesarean section and surgical repair (if type A and viable fetus) has been performed.
Amniotic fluid embolism	Shock; hypotension/hypoxia Respiratory distress and cyanosis Early and severe bleeding (disseminated intravascular coagulation [DIC])	CXR FBC, PT, APTT High-flow oxygen and respiratory and circulatory support Correct coagulopathy Consider peri-mortem section
Septic shock	Often rapid onset Temp >38 or <36°C HR >100/min RR >20 resps/min WBC <4 or>17 × 10^9/L Clinical signs – fever, rigors, abdominal pain, vomiting, headache, confusion, offensive vaginal discharge	Blood/urine cultures, plasma lactate, FBC, CRP, LFTs, U&Es, procalcitonin IV fluids Antibiotics HVS/LVS, throat swabs and MSU Imaging as appropriate Early transfer to level two critical care. Of note – group A strep is increasing in prevalence
Anaphylactic shock	As in non-pregnant.	Need senior anaesthetist early, as intubation in pregnancy is difficult.

Priorities

- Gather a thorough medical and obstetric history; establish the details of present and previous pregnancies, including the presence of any complications.
- Examination should include blood pressure, urinalysis and neurological examination, including fundoscopy.
- Pregnancy is not a contra-indication to computed tomography (CT), magnetic resonance imaging (MRI) or lumbar puncture.

Table 103.4 Differential diagnosis of headache in pregnancy.

Diagnosis	Key features	Management
Meningitis	As in non-pregnant population	Bloods: FBC, CRP, blood cultures Urgent antibiotics antivirals, consider acyclovir if suspicion of viral encephalitis
Subarachnoid haemorrhage	As in non-pregnant population	CT head Lumbar puncture to look for xanthochromia if CT head negative
Space occupying lesion **Benign intracranial hypertension**	As in non-pregnant population This can present for the first time in pregnancy Papilloedema and raised intracranial pressure (ICP) in the absence of another explanation	Depends on lesion and the presentation Imaging to exclude another cause for raised intracranial pressure Lumbar puncture to measure opening pressure; can be repeated for symptomatic relief Regular assessment of visual acuity and fields To reduce ICP, acetazolamide maybe used (avoid 1st trimester).
Migraine	Features as in non-pregnant population (see Chapter 15) Migraines may improve in pregnancy, however a significant number will still require acute treatment or prophylaxis. Women may develop aura for first time in pregnancy A post-partum exacerbation of headaches is frequently observed in the first 6 weeks	Analgesia Antiemetics Triptans can be used sporadically if they are the only successful treatment for an acute event Prophylaxis: low dose aspirin, propranolol, amitriptyline or greater occipital nerve (GON) block. Avoid ergotamine, pizotifen, valproate, gabapentin and topiramate
Pre-eclampsia or hypertension	Hypertension and proteinuria Other symptoms: visual disturbance, seizures, pulmonary oedema, oliguria, epigastric/right upper quadrant pain, oedema MRI may show posterior reversible encephalopathy syndrome (PRES)	Bloods: platelet count, renal and liver function, sFlt-1/PlGF ratio Antihypertensives IV magnesium sulphate if severe disease present (Table 103.8) Delivery depends on gestation and severity
Intracranial haemorrhage	Sudden onset headache Risk factors include pre-eclampsia or hypertension, trauma, vascular or coagulation abnormalities	Bloods: FBC and coagulation Imaging – CT or MRI Management is neurosurgical and depends on nature of the haemorrhage and underlying aetiology
Cerebral venous sinus thrombosis	Associated with pregnancy (can occur in any trimester) or the post-partum period May be associated with headaches, vomiting, photophobia, reduced conscious level, seizures or signs of raised intracranial pressure On examination focal signs may be present; a low-grade fever is also common	Bloods may show a raised white cell count Imaging – CT or MRI, and venography Thrombophilia screen LMWH or UFH can be used safely in pregnancy and during breastfeeding
Reversible Cerebral Vasoconstriction Syndrome	Thunderclap headache, visual changes, photophobia, vomiting, focal neurological deficit Hx of migraine/pregnancy common. Typically, immediately post-partum Risk of seizures/SAH/ischaemic stroke	Imaging: CT/MRI/angiography – widespread vasospasm Calcium channel blockers

(continued)

Table 103.4 (*Continued*)

Diagnosis	Key features	Management
Drug-related headache	Medication overuse headaches (MOH)- can be caused by regular analgesic use vasodilators such as calcium antagonists (e.g. nifedipine used in treatment of hypertension in pregnancy)	Review use of the likely causative drug
Post-dural puncture headache	Headache occurs within one to seven days of dural puncture Usually postural and is relieved on lying flat Other symptoms: neck stiffness, visual symptoms or seizures (rare)	Conservative management – analgesia, bed rest, maintain good hydration or a blood patch

Table 103.5 Differential diagnosis of seizures in pregnancy.

Diagnosis	Key features	Management
Epilepsy	Increased seizure frequency in ~1/3 patients (even if background of stable disease). Contributing factors include • AED dose reduction because of concerns re teratogenicity • Increased metabolism of AEDs • Precipitants such as sleep deprivation SUDEP Risks; seizure frequency, AED polytherapy, nocturnal seizures	Consider drug level to help guide dose adjustment- Lamotrigine and Levetiracetam may require increased dose (up to 50%) due to decreased plasma levels Management of status epilepticus as in non-pregnant patient Left lateral tilt or manual displacement of pregnant uterus
Eclampsia	May not have been preceded by hypertension, proteinuria or symptoms of pre-eclampsia	
Cerebral venous thrombosis	See headache section	
Intracranial haemorrhage	See headache section	
Thrombotic thrombocytopenic purpura	Features: microangiopathic haemolytic anaemia (MAHA), thrombocytopenia, AKI, fever, and neurological symptoms • often not all features are present	FBC/U+E/LFTs/LDH ADAMST13 levels Initiation of plasma exchange should be considered in all patients with MAHA and low platelets without another obvious cause
Hypoglycaemia	Usually in women taking exogenous insulin Less commonly: acute fatty liver of pregnancy, adrenal or pituitary disease, insulinomas	Parenteral glucose
Hypocalcaemia	Can be associated with magnesium sulphate therapy or hypoparathyroidism	Intravenous calcium (+ECG monitoring) Ensure Vit D replete
Hyponatraemia	Increasingly common Increased fluid intake during labour, oxytocin, pre-eclampsia, undiagnosed Addisons or NSAID use postnatally Headaches, nausea, confusion, reduced conscious levels	Defined as <130 mmol/L Volume status/fluid balance Risk of neonatal hyponatraemia
Drug or alcohol withdrawal	As in non-pregnant population	

Pre-eclampsia and acute fatty liver of pregnancy

The maternal death rate from pre-eclampsia is 0.44 per 100,000 maternities in the UK (MBRRACE-UK report 2023).

ISSHP diagnostic criteria: pre-eclampsia

Pre-eclampsia is gestational hypertension accompanied by one or more of the following **new onset** conditions at > 20 weeks gestation

1 **Proteinuria**
2 **Other maternal end-organ dysfunction, including**
   - Neurological complications (e.g. eclampsia, altered mental status, blindness, stroke, clonus, persistent headache or persistent visual scotoma)
   - Pulmonary oedema
   - Haematological complications (e.g. platelet count $\leq$ 150,000/uL, DIC, haemolysis)
   - AKI (creatinine $\geq$ 90umol/L or 1.1 mg/dL) or oliguria
   - Liver involvement (e.g. elevated transaminases such as ALT or AST $\geq$ 40 IU/L) with or without right upper quadrant or epigastric abdominal pain)
3 **Uteroplacental dysfunction (e.g. placental abruption, sFIT-1:PlGF, fetal growth restriction, abnormal umbilical artery Doppler waveform analysis, or intrauterine fetal death).**

The International Society for the Study of Hypertension in Pregnancy; 2021

Pre-eclampsia complicates 3–5% of all pregnancies and its course is unpredictable. Women with pre-eclampsia often present to maternity services. However, pre-eclampsia should be considered in any woman presenting to acute care services with signs and symptoms suggestive, as undiagnosed or concealed pregnancy is not uncommon.

Acute fatty liver of pregnancy (AFLP) is a distinct condition but it is likely to be related (Table 103.6). AFLP is rare but can cause fulminant liver failure (Chapter 42).

Priorities

Patients with pre-eclampsia or acute fatty liver of pregnancy should be admitted to hospital. If they show features of severe disease (Table 103.7), they should be managed on a high-dependency unit. Supportive resuscitation and prompt delivery are the cornerstone of management in AFLP.

Fluid balance: women with pre-eclampsia are often transiently oliguric but are at increased risk of pulmonary oedema, therefore use caution with fluid resuscitation.

Antihypertensive treatment: hypertension tends to peak three to five days post-partum. Calcium channel blockers, beta blockers and the ACE inhibitor enalapril can all be used while breastfeeding.

Organ dysfunction: in severe disease, organ support such as haemofiltration may be required, but renal function usually recovers. In acute liver impairment (i.e. AFLP) N-acetyl cysteine can be used.

Blood products: may be required depending on the severity of the anaemia, thrombocytopenia or coagulopathy.

Seizure prophylaxis: IV magnesium sulphate as treatment and prophylaxis for eclampsia (see Table 103.8).

Table 103.6 Acute fatty liver of pregnancy.

Element	Comment
Symptoms	Gradual onset (days) of nausea, anorexia and malaise, severe vomiting and/or abdominal pain, polyuria, polydipsia
Examination findings	Hypertension and proteinuria usually mild, RUQ/epigastric discomfort, jaundice or ascites, mild confusion
Blood tests	Leucocytosis, coagulopathy, acute kidney injury, elevated transaminases, hypoglycaemia, elevated urate, elevated ammonia, lactic acidosis
Swansea criteria for diagnosis	The presence of six or more features (in the absence of an alternative diagnosis): Vomiting — Leucocytosis Abdominal pain — Elevated transaminases Polydipsia/polyuria — Acute kidney injury Encephalopathy — Elevated ammonia Elevated bilirubin — Hypoglycaemia Elevated urate — Coagulopathy Ascites or bright liver on ultrasound — Microvesicular steatosis on liver biopsy

Table 103.7 Pre-eclampsia and HELLP syndrome (Haemolysis, Elevated Liver enzymes, Low Platelets).

Element	Comment
Risk factors	First pregnancy, multiple pregnancy, family history, medical conditions such as renal disease/HTN, > 40 years, BMI > 35
Symptoms	Headache, epigastric/RUQ pain, oedema of face or limbs, visual changes, seizures, pulmonary oedema
Examination findings	Blood pressure >140/90 mmHg, proteinuria either dipstick ≥1+, urinary protein:creatinine ratio >30 mg/mmol, oedema, RUQ/epigastric discomfort, hyperreflexia (NB: hypertension and proteinuria may be absent in HELLP syndrome)
Blood tests	Pre-eclampsia: raised uric acid, elevation in transaminases, elevation in creatinine, high sFlt/PlGF ratio, low PAPP-A HELLP (all or some): haemolysis (reduced Hb, increased reticulocytes, reduced haptoglobins, fragments on blood film), low platelets, raised transaminases +/− bilirubin, renal impairment, elevated LDH
Markers of severity	BP: SBP > 160 mmHg or DBP > 110 mmHg CNS: Seizures, visual disturbance, severe headache or >3 beats clonus Hepatic: RUQ/epigastric pain, nausea/vomiting, transaminases > twice ULN CVS: pulmonary oedema Renal: creatinine >100 umol/L; urine output <10 mL/h

Table 103.8 Use of intravenous magnesium sulphate.

Element	Comment
Loading dose	Magnesium sulphate 4 g by slow IV bolus over 5–10 min
Maintenance infusion	1 g/h magnesium sulphate for 24 h, or 24 h after last seizure Omit maintenance infusion if oligo-anuric
Therapeutic level	Aim for Mg level of 2–4 mmol/L
Caution	Caution with concurrent use of calcium antagonists as the use of both can lead to profound hypotension
Observation during infusion	Check reflexes (upper and lower limb) – before treatment, every 30 min for first two hours and then every hour
Management of suspected overdose	Overdose causes muscle weakness, and so if reflexes are absent the infusion should be stopped and an Mg level checked
Antidote	Calcium gluconate 1 g IV

Delivery: This is the only curative intervention for these conditions and should be expedited but only once the mother has been medically stabilized with coagulopathy corrected and blood pressure controlled.

Long-term issues: Lifetime risk of cardiovascular disease is increased in women who develop pre-eclampsia.

Further reading

Acute Care Toolkit- Managing acute medical problems in pregnancy. https://www.rcp.ac.uk/improving-care/resources/acute-care-toolkit-15-managing-acute-medical-problems-in-pregnancy.

Lim E, Mouyis M, MacKillop L. (2021) Liver diseases in pregnancy. *Clin Med (Lond)* 21(5), e441–e445. DOI: 10.7861/clinmed.2021-0497. PMID: 34507927; PMCID: PMC8439517.

Nelson-Piercy C. (2019) I067 Considering pregnancy complications: how to manage pregnancy morbidity in women with rheumatic disease. *Rheumatology* 58(3), kez109.066. DOI: 10.1093/rheumatology/kez109.066.

Nelson-Piercy C. (2020) *Handbook of Obstetric Medicine*, 6th edition. CRC Press. DOI: 10.1201/9780429330766.

Taylor E, Junaid F, Khattak H, *et al*. (2022) Care of pregnant women with epilepsy in the United Kingdom: a national survey of healthcare professionals. *Eur J Obstet Gynecol Reprod Biol* 276, 47–55. DOI: 10.1016/j.ejogrb.2022.06.021. Epub 2022 Jun 30. PMID: 35809458.

Terrault NA, Williamson C. (2022) Pregnancy-associated liver diseases. *Gastroenterology* 163(1), 97–117.e1. DOI: 10.1053/j.gastro.2022.01.060. Epub 2022 Mar 8. PMID: 35276220.

CHAPTER 104

Capacity and consent

KEZIA LANGE

It is an accepted principle that patients have a right to autonomy and self-determination with respect to choices in medical assessment, investigation and treatment (or lack thereof). The role of a physician is to ensure that patients are aware of this and present them with sufficient information, and in such a way, as to promote decision-making. This is at the heart of the physician-patient relationship. There is a competing right, which is that those patients who lack capacity to make a specific treatment decision must be treated in their best interests, ideally after consulting those close to the patient. To ignore the wishes of a patient who has capacity to make a decision, or not to treat a patient who lacks capacity in their best interests, could open the doctor to legal or professional misconduct claims.

Legislation and case law specific to England and Wales are used in this chapter to illustrate principles of capacity and consent which are relevant across a wide range of jurisdictions.

The General Medical Council of England and Wales (GMC) has outlined seven principles of decision-making and consent:

1 All patients have the right to be involved in decisions about their treatment and care and be supported to make informed decisions if they are able.

2 Decision-making is an ongoing process focused on meaningful dialogue: the exchange of relevant information specific to the individual patient.

3 All patients have the right to be listened to, and to be given the information they need to make a decision and the time and support they need to understand it.

4 Medical professionals must try to find out what matters to patients so they can share relevant information about the benefits and harms of proposed options and reasonable alternatives, including the option to take no action.

5 Medical professionals must start from the presumption that all adult patients have capacity to make decisions about their treatment and care. A patient can only be judged to lack capacity to make a specific decision at a specific time, and only after assessment in line with legal requirements.

6 The choice of treatment or care for patients who lack capacity must be of overall benefit to them, and decisions should be made in consultation with those who are close to them or advocating for them.

7 Patients whose right to consent is affected by law should be supported to be involved in the decision-making process and to exercise choice if possible.

There is helpful and specific guidance on how to support patients to make decisions (including the use of independent advocates), how to enlist the support of others in the multi-disciplinary team and how to record decisions.

Capacity

Capacity refers to the ability to make a decision. A patient's capacity may vary with age and circumstance, medical condition and time (even within hours), and so capacity is both time-specific and decision-specific. Patients can regain capacity rapidly (after treatment for hypoglycaemia, for instance) or be unlikely to (e.g. in advanced dementia). It is important not to presume that a person may (or may not) have capacity – a patient with schizophrenia with paranoid delusions may lack capacity to make decisions about their treatment for mental illness, but may have capacity to accept or reject specific treatment for their diabetes.

Although legislation and common law vary across jurisdictions, most follow the same basic 'test' for capacity:

A patient has capacity if they can:

1 Understand the information relevant to the specific decision in question and
2 Retain that information and
3 Use (weigh and balance) the information and
4 Communicate their decision.

In England and Wales, the Mental Capacity Act 2005 (MCA) has codified the common law and, together with its Code of Practice, protects the rights of people from the age of 16 years who lack the capacity to make decisions, and sets out the obligations of staff working with these patients.

It outlines a 'two-stage test':

Is there an impairment or disturbance in the functioning of their mind or brain? This could be anything from a head injury to encephalitis, overwhelming emotion, intoxication or dehydration. It may be temporary or permanent.

If so, has this caused the patient to be unable to make a decision? This is the case if the patient cannot understand, retain and use the information provided, or communicate the decision. An unconscious patient clearly cannot do any of these. A delirious patient might be able to communicate, but not retain or weigh the information. A patient with learning disability might be able to do all of the elements of the test, with appropriate support, time and facilitation of the discussion.

If the patient has an impairment that renders them, on the balance of probabilities, unable to make a decision, then that patient lacks capacity to make that decision.

How (and when) to assess capacity?

A systematic review by Lepping et al. looked at 23 studies that estimated the prevalence of patients lacking capacity to consent to treatment or admission in medical settings. The weighted average proportion of patients who lacked capacity was 34% (95% CI 25–44%). Raymont et al. studied 302 consecutively recruited acute medical in-patients and estimated that 40% did not have capacity to make treatment decisions. Clinical teams, however, tended not to recognise this. It is common that capacity is only assessed when a patient (or family) opposes the treatment suggested, and the MCA legislated to provide safeguards for the 'non-capacitous but compliant' group of patients. It is not unusual to be on an acute medicine ward with patients with dementia who clearly cannot consent to treatment, without any legal basis for their treatment being documented. All physicians should remind themselves to document capacity and make the necessary decisions based on that assessment, in order to comply with the law and professional standards.

Jayes et al. undertook a systematic review of mental capacity assessments undertaken by health and social care professionals in England and Wales which demonstrated that assessment practices varied widely and were not always consistent with the MCA. Capacity assessments were often 'general' rather than decision-specific, presumed lack of capacity based on diagnosis, and did not take into account patients' culture, ethnic or religious backgrounds which might have an effect on their decision-making.

Fundamental to an assessment of capacity is taking the time to speak to your patient (and sometimes others) to understand what support they might need to be able to make a decision and to have exhausted reasonable efforts to do so before concluding they are unable to make a decision (lack capacity). It is also necessary to take all contextual information into account, about their existing beliefs and background but also their physical health history, and their behaviour and expressed wishes since arrival in hospital and ideally before. Clearly, the requirement to consult or take time may well be superseded by a need to intervene immediately and the legislation accepts this necessity in a medical emergency.

Difficult capacity assessments

Whenever there are difficult capacity assessments, or clear disagreement with either patients or carers, colleagues with specialist expertise should be consulted. This might, for example, be a psychiatric liaison team, speech and language therapy team or learning disability specialist service.

Anorexia nervosa

Patients with anorexia who are admitted to acute medical wards are usually significantly medically and psychiatrically unwell. A core symptom of anorexia is the strong cognitive distortion that makes patients believe they are overweight, and that they should not take in calories. This might mean that the patient can understand and retain the information (for instance that they have deranged biochemistry or hypoglycaemia and that this may result in their death if untreated) but state that they would prefer to refuse treatment if it involved, for instance, glucose in their intravenous fluids. What must be recognised is that the core of their disease – the overvalued idea of being overweight – is strongly affecting their ability to use and weigh that information. If they were not suffering from anorexia, would they weigh the information in the same way? They are likely to lack capacity if anorectic cognitions are very prominent. The 'Medical Emergencies in Eating Disorders' (MEED) guidance may be helpful.

Substance misuse disorders

Patients may well lack capacity when acutely intoxicated, but regain capacity to make treatment decisions once they have sobered up. It is under-recognised that a proportion of patients with chronic substance misuse (particularly alcohol) may have significant cognitive impairment and may lack capacity with regards to decisions about issues which affect safe discharge – particularly around finances, accommodation and the decision to continue misusing substances. Social work colleagues are helpful in this situation.

Patients with emotional dysregulation/self-harm

All patients who have been admitted under medicine who have self-harmed, particularly those with a background of emotional dysregulation, should have their capacity assessed on admission and regularly as required. Those who are depressed may lack capacity if the strong negative cognitions common to this disorder affect the way they are able to weigh options (again, you can think of whether the patient would make the same choice if they were not depressed?). Some patients suffer from emotional dysregulation: this is a symptom experienced by many patients suffering from complex post traumatic stress disorder, attention deficit hyperactivity disorder, emotionally unstable personality disorder and autism spectrum condition. These patients may feel overwhelmed (triggered, for example, by sensory issues, memories or feelings of rejection) and may self-harm as a way of managing or wishing to escape these feelings. It is important to recognise that when such patients remain overwhelmed and acutely distressed, they may continue to be at risk of further self-harm, and may lack capacity to make treatment decisions until these feelings reduce in intensity. Complex presentations include patients who dissociate, so appear very calm and may appear to be understanding and using information, but their actions (tying ligatures on the ward, for instance) indicate their on-going distress. It is helpful to discuss such patients early with liaison psychiatry colleagues, or community clinicians who know the patient, if available.

How to manage a patient who lacks capacity

It is not sufficient to document that a patient lacks capacity to make treatment decisions: you should document what the proposed treatment is and when capacity should be reviewed. The MCA requires patients who lack capacity to be treated in their 'best interests'. The treating clinician is the decision-maker unless the patient has a valid Lasting Power of Attorney (LPA) for medical issues, a court-appointed Deputy or advance directive that applies to the current medication situation. There are requirements, other than in an emergency if it is impracticable, to consult the patient's carers and, where necessary, use an independent mental capacity advocate to help guide decision-making. Ill treatment or wilful neglect of a person who lacks capacity has been made a criminal offence under the MCA.

For patients who have longer-term conditions which mean they are unlikely to regain capacity to make treatment decisions, and their care is likely to involve a deprivation of liberty, a 'DoLS' (Deprivation of Liberty Safeguards) order will need to be applied for. The hospital safeguarding or social work team should work alongside the acute medicine team to ensure that there are appropriate procedures in place.

Consent

Consent is the process of obtaining permission from a patient before performing any treatment, examination or investigation. The patient must have capacity to make the decision, and the exchange of information between doctor and patient forms part of the capacity assessment, as well as the process of obtaining informed consent. The GMC provides detailed guidance and refers to providing patients with the 'information they want or need to make a decision', that the information is objective and that doctors should 'be aware of how your own preferences might influence the advice you give'. This is in line with the new medicolegal standard as set by the decision in the Montgomery v Lanarkshire Health Board (2015) case which shifted the test from the whether the doctor's conduct would be supported by a reasonable body of medical opinion (Bolam v Friern Hospital Management 1957) to the 'reasonable patient' test: whether, in the circumstances of the particular case, a reasonable person in the patient's position would be likely to attach significance to the risk, or the doctor is, or should reasonably be, aware that the particular patient would be likely to attach significance to it. Further case law has clarified the need to provide patients with both accurate information and 'adequate time and space' to make a decision as well as giving proper weight to patients' wishes, feelings, beliefs and values. There is an on-going trend in both regulatory and medicolegal advice to reduce medical paternalism and empower patients, with good communication between doctors and their patients being key to consent.

Mental Health Act (MHA)

The Mental Health Act (MHA) 1983 is legislation in England and Wales that provides safeguards for those patients who are detained for treatment of their mental illness, which cannot be provided outside of hospital due to the risks posed to the patient or others. The MHA does not authorise treatment of other illnesses, although there is provision for patients to be treated for the 'direct consequences' of their mental illness (such as in the treatment for anorexia nervosa) in certain circumstances. However, it is unusual for patients to be detained at an acute hospital under the MHA, and the MCA is more usually used. Patients may be transferred from a psychiatric hospital, while detained under the MHA for treatment of a medical illness, and the patient's capacity should be assessed as with any other patient. The effect of the patient's mental illness may or may not influence their capacity to make treatment decisions regarding their medical condition.

Further reading

General Medical Council (n.d.). The seven principles of decision making and consent. Retrieved from https://
www.gmc-uk.org/professional-standards/professional-standards-for-doctors/decision-making-and-consent/
the-seven-principles-of-decision-making-and-consent.

General Medical Guidance: Decision Making and consent Decision making and consent – professional
standards – GMC (updated-decision-making-and-consent-guidance-english-09_11_20_pdf-84176092.pdf).

Jayes M, Pamer R, Pamela Enderby AS. (2020) How do health and social care professionals in England and
Wales assess mental capacity? A literature review. *Disabil Rehabil 42*(19), 2797–2808. DOI: 10.1080/
09638288.2019.1572793.

Lepping P, Stanly T, Turner J. (2015) Systematic review on the prevalance of lack of capacity in medical and
psychiatric settings. *Clin Med (Lond) 15*(4), 337–343. DOI: 10.7861/clinmedicine.15-4-337.

Medical Emergencies in Eating Disorders: Guidance on Recognition and Management. (2023) Royal College
of Psychiatrists. https://www.rcpsych.ac.uk/docs/default-source/improving-care/better-mh-policy/
college-reports/college-report-cr233-medical-emergencies-in-eating-disorders-(meed)-guidance.pdf.

Office of the Public Guardian (2007) Mental Capacity Act 2005 Code of Practice. TSO (The Stationery Office)
2007. https://assets.publishing.service.gov.uk/media/5f6cc6138fa8f541f6763295/Mental-capacity-act-
code-of-practice.pdf.

Raymont V, Bingley W. (2004) Prevalence of mental incapacity in medical inpatients and associated risk
factors: cross-sectional study. *Lancet 364*(9443), 1421–1427. DOI: 10.1016/S0140-6736(04)17224-3.

Practical Procedures

CHAPTER 105

Airway management and upper airway obstruction

MATTHEW C. FRISE

Definitions

Management of the upper airway, which runs from the mouth and nose to the carina, has two fundamental aims
1 **Maintenance of a patent passage for free movement of gas** between the respiratory portion of the lungs and the atmosphere.
2 **Prevention of soiling of the lungs** by vomitus or other material.
   Upper airway obstruction (UAO) is a condition where functional or mechanical factors lead to loss of normal airway architecture and patency, compromising ventilation.

Overview

UAO is a life-threatening medical emergency. Precipitous deterioration may occur without warning, so treatment must be swift. Intervention may need to precede a definitive diagnosis.
   Airway compromise may be
- Functional: due to impairment of consciousness or neurological disease in a patient with an anatomically normal airway. This situation is commonly encountered by the Acute Physician. Simple interventions may be sufficient whilst the underlying problem is identified and treated.
- Mechanical: physical obstruction of the airway by a foreign body, tumour or oedema, for example. Critical care, anaesthetic and ENT expertise are often required, though temporising measures are important whilst help is awaited.
- Due to a combination of functional and mechanical factors: any functional cause of airway compromise may ultimately be complicated by mechanical obstruction, for example aspiration of vomitus in a patient intoxicated with alcohol. Likewise, uncorrected mechanical obstruction eventually results in exhaustion, asphyxia and loss of consciousness.

Obstruction tends to occur at sites of anatomical narrowing and the causes and clinical features differ according to the level, though no sign or symptom is pathognomonic. The time course and degree of obstruction are also important (Table 105.1).

Table 105.1 Clinical features of upper airway obstruction.

Acute partial obstruction

Respiratory distress – dyspnoea, tachypnoea, short sentences, agitation and diaphoresis

Coughing, choking, gagging and altered voice

Grunting and snoring – partial obstruction of pharynx by soft palate or epiglottis

Stridor

Drooling and gurgling

Paradoxical chest wall movements and supraclavicular retraction

Dermal ecchymoses and subcutaneous emphysema – if very forceful respiratory effort

Negative pressure pulmonary oedema – may be misdiagnosed as acute heart failure

Rapid decompensation and progression to complete obstruction

Subacute or chronic partial obstruction

May be almost asymptomatic at rest if develops gradually

Dyspnoea and tachypnoea

Stridor

Voice change

Hypercapnic ventilatory failure

Sudden progression to complete obstruction

Complete obstruction

Inability to breathe and speak

May clasp throat between thumb and index finger to indicate choking

Agitation and panic

Cyanosis

Vigorous respiratory effort becoming feeble as consciousness lost

Respiratory arrest, bradycardia and hypotension followed swiftly by cardiac arrest if not relieved

Differential diagnosis

Any medical cause of reduced consciousness may lead to UAO. Common examples include

- Intoxication: alcohol, opioids, benzodiazepines
- Intracranial haemorrhage, or extensive infarction leading to cerebral oedema
- Hepatic encephalopathy
- Seizures
- Meningitis or encephalitis
- Hypoglycaemia
- Severe sepsis

   Patients with existing **obstructive sleep apnoea** are at particularly high risk.

   Common mechanical causes of UAO are given in Table 105.2.

Priorities

The priority is to maintain or re-establish airway patency to permit adequate ventilation, whilst preventing aspiration.

1 In the specific situation where the patient is conscious and there are features suggestive of **acute severe airway obstruction by a foreign body** (choking), treat according to Adult BLS guidelines with alternating sequences of five intrascapular back blows and five abdominal thrusts.

Table 105.2 Some examples of mechanical causes of airway obstruction in adults.

Oedema
Anaphylaxis
Angioedema – angiotensin-converting enzyme inhibitors, C1 inhibitor deficiency
Post-extubation laryngeal oedema – typically a few hours after extubation
Extrinsic compression
Thyroid masses – benign or malignant
Lymphadenopathy of any cause
Neck haematoma, e.g. arterial puncture complicating central venous access
Tumours of the airway
Laryngeal carcinoma
Tracheal carcinoma
Infection
Retropharyngeal abscess
Ludwig's angina
Laryngitis and epiglottitis
Vocal cord paralysis
Recurrent laryngeal nerve palsy of any cause
Cricoarytenoid disease in rheumatoid arthritis
Trauma
Acute laryngeal trauma
Facial fractures and associated haemorrhage
Thermal inhalation injury to mucosa
Tracheal stenosis following intubation or tracheostomy
Foreign bodies

2 **Give high-flow supplemental oxygen via non-rebreathe mask** whilst making a rapid clinical assessment. The airway may be lost at any time leading respiratory and ultimately cardiac arrest, so do not withhold oxygen due to misplaced concerns about toxicity.

3 If there are any **features suggestive of anaphylaxis** give IM adrenaline 500 µg immediately and summon help. Treat according to Advanced Life Support (ALS) guidelines (Chapter 4). If there is cardiovascular instability raise the legs rather than laying the patient down and **do not instrument the airway** unless suitably experienced. If the patient becomes unresponsive or arrests in the meantime follow ALS guidelines (Chapter 1).

4 **Secure IV access**, ideally large bore. At least two IV access points should be available as rapid-sequence intubation (RSI) may be required.

5 **If the patient is conscious obtain a brief history**; yes/no answers may be all that is possible. Look closely at the thorax, head, and neck for swelling, masses, previous surgical scars (especially from tracheostomy or neck dissection), distended veins or distorted anatomy. **Listen carefully for stridor**. If the features suggest mechanical obstruction summon urgent ENT assistance. Optimise the patient's position and **stay at the bedside**.

6 If the patient is unconscious and has signs of obstruction such as snoring, check the airway is clear of debris, suction if necessary and **manipulate the airway to see if obstruction can be relieved**. Consider an oro- or nasopharyngeal airway. If the patient is breathing place them in the recovery position with adjuncts and supplemental oxygen in situ. If there is concern about a cervical spine injury, use manual in-line stabilisation, but the airway takes priority.

7 **If there is inadequate or absent respiratory effort despite relief of obstruction, ask for the arrest team to be summoned whilst commencing bag-mask ventilation** (BMV) using 100% oxygen. If this is ineffective, insert a supraglottic airway such as a laryngeal mask airway. If still ineffective and more experienced help is yet to arrive, attempt endotracheal intubation only if appropriately experienced. **If at any point cardiac output is lost, follow the ALS algorithm.**

It is essential not to make the situation worse
- Often **simple manoeuvres** are all that are required until more experienced help arrives.
- In certain situations, such as tracheal compression or laryngeal tumours, even **lying the patient flat can be enough to provoke complete UAO and respiratory arrest**. The conscious patient will often try to assume the position that best relieves obstruction - help the patient to do this.
- The use of airway adjuncts and attempted intubation in inexperienced hands may worsen the situation and make subsequent attempts at establishing a definitive airway more difficult. **Attempt the simplest and least invasive maneuverers first** and do so carefully. Use techniques with which you are experienced and confident.
- **Sedative drugs must be used with extreme caution** in patients with possible UAO; sedation before the airway is secured may precipitate respiratory arrest.

Non-invasive techniques
Manual manipulation of the airway
- **Head tilt and chin lift**: may be enough to relieve airway obstruction in a patient with reduced consciousness (Figure 105.1).
- **Jaw thrust**: preferred if there is concern over an unstable cervical spine (Figure 105.2).

Suction
- If vomit, secretions, or other debris are present in the oropharynx these can be removed with a **wide-bore rigid Yankauer sucker**, to relieve obstruction and prevent aspiration.

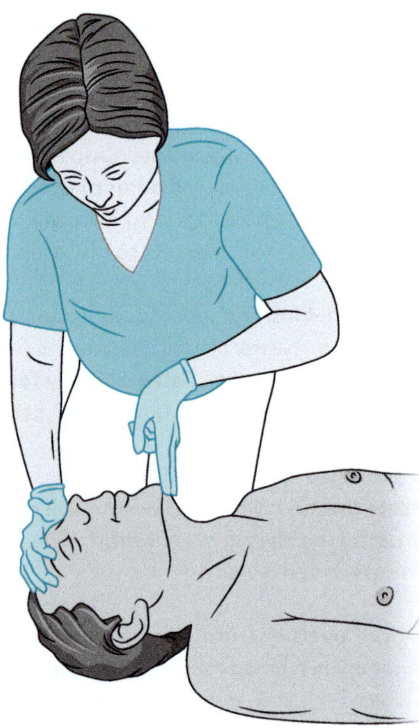

Figure 105.1 Head tilt and chin lift. Source: Taken from 4th edition.

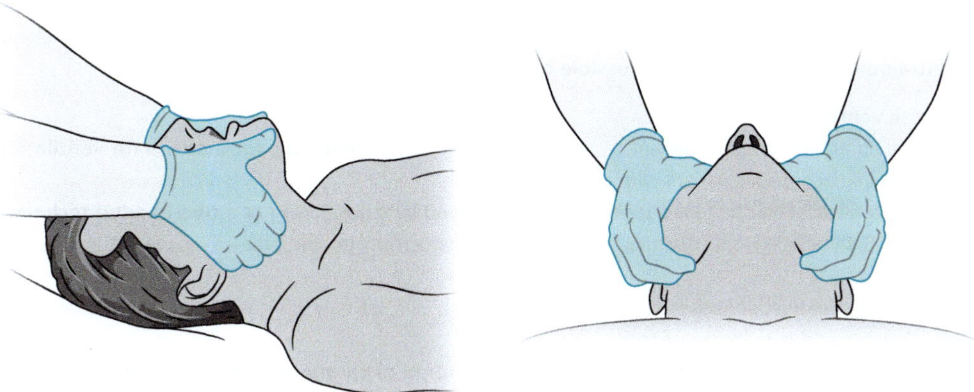

Figure 105.2 Jaw thrust. Source: Taken from 4th edition.

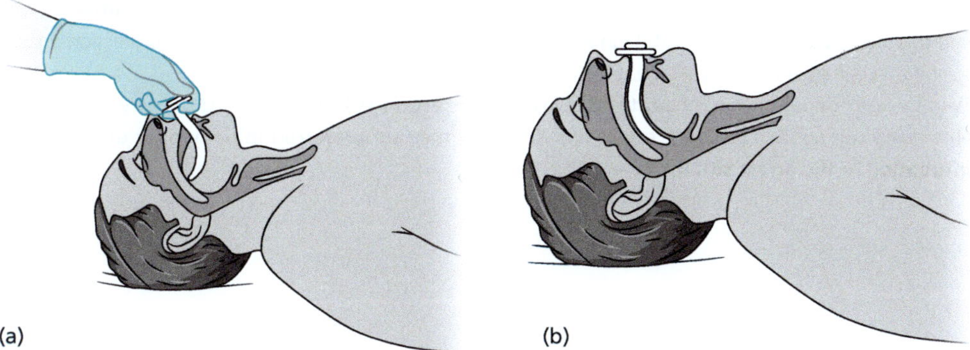

(a)

(b)

Figure 105.3 Insertion of an oropharyngeal (Guedel) airway. The device may be inserted upside-down (a) before rotation into final position (b). Source: Taken from 4th edition.

- A flexible suction catheter can also be passed through an oro- or nasopharyngeal airway.
- Care must be taken not to cause mucosal injury and bleeding; provoking vomiting or laryngospasm are also risks in semi-conscious patients.

Oropharyngeal airways

- **In unconscious patients, obstruction may occur in an anatomically normal airway** due to loss of muscle tone with collapse at the level of the soft palate, epiglottis or tongue base. An oropharyngeal (Guedel) airway may restore airway patency sufficient for spontaneous or bag-mask ventilation (BMV) to be effective.
- The length should be approximately that from the angle of the mandible to the incisors; insert with the concavity facing the palate and rotate 180° into final position (Figure 105.3).
- **Obstruction may be worsened** if the epiglottis is pushed against the laryngeal inlet or the tongue displaced posteriorly; laryngospasm may also result – try a smaller size or nasopharyngeal airway if so.

Nasopharyngeal airway

- As an alternative to the oropharyngeal airway, a soft lubricated tube may be inserted into the nostril. Remember that the floor of the nose is horizontal.

- Often **better tolerated in patients with disturbed consciousness** than the oropharyngeal airway.
- Epistaxis may result, and if too long, laryngospasm and vomiting are risks as with an oropharyngeal airway. **Contraindicated in those with a possible base of skull fracture**.

Bag-mask ventilation

- Rather than an airway management technique per se, this is **a treatment for inadequate ventilation**, usually in an unconscious patient with UAO.
- Inadequate ventilation due to a poor seal can be improved by repositioning or a **two-handed technique** (Figure 105.4); bearded and edentulous patients can be particularly troublesome – keep well-fitting dentures in place.
- Some devices feature a positive end-expiratory pressure (PEEP) valve which is very useful for managing airway obstruction due to laryngospasm.
- **Over-ventilation may cause barotrauma, pneumothorax or cardiovascular compromise** and should be avoided; gastric insufflation increases the risk of vomiting and aspiration. Aim for a tidal volume of 6–10 mL/kg.

Supraglottic airways: laryngeal mask airway (LMA™) and i-gel®

- The LMA is inserted blindly into the oropharynx to sit over the laryngeal inlet. **It is not a definitive airway** and does not allow ventilation with high airway pressures nor provide the same level of protection against soiling as a cuffed endotracheal tube (ETT).
- Even in inexperienced hands, the **rate of successful insertion is high**, making LMAs very useful in the emergency setting. ALS guidance now emphasises that they are **preferred initially over endotracheal intubation in the arrest situation**.

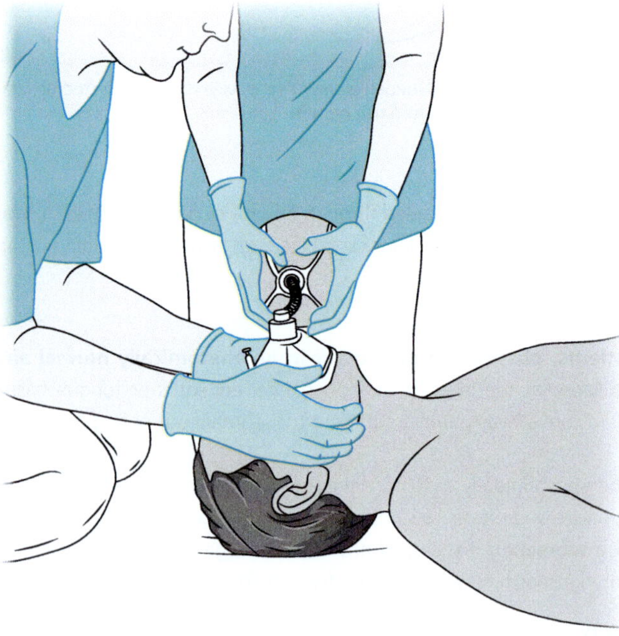

Figure 105.4 Two-person bag-mask ventilation with a two-handed mask technique to achieve a good seal. Note positioning of the patient's head and use of jaw thrust. Source: Taken from 4th edition.

- The i-gel® – like an LMA but with a soft, non-inflatable cuff – is increasingly used in preference to the classical LMA. **Familiarize yourself** with the particular supraglottic airways available on your cardiac arrest trolleys in advance of needing one.
- Supraglottic airways are **not helpful if the level of obstruction is at or below the larynx**.

Medical therapies for mechanical upper airway obstruction

Nebulised adrenaline – sometimes used to treat laryngeal oedema in patients with partial UAO who remain conscious and self-ventilating, based largely on case series in adults, rather than good evidence. A typical dose is 1 mL of a 1 : 1000 solution diluted with saline to 5 mL. It is **not a substitute for IM adrenaline in anaphylaxis**.

Corticosteroids – widely used in adults despite sparse evidence (even in the setting of anaphylaxis). Some studies suggest a reduction in post-extubation laryngeal oedema with prophylactic use. Typically used doses are hydrocortisone 100–200 mg IV or dexamethasone 10 mg IV or IM.

Heliox – a mixture of at least 70% helium in oxygen, heliox **reduces the work of breathing by diminishing turbulent flow** in the partially obstructed airway, but its use may be limited by concomitant lung disease requiring a higher fraction of inspired oxygen. Most research has involved patients with obstructive lung disease, rather than UAO. It is **only a temporising measure and does nothing to correct the underlying pathology**.

Endotracheal intubation

A GCS of ≤8 is often taken as an indication to intubate a patient for airway protection, but this threshold originates from work in trauma patients. Any degree of impairment of consciousness is associated with an increased risk of aspiration, though many medical patients in this category may reasonably be managed in a closely monitored environment with equipment and personnel on hand to intervene if necessary. **Testing the gag reflex is not useful for predicting aspiration risk**.

Endotracheal intubation provides a definitive airway permitting mechanical ventilation (with high airway pressures if needed) and protection from aspiration and is therefore considered a gold standard. However, there are several caveats

- Cardiac arrest: guidance now emphasises the harm that may result from interruption of cardiac massage by repeated intubation attempts; **the LMA is preferred** unless a Critical Care Physician or Anaesthetist is immediately on hand.
- Mechanical UAO: airway anatomy may be seriously distorted leading to **difficult intubation**. The advent of video laryngoscopy has probably improved rates of first-pass intubation, but the decision to sedate, paralyse and attempt endotracheal intubation with direct or video laryngoscopy should only be taken only by a clinician with appropriate expertise.
- The comatose patient: if airway protection is the primary aim, intubation may be straightforward, but **measures to reduce the risk of aspiration during the procedure should be considered**. These include cricoid pressure during an RSI and placement of a nasogastric tube to empty the stomach beforehand, although this has the potential itself to provoke vomiting and aspiration.

If intubation is performed it is essential to confirm correct tube placement by a combination of methods rather than any one in isolation

- Direct visualisation: the tube is seen to pass between the vocal cords.
- Measurement of expired carbon dioxide by capnography: resuscitation trolleys should include indicator devices that can be attached to the endotracheal tube to detect carbon dioxide. Beware false-positive results from initial breaths after oesophageal intubation with an insufflated stomach, and false-negative results in cardiac arrest.
- **Auscultation** over the epigastrium and bilaterally over the thorax.
- Portable CXR: to confirm where the tip of the tube lies and exclude complications such as pneumothorax.

Complications

- Failure
- Oesophageal intubation – devastating if unrecognised
- Laryngeal trauma
- Aspiration
- Cardiovascular instability from laryngeal stimulation and anaesthetic drugs
- Post-extubation airway obstruction
- Laryngeal and tracheal stenosis (late)

The Combitube (oesophageal–tracheal double-lumen airway) has been developed to have the benefits of a cuffed ETT but with easy insertion. It is blindly inserted into the oropharynx and ventilation can be delivered via either of two ports depending on where the device has settled. If unfamiliar with this device it is better to use an LMA.

Further management

Making a diagnosis

Once acute measures to control the airway are in place and any other resuscitation priorities addressed, investigations should be undertaken to determine the underlying diagnosis if this is not already evident. Disorders of consciousness that have compromised the airway should be managed as discussed in Chapter 3. For mechanical UAO several approaches are available

- Fibreoptic endoscopy: allows visualisation of the upper airway under local anaesthesia usually via the nose, but may also be performed orally or via an ETT or tracheostomy. It has the advantage of also permitting **awake fibreoptic intubation** of a patient with UAO who can sit up and cooperate, avoiding the risks of an RSI in this setting.
- Radiographs: plain films of the thorax and neck may be helpful initial tests for demonstrating the location of a foreign body or tracheal distortion and can be undertaken in the resuscitation room without the need to move the patient. These may also reveal evidence of complications such as aspiration, negative pressure pulmonary oedema or pneumothorax.
- CT: in a stable patient who can lie flat, or once a definitive airway has been secured, CT gives excellent cross-sectional imaging of the relevant anatomy and will reveal most pathologies of interest.

Surgical airway

Some causes of UAO, such as anaphylaxis, are reasonably quickly reversible and extubation can be attempted once the patient has recovered from the acute event. If the cause of UAO is one which is not likely to be quickly reversible, such as a laryngeal tumour or bilateral vocal cord paralysis, then it will be necessary to fashion a surgical airway. Formation of a tracheostomy is increasingly undertaken by critical care physicians percutaneously using the Seldinger technique. For the patient with UAO, anatomical considerations may make surgical formation in theatre preferable.

Problems

Transporting the patient

If a patient with a compromised airway and/or impaired consciousness requires transfer to another area, such as for diagnostic imaging, **careful consideration should be given to intubation** beforehand. Doing so in a controlled manner and well-resourced environment of the resuscitation room is far preferable to attempting advanced airway interventions in a CT scanner with limited equipment when the patient has vomited and aspirated. **If a patient with UAO needs to lie flat (and still) for imaging they may require intubation in any event**.

Aspiration of gastric contents

Aspiration pneumonitis is a chemical process resulting from lung injury by gastric acid. In the self-ventilating patient, this requires supportive therapy with supplemental oxygen and possibly continuous positive airway pressure (CPAP). If true aspiration pneumonia develops because of superinfection, antibiotic therapy should be instituted in line with local guidance. Evidence is lacking to support the use of empirical antibiotic therapy in all patients with evidence of aspiration. Aspiration is the commonest cause of death associated with airway management during anaesthesia.

Negative pressure pulmonary oedema

Occasionally the negative pressures generated by vigorous ventilatory effort in the face of UAO can cause pulmonary oedema. Confusingly, this **may develop some hours after relief of the obstruction**, and **misdiagnosis as acute cardiogenic pulmonary oedema or aspiration** is possible. Treatment is with supplemental oxygen and CPAP. Depending on volume status, loop diuretics may be helpful.

The patient with a tracheostomy

Following the national tracheostomy safety project, adult inpatients with a tracheostomy should all have **clear guidance at the bedside** indicating steps to be taken in the event of an emergency – follow these if called to an acutely unwell inpatient.

For patients presenting with signs of airway compromise and a tracheostomy, the priorities are to summon expert help and deliver oxygen by whatever means possible until assistance arrives. General steps are as follows:

1 Give high-flow oxygen **via the stoma and face.**
2 **Remove the inner tracheostomy tube and try to pass a suction catheter** – if it passes easily, suction and leave the outer tube in place. If respiratory effort is poor or lost, ventilate via the tracheostomy (the inner tube may need to be replaced to attach a circuit).
3 **If a suction catheter cannot be passed, deflate the tracheostomy cuff** and see if this relieves the obstruction. If so, leave the cuff down and continue to provide oxygen.
4 **If obstruction persists, remove the tracheostomy** altogether. Occlude the stoma and attempt ventilation from above using BMV with adjuncts or a supraglottic airway. If this fails try ventilation via the stoma using a bag and paediatric mask.

Patients with laryngectomies cannot be ventilated or intubated from above since they do not have an airway above the stoma. For this reason, supplemental oxygen applied to the face will not be helpful. The default position in the emergency setting where the exact anatomy may not be clear is to **apply oxygen to the stoma and the face**.

Can't intubate can't oxygenate

The situation where endotracheal intubation fails and oxygenation cannot be maintained despite ventilation with bag and mask and appropriate adjuncts is well recognised in anaesthetic practice and clear algorithms exist to manage such situations.

Emergency front-of-neck access (FONA) by means of scalpel **cricothyroidotomy** is the approach of choice to re-establish airflow if other interventions fail. A horizontal incision is made through the cricothyroid membrane and a small ETT inserted over a bougie allowing manual ventilation with 100% oxygen. A formal **surgical tracheostomy under local anaesthesia** is also an option if available without delay.

Further reading

Al-Qadi MO, Artenstein AW, Braman SS. (2013) The "forgotten zone": acquired disorders of the trachea in adults. *Respir Med* 107(9), 1301–1313. DOI: 10.1016/j.rmed.2013.03.017.

Eskander A, de Almeida JR, Irish JC. (2019) Acute upper airway obstruction. *N Engl J Med* 381(20), 1940–1949. DOI: 10.1056/NEJMra1811697.

Freund Y, Viglino D, Cachanado M, *et al.* (2023) Effect of noninvasive airway management of comatose patients with acute poisoning: a randomized clinical trial. *JAMA* 330(23), 2267–2274.

Higgs A, BA MG, Goddard C, *et al.*; Difficult Airway Society; Intensive Care Society; Faculty of Intensive Care Medicine; Royal College of Anaesthetists. (2018) Guidelines for the management of tracheal intubation in critically ill adults. *Br J Anaesth* 120(2), 323–352. DOI: 10.1016/j.bja.2017.10.021.

Lighthall G, Harrison TK, Chu LF. (2013) Videos in clinical medicine: laryngeal mask airway in medical emergencies. *N Engl J Med* 369(20), e26. DOI: 10.1056/NEJMvcm0909669.

Ortega R, Mehio AK, Woo A, Hafez DH. (2007) Videos in clinical medicine. Positive-pressure ventilation with a face mask and a bag-valve device. *N Engl J Med* 357(4), e4. http://www.nejm.org/doi/full/10.1056/NEJMvcm071298.

Patel A, Pearce A. (2011) Progress in management of the obstructed airway. *Anaesthesia* 66(Suppl 2), 93–100. DOI: 10.1111/j.1365-2044.2011.06938.x.

Penketh J, Nolan JP. (2023) Airway management during cardiac arrest. *Curr Opin Crit Care* 29(3), 175–180. DOI: 10.1097/MCC.0000000000001033.

CHAPTER 106

DC cardioversion

BOYANG LIU AND SANDEEP S. HOTHI

The management of arrhythmias is described in Chapter 13. Indications, contraindications and potential complications of DC cardioversion (DCCV) are summarised in Table 106.1. Equipment needed is given in Table 106.2. Haemodynamic compromise with tachyarrhythmias at rates less than 130/min should prompt consideration of other causes, such as hypovolaemia, sepsis, pulmonary embolism or heart failure.

Technique in haemodynamically stable patients

Preparation

1 Attach an electrocardiogram (ECG) monitor and record a 12-lead ECG. Check the arrhythmia. General aspects of patient preparation before cardioversion of atrial fibrillation or flutter are summarised in Table 106.3. Consult an anaesthetist for anaesthetic planning and timing. Discuss the procedure with the patient and obtain consent.
2 Insert a peripheral venous cannula, provide supplemental oxygen via nasal cannulae or a facemask, monitor arterial oxygen saturation and check blood pressure. Check that the defibrillator, resuscitation equipment and drugs are to hand.
3 Lay patient down, switch the ECG leads from bedside monitor to the defibrillator. Adjust the leads until R waves are significantly higher than T waves, ensuring that the synchronising marker consistently identifies the QRS complex but not the T wave. Place self-adhesive defibrillator pads over the sternum and cardiac apex. Elevate the bed to ensure easy airway accessibility.
4 The anaesthetist administers general anaesthesia or deep sedation.

Countershock

5 When the patient is anaesthetised, charge the defibrillator and deliver an appropriate charge to cardiovert the arrhythmia (Table 106.4). If initial shock fails, deliver second and if necessary, third shock at higher energy. Before delivering shock, notify all staff of defibrillator charging, instruct to remove oxygen source from patient's chest. Call out again once defibrillator is charged, and actively check that all team members have no direct or indirect contact with the patient before delivering shock.

Aftercare

6 Record a 12-lead ECG. Consider prophylactic antiarrhythmic therapy to maintain sinus rhythm. Document the procedure in the patient's record, including: indications, anaesthetic technique, shocks delivered, any complications, post-procedure rhythm and plan of management.
7 Continue anticoagulation for at least one month (or indefinitely if indicated) post-successful cardioversion of atrial fibrillation or flutter lasting over 48 h duration.

Acute Medicine: A Practical Guide to the Management of Medical Emergencies, Sixth Edition.
Edited by Mridula Rajwani, Leila Vaziri, and Ivie Gbinigie.
© 2026 John Wiley & Sons Ltd. Published 2026 by John Wiley & Sons Ltd.

Table 106.1 DCCV: indications, contraindications and potential complications.

Indications

Conversion of ventricular and supraventricular tachyarrhythmias

Contraindications

When another treatment is better (e.g. pharmacological cardioversion) or there is acceptance of supraventricular arrhythmia with rate control. Seek advice from a cardiologist about the management of haemodynamically stable tachyarrhythmias before cardioversion.
Paroxysmal tachyarrhythmia (arrhythmia will spontaneously resolve and return).
Digoxin toxicity.
Hypokalaemia (plasma potassium <3.5 mmol/L).
Thyrotoxicosis if in atrial fibrillation (cardioversion unlikely to be successful without correction of thyrotoxicosis).

Potential complications

Tachyarrhythmias:
- Ventricular: non-sustained ventricular tachycardia (VT) (5%); sustained VT; ventricular fibrillation (VF; especially if the shock is delivered during repolarisation: its delivery should be synchronized with the QRS complex to avoid R-on-T phenomenon).
- Atrial: SVT (30%), sinus tachycardia, atrioventricular nodal reentry tachycardia (AVNRT), atrial flutter.

Bradyarrhythmias (0.9%) – transient left bundle branch block (LBBB), high degree atrioventricular (AV) block, asystole. These may uncommonly require atropine or temporary pacing whether externally or transvenous. Risk factors: antiarrhythmic drugs.
ST elevation and T wave changes. These are non-specific and by themselves do not indicate an acute coronary syndrome.
Interference with settings of permanent pacemakers and implantable cardioverter-defibrillators (these should be checked post-cardioversion).
Thromboembolism – pulmonary or systemic. More likely in atrial fibrillation or flutter. Incidence is 5.3% if not anticoagulated and <1% if adequately anticoagulated (see Table 106.3). The cause can be dislodgement of exiting thrombus or more usually de novo thrombus due to atrial stunning.
Complications of general anaesthesia/sedation.
Skin burns from shocks – ensure good contact between skin and defibrillator pads; shave hair; consider prophylactic topical hydrocortisone or topical non-steroidal anti-inflammatory drugs (NSAID).
Myocardial necrosis –typically with higher energy levels; usually asymptomatic with mild troponin or creatine kinase-myocardial band (CK-MB) rise.
Myocardial dysfunction – global left ventricular systolic dysfunction (stunning), atrial stunning.
Pulmonary oedema (rare), transient hypotension (often fluid responsive).

Table 106.2 Assistance/equipment.

An anaesthetist and anaesthetic equipment
Defibrillator and resuscitation equipment
Availability of advanced life support medications
One assistant to monitor the patient and help with equipment

Considerations for specific arrhythmias and circumstances

Synchronized DCCV may not be possible (very rapid VT) or dangerous (polymorphic VT) with a risk of VF. In these situations, defibrillation should be performed as there is a risk of inducing VF with synchronized DCCV.

Patients with permanent pacemakers/implantable cardioverter-defibrillator (ICD)/cardiac resynchronisation therapy (CRT) devices – place pads in the antero-posterior position, at least 12 cm from the generator. Use the lowest indicated energy setting. Obtain a device check after DCCV.

Table 106.3 Checklist before DCCV of haemodynamically stable atrial fibrillation or flutter.

Anticoagulation

Arrhythmia reliably known to be of less than 48 h duration:
Moderate-to-high thromboembolic risk patients (CHA$_2$DS$_2$-VASc score ≥1 (males) or ≥2 (females)) should have IV heparin, low-molecular-weight-heparin (LMWH) or direct oral anticoagulant (DOAC) commenced before DCCV and continued long term.
Lower thromboembolic risk patients (CHA$_2$DS$_2$-VASc score = 0 (males) or 1 (females)) do not require anticoagulation prior to DCCV, and four weeks of anticoagulation following successful DCCV is recommended (but may be omitted due to lack of data). Perform bleeding risk vs thromboembolic benefit judgment for very high bleeding risk patients.

Arrhythmia of uncertain duration or more than 48 h duration:
Oral anticoagulation (warfarin with persistent INR ≥2.0, or DOAC) should be given for at least three weeks before, and at least four weeks after cardioversion.
Consider transoesophageal echocardiography (TOE) guidance for patients with under three weeks of pre-DCCV anticoagulation therapy. First commence anticoagulation with LMWH or unfractionated heparin (bolus + infusion for activated partial thromboplastin time (APTT, 1.5–2.0 times control) plus simultaneous oral warfarin initiation; or at least four doses dabigatran 150 mg bd or apixaban 5 mg bd; or a single loading dose of apixaban 10 mg 2 h prior to cardioversion; or five days of warfarin pre-TOE with INR 2.0–3.0 on procedure day. TOE can then guide DCCV after excluding thrombus in left and right atria, their appendages, and the LV. Post-procedural anticoagulation is continued for at least four weeks as per CHA$_2$DS$_2$-VASc score.
INR, international normalized ratio.

Plasma potassium
Check this is >3.5 mmol/L. Correct hypokalaemia before cardioversion (Chapter 52).

Digoxin
Check that there are no features to suggest toxicity (nausea, slow ventricular response, frequent ventricular extrasystoles) and that if the dose is high (>250 µgm/day), renal function is normal.

Thyroid function
Check that thyroid function is normal: cardioversion of atrial fibrillation due to thyrotoxicosis (which may be otherwise occult) is unlikely to be successful.

Tachybrady syndrome
Consider placing a temporary pacing lead or having an external pacing system on stand-by, as asystole or severe bradycardia may follow DCCV.

Nil by mouth
Water up to 2 h before anaesthesia.
Food and other drinks up to 6 h before anaesthesia.

Table 106.4 Cardioversion of arrhythmias: charges.

Arrhythmia	First shock (J)		Second and third shocks (J)	
	Monophasic	Biphasic	Monophasic	Biphasic
Ventricular arrhythmias				
Ventricular fibrillation or pulseless ventricular tachycardia	360	200	360	200
Other ventricular tachycardias	200	100–200	360	200
Atrial arrhythmias				
Atrial fibrillation	200	100–150	360	200
Atrial flutter	100	50–100	200	150
Other supraventricular arrhythmias	100	70–120	200	150

ICD/CRT-D – cardioversion may be performed via the device using a device programmer. This avoids the risk of injury to the device and of skin burns but consumes a significant device battery.

Digoxin toxicity-induced arrhythmias: digoxin toxicity increases the risk of adverse arrhythmias induced by DCCV; its presence is a relative contraindication to DCCV. Correct hypokalaemia, manage nodal or atrial tachycardia conservatively. SVTs: ideally defer DCCV until digoxin levels normalise and use the lowest indicated energy level. VT: consider IV lidocaine pre-shock and use the lowest indicated energy level. Use digoxin-specific antibody only for unstable, life-threatening arrhythmias.

Pregnancy – DCCV can be performed for the mother. Foetal heart rate monitoring is recommended.

Atrial fibrillation due to reversible causes (e.g. infection, pericarditis, post-operative state, pulmonary embolism and hyperthyroidism) may not benefit from immediate DCCV if the exacerbating factor persists, unless there is hemodynamic compromise, due to a higher risk of recurrence or failure.

Further reading

Page RL, Joglar JA, Caldwell MA, *et al.* (2016) 2015 ACC/AHA/HRS guideline for the management of adult patients with supraventricular tachycardia: a report of the American College of Cardiology/American Heart Association Task Force on Clinical Practice Guidelines and the Heart Rhythm Society. *J Am Coll Cardiol* 67, e27–e115.

The Task Force for the management of patients with ventricular arrhythmias and the prevention of sudden cardiac death of the European Society of Cardiology (ESC). (2015) 2015 ESC Guidelines for the management of patients with ventricular arrhythmias and the prevention of sudden cardiac death. *Eur Heart J* 36, 2793–2867. DOI: 10.1093/eurheartj/ehv316.

The Task Force for the management of atrial fibrillation of the European Society of Cardiology (ESC). (2024) 2024 ESC Guidelines for the management of atrial fibrillation developed in collaboration with EACTS. *Eur Heart J* 45, 3314–3414.

CHAPTER 107

Temporary cardiac pacing

CLEMENT LAU AND SANDEEP S. HOTHI

Temporary cardiac pacing is the electrical stimulation of the heart to induce contraction via several routes: transvenous, epicardial, transoesophageal and external (transcutaneous).

Temporary transvenous cardiac pacing

Indications, contra-indications and potential complications of temporary transvenous pacing are summarized in Table 107.1.
- Where permanent pacing is indicated, it should be performed instead, unless delay in achieving this is anticipated or contra-indications to early permanent pacing are present.
- Required equipment is given in Table 107.2. You will need at least one medical or nursing assistant and a radiographer.

Preparation

1 Confirm the indications. Check there is no major contra-indication to central vein cannulation. Decide on the route of venous access. Choose the femoral vein in preference to the internal jugular vein if the patient is haemodynamically unstable or has received thrombolysis. Ensure that a defibrillator and other resuscitation equipment are to hand.
2 Obtain consent, unless the situation precludes this.
3 Connect an electrocardiogram (ECG) monitor and put in a peripheral venous cannula. Give supplemental oxygen, with continuous monitoring of oxygen saturation by oximetry. If sedation is needed, give midazolam.
4 Put on mask, gown and gloves. Sterilise the skin and apply drapes to a wide area. Unpack the pacing lead and check that it will pass down the central venous catheter.

Cannulation of a central vein

5 See Chapter 108 for a detailed description of central vein cannulation.

Acute Medicine: A Practical Guide to the Management of Medical Emergencies, Sixth Edition.
Edited by Mridula Rajwani, Leila Vaziri, and Ivie Gbinigie.
© 2026 John Wiley & Sons Ltd. Published 2026 by John Wiley & Sons Ltd.

Table 107.1 Temporary cardiac pacing: indications, contra-indications and potential complications.

Indications

Bradycardia/asystole (sinus or junctional bradycardia or second/third-degree atrioventricular (AV) block) associated with haemodynamic compromise and unresponsive to atropine (Chapter 13).

After cardiac arrest due to bradycardia/asystole.

To prevent perioperative bradycardia. Temporary pacing is indicated in:

- Second-degree Mobitz type 2 AV block or complete heart block
- Sinus/junctional bradycardia or second-degree Mobitz type I (Wenckebach) AV block or bundle branch block (including bifascicular and trifascicular block) and a history of syncope or presyncope

Atrial or ventricular overdrive pacing to prevent recurrent monomorphic ventricular tachycardia or polymorphic ventricular tachycardia with preceding QT prolongation (torsade de pointes) (Chapter 13).

Contra-indications

Risks of temporary pacing outweigh benefits: for example complete heart block with a stable escape rhythm and no haemodynamic compromise. Discuss management with a cardiologist. Consider using standby external pacing system instead of transvenous pacing.

Prosthetic tricuspid valve.

Complications

Complications of central vein cannulation (Chapter 108).

Cardiac perforation by pacing lead (may rarely result in cardiac tamponade).

Arrhythmias (see below).

Infection of pacing lead.

Table 107.2 Temporary transvenous pacing: equipment.

Temporary pacing lead (a 6 French lead is easier to manipulate than a 5 French one, but its greater stiffness increases the risk of cardiac perforation)

Pacing box and connecting lead

Central vein cannulation pack, central venous sheath (one French size larger than the pacing lead to be used) and ultrasound device for central vein imaging

Suture

Local anaesthesia

X-ray screening equipment

Placement of the lead (Figures 107.1, 107.2 and 107.3)

6 Advance the lead into the right atrium and direct it towards the apex of the right ventricle: it may cross the tricuspid valve easily.

7 If you have difficulty, form a loop of lead in the right atrium. With slight rotation and advancement of the lead, the loop should prolapse across the tricuspid valve.

8 Manipulate the lead so that the tip curves downwards at the apex of the right ventricle and lies in a gentle S-shape within the right atrium and ventricle. Displacement of the lead may occur if there is too much or not enough slack.

9 Ask the assistant to attach the terminal pins of the pacing lead to the pacing box.

Checking the threshold

10 Set the box to 'demand' mode, with a pacing rate faster than the intrinsic heart rate. Set the output at 3 V. This should result in a paced rhythm. If it does not, you need to find a better position. Make sure the problem is not due to loose contacts.

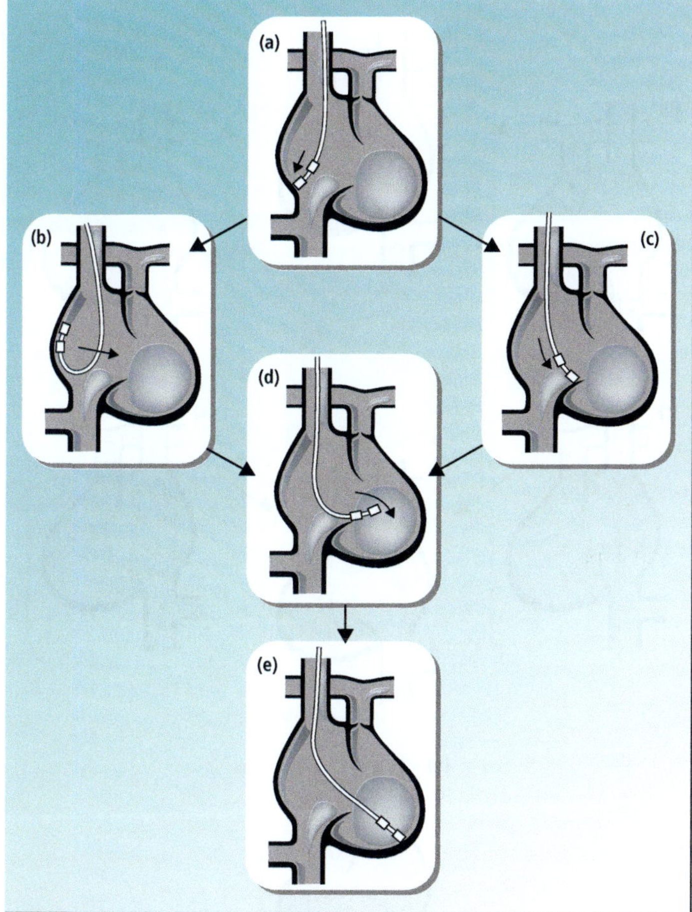

Figure 107.1 Placement of a ventricular pacing lead from the superior vena cava (via the internal jugular or subclavian veins). (a) The lead is advanced to the low right atrium. (b) Further advancement produces a loop or bend in the distal lead, which is then rotated medially. (c) Alternatively, the lead in low right atrium deflects off the tricuspid annulus directly into the right ventricle. (d) Superior orientation of the lead tip in the ventricle requires clockwise torque during advancement to avoid the interventricular septum. (e) Final lead position in the right ventricular apex. The catheter position in (b) is suitable for atrial pacing.

11 Progressively reduce the output until there is failure to capture A threshold of <1 V is ideal. A threshold a little above this is acceptable if the lead position is stable.

12 Check the stability of the lead position. Set the box at a rate faster than the intrinsic heart rate, with an output of 1 V (or just above threshold). Ask the patient to cough forcefully and breathe deeply. Watch the monitor for loss of capture.

13 Set the output at more than three times the threshold or 3 V, whichever is higher. Set the mode to 'demand'. If the patient is now in sinus rhythm at a rate of >50/min, set a back-up rate of 50/min. If there is atrioventricular block or bradycardia, set at 70–80/min (90–100/min if there is cardiogenic shock).

14 Remove the insertion sheath, with screening of the lead and counter-advancement if needed to prevent displacement.

15 Suture the lead (or sheath if left in place) to the skin close to the point of insertion and cover it with an air and water-occlusive dressing.

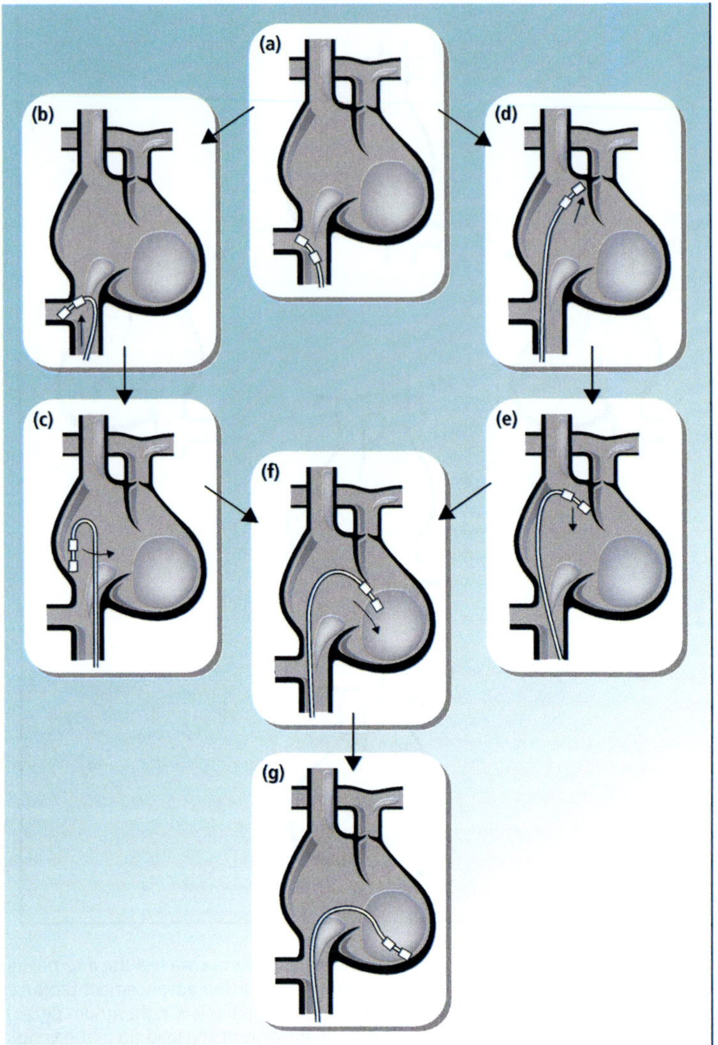

Figure 107.2 Placement of a ventricular pacing lead from the inferior vena cava (via the femoral vein). (a) The lead is advanced to the hepatic vein. (b) The lead tip engages in the proximal hepatic vein and is advanced further. (c) A loop or bend is formed in the distal lead, which is then rotated medially. (d) Alternatively, the lead is advanced to the high medial right atrium. (e) With advancement, a bend is formed in the lead, which is then quickly withdrawn or 'snapped' back to the level of the tricuspid orifice. (f) After crossing the tricuspid valve, the lead is advanced with counterclockwise torque to avoid the interventricular septum. (g) Final lead position in the right ventricular apex. The lead positions in (c) and (d) can be used for atrial pacing. Source: Ellenbogen KA (ed). Cardiac Pacing. Boston: Blackwell Scientific Publications, 1992; 178–9. Reproduced with permission of John Wiley & Sons.

16 Clear up and dispose of sharps safely. Arrange a chest X-ray to confirm satisfactory lead position and exclude a pneumothorax.

17 Document the procedure including: indications/access/threshold/final pacemaker box settings/any complications/post-procedure chest X-ray findings/plan of management.

18 Establish continuous ECG monitoring. Right ventricular (RV) apical pacing results in QRS complexes of left bundle branch block morphology with superior axis (positive in leads I and aVL).

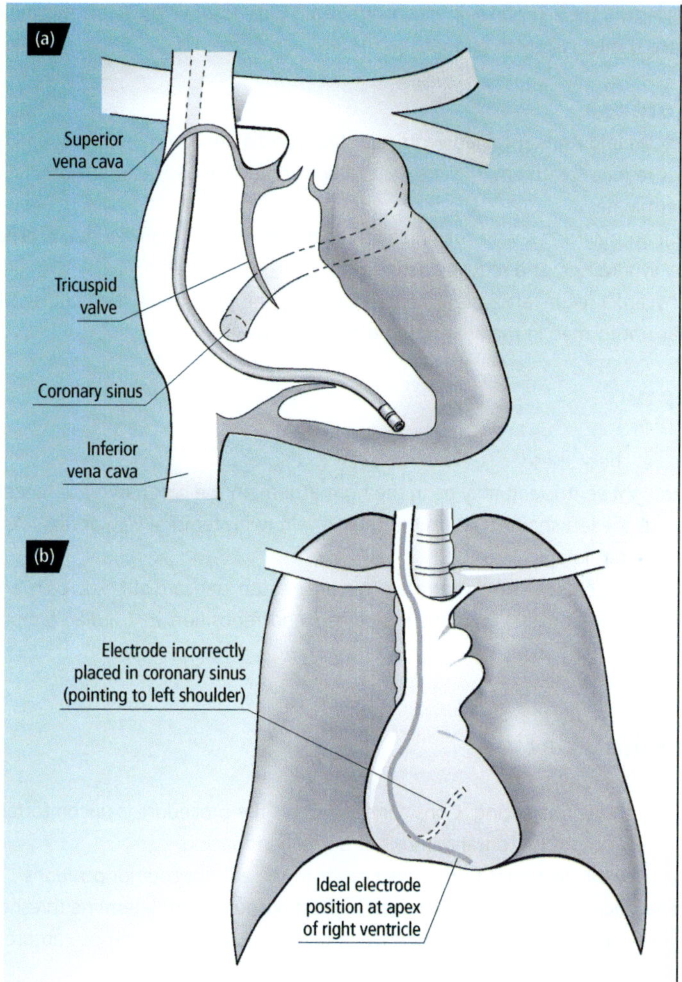

Figure 107.3 Lead position for temporary pacing: (a) anatomy and (b) screening.

Aftercare

19 Check the pacing threshold daily. The threshold usually rises to two to three times its initial value over the first few days after insertion because of endocardial oedema. The commonest reason for failure to capture and/or sense is lead displacement.

20 If infection related to the lead is suspected, seek advice from a cardiologist and microbiologist.

Troubleshooting

The pacing lead cannot be advanced into the heart

This can happen if you have cannulated the carotid artery: the pacing lead bounces off the aortic valve. Ask for advice from a senior colleague or cardiologist. Withdraw the lead and sheath and apply pressure over the vessel to achieve haemostasis.

A pacing lead placed via the femoral vein may keep diving into other veins. Reducing the curve on the end of the lead may make this less likely to happen.

Tachyarrhythmias

Ventricular extrasystoles and non-sustained ventricular tachycardia are common as the lead crosses the tricuspid valve and do not require treatment. If there is sustained ventricular tachycardia, withdraw the pacing lead and it will usually terminate.

Ventricular fibrillation may occur with manipulation of the lead in the right ventricle, especially in patients with acute coronary syndromes, and requires defibrillation.

If ventricular tachycardia recurs after placement, check that the position of the lead is still satisfactory and that excess slack has not formed in the area of the tricuspid valve.

Failure to capture

Causes include

- Contacts not secure: check these.
- Pacing lead not in right ventricle: it may be in the right atrium, in the coronary sinus (a lead in the coronary sinus points towards the left shoulder) or in the splenic vein (with femoral vein access). Ask for advice from a senior colleague or cardiologist.
- Pacing lead has perforated the right ventricle. This may cause pericardial chest pain and diaphragmatic pacing at low output (3 V or less). Withdraw the lead and reposition it. Cardiac tamponade may occur but is rare.

External cardiac pacing

Indications are as for transvenous pacing. Consider sedation as the procedure is uncomfortable: it is therefore more appropriate as a backup prior to transvenous or permanent pacing.

- Apply the large chest wall electrodes to the chest cavity in the anteroposterior positions.
- Connect to external pacing system. Commence at highest output. Then determine threshold by reducing in 5–10 mA steps until the loss of capture. The lowest current output that causes capture is the threshold. Ensure mechanical capture by palpating a pulse.
- Set the device to 5–10 mA above the threshold. Choose pacing mode: demand usually preferable to fixed.
- Change pads every 4–5 h to minimize skin burns.

Further reading

Glikson M, Nielsen JC, Kronborg MB, *et al.* (2021) 2021 ESC Guidelines on cardiac pacing and cardiac resynchronization therapy. *Eur Heart J* 42(35), 3427–3520.

CHAPTER 108

Central vein cannulation

Clement Lau and Sandeep S. Hothi

Indications, contra-indications and potential complications are given in Table 108.1.

Ultrasound should be used when available.

Equipment needed is given in Table 108.2. You will need at least one assistant to monitor the patient during the procedure and assist with the equipment.

Choosing the approach

The internal jugular, femoral and subclavian veins are the veins most commonly used for central access.

- Cannulation of the internal jugular vein is generally associated with fewer complications than with the subclavian vein and is the recommended approach in patients with a bleeding tendency or respiratory failure (greater risk of pneumothorax with subclavian access). The right internal jugular vein is preferable (contralateral to both the thoracic duct and the circulation of the dominant cerebral hemisphere in the right-handed).

- Femoral venous cannulation may be preferred if rapidity of access is paramount (e.g. temporary transvenous pacing lead in a haemodynamically unstable patient), or if central venous access is required during cardio-pulmonary resuscitation. Its drawbacks are a higher rate of infection, venous thrombosis and restricted mobility of the leg.

Ultrasound-guided cannulation of the internal jugular vein

Preparation

1 Confirm the indications for the procedure. Obtain informed consent.
2 Prepare the surroundings and your equipment.
3 Prepare the patient: connect electrocardiogram and oxygen saturation monitors; give oxygen via a mask (which will lift the drape off the face). Lie the patient supine with head-down tilt (Trendelenburg position) unless not tolerated. The head-down tilt is important to reduce the risk of air embolism, particularly for jugular venous access (as opposed to femoral access).
4 Visualize the internal jugular vein with ultrasound. The vein can be distinguished from the artery by compressibility and phasic change with respiration of the former (Figures 108.1 and 108.2). If the internal jugular vein is relatively flat (i.e. central venous pressure is low), head-down tilt or peripheral IV administration (if not contraindicated) may increase its calibre.
5 Open the procedure pack onto the trolley by the bedside. Use an aseptic, non-touch technique.

Table 108.1 Central vein cannulation: indications, contra-indications and potential complications.

Indications

Measurement of central venous pressure (CVP):

- Transfusion of large volumes of fluid required (the fluid itself can be given faster via a large-bore peripheral IV cannula)
- Fluid challenge in patients with oliguria or hypotension
- To exclude hypovolaemia when clinical evidence is equivocal

Monitoring venous oxyhaemoglobin saturation

Cardiac output monitoring with a pulmonary artery catheter

Insertion of a temporary pacing lead (see Chapter 107) or pulmonary artery catheter

Inferior vena cava (IVC) filter placement

Administration of some drugs (e.g. epinephrine, norepinephrine and dopamine) and IV feeding solutions, which must be given via a central vein

Renal replacement therapy and plasmapheresis

No suitable peripheral veins for IV infusion

Pacemaker/cardiac device placement

Contra-indications

Bleeding disorder (including platelet count $<50 \times 10^9$/L, international normalised ratio (INR) >1.5, receiving oral anticoagulant or anticoagulant-dose heparin, during or after thrombolytic therapy): discuss management with a haematologist. If central venous access is needed urgently, before the bleeding disorder can be corrected, use the femoral vein in preference to the internal jugular vein.

Prohibitive anatomic distortion

Local infection

Potential complications

During placement

Arterial puncture or laceration, which in the case of the carotid artery may lead to haematoma formation in the neck, with compromise of the airway. Seek vascular surgical advice.

Pneumothorax (via internal jugular or subclavian vein) or tension pneumothorax

Haemothorax

Cardiac tamponade (can be caused by central venous catheter introduced by any route, if its tip lies below the pericardial reflection and it perforates the vessel wall; least likely via internal jugular vein).

Injury to adjacent nerves

Air embolism

After placement

Infection

Venous thrombosis

Table 108.2 Central vein cannulation: equipment.

Ultrasound machine

Sterile sheath for ultrasound probe and sterile ultrasound gel

Central venous catheter set containing the appropriate catheter length, number of lumens and lumen diameters

6 Prepare the sterile sheath over the ultrasound probe.

7 Reconfirm the location of the internal jugular vein with the sheathed probe.

8 Anaesthetize the skin with 2 mL of lidocaine 1% using a 25 G (orange) needle. Then infiltrate a further 2–3 mL of lidocaine along the planned needle path.

9 While the local anaesthetic is taking effect, prepare the venous catheter. Flush all lumens with normal saline. Leave the central lumen open for passage of the guidewire but cap the other ports. Flush the dilator with normal saline. Ensure the guidewire flows freely from its coil.

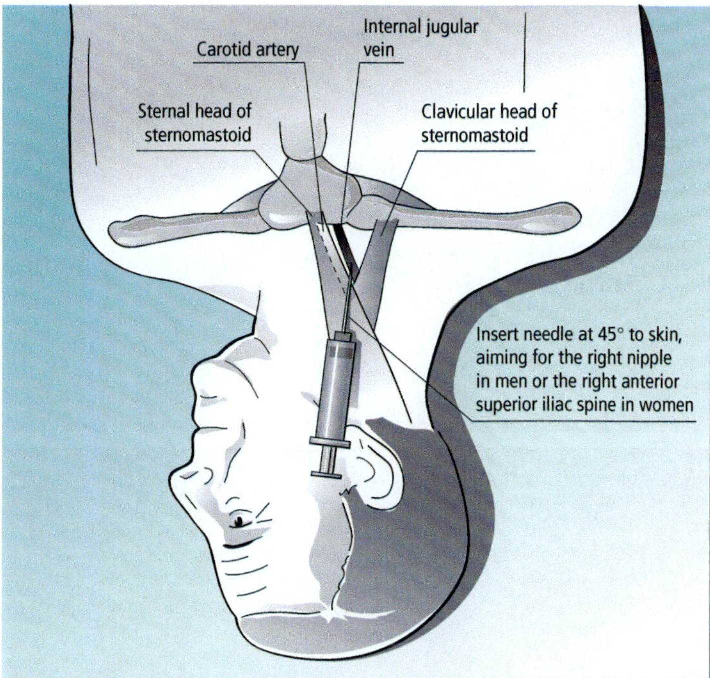

Figure 108.1 Relations of the right internal jugular vein. Ultrasound-guided puncture of the internal jugular vein is the recommended method. Landmark-guided puncture, as depicted, may be chosen in an emergency by an experienced operator.

Venepuncture

10 Mount the needle for the central vein puncture on a 10 mL syringe containing 5 mL of normal saline and flush it.

11 With the syringe and needle in your right hand, puncture the skin upstream of the probe and then stop. Angle the probe in your left hand towards the needle and identify the needle artefact. Slowly advance the needle with continuous gentle aspiration. Venepuncture is indicated by aspiration of venous blood or visualized puncture of the vein. Stop advancing the needle and re-aspirate to confirm you are in the vein.

12 Hold the needle steady in position. Remove the syringe while supporting the needle. Blood should drip from the needle. If it does not, then cover the hub of the needle with your thumb and use a clean syringe to aspirate venous blood. If blood cannot be aspirated, leave the needle in place and rescan the vein. Do not alter the angle of the needle while within the skin/soft tissue – doing so can result in laceration injuries. If you are not sure if the needle is in the vein or the artery, either aspirate blood and check oxygen saturation, or connect to a pressure transducer.

Placing the catheter

13 Having confirmed you are in the vein, pick up the guidewire and gently advance it (J end leading) into the needle and vein. Pass the guidewire to just beyond the 20 cm marking. Withdraw the needle over the guidewire and cover the puncture site with a piece of gauze.

14 Use the blade to make a short incision along the guidewire at the site of skin puncture.

15 Mount the dilator on the guidewire and advance it with gentle rotation and forward pressure to insert it to a depth of 3–4 cm. There is no need to insert its whole length: doing so risks perforation of the vein.

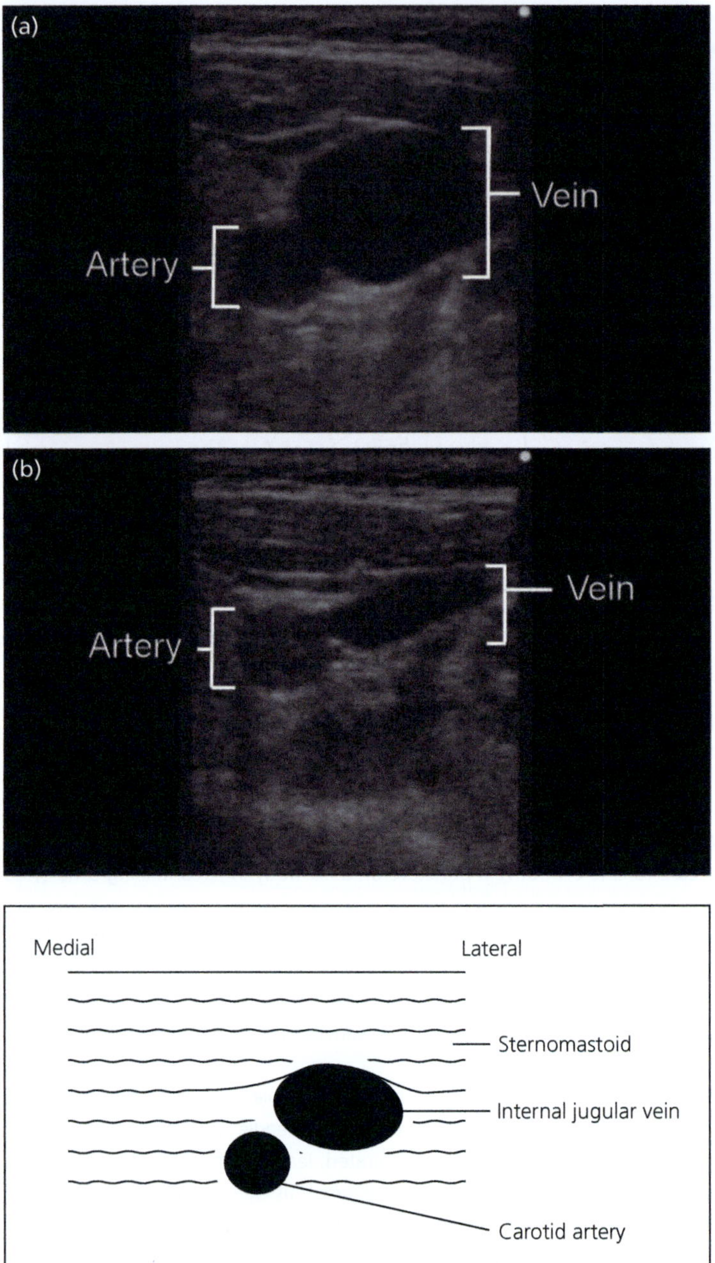

Figure 108.2 Ultrasonography of the right internal jugular vein. Ultrasonography of the right internal jugular vein, before (a) and after (b) compression by the ultrasound probe. The vein can be distinguished from the artery by its compressibility. The depth from the skin to the anterior wall of the vein averages 11 mm (range 6–18 mm). The vein is usually 10 mm in diameter, but its calibre is reduced in volume-depletion. Head-down tilt or volume loading increases the diameter of the vein and facilitates venepuncture.

16 Remove the dilator keeping the guidewire in place and cover the puncture site with gauze. Mount the catheter onto the guidewire and advance it with gentle rotation and forward pressure to an insertion depth of around 12 cm. Aspirate the central lumen to confirm venous blood then flush with normal saline. Close the port with a sterile bung.

17 Apply suture wings to the catheter as it exits the skin and suture in place.

18 Remove the sterile drape from around the catheter, clean the skin and apply a bio-occlusive dressing.

Final points

19 Clear up and dispose of sharps safely. Arrange a chest X-ray to confirm the position of the catheter. The tip of the catheter should be at or above the carina.

20 Document the procedure and post-procedure chest X-ray findings. If the catheter needs to be used immediately, use pressure monitoring to confirm the location is venous before starting any infusion.

Troubleshooting

Frequent ventricular extrasystoles or ventricular tachycardia during procedure may indicate that the tip of the guidewire has passed across the tricuspid valve into the right ventricle: draw it back.

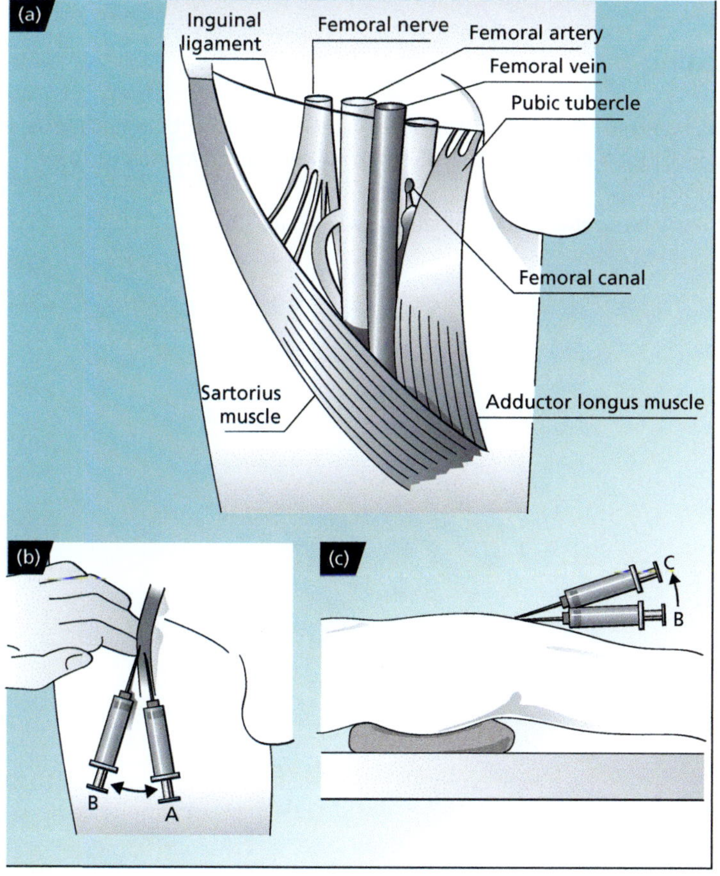

Figure 108.3 Right femoral vein puncture. Panel (a) depicts the anatomy of the femoral vein; and panels (b) and (c), the technique of femoral vein puncture. See text for details. Source: Rosen M, *et al.* (1993) *Handbook of Percutaneous Central Venous Catheterization*, 2nd edn. London: WB Saunders. Reproduced with permission of Elsevier.

Landmark-guided technique for cannulation of the femoral vein

1 Lie the patient flat. The leg should be slightly abducted and externally rotated. Identify the femoral artery below the inguinal ligament: the femoral vein usually lies medially (Figure 108.3). Prepare the skin and drape.

2 Infiltrate the skin and subcutaneous tissues with 5–10 mL of lidocaine 1%. Place two fingers of your left hand on the femoral artery to define its position. Holding the syringe in your right hand, place the tip of the needle at the entry site on the skin. Move the syringe slightly laterally and advance the needle at an angle of around 30° to the skin whilst aspirating for blood.

The above method can be easily performed with ultrasound guidance and this is recommended wherever possible.

Catheter infection

If the catheter is infected the catheter must be removed and the tip sent for culture. Take blood cultures (one via the catheter and one from the peripheral vein) and start antibiotic therapy. Seek a microbiologist's advice.

Further reading

Ortega R, Song M, Hansen CJ, Barash P. (2010) Videos in clinical medicine. Ultrasound-guided internal jugular vein cannulation. *N Engl J Med* 362, e57. http://www.nejm.org/doi/full/10.1056/NEJMvcm0810156.

Smith RN, Nolan JP. (2013) Central venous catheters. *BMJ* 347, f6570. DOI: 10.1136/bmj.f6570.

CHAPTER 109

Intraosseous access

ANN THOMPSON

- Where intravenous access is difficult or impossible in cardiopulmonary arrest the intraosseous route should be considered. The intraosseous route of drug administration achieves plasma concentrations in a time comparable with the intravenous route.
- There are three main insertion sites recommended for use in adults: the proximal humerus, proximal tibia and distal tibia.
- Training in the specific device to be used is essential. This information pertains to the use of the battery powered intraosseous device known as EZ-IO.

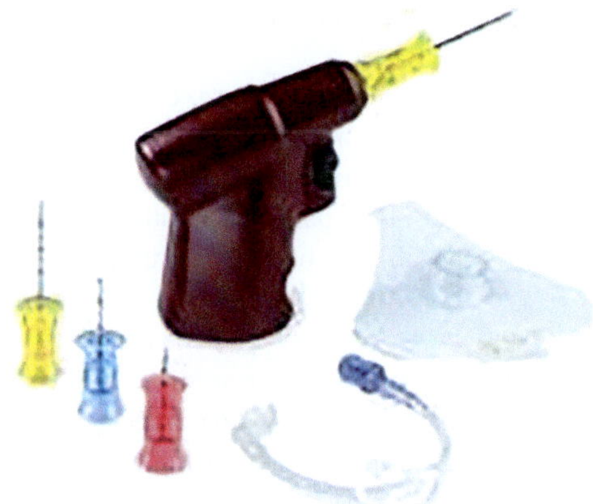

EZ-IO driver with needles, extension set and dressing.

Preparation

1 The IO device should be accessed once a cardiac arrest is declared in order that this is available without delay if needed.
2 The driver should be tested by activating it and ensuring the appearance of a green light on the display.
3 There are three sizes of EZ-IO needle 15, 25 and 45 mm. The selection of needles depends on the size of the patient and the location site. The 45 mm needle should be chosen if siting the needle in the humeral head.
4 The length of the needle to be used should be chosen based on the black graduations on the needle. Once inserted the last black 5 mm line should remain visible outside the skin, this should be estimated in choosing the needle prior to insertion.

Acute Medicine: A Practical Guide to the Management of Medical Emergencies, Sixth Edition.
Edited by Mridula Rajwani, Leila Vaziri, and Ivie Gbinigie.
© 2026 John Wiley & Sons Ltd. Published 2026 by John Wiley & Sons Ltd.

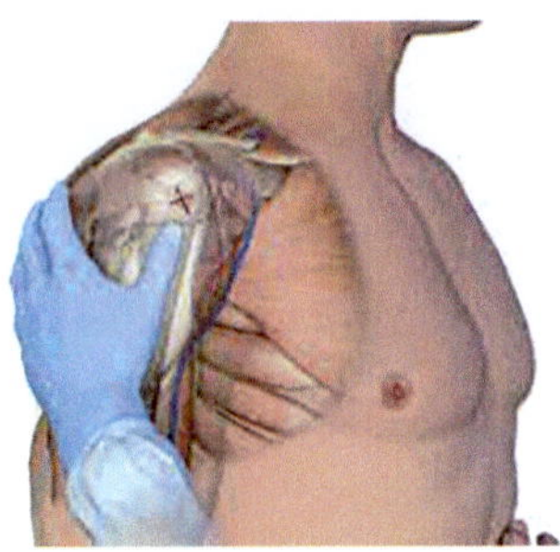 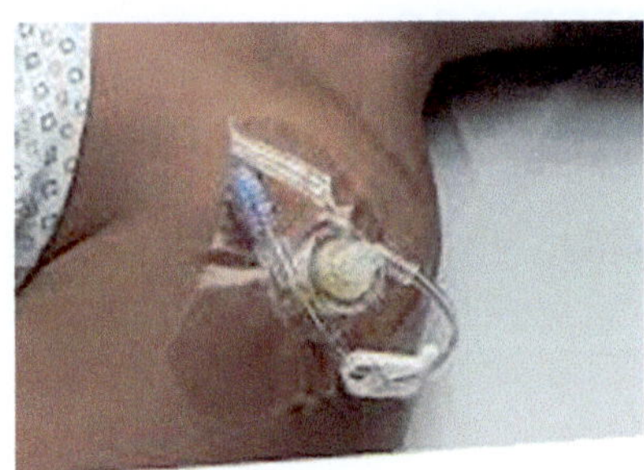

IO access proximal humerus

Technique

1 The chosen area should be cleaned using an alcohol-based solution and the limb stabilised.
2 The needle is attached to the driver, the needle should be inserted through the skin without activating the driver until bone is felt. Once the bone is felt the driver is activated, this is held steady allowing the driver to do the work until a 'give' is felt.
3 Once the give is felt the driver is removed from the needle, check the needle is standing firmly in the insertion site. The introducer is then removed. A syringe should be attached and an attempt made to aspirate fluid from the insertion site. If fluid is aspirated this can be used for blood cultures and a blood sugar. It should not be used for a blood gas. Check with local laboratories about the ability to use this sample for full blood count, the lab must be informed that this sample has been taken from an intraosseous device.
4 The IO is flushed with 10 mL of 0.9%NACL. There may be some resistance felt at this point. Once flushed observe for any swelling or signs of extravasation, if this is seen the needle should be removed.
5 A dressing is attached followed by the extension set. A name label confirming the location of the needle, the time and date of insertion should be attached to the patient's wrist.
6 In using an IO most fluids will need to be pushed in (if the proximal humerus is used fluid may free flow in). All fluids and drugs needed in the context of cardiopulmonary arrest can be administered via the IO route.
7 When removing an IO device a Luer lock syringe should be applied, alignment maintained the needle rotated clockwise while pulling straight up. An occlusive dressing can be placed over the site with the date and time of removal. If a further IO is needed the same limb cannot be used for a period of 48 h.

Contra-indications

Fracture of the bony site, burn on the affected limb, cellulitis or infection of the site, osteogenesis imperfecta, previous IO attempt within 48 h. The presence of osteoporosis is a relative contra-indication.

Complications

Extravasation into the tissues surrounding the insertion site, fracture or chipping of the bone during insertion, dislodgement of the needle, pain related to fluid or drug insertion, fat embolus and infection/osteomyelitis.

Further information and training opportunities

Teleflex Arrow EZ-IO System: https://teleflex.com

Reference

Teleflex Arrow EZ-IO System: https://teleflex.com.

CHAPTER 110

Insertion of an intercostal chest drain

John Corcoran and Adele Crapnell

Indications, contra-indications and potential complications of intercostal chest drain (ICD) insertion are summarized in Table 110.1. One assistant is required to monitor the patient and assist with the equipment (Table 110.2).

- You should only insert an ICD if you have received appropriate training or are being supervised by someone who has been appropriately trained. ICD insertion is potentially associated with significant morbidity and even mortality.
- Whenever possible, the decision to place an ICD, and the type of drain to be used, should be discussed with a chest physician or thoracic surgeon.
- Many patients with symptomatic pleural disease should be managed without an ICD. Often, simple pleural aspiration (thoracocentesis) will suffice and allow the patient to be managed as an outpatient or day case.
- Pleural interventions should not be performed out of hours unless it is a clinical emergency (i.e. a patient with significant physiological compromise and/or symptoms). If an out-of-hours intervention is necessary, it is worth considering whether thoracocentesis will provide adequate treatment and be safer than the insertion of an ICD.
- Pleural interventions should be performed using a full aseptic technique in a dedicated clean room (e.g. procedural suite, operating theatre) to reduce the risk of iatrogenic infection. A procedure should only be performed at the bedside in a clinical emergency when it is unsafe to move the patient elsewhere.
- Informed written consent should be taken from all patients undergoing any pleural intervention unless it is a clinical emergency and the planned treatment may be lifesaving.
- The use of thoracic ultrasonography is strongly recommended. The marking of a site remotely for subsequent thoracocentesis or chest drain insertion in a separate clinical area (e.g. 'X marks the spot' in radiology, prior to chest drain insertion on a medical ward) is not recommended, as it can provide false reassurance and is no more accurate than a 'blind' intervention.
- There is no evidence to support the routine use of thoracic ultrasonography prior to pleural intervention for a pneumothorax. The operator should utilize an anatomical landmark technique (i.e. 'triangle of safety' for ICD insertion, Figure 110.1).

Technique

Preparation

1 Confirm the indications for the procedure. Review the relevant imaging (e.g. chest X-ray) and if appropriate perform thoracic ultrasonography to define the location and anatomy of the effusion.

   Explain the procedure to the patient and obtain written consent where possible (see above).

Acute Medicine: A Practical Guide to the Management of Medical Emergencies, Sixth Edition.
Edited by Mridula Rajwani, Leila Vaziri, and Ivie Gbinigie.
© 2026 John Wiley & Sons Ltd. Published 2026 by John Wiley & Sons Ltd.

Table 110.1 Insertion of a chest drain: indications, contra-indications and potential complications.

Indications

Pneumothorax (see Chapter 28). Chest drain insertion is indicated as the first-line intervention for:
- Pneumothorax in any ventilated patient
- Tension pneumothorax (following on from initial needle decompression)
- Large symptomatic spontaneous secondary pneumothorax
- Large symptomatic recurrent or persistent pneumothorax (following thoracocentesis)

Consider thoracocentesis as the first-line intervention in:
- Symptomatic spontaneous primary pneumothorax of any size
- Small symptomatic spontaneous secondary pneumothorax in patients under 50 years

Pleural effusion (see Chapter 28). Chest drain insertion is indicated as the first-line intervention for:
- Pleural infection, i.e. complicated parapneumonic effusion or empyema (following diagnostic thoracocentesis)
- Symptomatic malignant pleural effusion where the intention is to perform a subsequent pleurodesis
- Traumatic haemothorax

Consider thoracocentesis as the first-line intervention in:
- Pleural effusion of unknown cause, for diagnostic purposes (small volume thoracocentesis, i.e. usually between 20 and 50 mL pleural fluid)
- Large symptomatic pleural effusion for therapeutic purposes (large volume thoracocentesis, i.e. usually up to 1.5 L pleural fluid depending on patient's symptoms)

Contra-indications

Uncertain diagnosis (e.g. emphysematous bulla misdiagnosed as pneumothorax; elevated hemidiaphragm, lung collapse or lung consolidation misdiagnosed as pleural effusion).

Evidence of lung adherent to the chest wall on imaging studies.

Coagulopathy including INR (international normalized ratio) >1.5, platelet count <50×10^9/L, recent use of thrombolytic or anticoagulant therapy; any concerns should prompt discussion with a haematologist before going ahead with the procedure.

Potential complications

Failure of treatment

Pain

Malposition of the ICD

Damage to viscera

Bleeding, including from intercostal vessels, during or following ICD insertion

Infection (wound or intrapleural) following ICD insertion

Drain dislodgement or blockage following ICD insertion

Re-expansion pulmonary oedema following ICD insertion and re-expansion of the collapsed lung

2 Assemble the equipment, including an appropriately sized chest tube, and ensure that any connections fit, e.g. for the underwater seal (Figure 110.2).

3 Connect the patient to appropriate monitoring, including ECG, blood pressure and pulse oximetry. Give supplemental oxygen via nasal cannulae or a mask if indicated. Ensure the patient has venous access.

4 Consider pre-medication with either an opioid analgesic (e.g. morphine 2.5 mg IV) or an anxiolytic (e.g. midazolam 1–2 mg IV), taking care particularly in patients who are elderly and/or at particular risk of respiratory compromise (e.g. chronic obstructive pulmonary disease). Reversal agents (i.e. naloxone or flumazenil) should be immediately available if required.

5 Ensure the patient is comfortable and in a position (Figure 110.3) that allows access to the site where the chest drain is to be inserted. This will usually be within the 'triangle of safety' (Figure 110.1).

6 Put on a surgical hat, mask, gown and gloves. Prepare the skin with chlorhexidine or povidone-iodine and apply drapes.

7 Draw up 20 mL of 1% lidocaine. Generous use of local anaesthetic (up to 3 mg/kg lidocaine), focusing on highly innervated areas such as the skin, periosteum and parietal pleura will reduce the risk of patient

Table 110.2 Insertion of a chest drain: equipment needed.

Surgical hat and mask
Sterile gloves and gown
Antiseptic solution for skin preparation (e.g. chlorhexidine in alcohol)
Sterile drapes
Sterile gauze swabs
Local anaesthetic (1% lidocaine)
Appropriate syringes and needles (18–25 G)
Sutures and dressings to secure the chest drain
Scalpel/surgical blade
Closed drainage system (e.g. connecting tubing, sterile water and kit for underwater seal)
Chest tube of appropriate size (see below) with equipment for insertion using either Seldinger technique or blunt dissection:
* Small-bore chest drains (8–14 French) are sufficient for most pleural conditions (including pleural infection, free-flowing pleural effusion and pneumothorax) and are associated with a lower risk of complications.
* Large-bore chest drains (>14 French) are specifically indicated in the context of, e.g. trauma and haemothorax, and may be useful in cases where the initial use of a small-bore drain has been unsuccessful.

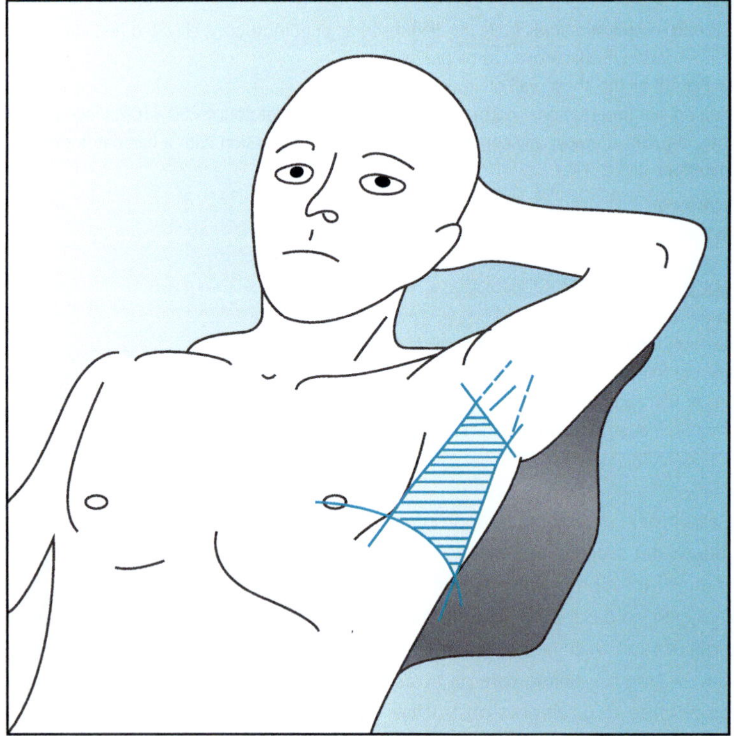

Figure 110.1 The 'triangle of safety'.
The triangle of safety is bordered anteriorly by the lateral edge of pectoralis major, laterally by the lateral edge of latissimus dorsi, inferiorly by the line of the fifth intercostal space and superiorly by the base of the axilla.
Source: BTS Pleural Disease Guidelines (2010) *Thorax* 65 (Suppl. II), ii61–76. Reproduced with permission of BMJ Publishing Ltd.

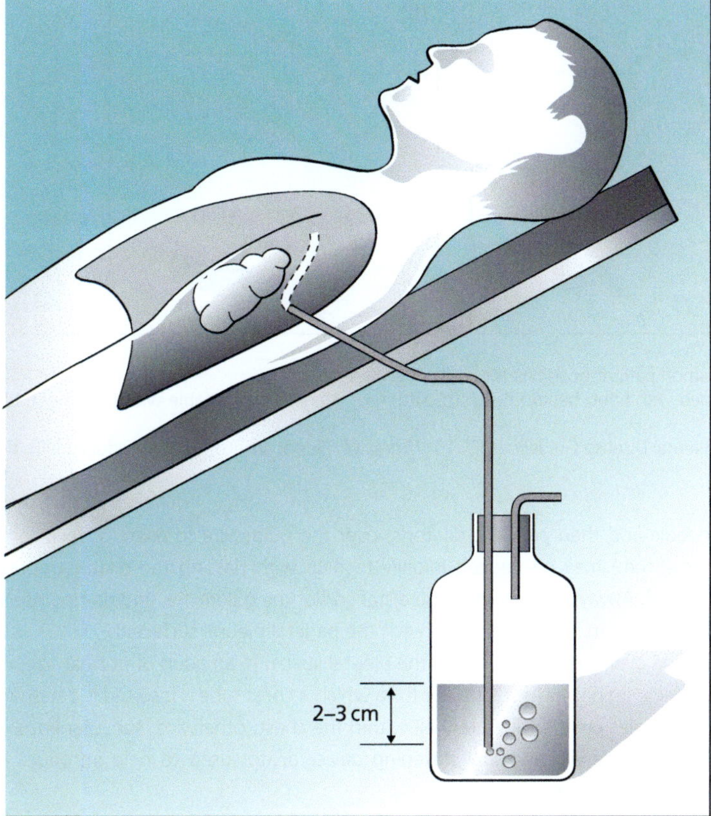

Figure 110.2 Intercostal chest drain attached to underwater seal.
The end of the tube is 2–3 cm below the level of the water in the bottle. If intrapleural pressure becomes negative, water rises up the tube, only to fall again when the intrapleural pressure falls towards atmospheric. The system operates as a simple one-way valve, allowing either air or fluid within the pleural space to drain out safely. Once a pneumothorax or effusion has resolved, the water level will generally be slightly negative throughout the respiratory cycle and reflect the normal fluctuation in intrapleural pressure. Source: Brewis RAL (1985)/John Wiley & Sons.

discomfort during the procedure. Infiltrate the skin with 3–4 mL using a 25 G (orange) needle, then change to an 18 G (green) needle in order to infiltrate the subcutaneous tissues.

8 Advance the needle into the thorax (passing just superiorly to the lower rib of the intercostal space) until air or fluid is aspirated, then withdraw slightly in order to infiltrate 5 mL at the parietal pleural surface. Withdraw the needle completely, infiltrating a further 5–10 mL in and around the needle track as you withdraw. If you have been unable to freely aspirate air or fluid from the pleural space, do not proceed further at this site and seek advice from a senior colleague.

Seldinger technique

9 Advance the introducer needle mounted on a 10 mL syringe into the pleural space (again, passing just superiorly to the lower rib of the intercostal space) and confirm free aspiration of air or effusion. Pass the guidewire, J end first, through the needle into the pleural space; ideally, this should be directed apically for a pneumothorax or posterobasally for an effusion.

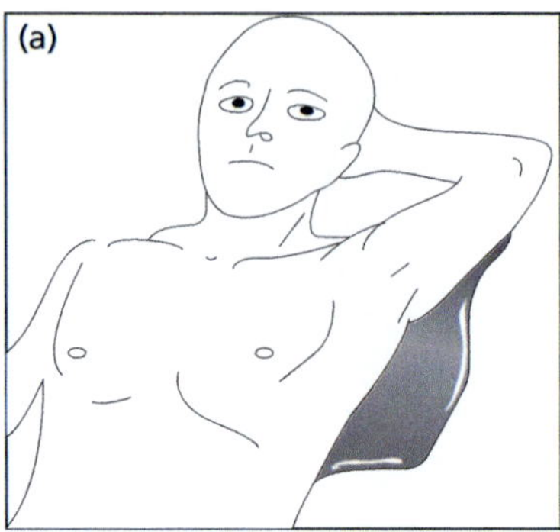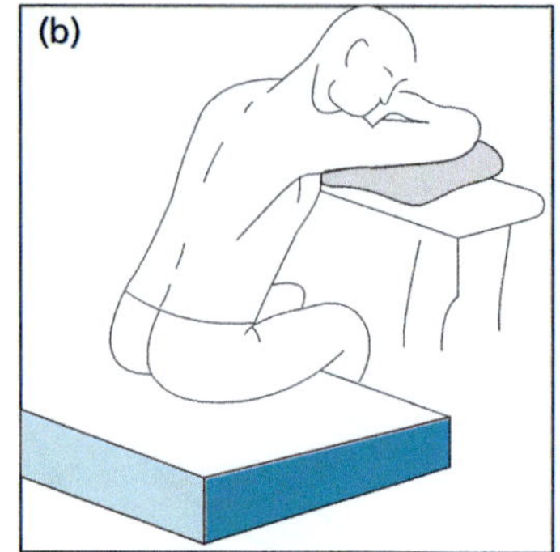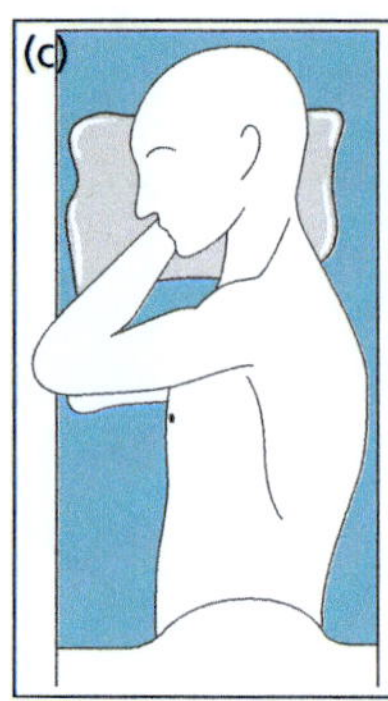

Figure 110.3 Common patient positions for chest drain insertion.
(a) Semi-reclined with hand behind head. (b) Sitting up leaning over a table with padding. (c) Lateral decubitus position.
Source: From BTS Pleural Disease Guidelines (2010) *Thorax* 65 (Suppl. II), ii61–76. Reproduced with permission of BMJ Publishing Ltd.

10 Remove the needle and then pass the dilator(s) over the guidewire to dilate a track for the chest tube. A small incision (5 mm) may be needed initially to help with passing the dilator through the skin and subcutaneous tissue. Always keep hold of the distal end of the guidewire, and do not insert the dilator any further into the chest than is necessary to breach the parietal pleural surface.

11 Pass the chest tube over the guidewire into the pleural space. In an adult of normal size, around 15 cm of drain will usually lie within the chest. The depth to which a chest tube is inserted is determined by the need to ensure the side holes on the tube are well within the chest; otherwise, subcutaneous emphysema will result. Remove the guidewire and any stiffening device/dilator used to help introduce the chest tube, leaving the tube itself in place.

12 Attach the underwater seal bottle to the chest tube.

13 Secure the chest tube in position using a non-absorbable 1/0 suture passed through the adjacent skin and subcutaneous tissues and then wrapped and tied several times around the tube (Figure 110.4). Place a pad of gauze between the patient's skin and the tube, then further anchor the tube to the chest wall using tape or other adhesive dressing.

Blunt dissection technique

The use of small-bore drains (8–14 French) inserted with a Seldinger technique is now the most common mode of chest drain insertion and is sufficient for most effusions and pneumothoraces. Large-bore drains (>14 French) inserted with a blunt dissection technique are used less frequently than before, but are still seen in emergency trauma or thoracic surgical cases.

9a Make a 1 cm incision with a scalpel in line with and just above the edge of the lower rib of the intercostal space. Place two interrupted 3/0 non-absorbable sutures across the incision. These should be left loose so the tube can pass and will be tied when the tube is removed. Place a separate 1/0 non-absorbable suture through the skin and subcutaneous tissues above the incision, which will be used to anchor the chest tube later (Figure 110.4).

10a Using a Spencer Wells or similar straight forceps, enlarge the track down to and through the pleura so that the tube will pass with a snug fit. Note that the forceps should always be removed in an open position during the process of blunt dissection to prevent accidental avulsion of any structures, e.g. blood vessels. Once a track has been created, this should be explored with a finger to ensure there are no underlying organs that might be damaged during subsequent chest tube insertion.

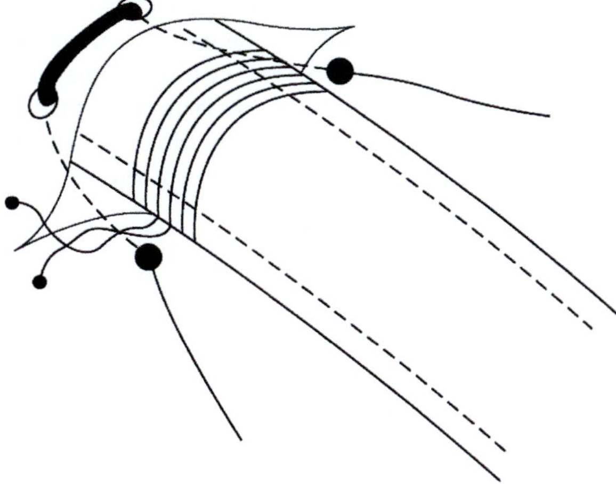

Figure 110.4 Stay and closing sutures for a chest drain. Source: BTS Pleural Disease Guidelines (2003)/BMJ Publishing Ltd.

11a Remove the chest tube from any trocar (a trocar should never be used to guide a chest tube due to the high risk of damaging underlying structures) and, holding the tip of the tube with the forceps, gently pass the tube into the pleural space. The tube should ideally be directed apically for a pneumothorax and posterobasally for an effusion. In an adult of normal size, around 15 cm of the chest tube will usually lie within the chest. The tube must be inserted far enough so that the side holes are well within the chest; otherwise, subcutaneous emphysema will result. Excessive force should never be required during drain insertion – if the tube does not pass easily then withdraw and seek advice from a senior colleague.

12a Attach the underwater seal bottle to the chest tube.

13a Secure the chest tube in position with the 1/0 suture wrapped and tied several times around it. Place a pad of gauze between the patient's skin and the tube, then further anchor the tube to the chest wall using tape or other adhesive dressing.

Final points

14 Remove the drapes and ensure the patient is able to sit up comfortably. Check that the chest tube is well anchored, all connections are secure and the dressings are satisfactory. Clear up and dispose of all sharps safely. Arrange a chest X-ray to check the position of the chest tube. The procedure should be fully documented in the patient's record, including as a minimum: indications; approach; chest tube size; technique used; pre-medication and local anaesthetic used; any complications; post-procedure chest X-ray findings; further management plan.

15 Ensure that the patient has regular analgesia prescribed whilst the chest drain remains in situ; assuming no contra-indications this should include regular paracetamol (1 g four times daily) and non-steroidal anti-inflammatory drugs as a minimum. Opioid analgesia may also be necessary on a regular or as required basis; this should be reviewed daily to ensure the patient is pain free.

Aftercare

16 Small-bore drains (8–14 French) require regular flushing (e.g. 20 mL normal saline three times daily) to prevent them from becoming blocked.

17 If draining a pleural effusion, no more than 1.5 L should be drained in the first hour. After one hour, the rest of the fluid may be drained slowly (e.g. a further 1.0 L every 2–3 h) as clinically indicated. Controlling the rate and volume of fluid drainage in this way is necessary to reduce the risk of causing re-expansion pulmonary oedema. Drainage of fluid should also be stopped immediately if the patient develops worsening cough, chest pain or breathlessness. These symptoms may indicate the presence of unexpandable lung, or predict an increased risk of developing re-expansion pulmonary oedema. Further medical assessment should occur before drainage of fluid is started again.

18 If draining a pneumothorax, the chest tube should never be clamped as long as it continues to bubble, due to the risk of potentially causing a tension pneumothorax. A chest X-ray should be repeated 24 h after chest tube insertion to assess for re-expansion of the lung.

- If the lung has re-expanded fully and the chest tube/underwater seal is no longer bubbling when the patient breathes and coughs forcefully, then this implies resolution of the pneumothorax with no ongoing air leak. It may therefore be appropriate to remove the chest tube in discussion with a chest physician or thoracic surgeon.
- If the lung has not re-expanded fully and/or the chest tube/underwater seal continues to bubble when the patient breathes and/or coughs forcefully, then this implies a continued air leak. In these circumstances it may be appropriate to apply low-pressure, high-volume suction (e.g. using a Vernon–Thompson pump) via the underwater seal at a level of 10–20 cm H_2O. This decision should be made by an experienced specialist clinician, i.e. a chest physician or thoracic surgeon.

19 When removing a chest drain, consider pre-medication with an opioid analgesic. Remove the dressings, then cut and remove the suture which has anchored the drain. The drain should be briskly withdrawn while the patient performs a Valsalva manoeuvre or during expiration. An assistant should apply a gauze swab to the drain site immediately after removal. Small-bore drains inserted using a Seldinger technique do not usually require a suture to close the incision at the insertion site and a simple sterile adhesive dressing will suffice. For large-bore drains inserted using blunt dissection, the two interrupted 3/0 sutures should be tied to close the incision before covering it with a simple sterile adhesive dressing. These closing sutures should be removed after one week.

20 The patient should have specialist follow-up with either a chest physician or thoracic surgeon, ideally within two weeks of discharge from hospital and with a repeat chest X-ray taken prior to the appointment.

Troubleshooting

Pain

- Pain around the site of chest drain insertion is common post-procedure and should be managed with regular analgesia (see above).
- If the pain is distant to the insertion site (e.g. referring to the ipsilateral shoulder) this may relate to the drain tip position. A chest X-ray should be reviewed and if appropriate (e.g. chest tube tip seen to lie against the mediastinum) the tube should be withdrawn slightly.

Fluid level in underwater seal does not move with breathing (not 'swinging')

- Check for kinking of the tube, usually seen due to angulation of the ribs where the tube enters the chest, and if necessary, release the dressings or withdraw the tube slightly.
- Small-bore chest tubes should be flushed regularly as part of routine aftercare (see above) to prevent blockage. Occasionally it may be appropriate to replace a small-bore chest tube that has become blocked with a larger tube, although this should be discussed with a specialist beforehand.

- The drain may be in the wrong position or dislodged – this can be confirmed on either chest X-ray or clinical assessment (e.g. drainage holes may be partially or wholly extrapleural), in which case the tube should be removed and replaced with another if clinically necessary.

Surgical emphysema

- It is normal to have a small amount of localized subcutaneous air at the drain insertion site.
- Increasing surgical emphysema may indicate malposition of the tube with a drainage hole in a subcutaneous position; if so, a new tube must be inserted.

Non-resolving pneumothorax

- This may present as failure of the lung to re-expand following chest tube insertion and/or continued bubbling from the chest tube/underwater seal. Assuming the chest tube is well positioned and patent, this indicates an ongoing air leak from the underlying lung parenchyma.
- Some cases may resolve with application of suction (see above), but all patients with a non-resolving pneumothorax should be discussed with an appropriate specialist (chest physician or thoracic surgeon).

Further reading

British Thoracic Society Clinical Statement on pleural procedures, published in 2023 - please see https://thorax.bmj.com/content/78/Suppl_3/s43.long and/or https://www.brit-thoracic.org.uk/document-library/clinical-statements/pleural-procedures/bts-clinical-statement-on-pleural-procedures/.

Corcoran JP, Hallifax RJ, Talwar A, *et al.* (2015) Intercostal chest drain insertion by general physicians: attitudes, experience and implications for training, service and patient safety. *Postgrad Med J* 91, 244–250.

CHAPTER 111

Aspiration of the knee joint

Kehinde Sunmboye

The indications, contraindications and potential complications of knee joint aspiration are summarized in Table 111.1. If you are not familiar with joint aspiration, ask the help of a rheumatologist or orthopaedic surgeon.

Technique

1 Confirm the indications for joint aspiration. Explain the procedure to the patient and obtain consent. Verbal consent is sufficient.
2 The patient should lie down with the knee slightly flexed. The knee joint can be aspirated from the medial or lateral side. The needle should pass from a skin entry point 1 cm medial or lateral to the superior, middle or inferior third of the patella (see Figure 111.1). Points marked with X medially and laterally are the preferred entry sites due to the proximity to the suprapatellar pouch where effusions usually accumulate. Check the bony landmarks and mark the skin entry point with the tip of the needle cover.
3 Put on gloves. Prepare the skin with chlorhexidine or povidone-iodine. Anaesthetize the skin with 2 mL of lidocaine 1% using a 25 G (orange) needle. Then infiltrate a further 5 mL of lidocaine along the planned needle path.

Table 111.1 Aspiration of a knee joint: indications, contraindications and potential complications.

Indications
To confirm or exclude septic arthritis
To establish the diagnosis of acute mono- or polyarthritis
To relieve symptoms from a tense effusion by draining the joint

Contraindications
Cellulitis of overlying skin
Bleeding disorder (including platelet count $<50 \times 10^9$/L, INR >2 or receiving anticoagulant-dose heparin).
Liaise with haematologist as indicated.

Potential complications
Introduction of infection rarely occurs (<1/10,000) with appropriate sterile technique
Bleeding into the joint in patients with bleeding disorder
Cartilage injury

INR, international normalized ratio.

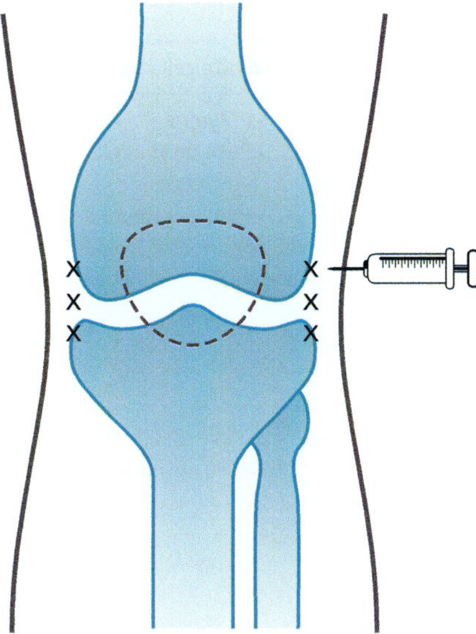

Figure 111.1 Points of needle entry (marked X) for aspiration of the knee joint.

4 Give the local anaesthetic time to work. Mount a 21 G (green) needle on a 20 mL syringe and then advance along the anaesthetized path, directing the needle perpendicularly behind the patella. Aspirate as you advance.

5 When you enter the effusion, hold the needle steady and aspirate to dryness (two syringes may be needed if the effusion is large). Remove the needle and place a small dressing over the puncture site. Send samples of the effusion for analysis: ethylene diaminetetra-acetic acid tube for white cell count; plain sterile container for Gram stain and culture; plain sterile container for microscopy for crystals.

6 Clear up and dispose of sharps safely. Write a note of the procedure in the patient's record: approach/appearance of synovial fluid/volume aspirated/samples sent. Ensure the samples are sent promptly for analysis.

Troubleshooting dry tap

- This may be due to misdiagnosis of effusion, or obesity with resulting difficulty in accurately identifying the bony landmarks.
- Try again from the lateral approach if the medial approach was used, and vice versa.
- If you still cannot obtain fluid, and septic arthritis needs to be excluded, use ultrasound to confirm the presence of the effusion and identify the appropriate puncture site and depth of needle insertion.

Interpreting the results

See Table 111.2.

Table 111.2 Findings on analysis of synovial fluid.

Classification of effusion	Features	White cell count	Causes
Normal synovial fluid	Clear colourless, viscus	<200/mm³ <25% polymorphs	
Non-inflammatory	Cloudy, yellow, viscus	200–2000/mm³ <25% polymorphs	**Common** • Osteoarthritis • Trauma **Uncommon** • Early or subsiding inflammation, osteochondritis dissecans • Neuropathic arthropathy • Pigmented villonodular synovitis
Inflammatory	Cloudy, yellow, watery	2000–100,000/mm³ >50% polymorphs	**Common** • Rheumatoid arthritis • Crystal arthropathies • Psoriatic arthritis **Uncommon** • Reiter syndrome • Ankylosing spondylitis • Arthritis associated with inflammatory bowel disease • Rheumatic fever • Systemic lupus erythematosus • Hypertrophic osteoarthropathy • Scleroderma
Septic	Purulent	>80,000/mm³ >75% polymorphs	**Common** • Bacterial • Mycobacterial **Uncommon** • Fungal

Further reading

Douglas RJ. (2014) Aspiration and injection of the knee joint: approach portal. *Knee Surg Relat Res.* 26(1), 1–6. doi: 10.5792/ksrr.2014.26.1.1. Epub 2014 Feb 27. PMID: 24639940; PMCID: PMC3953519.

Villa-Forte A (2023) How to do knee arthrocentesis – musculoskeletal and connective tissue disorders. MSD Manual Professional Edition. Available from: https://www.msdmanuals.com/en-gb/professional/musculoskeletal-and-connective-tissue-disorders/how-to-do-arthrocentesis/how-to-do-knee-arthrocentesis. [Accessed: 8 May 2024].

CHAPTER 112

Abdominal paracentesis

AJMAL MEMON AND KIRN SANDHU

Abdominal paracentesis is an efficacious diagnostic procedure used to assess and manage patients with ascites. Ascites is the accumulation of fluid in the peritoneal cavity. The commonest cause of ascites is cirrhosis of the liver. Abdominal paracentesis can help differentiate between the several causes of ascites and thus guide the management of these patients.

Ascites can be exudative or transudative. This can be established by measuring the total protein in the ascitic fluid. The preferred method to evaluate ascitic fluid is by calculating the serum ascitic albumin gradient (SAAG), which is directly associated with the portal pressure. Using a cut-off value of 11 g/L or 1.1 g/dL can help divide the different causes of ascites as shown in Table 112.1. Abdominal paracentesis is also a vital therapeutic intervention in patients with significant ascites causing pain and respiratory distress.

Indications

These can be divided into diagnostic and therapeutic.

Diagnostic indications

- Identify the cause of recently developed ascites.
- To rule out spontaneous bacterial peritonitis in a patient with known ascites who has had a clinical deterioration.

Table 112.1 Cause of ascites based on serum albumin ascites gradient (SAAG).

SAAG >11 g/L indicates portal hypertension and transudative ascites
- Cirrhosis of liver
- Alcoholic hepatitis
- Hepatic vein obstruction (Budd–Chiari syndrome)
- Portal vein thrombosis
- Schistosomiasis
- Cardiac failure
- Hypothyroidism

SAAG ratio <11 g/L indicates exudative ascites
- Malignancy (primary peritoneal malignancy and peritoneal metastasis)
- Pancreatitis
- Peritoneal tuberculosis
- Bowel perforation
- Nephrotic syndrome

Acute Medicine: A Practical Guide to the Management of Medical Emergencies, Sixth Edition.
Edited by Mridula Rajwani, Leila Vaziri, and Ivie Gbinigie.
© 2026 John Wiley & Sons Ltd. Published 2026 by John Wiley & Sons Ltd.

Therapeutic indications
- Abdominal paracentesis can be performed to help provide comfort to patients with a large amount of ascites causing pain and breathing difficulties.
- It can be used to manage refractory ascites or in patients not responding/poorly tolerant to diuretics.

Contraindications

Although on most occasions, the benefits outweigh the risks of abdominal paracentesis, there are some occasions that can put the patient at a higher risk of complications.
- Disseminated intravascular coagulation
- Skin infection at the proposed puncture site
- Massive ileus with bowel distention: There is a higher risk of bowel perforation with this. If necessary, then abdominal paracentesis should be performed under ultrasound guidance.
- Pregnancy

Complications of paracentesis

Paracentesis does carry complications and should ideally not be performed out of hours unless it is a clinical emergency. It is important that the below-mentioned complications are discussed with the patient whilst consenting for the procedure.
- Infection: where the drain is placed.
- Bleeding: it is important that patient's full blood count (FBC) and INR are checked prior to performing the procedure. INR >1.5 and platelets <50 places the patient at higher risk of bleeding and may require vitamin K, Fresh Frozen Plasma (FFP) and platelet cover.
- Leakage: at paracentesis site post procedure.
- Perforation: increased risk in patients with concerns regarding bowel obstruction, altered anatomy and previous surgery.
- Circulatory collapse: especially in patients whose large volumes of ascites >10 L have been drained.

Pre-procedure
A few things to keep in mind before performing the procedure
- Bloods: check FBC, clotting, renal and liver profile. If FBC and clotting are deranged the patient is at increased risk of bleeding.
- Informed written consent.
- Ultrasound to confirm fluid and mark insertion site (especially in patients where there are concerns regarding obstruction, loculated ascites and hepatosplenomegaly).
- Review drug chart: ensure anticoagulants and antiplatelets have been stopped at least 48 hours before the procedure.
- Ensure there is secure intravenous access.
- Set up the sterile trolley.
  Patients routinely do not need to be fasted for the procedure or require prophylactic antibiotics.

Equipment required
- Dressing trolley and sharps bin
- Sterile dressing pack and sterile gloves
- Surgical mask and apron
- 2% chloraprep 3 mLs applicator
- Local anaesthetic (1% or 2% lidocaine)

- Green and orange needles
- 10 and 20 mL syringes
- Paracentesis needle
- Drain attachment device
- Drainage bag
- Three standard universal containers
- Two blood culture bottles
- EDTA blood bottle

Procedure

Abdominal paracentesis is a sterile procedure and therefore strict aseptic technique should be maintained throughout the procedure. Ensure the patient has an empty bladder before starting the procedure.

1 Position: patient should be positioned supine with the bed flat and head slightly raised.
2 Landmark: ideally an ultrasound should have been performed including marking the site for insertion. However, the safe approach to performing abdominal paracentesis is lateral to the rectus abdominis muscle, at least 2–4 cm above and medial to the anterior superior iliac spine (as marked x on Figure 112.1). These landmarks avoid rupturing the inferior epigastric vessels. It is important any surgical scars or visible abdominal veins are avoided.
3 Clean: patient's skin should be cleaned with a chloraprep applicator and a sterile drape placed.
4 Local anaesthetic: 5–10 mL of 1% lidocaine should be used. Firstly, an orange needle should be used for subcutaneous infiltration over the marked site. After a few minutes, a green needle should be used to infiltrate deeper tissues until ascitic fluid is aspirated. The green needle should be inserted at an oblique angle.
5 Paracentesis: Using the same trajectory as the anaesthetic needle, the paracentesis needle is advanced while applying negative pressure with the syringe. Insert the needle using a Z-track – this reduces the risk of leakage at the puncture site. Initially puncture the skin perpendicularly, then perforate the subcutaneous tissue obliquely for 1–2 cm followed by puncturing the peritoneal cavity perpendicularly. As soon as ascites start to drain the needle should be stabilised in that position. If you are using a catheter kit then you may need to

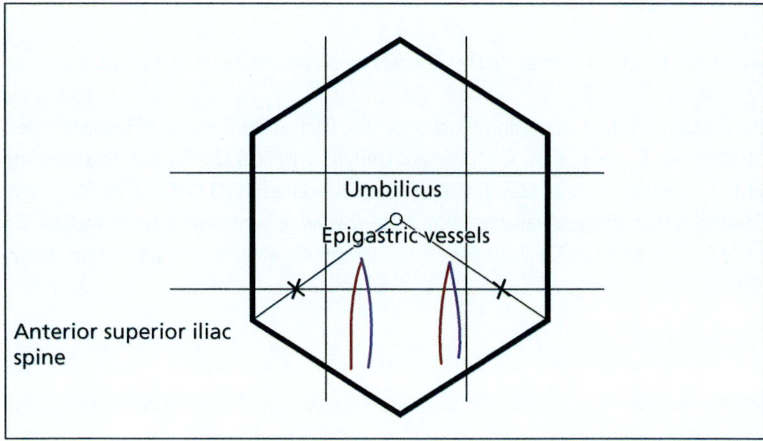

Figure 112.1 Depicting the safe anatomical landmarks for paracentesis **x** which lies 2–4 cm superomedial to the anterior superior iliac spine.

Table 112.2 Tests that can be requested on ascitic fluid.

- Cell count and differential
- Culture
- Ascitic albumin (to calculate SAAG)
- Glucose concentration
- Lactate dehydrogenase
- Cytology
- Adenosine deaminase
- Amylase
- Triglycerides and chylomicrons

make a small cut using a scalpel. A drainage catheter should be inserted if moderate to large amounts of ascites are drained.

6 Removal: Once the desired amount of ascitic fluid is drained, safely remove the needle and apply a sterile dressing at the puncture site. Ideally, the drain should be removed by 6 h.

7 Dispose: make sure to dispose of sharps safely in the sharps bin.

Post-procedure instructions

- Drained fluid should be sent for biochemical and microbiological analysis. All the tests that can potentially be done on the ascitic fluid are summarised in Table 112.2.
- Patient should lie opposite the site of drain insertion
- Review pain and prescribe analgesia
- Review the site for any ascitic fluid leakage or haematoma
- Regular observations and document amount drained
- If more than 5 L of ascitic fluid is drained this will need replacement with 20% HAS (human albumin solution). Patients with acute or chronic liver failure or high risk of kidney injury may require 20% HAS even if <5 L are drained.

Further reading

Aithal GP, Palaniyappan N, China L, *et al.* (2021) Guidelines on the management of ascites in cirrhosis. *Gut* 70(1), 9–29.

Abdominal paracentesis Standard Operating Procedure UHL (University Hospital of Leicester) Department (LOCSSIPS), Delahooke T, Li K-K, Kent C *et al.* Approved by CHUGGS Quality & Safety Meeting 2023.

Aponte EM, Katta S, Kurapati R, *et al.* (2024) Paracentesis. [Updated 2023 Oct 27]. In: StatPearls. Treasure Island (FL): StatPearls Publishing. Available from: https://www.ncbi.nlm.nih.gov/books/NBK435998.

Harvey JJ, Prentice R, George J. (2023) Diagnostic and therapeutic abdominal paracentesis. *Med J Aust* 218(1), 18–21.

CHAPTER 113

Non-invasive ventilation

IVAN TANG AND CHRISTOPHER TURNBULL

Non-invasive ventilation (NIV) refers to systems that support gas delivery between the atmosphere and the lungs without the need for invasive ventilation via either endotracheal intubation or tracheostomy.

The two main uses of NIV in acute medicine are:

- Management of acute type 2 respiratory failure (T2RF) complicating an exacerbation of chronic obstructive pulmonary disease (COPD) (Chapter 23), when it can reduce the need for invasive ventilation and improve survival.
- Management of patients with chronic T2RF maintained on home NIV presenting with worsening respiratory failure.

Less commonly, acute decompensated T2RF is the first presentation of chronic diseases causing T2RF (kyphoscoliosis, spinal injuries, neuromuscular diseases, e.g. motor neuron disease, or morbid obesity) and may require similar management with NIV.

Contraindications to the use of NIV are summarized in Table 113.1. When a relative contraindication is present, NIV may be considered on the ward, if invasive ventilation and intensive care unit (ICU) care is inappropriate.

NIV is often ineffective in treating severe hypoxaemia, as oxygen delivery may not be controlled. American Thoracic Society guidelines suggest using NIV on a trial basis, before invasive ventilation. Liaise with intensive care colleagues.

Non-invasive ventilation in acute hypercapnic respiratory failure

NIV should be considered for respiratory acidosis which persists despite maximal medical therapy given within 60 min of admission (pH 7.25–7.35, $PaCO_2$ >6 kPa (>45 mmHg)), where controlled oxygen is administered to target peripheral saturations 88–92% using a Venturi system. The patient should be conscious and cooperative, and the treatment should be in keeping with the patient's wishes. The underlying respiratory condition and precipitant should be treated and optimised:

- In COPD, administration of bronchodilators (nebulised salbutamol 2.5–5 mg, ipratropium 500 mcg), steroids if indicated (prednisolone 0.5-mg/kg or IV hydrocortisone 100 mg if no oral route), and antibiotics if indicated.
- In other conditions, treat the underlying cause, for example giving naloxone for opiate toxicity, antibiotics if suspected bacterial infection, or drainage of pneumothorax.

Acute Medicine: A Practical Guide to the Management of Medical Emergencies, Sixth Edition.
Edited by Mridula Rajwani, Leila Vaziri, and Ivie Gbinigie.
© 2026 John Wiley & Sons Ltd. Published 2026 by John Wiley & Sons Ltd.

Table 113.1 Contraindications to NIV.

Absolute contraindications to NIV	Relative contraindications to NIV
Impending respiratory arrest*	Confusion or agitation
Upper airway obstruction*	Diagnosis of pneumonia
Glasgow Coma Scale score <8*	Severe hypoxaemia
Respiratory rate <8 breaths/min*	Haemodynamic instability
Acute asthma*	Copious respiratory secretions
Guillain-Barré syndrome with bulbar palsy*	Vomiting
Undrained pneumothorax	Bowel obstruction
	Facial burns or trauma
	Upper airway or upper GI surgery
	Arterial pH < 7.25

* In all these settings invasive ventilation should be considered.

- If immediate mechanical ventilation is not indicated, a plan of management and escalation should be decided with consultant involvement and documented before starting NIV. Scenarios could include:
  - Suitable for NIV and suitable for escalation to intensive care treatment/intubation and ventilation, if required. Inform the local critical care outreach team, if available.
  - Suitable for NIV but not suitable for escalation to intensive care treatment/intubation and ventilation
  - Not suitable for NIV but for full active medical management
  - Palliative care agreed as the most appropriate management

Set-up of non-invasive ventilation

NIV should be prescribed by a doctor trained in the use of NIV, and delivered in a setting where it can be managed by experienced staff (e.g. nurses and/or NIV physiotherapists working in resus, ICUs, high-dependency units (HDUs), acute medical units or respiratory support units).

NIV typically refers to bi-level ventilation delivering two set pressures:

- The expiratory positive airway pressure (EPAP) that recruits under-ventilated areas of the lungs, splints the upper airway open, and reduces work of inspiration.
- The inspiratory positive airway pressure (IPAP) that delivers a driving pressure above EPAP, which is proportional to tidal volume.

The set-up of bilevel NIV is summarized in Table 113.2.

Continuous positive airway pressure (CPAP) is another form of NIV that provides one fixed pressure and is used mainly to improve oxygenation in type 1 respiratory failure due to cardiogenic pulmonary oedema (Chapter 14) and COVID-19 pneumonitis.

Up to 30% of patients are unable to tolerate NIV; the set-up is crucial to its success. Time spent with the patient in the first 30 min helps to reassure the patient and prevents future problems.

Management of the patient receiving non-invasive ventilation

Patients receiving NIV outside HDU/ICU should have continuous electrocardiogram and pulse oximetry monitoring for the first 12 h, and physiological observations recorded every 15 minutes for the first 2 h.

- Repeat arterial (or arterialised capillary) blood gas sampling should be done an hour after achieving the target settings. Further sampling should be performed at 4 h, sooner if significant changes are made to the

Table 113.2 Checklist for set-up of NIV (bi-level NIV).

Explain the treatment to the patient.

Use a well-fitting full-face mask (sized to the patient: small, medium or large).

Start at low pressures tolerated by most patients: IPAP of $10\,cmH_2O$, EPAP of $5\,cmH_2O$

Other settings at default levels.

Allow the patient to hold the mask over their face without the straps tightened.

Tighten the straps to form a seal around the face, but not so tight as to squash the membranes of the mask.

Increase the IPAP by increments of $2\,cmH_2O$, as tolerated by the patient, to target a tidal volume of 6–8 mL/kg (ideal body weight). It should not take long to reach the target pressure.

In general, lower EPAPs ($5\,cmH_2O$) are adequate for patients with COPD due to intrinsic resistance to expiration, whereas with obesity hypoventilation and obstructive sleep apnoea higher EPAPs (8–$10\,cmH_2O$) may be required for recruitment and splinting. Changes in EPAP should trigger a change in IPAP to maintain the driving pressure (IPAP-EPAP).

Entrain oxygen to the circuit (or in newer ventilators, change FiO_2) to a prescribed target (e.g. 88–92%).

Ensure correct equipment available, e.g. Venturi systems for breaks, T-pieces for nebulisers via NIV.

settings. If improvement is inadequate, or if there is deterioration, it may be necessary to escalate to intensive care for consideration of invasive ventilation.

- Problem solving is summarized in Table 113.3.

Weaning of non-invasive ventilation

- In general, patients require acute NIV for 48–72 h after presentation.
- Day 1 continual NIV with breaks for meals, drinks, administration of medications by mouth or nebulizer, reducing the NIV time by 4–6 h/day (though continuing with overnight therapy).
- Some patients will self-wean earlier, and others may need longer. Weaning should be guided by clinical impression and blood gases.
- Patients who cannot be fully liberated from NIV or those who remain hypercapnic should be referred to a specialist for consideration of home NIV.

Problems

Table 113.3 Problem-solving in NIV.

If the patient receiving NIV is not improving, consider:

Ventilator issues

- Check the ventilator is connected to mains, switched on and connected
- Check for alarms

Circuit and mask issues

- Check that pressure is being delivered at the mask end; are respiratory secretions blocking any ports? If using a non-vented system is there an expiratory port correctly sited in the circuit?
- Check for kinks in tubing, e.g. in bedrails
- Check for mask leaks and adjust by loosening and reseating. Over-tightening can lead to skin ulceration. Nasogastric tubes, if needed, should be fine-bore to reduce mask leak

Suboptimal medical management

- Consider chest physiotherapy, nebuliser administration via NIV circuit
- Incorrect oxygen target

Complications arising from NIV

- Check for the development of pneumothorax or aspiration

Persistent hypercapnia, when none of the above applies, is likely to be due to inadequate ventilation. If continuing with ward-based NIV, in general the next step would be to increase the IPAP by an increment of 2–$5\,cmH_2O$ (most machines deliver a maximal IPAP of $\sim30\,cm\,H_2O$).

Breathing asynchrony

Breathing asynchrony, one of the commonest reasons for patients failing on NIV, is when the ventilator delivers breaths outside of the patient's intrinsic breathing rate, ergo causing discoordination. From the end of the bed, look for chest wall movements and timing of breathing with NIV. If asynchrony is detected, seek expert help. Changes can be made to trigger sensitivity, inspiratory and expiratory times and back-up breathing rate as appropriate.

Nasal bridge ulceration

Ulceration of the skin of the nasal bridge from a tightly or poorly fitting mask is a common problem. Regular checks of skin integrity should be performed, as well as checking for mask leak, as air leaks can cause corneal injury. If there is incipient ulceration, consider changing to a different mask interface such as a low-profile full-face mask, using gel pads, and seeking advice from a tissue viability team.

Admissions in patients on long-term home NIV

Increasing numbers of patients are being cared for in the community with home NIV. There may be features of inadequate treatment, such as daytime sleepiness (indicative of sleep fragmentation), morning headaches suggestive of persisting hypercapnia or snoring while on NIV. There should be a low threshold to check arterial or capillary blood gases and seek specialist advice. Home ventilation teams can often interrogate the ventilator for usage data.

When admitted with unrelated problems, patients have occasionally had their NIV omitted in error. Ongoing NIV is crucial to prevent decompensation and should be continued unless a contraindication has developed.

Use the patient's own NIV where possible. Inform the respiratory team/team responsible for their NIV therapy. In those who have presented with worsening/decompensated T2RF, both the respiratory and intensive care teams should be involved as appropriate. The reasons for deterioration include:

- Presenting condition worsens respiratory function, for example pneumonia.
- Decreased use of NIV prior to admission, for example because of vomiting.
- NIV not tolerated.
- NIV interface no longer adequate due to patient factors, i.e. excessive facial hair, or equipment degradation.
- Settings no longer adequate, for example following weight gain.
- Worsening of underlying condition.
  Identify and treat the underlying cause if possible and consider either increasing the NIV pressure settings if inadequate tidal volumes (target usually 6–8 mL/kg ideal body weight) or increasing the hours of NIV usage.
  Many patients on NIV have a poor prognosis because of the underlying diagnosis
- Check if they have advanced care plans.
- Check current or previously expressed wishes about future treatments, such as 24 h-a-day NIV use, invasive ventilation, and resuscitation.
- Consider palliative care involvement.
- NIV can be weaned in end-of-life care if wished by the patient. An individualised approach is suggested, and it may be useful to seek advice from experienced respiratory and palliative care colleagues.

Further reading

Davidson AC, Banham S, Elliott M, *et al.* (2016) British thoracic society/intensive care society acute hypercapnic respiratory failure guideline development group. 2016 BTS/ICS Guidelines for the ventilatory management of acute hypercapnic respiratory failure in adults. *Thorax* 71, ii1–ii35. https://www. britthoracic.org.uk/document-library/clinical-information/acute-hypercapnic-respiratory-failure/bts-guidelinesfor-ventilatory-management-of-ahrf/.

Ergan B, Oczkowski S, Rochwerg B, *et al.* (2019) European respiratory society guidelines on long-term home non-invasive ventilation for management of COPD. *Eur Respir J* 54(3), 1901003. DOI: 10.1183/13993003. 01003-2019.

Kelly CR, Higgins AR, Chandra SN. (2015) Videos in clinical medicine. non-invasive positive-pressure ventilation. *N Engl J Med* 372, e30. http://www.nejm.org/doi/full/10.1056/NEJMvcm1313336.

Murphy PB, Rehal S, Arbane G, *et al.* (2017) Effect of home noninvasive ventilation with oxygen therapy vs oxygen therapy alone on hospital readmission or death after an acute COPD exacerbation: a randomized clinical trial. *JAMA* 317(21), 2177–2186. DOI: 10.1001/jama.2017.4451.

Rochwerg B, Brochard L, Elliott MW, *et al.* (2017) Official ERS/ATS clinical practice guidelines: noninvasive ventilation for acute respiratory failure. *Eur Respir J* 50(2), 1602426. DOI: 10.1183/13993003. 02426-2016.

CHAPTER 114

Arterial line insertion

Tom Cibulskas

Introduction

An 'arterial line' is an intravascular catheter placed into a peripheral artery. This is a common procedure in the emergency department and critical care units and is also used for monitoring acutely unwell patients prehospitally. Some wards providing increased care (e.g. medical high-dependency units) may support arterial line usage; most low-dependency medical wards in the United Kingdom are not able to care for patients requiring arterial line insertion and monitoring.

Indications

1 Haemodynamic monitoring

Transduction of the arterial pressure waveform allows real-time monitoring of blood pressure (BP) in critically unwell patients. It can also be used to secure reliable BP readings in patients at extremes of body size and with arrhythmias (e.g. atrial fibrillation with fast ventricular rate) which can make non-invasive blood pressure monitoring less accurate.

Beat-to-beat BP monitoring is used to titrate and monitor the resuscitation of shocked patients. In critical care, computer analysis of the waveform is used to estimate cardiac stroke volume and stroke volume variation as a marker of volume status.

2 Blood sampling

Aspiration of arterial blood from the line can be performed, which can be used for arterial blood gas analysis as well as standard lab tests. This has the advantage of minimising painful peripheral blood samples, particularly in patients needing several tests done in a short time (e.g. ventilatory support or during the acute phases of Diabetic Keto Acidosis [DKA]). Arterial line aspiration can be an alternative in patients with poor peripheral IV access. Care should be taken to ensure that any saline present in the tubing between the patient and the aspiration port is removed and disposed of before the blood is aspirated with a fresh syringe.

Arterial lines are NOT used for the administration of drugs, and the accidental administration of vasoactive or vaso irritant substances via the intra-arterial route can result in severe distal ischaemia and limb loss.

Acute Medicine: A Practical Guide to the Management of Medical Emergencies, Sixth Edition.
Edited by Mridula Rajwani, Leila Vaziri, and Ivie Gbinigie.
© 2026 John Wiley & Sons Ltd. Published 2026 by John Wiley & Sons Ltd.

Contraindications

1 High risk of limb ischaemia: for example, known severe arterial disease in the artery intended for cannulation. Allen's test can be used to assess collateral perfusion of the hand in radial artery cannulation (see below).
2 Infection (e.g. cellulitis) in the peri-arterial soft tissues.
3 Known or suspected aneurysm/pseudoaneurysm at the site of intended cannulation.
4 Future planned procedure at the same site (e.g. radial artery cannulation for percutaneous coronary intervention).
5 Coagulopathy: a relative contraindication; the risk of bleeding and time needed to correct coagulopathy should be weighed against the urgency of line insertion.

Complications

- Vasospasm: rarely causes long-term complications, but reduces the chance of subsequent successful attempts at the same site.
- Bruising/bleeding.
- Infection.
- Injection of intra-arterial air (air embolism) or vasoactive drugs leading to distal ischaemia.
- Damage to local structures – typically nerves running adjacent to arteries causing neuropraxia. Long-term nerve injury is rare.
- Formation of aneurysm, pseudoaneurysm or arteriovenous fistula.
- Loss of guidewire into circulation when using Seldinger technique – often requiring surgical or radiological retrieval.

Equipment

- Arterial catheter: usually 20G or 22G. Both Seldinger (guidewire) and cannula-type (plastic catheter over a rigid needle) catheters are commonly used.
- Sterile procedure pack including a drape, skin prep, needles and syringes for local anaesthetic administration.
- Sterile dressing: specific arterial line dressings are commonly available; however a standard intravenous cannula dressing can be used if unavailable.
- Sterile gloves.
- Arterial line transducer set: usually a specific tubing system attached to a 500 mL bag of 0.9% saline, which is flushed before connection to the patient to avoid air embolism and give the most relative pressure trace. Most commercially available sets have a built-in transducer wiring to allow connection to compatible bedside monitoring systems.
- Pressure bag: pressurises the saline to 300 mmHg, allowing the transducer to function. Most transducer sets will also incorporate a flushing device to allow catheter patency to be checked and to ensure no blood is left to clot inside the tubing after aspiration.
- Local anaesthetic: usually 2 mL 1% or 2% lidocaine.

Most arterial line insertion is performed using an aseptic non-touch technique (ANTT). In certain settings (e.g. theatre and critical care) demanding full asepsis a sterile gown, mask and surgical hat can also be worn.

Technique

- Wash hands; don sterile gloves. Apply skin prep whilst ensuring ANTT. Apply drape to skin once fully dry.
- Palpate the target artery (most commonly radial) and inject 1–2 mL of local anaesthetic subcutaneously. Be sure to aspirate first to avoid intra-arterial local anaesthetic injection.
- Insert the tip of the chosen device through the anaesthetised skin and into the artery. An ultrasound probe can be used if needed (see below). A shallow angle of approximately 30° to the skin is ideal.

If using a Seldinger-type set

- Vascular cannulation is confirmed by a strong flashback of bright red arterial blood through the introducer needle. The arterial pulsation should be obvious and blood will flow freely until the needle is occluded (most sets include a bung which can be used to temporarily occlude the proximal end of the needle). Poor flow of darker blood indicates likely venous cannulation; if this occurs the needle should be removed and flushed before further attempts.
- Advance the guidewire through the introducer needle into the artery. It should pass freely; significant resistance indicates that the tip of the needle is lying in the subcutaneous tissue and should be withdrawn or relocated. Care must be taken to NOT advance the wire too far and a grip should always be maintained on the wire to minimise the risk of this.
- Remove the introducer needle over the guidewire, taking care to not dislodge or advance the wire in the process.
- Advance the catheter over the guidewire; it should pass into the vessel without significant resistance.
- Remove the guidewire; flashback of bright red arterial blood confirms the correct location.

If using a cannula-type set

- Advance the cannula tip into the artery; flashback or bright red blood into the chamber (similar to the flashback when using a *venflon*-type intravenous cannula) confirms arterial positioning.
- Advance the plastic cannula into the vessel whilst keeping the needle still. It is easy to withdraw the needle rather than advance the cannula at this stage, which can result in the cannula inadvertently being advanced into the subcutaneous tissues. The risk of this can be reduced by advancing the needle a further 2–3 mm after flashback is first achieved. The cannula should advance without significant resistance.
- Once the cannula is fully advanced, remove the needle. Aspiration of arterial blood from the proximal end of the cannula confirms intra-arterial positioning.

Final steps

- Connect the appropriate, flushed transducer tubing to the cannula.
- Use a sterile swab to remove any blood from the surrounding skin.
- Some cannulas have small holes to allow suturing to the underlying skin, which is common practice to increase the lifespan of arterial lines in critical care.
- A sterile dressing should be applied, ideally with a transparent section to allow direct observation of the insertion site for bleeding, kinks or signs of infection.

Allen's test

Allen's test is used to assess patency of the collateral circulation (ulnar artery) to the hand prior to radial artery cannulation. It is good practice to perform it before starting, although the risk of hand ischaemia secondary to arterial line insertion is very low. It may be appropriate to omit Allen's test in emergency situations involving the resuscitation of a shocked patient.

- Occlude both the radial and ulnar arteries of the same wrist with firm pressure.
- The patient should open and close their fist several times. If the arterial supplies are properly occluded, the palm with appear pale.
- The ulnar pressure is released, whilst radial pressure is maintained. In a normal result, the collateral ulnar circulation perfuses the palm and it becomes pink.

Use of ultrasound

Ultrasound can be used to help locate the peripheral arteries, which can be helpful in patients in shock or with significantly raised BMI. With an appropriate probe cover, real-time ultrasound-guided cannulation of arterial vessels can be accomplished. As with intravenous access, both in-plane and out-of-plane views can be used to aid in choice and localisation of a target vessel (US images below).

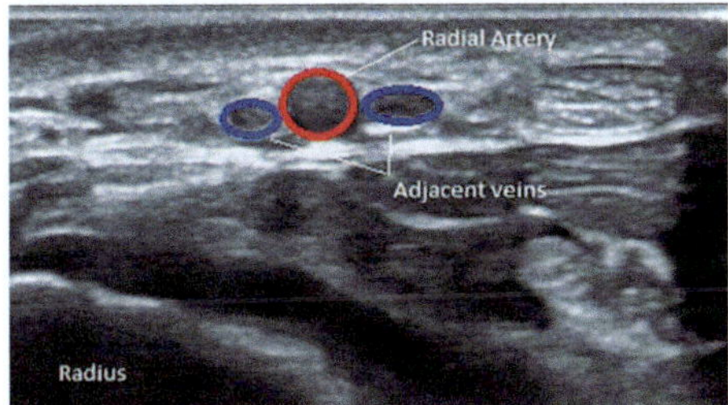

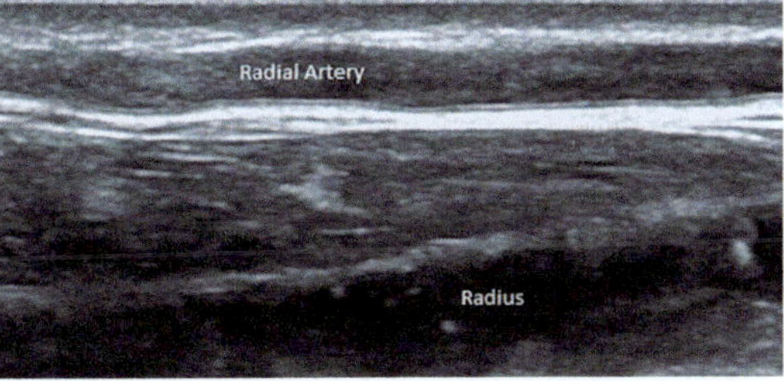

CHAPTER 115

Point-of-care ultrasound

SILVIA SBARDELLA AND BEN MILLETTE

- Acute medicine is one of the first medical specialties to adopt point-of-care ultrasound (POCUS) within its core curriculum competencies.
- Portable and hand-held devices allow ultrasonography to be used as an extension of the clinical examination, providing bedside information about the heart, lungs and abdomen.
- These scans guide immediate management and the need for further tests.
- They do not replace definitive ultrasound scans and are potentially dangerous if the operator is not adequately trained or supervised.
- Emergency ultrasonography is useful for the presentations outlined in the table below (Table 115.1).
- A thorax POCUS exam is more accurate than a chest X-ray for the detection of pleural fluid. It can be used to guide chest drain insertion for those who have approved British Thoracic Society training or equivalent certification (Chapter 110).
- A bladder scan can assess the amount of urine in the bladder pre- and post-voiding to diagnose acute and chronic urinary retention.
- A scan of the kidneys can help diagnose hydronephrosis and grade its severity in the patient presenting with undifferentiated acute kidney injury.
- Ultrasonography can also be used to identify peripheral veins for venepuncture or cannulation, or central veins for the insertion of central lines (Chapter 108).
- Practical aspects are summarized in Table 115.2.

Surgical applications (e.g. diagnosis of ruptured abdominal aortic aneurysms or traumatic intraperitoneal bleeds) are not described in this chapter.

Cardiac scan

- A focused echocardiography exam should be considered for all patients presenting with shock, it can help correctly identify the underlying mechanism of shock and guide initial management.
- Table 115.3 summarises the potential causes of shock and echocardiographic findings associated with these.
- In a cardiac arrest the cardiac scan can be performed in the 5 s pulse check of the Advanced Life Support Resuscitation Council algorithm of 'non-shockable' rhythms.
- A motionless, asystolic heart at Cardio Pulmonary Resuscitation (CPR) is associated with a positive predictive value of 97% death.

Acute Medicine: A Practical Guide to the Management of Medical Emergencies, Sixth Edition.
Edited by Mridula Rajwani, Leila Vaziri, and Ivie Gbinigie.
© 2026 John Wiley & Sons Ltd. Published 2026 by John Wiley & Sons Ltd.

Table 115.1 Indications for emergency ultrasonography.

Clinical scenario	Cardiac scan	Thoracic scan	Abdominal scan
Undifferentiated shock (Systolic Blood Pressure [SBP]<90)	+	(+)*	(+)[†]
Respiratory failure	+	+	
Acute kidney injury with sepsis			(+)**
Lower respiratory tract infection	+	+	
Chest pain	+	(+)	
Abdominal pain			+[†]

* To exclude tension pneumothorax.

** To exclude pyelonephrosis.

[†] In suspected rupture of abdominal aortic aneurysm.

Table 115.2 Practical guide to emergency ultrasonography.

Cardiac scan	Abdominal scan
Probe • Phased array	**Probe** • Curvilinear
Positioning • Left lateral • Supine (subcostal view)	**Positioning** • Supine
Views • Parasternal long-axis • Parasternal short-axis • Apical four-chamber • Subcostal	**Views** • Central abdominal • Right and left iliac fossa (free fluid) • Right and left subphrenic spaces
Uses • Identifies critical pathology and major causes of shock • Pericardial effusion assessment • Left ventricular dysfunction • Right ventricular dysfunction • Surrogate assessment of intravascular fluid status	**Uses:** • Ascites and paracentesis • Hydronephrosis

Thoracic scan	Bladder scan
Probe: • Linear: for pleura and detect pneumothorax • Curved: for all purposes	**Probe:** • Curved
Positioning: • Seated forward with arms folded on pillow for pleural effusion • Supine/near-to-supine for pneumothorax • Any position for pulmonary oedema	**Positioning:** • Supine with full bladder
Views: • Posterior approach for pleural effusion • Anti-dependent zones for pneumothorax (anterior sagittal, second intercostal space, mid-clavicular line)	**Views:** • Pelvis – sagittal • Transverse
Uses: • Pneumothorax • Pleural effusions • Pulmonary oedema (cardiogenic and non-cardiogenic) • Consolidation	**Uses:** • Incomplete voiding • Reduced urine output vs catheter blockage

(continued)

Table 115.2 (*Continued*)

Vascular scan
Probe: • Linear
Positioning: • Supine, Prone
Uses: • Intravascular access • Rule in Deep Vein Thrombosis (DVT) • Jugular Venous Pressure (JVP) assessment

- In suspected pulmonary embolism (Chapter 31):
  - The signs in Table 115.3 can be used to prove the working diagnosis sufficient to give immediate thrombolysis in a critically ill patient.
  - Sometimes the presence of RV dilatation/ultrasound signs of RV strain can suggest the need for inpatient care in patients apparently suitable for outpatient care using clinical scoring systems.
- In hypotension (Chapter 2), a cardiac scan is not only useful to detect hypovolaemia (small, flat collapsing IVC) but it can also detect patients in whom fluids are unlikely to provide benefit (large circular fixed IVC).
- In patients with suspected exacerbation of Chronic Obstructive Pulmonary Disease (COPD) (Chapter 23), LV systolic dysfunction is either the correct diagnosis or an associated diagnosis in up to 20% of cases.

Table 115.3 POCUS applications and findings in multifactorial shock and cardiac arrest.

Recognised conditions presenting with shock	Findings on point of care ultrasound
Massive pulmonary embolism	• Dilated Right Ventricle (RV) • RV systolic dysfunction (Tricuspid Annular Plane Excursion [TAPSE] <16 mm) • Interventricular septal flattening • Mc Connel's sign (RV akinetic free wall with hyperdynamic apex) • Distended Inferior Vena Cava (IVC), non-collapsing • Thrombus may rarely be visible in the right heart or pulmonary artery
Pericardial tamponade	• Pericardial fluid collection (ends anterior to the descending thoracic aorta) • RA collapse during systole • RV collapse during diastole • Heart 'swinging' during cardiac cycle • Dilated IVC with <50% collapse
Hypovolemic shock	• Markedly reduced end-diastolic chamber size reflecting reduced filling • Hyperdynamic wall motions of both ventricles with ventricular walls 'kissing' during systole • Flat inferior vena cava, with >30% variability during the respiratory cycle
Cardiogenic shock	**Direct results of myocardial infarction** • Regional Left Ventricle (LV) wall-motion abnormality* • Global LV dysfunction **Acute complications of myocardial infarction** • Flail mitral valve* • Ventricular septal rupture*

Table 115.3 (*Continued*)

Recognised conditions presenting with shock	Findings on point of care ultrasound
	Aortic root dissection • Dilated aortic root * • Severe aortic regurgitation* • Intimal tear sometimes visible **Structural abnormalities** • Hypertrophic cardiomyopathy* • Obstructed or regurgitant prosthetic valve* • Severe valve lesions such as severe aortic stenosis* • Dynamic left ventricular outflow tract obstruction* • Takotsubo cardiomyopathy*
Septic shock	• A distributive shock usually characterised by ultrasound signs of euvolaemia. This may coexist with signs of LV/RV dysfunction (septic cardiomyopathy)

* These findings should be picked up by an expert ultrasonographer and do not pertain to point-of-care echocardiography learning outcomes.

Thoracic scan

- A thoracic emergency scan does not substitute for a standard thoracic ultrasound scan for pleural diseases as defined by British Thoracic Society (BTS) guidelines.
- A BTS-approved ultrasound course or equivalent certification (FAMUS thorax/FICE Lung) is mandated before performing interventions such as chest drain insertion under real-time ultrasound.
- The Bedside Lung Ultrasound in Emergency (BLUE) protocol for the assessment of undifferentiated respiratory failure carries 90.5% diagnostic accuracy.
- A thoracic scan can aid management by the detection of:
  - Pleural effusion. Ultrasound is more accurate than a chest X-ray on which lobar collapse and elevated hemidiaphragm may mimic a pleural effusion. Specific features outlined in Table 115.4 can help distinguish a simple from a complicated pleural effusion
  - Consolidation.
  - Pneumothorax.
  - Pulmonary oedema.
- Normal aerated lung reflects ultrasound poorly and is characterized by A lines (Table 115.5, Figure 115.1a). The scatter of ultrasound causes a 'snow-storm' appearance.
- A wet lung reflects ultrasound and is characterized by 'B-lines' (Table 115.5, Figure 115.1b):
  - Identifying whether A or B lines are present helps differentiating between COPD and heart failure with pulmonary oedema.

Table 115.4 Ultrasound signs of empyema.

Appearance	Interpretation
• Echogenic debris visible in pleural fluid	• High probability of exudative effusion
• Fibrin strands visible in pleural fluid	• High probability of exudative effusion, increasing probability of empyema
• Separate loculations of pleural fluid and lung that are stuck down and not moving freely within pleural fluid	• High probability of empyema

Table 115.5 Appearances of A- and B-lines on thoracic scan.

	A-lines (Figure 115.1a (left))	B-lines (Figure 115.1b (right))
Appearance	Normal horizontal reverberation artefact, parallel to the pleural line	Pathological vertical reverberation artefact, arising from the pleural line
Interpretation	Normal lung asthma COPD	Fluid-thickened interstitium: pulmonary oedema; or collagen-thickened interstitium: pulmonary fibrosis

(a)   (b)

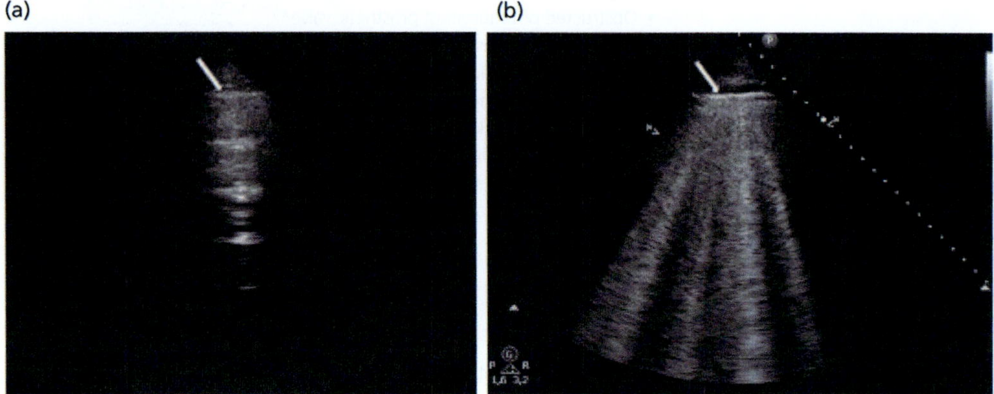

Figure 115.1 Appearances of A-lines (a) and B-lines (b) on thoracic scan. The bright white line (arrowed) is the visceral pleura. A-lines are normal horizontal reverberation artefacts, and B-lines are pathological vertical reverberation artefacts. See also Table 115.6.

- The absence of multiple bilateral B lines excludes cardiogenic pulmonary oedema with negative predictive value of 100%.
- Acute respiratory distress syndrome/acute lung injury (Chapter 14) is characterized by non-homogeneously distributed B-lines and lung consolidations.

Abdominal scan

- In a tense distended abdomen, ultrasound can confirm the presence of ascites immediately (Figure 115.2).
- Points on the examination are given in Table 115.6.
- Unless there is marked splenomegaly, the left lateral flank is the preferred site for a diagnostic ascitic tap or paracentesis, aiming for an area between the anterior abdominal wall and the dark hypoechogenic fluid, and having confirmed that there is no bowel or other organ in the proposed track.
- In patients presenting with reduced urine output and acute kidney injury, an ultrasound assessment of the renal tract can identify obstruction (hydronephrosis) and grade its severity with 90% sensitivity and specificity.

Bladder scan

- The bladder produces a posterior acoustic shadow. Scan superior to the pubic bone in midline both longitudinally and transversely.

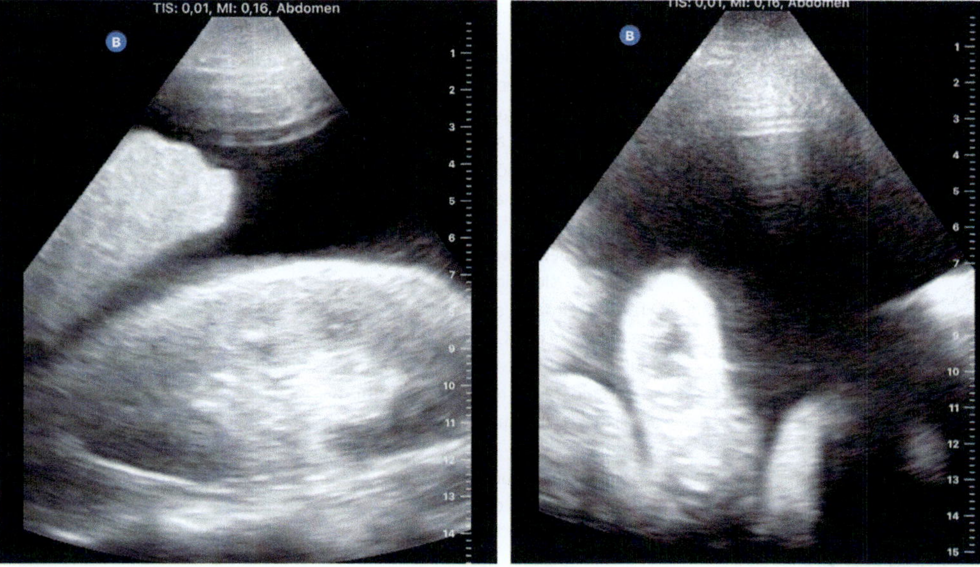

Figure 115.2 Ultrasonographic appearance of abdominal ascites.

Table 115.6 The abdominal scan in suspected ascites (Chapter 36).

Suggests ascites
- Dark and hypo-echoic appearances in the flanks
- Loops of gas-filled bowel afloat around the centre/periumbilical region

Points of concern before ascitic tap
- Hepatomegaly or enlarged gallbladder
- Splenomegaly
- Full bladder. A common mistake is to insert a needle into the fluid of the bladder, so ensure several planes of view are evaluated before proceeding in real-time. It is also sensible to ask the patient to void beforehand.
- Measure the fluid in two planes to get a better idea of depth.

A bladder scan is useful for
- Obese elderly males where clinical assessment for urinary retention due to prostatic hypertrophy can be difficult.
- Post-voiding volumes when uncertainty about incomplete bladder emptying exists.
- Confused patients who cannot tell you when they were last able to pass urine.
- In acute kidney injury (Chapter 86).

Point of care ultrasound governance

- Point-of-care ultrasound has gained significant popularity over recent years, attracting a large number of non-radiologist users and welcoming new technologies in the form of hand-held, portable devices.
- In response to this growing trend, the Royal Society of Radiologists in collaboration with the British Society of Medical Ultrasound published a set of recommendations offering a framework for good clinical ultrasound practice and governance.
- The main aspects of POCUS governance are summarised in Table 115.7.

Table 115.7 Point of care ultrasound governance.

Ultrasound equipment and safety	• Dedicated group or lead overseeing purchase of equipment and maintenance • Periodic assessment of image quality • SOPs (standard operating procedure) for scan types • Equipment cleaning and decontamination
Ultrasound user	• Training and education • Engagement in CPD activities • Audit

Reporting	• Contemporaneous written reporting, to include a minimum of:
	  • Time, date &location.
	  • Practitioner name and grade.
	  • Exam type (e.g. FICE echo, lung or abdomen)
	  • Outcome, complications and recommendation if appropriate.
	• Use of standardised reporting proforma across departments

Images storage	• Compliance with patient data security as per National Health Service (NHS) digital requirements. • Integration into Picture Archiving and Communication System (PACS) systems or similar data-secured-cloud-based systems.

Further reading

Flower L, Olusanya O, Madhivathanan PR. (2021) The use of critical care echocardiography in peri-arrest and cardiac arrest scenarios: pros, cons and what the future holds. *J Intensive Care Soc* 22(3), 230–240. DOI: 10.1177/1751143720936998. Epub 2020 Jun 25. PMID: 34422106; PMCID: PMC8373287.

Gargani L, Volpicelli G. (2014) How I do it: Lung ultrasound. *Cardiovasc Ultrasound* 12, 25. http://www.cardiovascularultrasound.com/content/12/1/25.

Hothi SS, Sprigings D, Chambers J. (2014) Point-of-care ultrasound in acute medicine – the quick scan. *Clin Med* 14, 608–611.

Lancellotti P, Price S, Edvardsen T, *et al.* (2015) The use of echocardiography in acute cardiovascular care: recommendations of the European association of cardiovascular imaging and the acute cardiovascular care association. *Eur Heart J* 16, 119–146. http://ehjcimaging.oxfordjournals.org/content/ejechocard/16/2/119.full.pdf.

Lichtenstein DA, Mezière GA. (2008) Relevance of lung ultrasound in the diagnosis of acute respiratory failure: the BLUE protocol [published correction appears in Chest. 2013 Aug;144(2):721]. *Chest* 134(1), 117–125. DOI: 10.1378/chest.07-2800.

Nepal S, Dachsel M, Smallwood N. (2020) Point-of-care ultrasound rapidly and reliably diagnoses renal tract obstruction in patients admitted with acute kidney injury. *Clin Med (Lond)* 20(6), 541–544. DOI: 10.7861/clinmed.2019-0417.

Royal College Radiologists. (2023) *Recommendations for specialists practising ultrasound independently of radiology departments*. Safety, governance and education.

Index

Note: *Italic* page numbers refer to *figures* and **Bold** page numbers reference to **tables**

Acute Medicine: A Practical Guide to the Management of Medical Emergencies, Sixth Edition.
Edited by Mridula Rajwani, Leila Vaziri, and Ivie Gbinigie.
© 2026 John Wiley & Sons Ltd. Published 2026 by John Wiley & Sons Ltd.